Pediatric Gastrointestinal Motility Disorders

EDITOR

Paul E. Hyman, MD

ASSOCIATE EDITOR

Carlo Di Lorenzo, MD

Library of Congress Cataloging in Publication Data

Main Entry Under Title:
Pediatric Gastrointestinal Motility Disorders

Published by
Academy Professional Information Services, Inc.
116 West 32nd Street
New York, NY 10001 USA

Library of Congress Catalogue Card Number: 94-072608

ISBN 0-934205-12-4

The publishers have made every effort to trace the copyright holders for borrowed material. If they have inadvertently overlooked any, they will be pleased to make the necessary arrangements at the first opportunity. The editorial content reflects only the opinions of the contributors and not of the publisher.

CONTRIBUTORS

Susan Arnoult, BS
Medical Student
University of Maryland
School of Medicine
Baltimore, Maryland

J. Boix-Ochoa, MD
Professor of Pediatric Surgery
Universidad Autònoma
Head of the Pediatric Surgery
Department
Hospital Materno-Infantil Vall d'Hebron
Barcelona, Spain

J. Timothy Boyle, MD
Chief, Division of Pediatric
Gastoenterology and Nutrition
Rainbow Babies and Children's Hospital
Cleveland, Ohio

Samy Cadranel, MD
Head of Department of
Gastroenterology-Hepatology
Queen Fabiola Children's Hospital
Free University of Brussels
Brussels, Belgium

Josep M. Casasa, MD
Head of the Surgical
Gastroenterology Department
Hospital Materno-Infantil Vall d'Hebron
Barcelona, Spain

Salvatore Cucchiara, MD
Associate Professor of Pediatrics
Gastrointestinal Motility and
Endoscopy Unit
University of Naples
Naples, Italy

Steven DeLaura, BS
Department of Psychobiology
University of California, Los Angeles
Los Angeles, California

Carlo Di Lorenzo, MD
Visiting Assistant Professor
Division of Pediatric Gastroenterology
University of Pittsburgh
School of Medicine
Children's Hospital of Pittsburgh
Pittsburgh, Pennsylvania

Andre Dubois, MD, PhD
Departments of Medicine and Surgery
Uniformed Services University of the
Health Sciences
Bethesda, Maryland

David R. Fleisher, MD
Associate Professor
Department of Child Health
University of Missouri
School of Medicine
Columbia, Missouri

Alejandro F. Flores, MD
Attending Pediatric Gastroenterologist
Pediatric GI Unit
Newton-Wellesley Hospital
Newton, Massachusetts

Josep M. Gil-Vernet, MD
Head of the Surgical Digestive
Physiology Department
Hospital Materno-Infantil Vall d'Hebron
Barcelona, Spain

Bruce B. Grill, MD
Associate Professor of Pediatrics
Loma Linda University
School of Medicine
Medical Director
Inland Pediatric Specialties
Medical Group
San Bernardino, California

Alison Hamilton, BA
Senior Research Associate
Pediatric Pain Program
University of California, Los Angeles
School of Medicine
Los Angeles, California

Sydney Heyman, MD
Director, Division of Nuclear Medicine
Department of Radiology
Children's Hospital of Philadelphia
Philadelphia, Pennsylvania

Paul E. Hyman, MD
Associate Professor of Pediatrics
University of California, Los Angeles
School of Medicine
Los Angeles, California
Chief, Division of Pediatric
Gastroenterology
Harbor-UCLA Medical Center
Torrance, California

Takayoshi Kuroume, MD
Department of Pediatrics
Gunma University School of Medicine
Maebashi, Gunma, Japan

Vera Loening-Baucke, MD
Professor of Pediatrics
Department of Pediatrics
University of Iowa Hospitals and Clinics
Iowa City, Iowa

Claudia Marhuenda, MD
Pediatric Surgeon
Surgical Digestive Physiology Department
Hospital Materno-Infantil Vall d'Hebron
Barcelona, Spain

Peter J. Milla, MSc, MBBS, FRCP
Senior Lecturer in Child Health
Department of Child Health
University of London
Honorary Consultant Paediatric
Gastroenterologist
The Hospital for Sick Children
London, England

Susan R. Orenstein, MD
Associate Professor of Pediatrics
Division of Pediatric Gastroenterology
University of Pittsburgh
School of Medicine
Children's Hospital of Pittsburgh
Pittsburgh, Pennsylvania

Alberto Peña, MD
Professor of Surgery and Pediatrics
Albert Einstein College of Medicine
Chief of Surgery
Schneider Children's Hospital
Long Island Jewish Medical Center
New Hyde Park, New York

Marjolain Pineault, PhD
Parenteral Nutrition Service
Hôpital Ste-Justine
Associate Professor
Faculty of Pharmacy
Université de Montréal
Montreal, Canada

Victor M. Piñeiro-Carrero, MD
Assistant Professor of Pediatrics
*Uniformed Services University
of the Health Sciences
Bethesda, Maryland*
Attending Physician
*Division of Pediatric Gastroenterology
Walter Reed Army Medical Center
Washington, DC*

S. Narasimha Reddy, PhD, PEng
Director, Sriram Motility Center
Hyderabad, India
Associate Director
*Gastrointestinal Motility
Long Beach Memorial Medical Center
Long Beach, California*

Colin D. Rudolph, MD, PhD
Assistant Professor of Pediatrics
Director, Children's Center for
Motility Disorders
*Division of Gastroenterology
and Nutrition
Children's Hospital Medical Center
Cincinnati, Ohio*

Michele Scaillon, MD
*Department of Gastroenterology-
Hepatology
Queen Fabiola Children's Hospital
Free University of Brussels
Brussels, Belgium*

Michael D. Schuffler, MD
Professor
*University of Washington School of
Medicine*
Chief of Gastroenterology
*Pacific Medical Center and Clinics
Seattle, Washington*

Ernest Seidman, MD
*Division of Pediatric Gastroenterology
and Nutrition
Hôpital Ste-Justine*
Associate Professor
*Department of Pediatrics
Université de Montréal
Montreal, Canada*

Annamaria Staiano, MD
*Department of Pediatrics
Universita Federico II
Naples, Italy*

Takeshi Tomomasa, MD
*Department of Pediatrics
Gunma University School of Medicine
Maebashi, Gunma, Japan*

Yvan Vandenplas, MD
*Academic Children's Hospital
Free University of Brussels
Brussels, Belgium*

Lonnie K. Zeltzer, MD
Professor of Pediatrics
Director, Pediatric Pain Program
*University of California, Los Angeles
School of Medicine
Los Angeles, California*

◆ ◆ ◆ ◆ ◆ ◆ ◆ ◆ ◆ ◆ ◆ ◆

This book is dedicated to

Bev and Sammy Hyman

and

Daniela and Mario Di Lorenzo

◆ ◆ ◆ ◆ ◆ ◆ ◆ ◆ ◆ ◆ ◆ ◆

We are grateful to our mentors, Thomas Q. Garvey III and Marvin E. Ament (for Paul E. Hyman), Jorge Valenzuela (for Carlo Di Lorenzo), and William J. Snape, Jr., (for both of us), for introducing us to the art and science of gastrointestinal motility. We appreciate Edelmira Darna for coordinating the efforts of the contributors, editors, and publishers in timely fashion.

We also appreciate all the efforts of Judith Lerner, Alison Marek, and the staff at Academy Professional Information Services, Inc.

FOREWORD

A valuable text on pediatric gastrointestinal motility disorders will provide more than an encyclopedic listing of disorders that affect children and a summary of diagnostic and therapeutic modalities. The explosion of medical information seen in recent years certainly warrants such an effort, but a text such as this goes further. It highlights the developmental issues and physiologic processes that cause the discipline of pediatrics to be more than the study of "small adults." Many gastrointestinal motility disorders in children have the same names as adult disorders (ie, gastroesophageal reflux, abdominal pain, intestinal pseudo-obstruction), but have markedly different clinical presentations, epidemiologies, and responses to therapy.

The reason behind the uniqueness of the clinical disorders that occur in children when compared with adults frequently has to do with the developmental physiology which underlies the disorder. For example, chronic intestinal pseudo-obstruction in adults is usually secondary to a life-long process such as progressive systemic sclerosis, diabetes, neuromuscular disease, or a familial degenerative disorder. Congenital pseudo-obstruction in children is often primary. Our previous lack of understanding of the pathophysiology involved in this disorder resulted in suboptimal care for some children. The decision of when and where to place enteral feeding tubes and how best to utilize parenteral nutrition will improve as we continue to expand our knowledge of chronic intestinal pseudo-obstruction.

Recognition of other specific pediatric enteric neuromuscular disorders is increasing as techniques of histochemical analysis improve. These techniques have increased our understanding of the embryologic processes that contribute to the development of the gastrointestinal tract and the developmental abnormalities that cause disorders such as Hirschsprung's disease. Detailed descriptions of the neuropathology in Hirschsprung's disease are particularly helpful to those interested in understanding the pathophysiology of this disorder.

Gastroesophageal reflux is an example of a motility disorder that has different clinical symptoms in children than in adults. The adult with gastroesophageal reflux will often complain of heartburn but rarely has emesis, while the infant with significant gastroesophageal reflux will usually have emesis and may have associated failure to thrive or respiratory symptoms. Despite considerable clinical investigation, it is not clear whether the pathophysiology of this disorder is similar in adults and children. Early motility studies suggested that decreased basal lower esophageal sphincter pressure was not a sufficient explanation for gastroesophageal reflux in most infants. The wide use of intraesophageal pH monitoring led to a much better quantitation of reflux but has failed to improve our understanding of the disease process. A thoughtful and coordinated approach to this problem utilizing the concepts laid out in this textbook will enable future investigators to determine if conditions such as inappropriate relaxation of the lower esophageal sphincter during infancy are secondary to an enteric reflex, which is enhanced during the newborn period.

Chronic abdominal pain occurs during both childhood and adulthood, but its effects on quality of life differ. There is considerable evidence to suggest that perception of pain may have physiologic differences between the young and elderly. The threshold for pain perception and ability to tolerate pain may vary through development and is based on biopsychosocial factors. Children are more vulnerable to coping with chronic abdominal pain in a dysfunctional manner. While most adults would not tolerate their own absence from work for extended periods of time, they often will encourage their child to be absent from school for long periods secondary to ill-defined abdominal pain.

During childhood, the management of chronic problems such as abdominal pain or cyclic vomiting in children usually requires psychosocial intervention at the family level— a form of therapy which is not often pursued in adult patients. Munchausen's syndrome-by-proxy, in which a caregiver reports fictitious symptoms, is often associated with fabricated digestive complaints. A clinician who is unaware of these possibilities will be unable to provide appropriate care to some pediatric patients.

The role of development and learned behavior in motility disorders is probably most often and clearly demonstrated in toilet learning and its role in functional constipation. The child who has not learned to respond appropriately to the sensations that signal readiness for defecation will often develop functional fecal retention, a syndrome characterized by constipation and soiling. Functional fecal retention is not seen in nonpsychotic adults. Fortunately, a comprehensive understanding of this common clinical pediatric problem will lead to speedy, successful management in many cases.

This textbook will not only help the reader understand the uniqueness of these pediatric motility disorders, it also covers what diagnostic studies are of greater or lesser value in the pediatric patient. Esophageal manometry probably has less of a role in the clinical evaluation of gastroesophageal reflux during infancy than during the adult years. However, colonic manometry may be more useful and easily interpreted during childhood because of age-related changes in high-amplitude propagated contractions (HAPC) frequency. In vivo manometric studies combined with the ability to look at intestinal transit with nuclear scintigraphy will greatly increase our understanding of such common disorders as recurrent abdominal pain, gastroesophageal reflux, and cyclic vomiting. It is likely that further development of these techniques will allow us to determine which of these disorders are primary defects in intestinal motility and which are secondary manifestations of other systemic disorders. The role of the central nervous system in modulating intestinal motility will be more clearly defined through clinical applications of these tools.

This text represents an exciting opportunity to summarize the growth of knowledge in clinical pediatric enteric neuromuscular disorders, an area which has expanded from initial descriptive studies just a decade ago to search for the pathophysiologic mechanisms of diseases that affect children. In the future, there will be explanations for the genetic bases for congenital motility disorders, and our fuller understanding of childhood motility disorders may provide insight towards understanding functional bowel disorders in adults.

A. Craig Hillemeier, MD
Associate Professor of Pediatrics
Director of Pediatric Gastroenterology
University of Michigan Medical Center
Ann Arbor, Michigan

CONTENTS

Introduction to Pediatric Gastrointestinal Motility

Clinical Spectra of Chronic Enteric Neuromuscular Disorders

Motility Testing

Treatment of Enteric Neuromuscular Disorders

Introduction to Pediatric Gastrointestinal Motility

1

Developmental Physiology

TAKESHI TOMOMASA, TAKAYOSHI KUROUME

ONTOGENY OF ESOPHAGEAL MOTILITY

Structural Development

The gastrointestinal tract appears in approximately the fourth week of gestation as a hollow, tubular structure extending from the mouth to the cloaca. The most proximal part of this tube forms the esophagus, which is separated by the diaphragm from the developing abdominal cavity. The total length of the esophagus is 2.5 mm in a 13.5-mm embryo and 6.3 mm in a 37-mm embryo. Its absolute length increases at a more rapid rate than does the fetus as a whole.[1]

At birth, the esophagus measures approximately 8 to 10 cm in length from the cricoid cartilage to the diaphragm. This length doubles in the first 2 to 3 years of life. During growth, its upper and lower margins move caudally. The vertebral levels of the upper and lower ends of the esophagus in the neonate are approximately two vertebral levels higher than in the adult.[2] After birth, there is a linear correlation between the distance from the nose to the diaphragm and both body length and crown to rump length.[3]

The abdominal esophagus is as large as the stomach in the 8-week-old fetus. It gradually becomes very short, until it is only a few millimeters in length at term. It then lengthens over a period of a few years to reach a final length of 3 to 6 cm.[2] This process is essential to understanding the pathophysiology of gastroesophageal reflux in young infants. The presence of an intra-abdominal esophagus is one of the most important antireflux mechanisms. An increase in intra-abdominal pressure causes

compression of this part of the esophagus. When coughing, the increase in intra-abdominal pressure is as high as 85 mm Hg in adults, clearly higher than the sphincter pressure alone. Thus, this compression of the intra-abdominal esophagus, which occurs immediately and with a strength equal to the intra-abdominal pressure, must play a critical role in the antireflux mechanism.

Esophageal muscles have two origins. The upper third of the esophagus contains the mainly striated muscles derived from the caudal bronchial arches. The smooth muscle of the lower esophagus is derived from the splanchnic mesoderm.[2] The myenteric plexus of Auerbach demonstrates cholinesterase activity by 9½ weeks' gestation, and ganglion cells are differentiated by week 13 of gestation.[1] Immunoreactivities for nerve and glial cell protein first appear in the esophagus by week 8 of gestation, and immunoreactivities for regulatory peptides, such as VIP, bombesin, and neuropeptide Y, appear by week 11.[4]

Functional Development

Swallowing. Several studies have demonstrated that the intrauterine human fetus swallows amniotic fluid. In 1963, McLain[5] first demonstrated by means of amniography the swallowing of contrast medium in the human fetus as early as the 30th week. Three years later, Pritchard[6] used a radioisotope to measure the volume of amniotic fluid swallowed by the fetus. He showed effective swallowing by the fetus at 16 to 17 weeks' gestation. In weeks 20 and 21, the fetus swallows 13 to 16 ml of amniotic fluid per day. Although animal studies have demonstrated peristaltic movement in the esophagus of the fetus, there is no data on peristalsis in the esophagus of the human fetus.

Early studies with cineradiography showed that esophageal peristalsis in the first few hours of life appears to be the same as in adults.[7] Later, however, a manometric study revealed that normal newborns under 12 hours of age show a poorly coordinated response to deglutition, with an extremely rapid peristalsis, and at least 20% nonperistaltic, simultaneous contractions along the entire length of the esophagus in response to deglutition. Biphasic contractions were present occasionally at this age. Repeated observation of these infants showed that those who had demonstrated a rapid propagation velocity when under 12 hours of age had a slower propagation speed on the third day of life. Those infants who had a less rapid propagation velocity when under 12 hours of age showed no change on the third day.[8]

Secondary peristalsis, or peristalsis unrelated to deglutition, is frequent in young infants.[8] Secondary peristalsis may be important for the clearance of spontaneous reflux of gastric contents, and for the prevention of peptic esophagitis.[9]

Lower esophageal sphincter. The high-pressure zone generated in the lower end of the esophagus by the lower esophageal sphincter (LES) is believed to be an important antireflux mechanism. In humans, the LES is not a distinct muscle but is an extension of the esophageal body circular muscle. The LES in newborns is several times shorter than in adults. Lower esophageal sphincter pressure measured manometrically is lower in infants than in adults. The LES pressure in infants increases with age, reaching adult levels in 3 to 6 weeks.[10] Measured at rest, however, it does not accurately predict which infants will suffer from gastroesophageal reflux, suggesting that resting LES pressure is not the sole determinant.[11,12]

In addition to its function as an antireflux barrier, appropriate relaxation is another important function of the LES. Lower esoph-

ageal sphincter relaxation occurs 2.5 seconds after the initiation of swallowing, before the arrival of the bolus in the lower esophagus. The LES remains open for 10 to 12 seconds, until the peristaltic wave enters the sphincter.[13] This relaxation has been observed in infants less than 12 hours of age.[8] Inappropriate relaxation or relaxation that occurs in the absence of a peristaltic sequence in the esophageal body has been reported not only in adult patients with reflux esophagitis,[14] but also in infants with the same condition.[9,11,15,16]

Lower esophageal sphincter function is regulated by a complicated mechanism involving neural and hormonal controls. Serum and tissue concentrations of regulatory peptides and other neurotransmitters change during perinatal development. For example, fasting serum concentrations of gastrin, a potent hormone that increases LES pressure, is three times higher in cord blood than in adult serum.[17] Other gastrointestinal hormones exhibit age-related change in the postnatal period.[18] The physiologic implications of these phenomena are not clear. Although an age-dependent rise in the sensitivity of LES to gastrin has been demonstrated in the opossum, there are no studies of LES pressure responses to hormone infusions in human neonates.

ONTOGENY OF GASTRIC MOTILITY
Structural Development

The stomach appears as a fusiform dilation of the foregut in the neck of the embryo in approximately week 4 of gestation. By the end of week 7, it has descended into the abdomen. The dorsal border enlarges more rapidly than the ventral border, producing a convexity that later becomes the greater curvature. At about 6 weeks, the stomach undergoes a 90° clockwise rotation.[1]

Following a craniocaudal pattern of development, circular smooth muscle appears in weeks 8 to 9 of gestation. By about 3½ months, the circular muscle is arranged into definite bundles in the stomach. Circular muscle is fully organized in the pylorus in the fourth and fifth months. The outer longitudinal muscle appears at week 11 or 12. By about the seventh month of gestation, the stomach musculature appears mature, both morphologically and histologically. Even at birth, however, the thickness of the muscular layer is thinner than that of the adult stomach.[19] In animals such as cats and rabbits, gastric myocytes in newborns are smaller in size compared with those in mature animals.

Vagal and sympathetic fibers have innervated the entire stomach by about week 9 of gestation.[20] Neuroblasts are seen in the stomach in the seventh week.[21] Catecholamines have been demonstrated in sympathetic fibers in Auerbach's plexus by week 10 and in Meissner's plexus by week 13.[22]

Functional Development

Gastric motility can be evaluated from several different perspectives: contraction and relaxation of the muscle, transit of luminal contents, and regulating mechanisms.

Motility. One of the functions of the gastric fundus is receptive relaxation. When the stomach accepts a meal and gastric volume increases, only a slight rise in intraluminal pressure occurs, due to the relaxation of the fundic smooth muscle. Recent studies using a barostat revealed that gastric wall compliance in newborns under 36 hours old was less than that in adults, and that the receptive relaxation seems negligible in newborn infants.[23] These facts might explain in part why gastroesophageal reflux is more common in newborns than in older subjects.

Tonic intraluminal pressure increases in the fundus are necessary for the emptying of liquid meals, whereas antral peristalsis is important for the emptying of solid meals.[24] It follows that functions of the fundus might be very important in infants whose diet consists of nothing but milk. Using cineradiography, Tornwell et al[7] found that there are no peristaltic contractions in the stomach during the first 2 to 4 days of life, and speculated that within that time the stomach empties mainly by fundic contraction.

In the distal half of the stomach, gastric peristalsis, (propagating phasic contraction) plays two roles in coordination with the pylorus: mixing and emptying. Gastric peristaltic waves originate in the body of the stomach and propagate toward the pylorus as a ring that sweeps the intraluminal contents. In the postprandial period, the pylorus contracts as the peristaltic wave approaches the antrum, causing a rise in intragastric pressure and pushing undigested foods greater than 0.2 mm in phasic diameter back behind the ring. Gastric contractions have not been observed in infants younger than 2 days old.[8]

During fasting, there is a cycle of gastrointestinal motility patterns called the migrating motor complex (MMC). Three distinctive patterns or phases appear in sequence (Fig. 1.1). Phase 1 is a pattern of quiescence that always follows phase 3 and precedes phase 2. Phase 2 is a period of irregular contractions, varying in amplitude and periodicity. Some contractions in phase 2 are propagated, but not as often as those in phase 3. Phase 3 is a distinctive pattern of regular high-amplitude contractions repeating at a maximal rate for 3 to 10 minutes and migrating from proximal to distal.[25-27]

Phase 3 begins anywhere from the esophagus to the ileum. In the human, about half of phase 3s begin in the esophagus or the gastric body and migrate downwards, often but not always reaching the terminal ileum. The rest start in the small intestine.[27] Motilin, a 22-amino acid peptide, is responsible for initiating phase 3s that begin in the stomach. It is unclear how phase 3 is initiated in the small bowel. Somatostatin,[28] the intrinsic nervous system of the gastrointestinal tract,[29] and Cajal cells in the intestine[30] might be involved. The regulating mechanisms of phase 3 and their physiologic significance will be discussed in Chapter 12.

Intravenous erythromycin, a motilin receptor agonist, induced phase 3-like clusters of contractions in the stomach[31,32] (Fig. 1.2). These clusters, however, did not migrate caudally as they did in older children and adults.[33] It is therefore speculated that premature infants have a functioning motilin

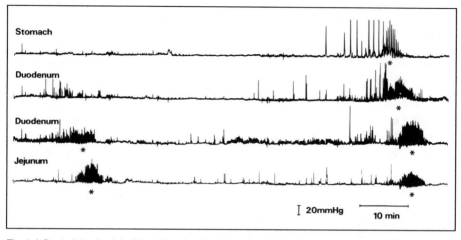

Fig. 1.1 Gastrointestinal motility pattern in a healthy adult. Note the cyclic occurrence of each phase of the migrating motor complex (MMC). The most recognizable motor pattern in the digestive tract is phase 3 (asterisks), which is distinguished by a band of repetitive contractions. It is followed by phase 1, motor quiescence, and then phase 2, which is characterized by periodic irregular contractions. Phase 3 starts either in the stomach or in any part of the small intestine.

receptor, but the mechanisms responsible for the propagation of phase 3 are immature. Whether motilin serum concentrations fluctuate in premature babies who do not have phase 3 as they do in adults has not been investigated.

Gastric and duodenal MMCs are present in term newborns and preterm infants older than 32 to 35 postconceptional weeks (Fig. 1.3). Approximately 30% of phase 3s begin in the stomach and 70% in the duodenum or small intestine in premature and term infants. In younger preterm infants, only uncoordinated sporadic single contractions and nonmigrating clusters of contractions are present (Fig. 1.4). These nonmigrating clusters of contractions have the same number of phasic contractions per minute (range: 2.6-3.6/min in the gastric antrum) as phase 3s, but they do not migrate aborally.[34]

The mean duration of gastric phase 3 in term and preterm infants is 3.5 to 4 minutes[34,35] and does not significantly differ from older children,[36] adolescents,[37] or adults.[34] The interval of gastric phase 3s in newborns has not been reported. However, since intervals of duodenal phase 3s are about 25 to 75 minutes[34,35,38] and 30% of them originate in the stomach, the periodicity of gastric phase 3 is estimated at approximately 150 minutes. This interval is shorter than in adults.

The clinical implications of the absence of gastric phase 3, or absence of its migration, are unknown. It may have little to do with feeding problems, because emptying of milk is mainly related to the function of the fundus, not to antral peristalsis. Or it may represent some prematurity in gastroduodenal coordination and be related to feeding problems, which are not uncommon in premature babies.

The contractile pattern in phase 2 of the MMC does not differ qualitatively from the postprandial pattern. The overall motility pattern in preterm infants who are too young to have phase 3 (28 to 32 weeks' gestational age) also appears similar. These patterns include sporadic contractions and clusters of contractions. The clusters have the same frequency of contractions per minute as that of phase 3. The absence of migration to the duodenum differentiates them from phase 3. These nonmigrating clusters occur 2 to 4 times per hour and last 3 to 5 minutes.[34,39] Contractions in these clusters comprise more than half the total contractions in the antrum of infants. They appear to be the dominant motor pattern in infants, whereas they are present only after meals in adults. As mentioned above, similar clusters of contractions are induced by intravenous erythromy-

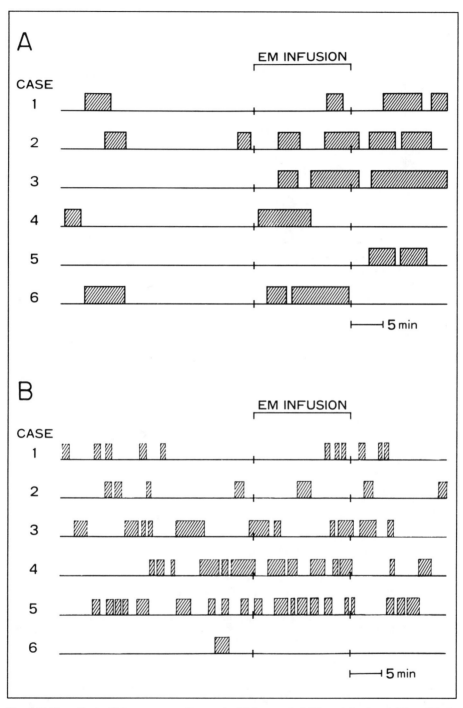

Fig. 1.2 The effect of intravenous erythromycin (EM) on antral (**A**) and duodenal (**B**) motility in premature infants who do not have phase 3s. Clusters of antral and duodenal contractions that are similar to phase 3 are indicated by shaded squares. After erythromcyin, many clusters are noted in the antrum. However, none of these migrated aborally. The frequency of clusters did not change after erythromycin infusion in the duodenum.

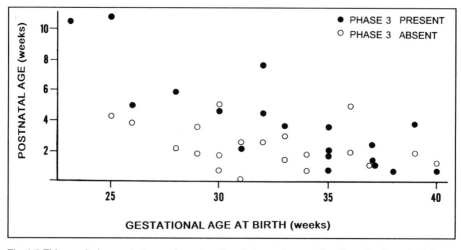

Fig. 1.3 This graph demonstrates a phase 3 pattern in neonates as a function of both postnatal age and length of gestation. There are phase 3s in the neonate whose postconceptual age is more than 35 weeks.

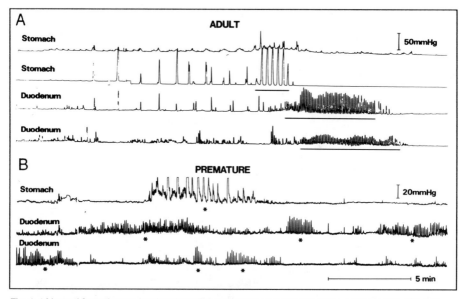

Fig. 1.4 Normal fasted antroduodenal motility pattern in an adult **(A)** and a neonate **(B)**. After phase 2, the regular, repetitive, strong contractions of phase 3 occur in the stomach and migrate down to the duodenum (underlines). Phase 3 is followed by a motor quiescence, or phase 1. In the neonate, no phase 3s occur, and nonmigrating clusters of contractions (asterisks) are present in both the antrum and duodenum. These clusters are the dominant motility pattern in newborns during the fasted and fed periods.

cin. The physiologic role of clusters in the transit of milk is unclear. The mean amplitude of both sporadic and clusters of antral contractions in infants is about 20 mm Hg,[33,39] or less than a tenth of the amplitude of antral contractions in adults.

The function of the pylorus must be important in regulating gastric emptying. Recent technical developments have made monitoring pyloric motility possible in human adults.[40,41] However, direct measurement of pyloric contraction has not yet been accomplished in neonates or children.

Gastric emptying. Amniographic studies performed 30 years ago showed that contrast medium moved beyond the stomach in a fetus as young as 31 weeks.[5] Gastric emptying, plotted as gastric volume as a function of time, best fits a monoexponential curve in healthy adults given a liquid meal. The pattern of gastric emptying in milk-fed neonates is similar to that in adults.[42] It seems clear from clinical experience that gastric emptying is slower in neonates than in adults, especially in premature infants. This conclusion has been difficult to document, however, because decisions on how much milk should be given to each age group for a fair comparison are arbitrary. In comparisons between term and preterm infants, where the same volume of milk per body weight was given, there was no significant difference in half emptying time ($T_{1/2}$) between groups.[43,44] Gastric emptying immediately after birth was delayed. Gastric retention 30 minutes after feeding was greater in infants during the first 12 hours of life than in infants who were 22 to 36 hours old.[45]

ONTOGENY OF SMALL INTESTINAL MOTILITY

Structural Development

At week 4 of gestation, the intestine is a simple tube. It subsequently elongates more quickly than the body does, and is approximately four times the crown to heel length at birth.[46] After transient herniation into the umbilical cord, the intestine reenters the abdominal cavity, rotating 270° at about 10 weeks.[1] After birth, the small intestine continues to elongate from approximately 2.5 m at birth to 6 m in the adult. Elongation is rapid until the crown to heel length is 60 cm, but the growth rate then proceeds more slowly and constantly.[47]

Separate circular and longitudinal muscle layers are recognizable in 10-week-old fetuses, although at this age the longitudinal muscle appears as essentially undifferentiated mesenchyma.[22]

Neuroblasts are present in the duodenum at 6 to 7 weeks' gestation,[48] and migrate craniocaudally through the alimentary tract, preceding the formation of the longitudinal muscle layer. As with the esophagus, Auerbach's plexus appears in the small intestine at week 9 of gestation and Meissner's plexus is evident at week 13.[1]

Functional Development

The function of the small intestine is to absorb nutrients and to transport indigestible residue, toxic substances, and bacteria into the colon for elimination. The motility of the intestine, therefore, is a series of preprogrammed, coordinated movements capable of adjustments and modifications related to the digestive or pathologic state (eg, fasted or fed, ileum full or empty, etc). These motility patterns are controlled by a hierarchical coordination of functions, including myocytes, intrinsic gut nerves, hormones, and the central nervous system.

The small intestine of the 8-week-old fetus responds to adrenaline by relaxing in vitro.[49] Microscopic cinematography showed peristaltic waves of the small intestinal walls in the fetus as early as the 12th week. These peristaltic contractions, however, propagate orally as well as aborally until the 30th fetal week.[48]

As described in the gastric motility section, a cyclic motor pattern, or MMC, is the characteristic motility pattern during fasting. In the small intestine, phase 3 is followed by phase 1, then phase 2, and another phase 3. As with gastric phase 3, small intestinal phase 3 is not present in preterm infants younger than 32 to 35 weeks of postconceptional age (see Fig. 1.2). Several other studies have shown similar results.[35,39] Before phase 3 appears, the small intestinal motility pattern consists of sporadic bands of nonmigrating repetitive contractions.[50]

There are several age-related differences in the characteristics of intestinal phase 3. The mean interval between episodes of duodenal phase 3s increases with age. It is 25 to 45 minutes in newborns,[34,35,51] 60 minutes in older children (mean age, 20 months),[36] 100 minutes in adolescents (17 to 19 years),[37] and 100 to 150 minutes in adults.[27] The mean duration of phase 3 does not change significantly with age.[34,36,37,52] Migration velocity and mean amplitude of contractions in newborns average 2 to 4 cm per minute and 20 mm Hg, respectively. These figures nearly double in adults.[34,35]

During phase 2 and the postcibal period, many clusters of contractions are present in infants. These contractions have the same frequency of contraction as phase 3, but do not migrate caudally. These clusters are absent or, if present, last less than 2 minutes in the healthy adult proximal intestine. It is not known by what age these clusters disappear.

Morris et al[53] reported that the number and amplitude of duodenal contractions increased markedly between 29 and 32 weeks. They also showed that these elements increased in infants whose mothers were treated with antenatal betamethasone, suggesting that maturational changes in duodenal motility may be induced before 29 weeks by corticosteroid administration. Others,[32,52] however, have shown gradual maturation in these variables throughout the perinatal period (Fig. 1.5).

In two controlled studies by Berseth,[52,54] premature infants who received enteral feeding within 2 weeks of age developed a more mature intestinal motility pattern, with more phase 3s, and fewer nonmigrating clusters, as compared with age-matched infants who received no enteral feedings.

In adults, the absence of intestinal phase 3s is associated with bacterial overgrowth.[55] In utero, however, the small bowel is sterile, so that absence of phase 3s is irrelevant. After birth, bacterial overgrowth of the small bowel might cause excessive gas production, nutrient malabsorption, pooling of secretions, luminal distention, and mucosal inflammation. Consequently, the release of inflammatory mediators and stretching of the bowel wall might result in ischemia, and cause a cascade of events leading to necrotizing enterocolitis. No similar data are available in children. Morris et al[56] measured small-intestinal motility in preterm infants and later analyzed the data based on whether the baby developed necrotizing enterocolitis after the motility study. They found no remarkable difference between the two groups

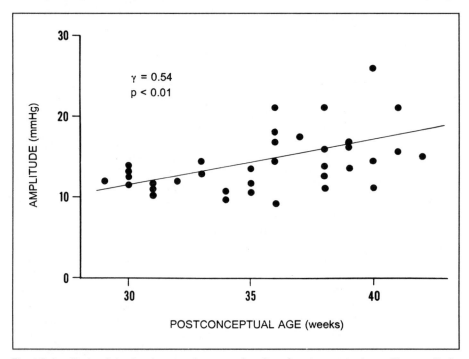

Fig. 1.5 Amplitude of duodenal contractions as a function of postconceptual age. The amplitude increases with maturation and reaches about half of adult values at term.

in terms of number of contractions per minute or amplitude of contractions. They could not, however, evaluate if the MMC was present, because they recorded intraluminal pressures using a catheter with only a single recording site, which could not detect migration.

Peristaltic reflex. Nearly 100 years ago, Bayliss and Starling[57] described the peristaltic reflex as contractions above and relaxation below that point of the intestine stimulated by mucosal contact or luminal distention. This local reflex is presumably mediated by neural currents within the myenteric plexus. Acetylcholine and substance P are the likely excitatory neurotransmitters.[58] Nitric oxide, vasoactive intestinal polypeptide, somatostatin, and CGRP may mediate relaxation. Substance P and CGRP are likely to be among the sensory neurotransmitters. Although this reflex seems very important for the control of small-intestinal motility, its ontogeny has not yet been investigated.

Frequency plateau. Each myocyte has its own cyclic rhythm of excitement that triggers contraction. This intrinsic rhythm of excitement (frequency of depolarization) is highest in the duodenum (10-13/min) and decreases continuously along the length of the small intestine until its lowest point in the ileum (7-9/min). This frequency gradient,[59] however, is not observed in the intact or in vivo duodenum and proximal jejunum. There is no change in the frequency until 10 to 15 cm beyond the ligament of Treitz. The electrical cell-to-cell contact is very tight in this region, thus the frequency of the proximal duodenum prevails. Together, these phenomena—frequency gradient and frequency plateau—explain why contractions in the region often propagate and why they almost always do so aborally. Since propagating contractions produce effective transport of the intraluminal contents, these mechanisms should quickly spread food that exits through the pylorus along the duodenum and proximal jejunum, ensuring that it quickly contacts

a wide surface of mucosa. Inversion of the frequency gradient is reported in symptomatic patients with Roux-en-Y anastomosis.[60]

When the frequency gradient and plateau are established in humans is unknown. Until week 30 of gestation, however, small intestinal contractions in the fetus propagate both orally and aborally,[48] suggesting that at least one of these mechanisms has not been established at that time. In preterm infants at weeks 28 to 30, the maximal frequencies of contractions—with or without clustering—in the proximal duodenum did not appear to differ between two motility recording sites that were 5 to 10 cm apart. The frequency plateau, therefore, could have appeared by week 30 (unpublished data).

Ileal brake. Infusion of nutrients into the ileum of healthy adults slows gastric emptying and small-bowel transit. This mechanism may contribute to preventing a volume overload in the distal intestine and to the efficient absorption of nutrients. The pathway of this reflex might involve hormonal regulation.[61] Whether this reflex is operative in human babies is unknown.

REFERENCES

1. Grand RJ, Watkins JB, Torti FM. Development of the human gastrointestinal tract: a review. *Gastroenterology* 1976;70:790-810.

2. Vandenplas Y, Heymans H. Development of the upper gastrointestinal tract. In: Vandenplas Y, ed. *Oesophageal pH Monitoring for Gastro-oesophageal Reflux in Infants and Children.* Chichester, England: J Wiley & Sons, 1992;3-26.

3. Putnam PE, Orenstein SR. Determining esophageal length from crown-rump length. *J Pediatr Gastroenterol Nutr* 1991;13:354-9.

4. Hitchcock RJI, Pemble MJ, Bishop AE, Spitz L, Polak JM. The ontogeny and distribution of neuropeptides in the human fetal and infant esophagus. *Gastroenterology* 1992;102:840-8.

5. McLain CR Jr. Amniography studies of the gastrointestinal motility of the human fetus. *Am J Obstet Gynecol* 1963;86:1079-87.

6. Pritchard JA. Fetal swallowing and amniotic fluid volume. *Obstet Gynecol* 1966;28:606-10.

7. Tornwall L, Lind J, Peltonen T, Wegelius C. The gastro-intestinal tract of the newborn. *Ann Paediatr Fenn* 1958;4:209-26.

8. Gryboski JD. The swallowing mechanism of the neonate: esophageal and gastric motility. *Pediatrics* 1965;35:445-52.

9. Cucchiara S, Staiano A, Di Lorenzo C, et al. Pathophysiology of gastroesophageal reflux and distal esophageal motility in children with gastroesophageal reflux patients with reflux esophagitis. *J Pediatr Gastroenterol Nutr* 1988;7:830-6.

10. Boix-Ochoa J, Canals J. Maturation of the lower esophagus. *J Pediatr Surg* 1976;11:749-56.

11. Moroz SP, Espinoza J, Cumming WA, Diamant NE. Lower esophageal sphincter function in children with and without esophageal reflux. *Gastroenterology* 1976;71:236-41.

12. Herbst JJ. Gastroesophageal reflux. *J Pediatr* 1981;98:859-70.

13. Pope CE. A dynamic test of sphincter strength: its application to the lower esophageal sphincter. *Gastroenterology* 1967;52:779-83.

14. Dodds WJ, Dent J, Hogan DJ, et al. Mechanism of gastroesophageal reflux in patients with reflux esophagitis. *N Engl J Med* 1982;307:1547-52.

15. Werlin SL, Dodds WJ, Hogan WJ, et al. Mechanisms of gastroesophageal reflux in children. *J Pediatr* 1980;97:244-9.

16. Dent J, Davidson GP, Baarnes BE, et al. The mechanism of gastroesophageal reflux in children. *Aust Paediatr J* 1981;17:125.

17. Euler AR, Ament ME, Walsh JH. Human newborn hypergastrinemia: an investigation of prenatal and perinatal factors and their effects on gastrin. *Pediatr Res* 1978;12:652.

18. Lucas A, Bloom SR, Aynsley-Green A. Development of gut hormone response to feeding in neonates. *Arch Dis Child* 1980;80:678-82.

19. Deren JJ. Development of structure and function in the fetal and newborn stomach. *Am J Clin Nutr* 1971;24:144-59.

20. Indir J. The development of the nerve supply of the human oesophagus and stomach. *J Anat Sco India* 1955;4:55-68.

21. Okamoto E, Ueda T. Embryogenesis of intramural ganglia of the gut and its relation to Hirschsprung's disease. *J Pediatr Surg* 1967;2:437-43.

22. Read JB, Burnstock G. Development of adrenergic innervation and chromaffin cells in the human fetal gut. *Dev Biol* 1970;22:513-34.

23. Di Lorenzo C, Mertz H, Alvarez S, Mori C, Mayer E, Hyman PE. Gastric receptive relaxation is absent in newborn infants. *Gastroenterology* 1993;104:A498.

24. Kelly KA. Gastric emptying of liquid and solids: roles of proximal and distal stomach. *Am J Physiol* 1980;239:G71-6.

25. Code CF, Schlegel JF. The gastrointestinal interdigestive housekeeper: motor correlates of the interdigestive myoelectric complex of the dog. In: Daniel EE, ed. *Proceedings of the 4th International Symposium on Gastrointestinal Motility.* Vancouver, Canada: Mitchell Press, 1974:631-4.

26. Wingate DL. Backwards and forwards with the migrating complex. *Dig Dis Sci* 1981;26:641-66.

27. Kellow JE, Borody TJ, Phillips SF, Tucker RL, Haddad AC. Human interdigestive motility: variations in patterns from esophagus to colon. *Gastroenterology* 1986;91:386-95.

28. Soudah HC, Hasler WL, Owyang C. Effect of octreotide on intestinal motility and bacterial overgrowth in scleroderma. *N Engl J Med* 1991;325:1461-7.

29. Itoh Z, Aizawa I, Takeuchi S. Neural regulation of interdigestive motor activity in canine jejunum. *Am J Physiol* 1981:240:G324-30.

30. Suzuki N, Prosser CL, Dahms V. Boundary cells between longitudinal and circular layers: essential for electrical slow waves in cat intestine. *Am J Physiol* 1986;250:G287-94.

31. Tomomasa T, Kuroume T, Arai H, Wakabayashi K, Itoh Z. Erythromycin induces migrating

motor complex in the human gastrointestinal tract. *Dig Dis Sci* 1986;31:157-61.

32. Peeters T, Matthijs G, Depoortere I, Cachet T, Hoogmartens J, Vantrappen G. Erythromycin is a motilin receptor agonist. *Am J Physiol* 1989;257:G470-4.

33. Tomomasa T, Miyazaki M, Koizumi T, Kuroume T. Erythromycin increases gastric antral motility in human premature infants. *Biol Neonate* 1993;63:349-52

34. Tomomasa T, Itoh Z, Koizumi T, Kuroume T. Nonmigrating rhythmic activity in the stomach and duodenum of neonates. *Biol Neonate* 1985;48:1-9.

35. Bisset WM, Watt JB, Rivers RPA, Milla PJ. Ontogeny of fasting small intestinal motor activity in the human infant. *Gut* 1988;29:483-8.

36. Cucchiara S, Bortolotti M, Colombo C, et al. Abnormalities of gastrointestinal motility in children with nonulcer dyspepsia and in children with gastroesophageal reflux disease. *Dig Dis Sci* 1991;36:1066-73.

37. Pineiro-Carrero VM, Andres JM, Davis RH, Mathias JR. Abnormal gastroduodenal motility in children and adolescents with recurrent functional abdominal pain. *J Pediatr* 1988;113:820-5.

38. Berseth CL, Nordyke CK, Valdes MG, Furlow BL, Go VLW. Responses of gastrointestinal peptides and motor activity to milk and water feedings in preterm and term infants. *Pediatr Res* 1992;6:587-90.

39. Ittmann PI, Amarnath R, Berseth CL. Maturation of antroduodenal motor activity in preterm and term infants. *Dig Dis Sci* 1992;37:14-9.

40. Dent J. A new technique for continuous sphincter pressure measurements. *Gastroenterology* 1976;71:263-7.

41. Houghton LA, Read NW, Heddle R, et al. Motor activity of the gastric antrum, pylorus, and duodenum under fasted conditions and after a liquid meal. *Gastroenterology* 1988;94:1276-84.

42. Siegel M, Lebenthal E. Development of gastrointestinal motility and gastric emptying during the fetal and newborn periods. In: Lebenthal

E, ed. *Human Gastrointestinal Development.* New York, NY: Raven Press, 1989;277-98.

43. Signer E, Fridrich R. Gastric emptying in newborns and young infants. *Acta Paediatr Scand* 1975;64:525-30.

44. Blumenthal I, Pildes RS. Effect of posture on the pattern of stomach emptying in the newborn. *Pediatrics* 1979;63:532-6.

45. Gupta M, Brans YW. Gastric retention in neonates. *Pediatrics* 1978;62:26-9.

46. Reiquim CW, Allen RP, Akers DR. Normal and abnormal small bowel length. *Am J Dis Child* 1965;109:447-51.

47. Siebert JR. Small-intestine length in infants and children. *Am J Dis Child* 1980;134:593-5.

48. Takita S. Automaticity of the alimentary tract: observation on the fetal alimentary tract, the so-called ganglion-free intestine, and the anastomosed organ. *Jpn Smooth Muscle Res* 1979;6:79-86.

49. Hart SL, Mir MS. Adrenoceptors in the human foetal small intestine. *Br J Pharmacol* 1970;41:567-9.

50. Milla PJ, Fenton TR. Small intestinal motility patterns in the perinatal period. *J Pediatr Gastroenterol Nutr* 1983;2(suppl 1):S141-4.

51. Amarnath RP, Berseth CL, Malagelada J-R, Perrault J, Abell TL, Hoffman AD. Postnatal maturation of the small intestinal motility in preterm and term infants. *J Gastrointest Motil* 1989;1:138-43.

52. Berseth CL. Gestational evolution of small intestine motility in preterm and term infants. *J Pediatr* 1989;115:646-51.

53. Morris FH, Moore M, Weisbrodt NW, West MS. Ontogenic development of gastrointestinal motility: duodenal contractions in preterm infants. *Pediatrics* 1986;78:1106-13.

54. Berseth CL. Effect of early feeding on maturation of the preterm infant's small intestine. *J Pediatr* 1992;120:947-53.

55. Vantrappen G, Janssens J, Hellemans J, Ghoos Y. The interdigestive motor complex of normal subjects and patients. *J Clin Invest* 1977;59:1158-66.

56. Morris FH, Moore M, Gibson T, West MS. Motility of the small intestine in preterm infants who later have necrotizing enterocolitis. *J Pediatr* 1990;117:S20-3.

57. Bayliss WM, Starling EH. The movements and innervation of the small intestine. *J Physiol (Lond)* 1989;24:99-143.

58. Grider JR. Identification of neurotransmitters regulating intestinal peristaltic reflex in humans. *Gastroenterology* 1989;97:1414-9.

59. Diamant NE, Bortoff A. Nature of the intestinal slow-wave frequency gradient. *Am J Physiol* 1969;216:301-7.

60. Vantrappen G, Coreman G, Janssens J, Mantides A, Vanden Borre F. Inversion of the slow-wave frequency gradient in symptomatic patients with Roux-en-Y anastomosis. *Gastroenterology* 1991;101:1282-8.

61. Soper NJ, Chapman NJ, Kelly KA, Brown ML, Phillips SF, Go VLW. The "Ileal brake" after ileal pouch-anal anastomosis. *Gastroenterology* 1990;98:111-6.

2

Integration of Biomedical and Psychosocial Management

DAVID R. FLEISHER

Two concepts helped and hindered clinicians throughout the 20th Century: 1) the most important and legitimate use of physicians' time is in the diagnosis and cure of disease; and 2) patients are cured of illness through cognitive learning and compliance with rational prescriptions based on biomedical science. What has made these concepts a hindrance is that they exclude most of what doctors and patients do together.

The majority of patients referred to pediatric gastroenterologists have functional disorders, including toddler's diarrhea, gastroesophageal reflux, functional fecal retention, and recurrent abdominal pain (RAP). Toddler's diarrhea is incurable, but is self-limited. Functional fecal retention can be cured by the child, with the aid of physicians and parents. Recurrent abdominal pain and gastroesophageal reflux have no cure and may not be self-limited. Other disorders, such as inflammatory bowel disease, cystic fibrosis, and chronic liver disease, are managed with drugs and surgery, none of which completely restores the child's health.

Every clinician encounters patients who want to get well but are unable to recognize or change behaviors that limit the success of optimal medical treatment. Helping patients who feel troubled by illnesses that may not be amenable to diagnosis or cure, and helping them overcome self-inflicted impediments to recovery will remain the clinician's greatest challenge and, perhaps, most noble achievement.

The doctor-patient relationship is where clinical care and research begins and—ultimately—succeeds or fails. What follows is an attempt to review the nature and dynamics of that relationship and the clinical process that begins the moment a patient and physician engage in it. Recurrent abdominal pain, perhaps the most common condition encountered in pediatric gastroenterology, is used in the following discussion. However, the validity of the concepts put forth rests on their applicability to almost any disorder encountered in clinical practice.

DISEASE, ILLNESS, AND THE ROLE OF THE PHYSICIAN

Criteria for successful management for RAP have yet to be clarified or tested.[1-6] If therapeutic goals extend beyond rigorous diagnostic elimination of organic disease[7,8] and success is viewed as keeping the symptom from impairing the ability of the child to function normally, then sophistication in the use of the doctor-patient relationship becomes necessary.[1,9-11] If the physician's role is limited to the diagnosis and treatment of disease,[12-14] how does a clinician help someone troubled by symptoms that cannot be reduced to physicochemical terms or "cured" by technologic means?[12]

An alternative role for the clinician is based on the distinction between "disease" and "illness." Disease is objectively demonstrable tissue damage and organ malfunction. Illness is the subjective sense of feeling unwell, suffering, or being disabled.[15] An alternative role, then, defines the clinician as one who views the diagnosis and treatment of disease as important, but only part of what is needed to overcome illness.

Basic Values of Clinical Practice

Patient-oriented practice requires conceptual tools that aid the doctor-patient relationship, as well as communication skills.[13,16-18] The clinical process is predicated on three values: the intrinsic worth of the individual, acceptance, and the patient's right to self-determination.[19]

A belief in the intrinsic worth of the individual allows the doctor to care about the individual who needs help. It leads to a more conservative approach to health care and allows the patient to trust the physician.

The value of acceptance implies that the doctor is committed to try to help the patient regardless of whether the patient is attractive or unpleasant, or the disease is interesting or mundane.[20] Acceptance is the basis of professionalism—the value that helps the clinician be nonjudgmental.

The patient's right to self-determination implies that physicians do not own patients. We are hired by patients to engage in a collaborative effort aimed at overcoming their illness. If we want patients to follow our recommendations, we must use language the patient understands and explain the reasons for recommendations so that the patient can make a rational choice.

The Doctor-patient Relationship

Three models of the doctor-patient relationship have been proposed.[16] *The activity-passivity* model is one in which the physician ministers to the patient, who passively receives these actions and whose participation is not required. This model is appropriate for patients in coma or who are otherwise unable to respond. Responsibility for outcome rests solely with the physician. In the *guidance-cooperation model,* the physician tells the patient what to do. It is the patient's responsibility to answer the doctor's questions and comply with the doctor's orders. The *mutual participation model,* however, is based on a partnership of experts: the physician, whose expertise is in the knowledge of illness and disease, and the patient, whose expertise is in his or her unique personal experience with illness and disease. The importance of their respective roles is equal.

In collaborating, the physician helps the patient overcome illness and, in return, receives compensation.[21]

The doctor-patient relationship malfunctions when inappropriate models are utilized. For example, a child with RAP is brought to a physician who only allots a few minutes of time to each patient. The history is taken by the nurse. It is read by the doctor, who enters the examining room, asks few questions, palpates the child's abdomen, prescribes an antispasmodic, then leaves. The activity-passivity model thus applied is not likely to ease the child's pain or satisfy the parents.

Another example of malfunction can be seen when parents bring their child with RAP to a pediatric gastroenterologist. The consultant spends 30 minutes obtaining a history. The chronology of the child's pain is obtained, and questions searching for causes of abdominal pain are asked from a differential diagnostic list. There are no open-ended questions, questions about what the parents have been told previously, or description of parental fears or concerns regarding the child's symptoms. This illustrates the use of the paternalistic guidance-cooperation model of doctor-patient relationships. The physician determines "what's wrong," but he misses the opportunity to discover "what's going on." What are the present concerns? What may have caused the child's pains to have become problematic at this time? What feelings and attitudes may either impede or facilitate reassurance and compliance with treatment?

Dane Prugh stated that any of these three models can be appropriate, depending on the individual situation:

> Sometimes the doctor-patient relationship passes through all three phases. For example, if the physician is called upon to treat a late adolescent in a diabetic coma, an active and authoritative approach to immediate diagnosis and treatment is vital, and can be most assuring to the parents and the patient. Later, as the patient learns to control his diabetes, the guidance of the physician becomes paramount, and the mutual participation phase gradually evolves.[22]

Some patients are only comfortable with

the activity-passivity or guidance-cooperation models for personal or cultural reasons. Although these models place less responsibility on parents and child, the mutual participation model is more realistic when coping with clinical problems that elude total understanding and control, requiring mature participation by all members of the doctor-patient relationship for optimal results.[23]

Rapport. Good rapport promotes disclosure. Rapport is built when the physician is perceived as professionally competent, conveying an attitude of concern, respect, and trustworthiness. Rapport is not bedside manner—a bag of conversational or behavioral tricks by which patients can be charmed and manipulated. It is the conduit through which the patient reveals illness and enables treatment to be maximally effective.[23]

Assessing pain and pain behavior. A child's complaint of pain is determined by many factors: the intensity of sensory input, pain threshold, level of development, capacity to filter the environment, the child's emotional state and its influence on pain tolerance, cultural context, the expectation of response (or lack of response) from others, models of pain behavior in the environment, and the degree to which pain is used for somatizing (see page 17).[10,24,25]

Childrens' ability to differentiate between emotional distress and bodily pain is limited.[26] They may complain of a "tummy ache" when most or all of the distress is fear or anxiety.[24] Children may use "tummy ache" to mean hunger, the urge to stool, or nausea. Children can not accurately describe subjective phenomena. Their statements require objective corroboration.

Effects of a child's illness on parenting. The parent-child relationship normally requires parents to set limits and place expectations on the child that foster development and protect from harm.[27-30] When the child becomes ill, obligations of school and chores are put aside. Parents become more attentive and compliant with the child's wishes. If the illness is prolonged or perceived as potentially tragic, the parent-child relationship

tends to change. The child begins to ask for—and often receives—what he would never have asked for or gotten when well. The parents find themselves accepting limits, eg, cancelling vacations, taking time off from work, or tolerating behavior they would not have put up with previously. These changes are driven by parents' realistic or unrealistic fears and guilt that they have failed to preserve their child's well-being, notwithstanding that there may have been nothing they could have done to prevent the illness. When the diagnosis and cure are not forthcoming, parents go to increasing lengths to find a cure. The child's anxiety may increase as parents' control over attitudes and behavior weakens, and he may be exposed to increasingly stressful diagnostic procedures by a succession of physicians. In the process, the child's suffering intensifies. When a clinical presentation is dramatic and alarming, clinicians may jump to procedures that are unwarranted or even harmful. Children with RAP may develop incapacity and invalidism out of proportion to objective evidence of pain. To help the child and family, the clinician must address the child's exaggerated incapacity as a related but separate issue, with respect to abdominal symptoms.

The form and content of consultations. It is important to elicit the history from the parents in the absence of the child to allow them to speak freely and not expose the child to adult-level concerns.[31-33] At the end of history taking, the parent is asked: 1) "What have you been told by other physicians regarding your child's abdominal pain?" 2) "What are your concerns, your worst fears?" 3) "What are your spouse's concerns?" In answering these questions, the parent may reveal misconceptions derived from statements by other physicians as well as realistic or irrational fears derived from their own experiences and thoughts. The answer may provide clues about one parent's view of the other's concerns, parenting abilities, and the quality of their relationship.

A private chat with the child provides the opportunity to elicit the child's description of symptoms. It demonstrates the physician's respect for the child, respect that permits the physician to require the child's participation in understanding and coping with pain. Sometimes, the child discloses information that neither the physician nor the parents knew.[34] This chat might be the only opportunity the physician will have to discreetly question the child about possible abuse.

After the examination, the doctor and parents confer. What transpires during this conference largely determines whether management succeeds or fails. Success depends on three essential communications[2]: 1) an understanding of the child's symptoms; 2) effective reassurance; and 3) an offer of continuity and accessibility by the physician until the child's problem resolves.

Understanding the Symptom

Parents want to know: 1) What is the diagnosis, and what creates pain? 2) Is the condition safe or dangerous? 3) What can be done to relieve the pain? 4) Can the condition be cured? Will it resolve quickly or will recovery take time?

They can be told that the pains result from the most common cause of pain in healthy school-aged children, namely, the recurrent abdominal pain syndrome. Apley's prevalence data[4] are used to convince the parents that the condition is recognizable, occurs in other children, and is therefore not unique, puzzling, or ominous. The relationship of gut motility to pain can be explained in nontechnical terms. An analogy between gut spasm and leg cramps lessens the mystery surrounding the abdominal cramp. Although both may be painful, neither is caused by disease and both are self-limited. This speaks to the safety of the symptom.

Parents want to know what can be done to alleviate the abdominal pain when it occurs. If gut pain is likened to skeletal muscle spasm, it follows that the first remedy to relieve pain is for the child to lie or sit in a peaceful, quiet place, perhaps apply a heating pad, and expect the brunt of the pain to pass within 30 minutes. If the pain does not subside within that time, an antispasmodic, (eg, propantheline or hyoscyamine) may be taken. Parents are told that medication may help a great deal, only a little, or not at all.

They should not expect the medicine to immediately eliminate the pain. They should not administer the medicine for mild abdominal discomfort.

If an hour has passed and, despite these measures, the pain is the same or worse, the doctor should be called. Parents worry that a serious cause of pain may have supervened, (eg, appendicitis), or that a serious disease may have been missed and is now declaring itself. It would be ill-advised for the physician not to share these concerns about an unusually severe or prolonged episode of pain. The appropriate response is to reassess the child by phone, by examination in the office or emergency room, or by hospitalization, depending on the presentation.

The parents and child should understand that although RAP neither results from nor causes disease and tends to diminish with time,[35] there is no cure. Any disappointment caused by this statement is, with few exceptions, outweighed by the clarity gained during the consultation and the partnership established between the child, parents, and physician.

Effective Reassurance

Explanations transmit information on a cognitive level, but information alone may not enable parents to change their focus from the illness to the need for the child to proceed with development. To change their behavior, parents must shift emotionally, from being worried to feeling safe. The medical data are different from the parents' subjective reality, which may hold unrecognized, irrational, or displaced fears. Such unspoken fears may cause them to seek yet another "second opinion" and more diagnostic intervention. It is when we speak to their feelings that reassurance becomes effective.[36] How can the clinician discover the patient's unstated fears? An open ear can discern clues during the history taking. These clues are often seemingly unimportant statements about events and experiences that were deeply painful, eg, a parent who had surgery as a young child, or lost a sibling or parent during childhood or more recently, or whose favorite aunt developed abdominal pain, was told by her doctor that it was nothing to worry about, and then turned out to have colon cancer. When parents are asked what their worst fear is regarding their child's pain, they often mention cancer or the loss of their child. Once this emotional burden is uncovered, it may be easily relieved by, in this case, telling them that cancer of the colon is extremely rare in children.

The moment reassurance becomes effective is signaled by a change in the parents' mood, from frustration and worry to perceptible relief. The value of effective reassurance is that it enables the parent to once again expect their child to cope with symptoms and the tasks of growing up.

Continuity and Accessibility

"If Jenny is still having pain a month from now, bring her back for a follow-up visit. Let me see her again to determine if something has been missed or if we are still on the right track. In the meantime, should her symptoms become worrisome, call me anytime, day or night."

Individuals cope more confidently and independently when they know that support is available. The offer of continuity does not oblige the family to return for unnecessary visits. The need for follow-up visits varies widely. The physician's offer of ongoing availability is a warranty for the diagnosis, plan of management, and open-mindedness. The offer allows the use of time as a diagnostic and therapeutic tool and may substitute for stressful, costly diagnostic procedures.

THE ETIOLOGY OF RAP: SEMANTIC CONSIDERATIONS

Is RAP organic, functional, psychosomatic, or psychogenic? There is a great deal of semantic confusion regarding RAP and other disorders in which patients' emotions influence symptoms. The terms we use may aid or impede our understanding and enhance or destroy the therapeutic effects of what we say to patients.

Zighelboim and Talley contend:

Because of the overwhelming evidence that pathophysiologic and psychophysiological disturbances exist in patients with irritable bowel syndrome who present for medical care, and because of the real distress that patients with IBS endure, we conclude that this condition must be considered a disease.[37]

The reasons given by these authors for calling IBS a disease are sound, but the usefulness of classifying as "diseased" 10% of otherwise healthy schoolchildren (28% of fourth-grade girls)[4] is dubious. A diseased child is handicapped, vulnerable, and less capable of tolerating the stresses and enjoying the fun inherent in normal development.[29] Parents have a need to view their child as sound, and symptoms as discomfort, rather than disease.[27,28] Although identifying IBS as a disease may make physicians take it more seriously, the suffering and monetary costs of RAP in children are more than enough to justify its seriousness.[38]

Conditions in which organ malfunction is secondary to tissue damage are appropriately called disease. In contrast, symptoms caused by events that are in the repertoire of responses inherent in healthy organs are called "functional." The term is useful when explaining the mechanism of gut pain and its relationship to physical and emotional phenomena if the presumption of psychopathology is explicitly avoided in discussion with parents.[1]

The term "psychosomatic" has been applied to children with nonorganic recurrent abdominal pain.[39,40] Psychosomatic symptoms are the demonstrable and measurable physical accompaniments of primary neurotic illness.[41,42] Again, the presumption of psychopathology inherent in this term is unwarranted in the absence of neurosis.

The term "psychogenic" has similar implications and creates the same obstacles.[43,44] Psychogenic symptoms are those that the patient feels are located in the body, but are actually the result of disordered perception such as that which occurs in conversion disorder or somatoform pain disorder.[45]

SOMATIZING

Somatizing is defined as the conscious or unconscious use of physical symptoms for psychologic purposes or personal advantage.[15] Attention is shifted away from distressing thoughts or emotions towards bodily symptoms and concerns about disease for the purpose of keeping anxious feelings out of awareness. The following vignette illustrates somatization.

Case 1. A 19-year-old man with Crohn's disease returned for an unscheduled visit. He was distressed by increased abdominal pain and diarrhea, which he identified as an exacerbation of his inflammatory bowel disease (IBD). His agitation seemed out of proportion to his symptoms. He was afebrile, had gained a pound since the previous visit, and had no new abdominal findings. Although he seemed more anxious than usual, a 35-minute discussion failed to reveal any external cause of anxiety. "Honest, Doc, nothing's bothering me. It's just my stomach!" he insisted. The physician was ready to accept that the new complaints were caused by increased Crohn's disease activity, attribute the anxiety to it, and raise the dose of prednisone. As the patient was going out the door, he mentioned that he had been speeding the day before and was stopped by a policeman. On further questioning, the patient said that he had been surly with the officer, who responded by forcing him to undergo a humiliating search of his car and his person.

Comment: This patient's distress was not caused by a flair of Crohn's disease, but by the upsetting experience of the day before. He had a characteristic common to individuals who somatize: he was not aware of his emotions.[15,46] In somatizing, he unwittingly used his Crohn's disease and his transient increase in stooling to deny the existence of his emotional distress. As soon as the physician recognized the somatization, he was able to help the patient discover the emotional distress, validate it by reflecting on how upsetting such an experience would be for anyone, provide an alternative explanation for the increased symptoms, allow the patient to stop worrying about an exacerbation of Crohn's disease, enable the patient to ameliorate his anxiety by resolving not to repeat the behavior that caused the trouble, and avoid an unnecessary increase in prednisone.

Another use of physical symptoms is to manipulate an interpersonal relationship or communicate a need that would be unacceptable if asked for directly.

Case 2. A 10-year-old girl with sickle cell disease was experiencing frequent abdominal pain crises and spending more time in hospital than at home. Diagnostic interviews with each parent revealed that their marriage, the mother's third, had become stormy and that the "sickle crises" had increased in frequency at about the time the parents' arguments had become violent. No matter how intensely the parents fought, the fracas stopped the moment the patient pitched over in pain and they rushed her to the hospital.

Because somatizing usually occurs without patient awareness, the physician needs to recognize its presence. Confronting parents with the observation that their child is somatizing will cause them to feel that the doctor does not understand. It is usually necessary to start from the parents' view and not insist on our view of the problem before they are ready to hear it.

Somatoform Disorders

It is necessary to clarify the distinction between ordinary somatizing and somatoform disorders. Ordinary somatizing is encountered in everyday practice as part of the larger clinical picture of illness in many patients. The somatoform disorders are a group of five psychiatric syndromes, each consisting entirely of somatization.[45] Four of these sometimes present to pediatric gastroenterologists. *Conversion disorder* (300.11DSM-III-R) is marked by "an alteration or loss of physical function that suggests physical disorder, but that instead is apparently an expression of psychological conflict or need." *Hypochondriasis* (300.70, DSM-III-R) is a morbid "preoccupation with the fear of having, or the belief that one has a serious disease based on the person's interpretation of physical signs or sensations as evidence of physical illness." *Somatization disorder* (300.81, DSM-III-R) is often encountered in adolescent girls who present with "recurrent and multiple somatic complaints of several years duration, for which medical attention has been sought...from a number of physicians, sometimes simultaneously...but apparently are not due to any physical disorder...Complaints are often presented in a dramatic, vague, or exaggerated way, or as part of a complicated medical history in which many physical diagnoses have been considered." *Somatoform pain disorder* (307.80, DSM-III-R) is defined as a "preoccupation with pain in the absence of adequate physical findings that would account for the pain or its intensity."

Patients with somatoform disorders believe that their symptoms result from organic disease. They pressure physicians to pursue extensive diagnostic studies and therapeutic adventures. In some instances, the patient's relentless pursuit of medical procedures prompts suspicion of factitious disorders such as Munchausen's syndrome or Munchausen's syndrome-by-proxy.

Three categories of psychiatric illness in addition to the somatoform disorders are important in pediatric gastroenterology. In the section of DSM-III-R entitled, "Disorders Usually First Evident in Infancy, Childhood, or Adolescence,"[45] two disorders are mentioned that frequently present with abdominal pain: *separation anxiety disorder* (309.21, DSM-III-R), and *over-anxious disorder* (313.00, DSM-III-R). The section entitled "Factitious Disorders"[45] contains Munchausen's syndrome and Munchausen's syndrome-by-proxy. The section entitled "Codes for Conditions Not Attributable to Mental Disorders That Are a Focus of Attention or Treatment" contains malingering—the intentional production of false symptoms for the purpose of personal gain or advantage.[45]

Three somatizing disorders are frequently confused with each other: conversion disorder, factitious disorder, and malingering.[15] In conversion disorder, physical symptoms are not intentionally produced but are motivated by unconscious conflicts, which are "converted" to physical symptoms. In factitious disorder, the symptoms are intentionally produced, but are driven by psychologic forces that the patient does not understand and cannot control. When the factitious nature of the symptoms is disclosed, the patient cannot stop producing them, moves to another medical facility, and repeats the behavior. In malingering, symptoms are premeditated and intentionally produced for consciously manipulative purposes. The malingerer can discontinue symptoms as soon as they lose their desired effect.

By gaining familiarity with psychiatric disorders that entail somatizing, the physician's recognition of somatization is enhanced and inappropriate procedures are avoided. Such knowledge should not devalue the importance of a thorough database regarding the somatic health of somatizing patients, but will assist the physician in avoiding endless quests for the diagnosis and cure of nonexistent organic disease.[47]

REFRACTORY RAP

Management succeeds when parents feel reassured of their child's health, let go of the responsibility for "taking away" all pain from their child, and then place a clear expectation on the child to cope with the pain and not allow it to interfere with accomplishing important tasks. The child responds by rising to the parents' expectations, functioning better, and complaining less or not at all.[1,33,48,49] In some cases, however, the patient continues to complain of symptoms and the parents remain focused on the pain, their fears regarding its origin, and their helplessness in not being able to relieve their child's suffering. In most cases, treatment failure in children with incapacitating RAP is due to failure to recognize or effectively manage the accompanying somatizing.

The following vignette illustrates the use of the doctor-patient relationship, communication skills, and a hospital experience to understand a child's RAP and the family crisis that accompanied it. The parents rejected suggestions that their child be evaluated by a psychiatrist. They were willing, however, to work with the pediatric gastroenterologist, whose efforts included individual diagnostic interviews of each parent.[50]

Case 3. Donald, 12 years old, presented with incapacitating RAP in October. The previous summer he was sent home early from music camp because of "the worst case of home sickness they had ever seen," according to his parents. On a Monday morning 10 days prior to the consultation, he had one of many recurrences of sore throat. That was also the day his mother was to have begun working—her first job outside the home. Instead of going to work, she took Donald to his allergist, who prescribed amoxicillin. On the way home, the patient ate a hamburger that "tasted funny" and began complaining of abdominal pain. Two days later, still in pain, he was examined by his pediatrician, who diagnosed a viral illness, discontinued amoxicillin, and prescribed an antispasmodic, an antacid, and a bland diet. Donald's pains worsened, although there were no new physical findings. First, acetaminophen, then oxycodone were prescribed. The oxycodone caused Donald to nap for 45 minutes, after which he resumed his complaints of abdominal pain. Continued use of oxycodone seemed to make him more talkative and have nightmares; he began waking up during the night with "pains." His temperature rose to 99.8°. He was given milk of magnesia for constipation.

At the time of the gastroenterology consultation, he had spent the previous 8 days at home, moaning, holding his abdomen, but able to watch TV and eat normally. It became obvious that the parents' concerns were focused on their son's abdominal pain. They showed no recognition of his anxiety and therefore had no motivation to pursue psychologic issues. The consultant, therefore, did not insist on a psychiatric evaluation, but addressed the parents' concerns about their son's abdominal pain. After discussing the diagnosis of RAP, attempting to effectively reassure them, and committing himself to their service until the illness resolved, the physician stated that the greatest danger to Donald's well-being was not whatever was causing his abdominal pain, but continued school absence. The parents were urged to get their boy into school even if he were in pain. A liaison was established with the school nurse to keep Donald in school even when he might be too uncomfortable to sit in class some of the time.

Donald was in too much pain to go to school the next day and his mother was desperately worried. No alternative was apparent, so the patient was hospitalized for 5 days. His complaints subsided within 24 hours of admission. He assured the doctor that he was well, that he saw no purpose in continuing the in-patient assessment, and stated that he wanted to go home to prepare for Halloween. Interviews with each parent revealed stress within the family. The patient's 22-year-old half brother, the mother's child by a previous marriage, still lived at home, showed no desire for gainful employment or independence, and was causing increasing marital discord. In her interview, the mother described herself as someone who worried too much. "I'm very conscientious, maybe too much so. I want everybody to be happy. I hate arguments. I can't stand to have people mad at me." In his interview, the father said, "Ninety percent of our arguments are about Steve (the older boy). When Steve gets mad, she feels bad, unsure of herself."

Donald had been surprisingly symptom-free for 4 days and diagnostic studies had confirmed the absence of organic disease, supporting the diagnosis of RAP. The physician suggested that Donald be discharged that evening and that the family return to the office the next afternoon. "He'll be ecstatic when he hears that he can go home tonight instead of tomorrow," the father said. The physician went to the patient's room and told him, in the presence of his mother, that he could go home so as not to miss another day of school or the opportunity to carve his pumpkin. Surprisingly, Donald suddenly became agitated, saying that he preferred to stay in the hospital and not have to make the trip back to the doctor's office the next day. The physician and the mother had to insist that he go home.

The patient and his parents returned as planned the next afternoon. Donald had been unable to go to school that morning. He entered the office holding his head and moaning in much the same way he had moaned while holding his abdomen the week before. He assured the doctor that he no longer had abdominal pain, only a terrible headache. Donald and his parents were separated for consultation. His parents had become skeptical of his complaints and were now ready to insist that he return to school, even though he might be uncomfortable. Donald had no more absences from school and became free of complaints within 2 or 3 days.

Comment: Separation anxiety disorder most commonly occurs in school-age children; onset during adolescence is rare. The families are close-knit and caring. This kind of "school phobia" is unlikely in neglected children.[51] Diagnosing this disorder requires that the clinician search for the elements of the diagnosis: 1) symptoms of anxiety in the child, eg, the history of extraordinary home sickness; 2) recent stress, in this case the parents' heightened marital discord; 3) a triggering event, eg, the mother's new job outside of the home; 4) "receptor sites" in the parents that could foster the child's use of physical symptoms, such as the mother's guilt-prone, indulgent attitude towards her sons.

The success in managing Donald's case was limited. The parents did not acknowledge their son's psychiatric disorder or seek psychologic help; they did not use family therapy to help resolve their marital and family problems. It could not be said that Donald would avoid somatizing when confronted with future circumstances that exacerbate his anxiety. Nevertheless, the present episode resolved, inappropriate utilization of medical resources ended, and the child returned to school. Perhaps the family learned from the experience and might thereby better cope with future difficulties.[52]

Why Somatizing Patients Are Difficult to Manage

Society assigns three rights and three obligations to anyone deemed sick.[20] The rights are: 1) to be held blameless for the affliction; 2) to receive help and care from others; and 3) to be released from normal responsibilities. The obligations include: 1) a desire to get well; 2) a search for competent care; and 3) cooperation with care givers. A patient who discharges these obligations has normal illness behavior,[15] which physicians assume all patients should have. Although somatizing patients feel entitled to the rights accorded the sick, they are unable to live up to their obligations. They may seek competent care, but prevent its benefits by going to too many doctors for any of them to be effective. They are often noncompliant and engage in abnormal illness behavior.

Donald's case was challenging because his complaints seemed false from the start. This created a pitfall that could have been catastrophic to successful management. Implying or frankly stating that Donald was malingering would have destroyed the clinical effort in two ways: First, it would have been judgmental and caused his parents to defend their suffering child from insult. Second—and perhaps more important—a diagnosis of malingering would have precluded any opportunity to discover what was really troubling this boy. He would not be complaining, thereby bringing on himself so many distressful experiences, if there were not some hidden source of emotional pain. It is the clinician's task to suspect and discover this "pain underneath the pain," even if the patient cannot acknowledge it. This can be achieved by recognizing the anger that may be triggered in us by the patient who distorts symptoms, by avoiding judgmental pronouncements, and by searching for the unrecognized suffering that is at the heart of the clinical problem.[15] Discovering and coping with it, even if this means little more than not compounding it, is a test of clinical skill. Abnormal illness behavior is a legitimate clinical problem that provides opportunities for learning and therapeutic success.

THE GAP BETWEEN PEDIATRICS AND CHILD PSYCHIATRY

To care for a patient, a clinician must care about the patient,[53] and be honest and empathic.[54] Arguably, these characteristics require no special training or theory.[55] However, they may not be sufficient to deal with many somatizing patients, whose attitudes and behaviors may be frustrating to physicians and mental health professionals.[47,56] In discussing how to convince the doubting parent of the need for psychologic treatment, Lask & Fosson[56] designate those families who ultimately reject all psychologic treatment as choosing the "chronic illness option." Although their "choice" creates an impasse to clinical progress, such families nevertheless do seek further care for their physical complaints.

There are several role options available to the pediatric gastroenterologist when encountering such patients. The physician can avoid the mental health issue by opting to define his or her responsibility as the diagnosis and treatment of disease, not psychologic issues.[13] The physician could recognize the presence of a psychologic component to the patient's illness, feel inadequately trained to deal with it, and refer the family to a mental health professional. However, the referral would then be based on the physician's need to procure expert care, not the family's readiness for such a referral. The physician might attempt to compel reluctant parents toward a mental health referral by warning them that not doing so would prevent their child from "getting the treatment she needs,"[56] or by threatening to withdraw medical care if they do not comply.[30] Parents who feel judged or coerced might counter by blaming the physician for not being able to find the organic disease that caused their child's symptoms.[57] In an attempt to prove the absence of disease, the physician might subject the child to more invasive tests. It is impossible, however, to prove the absence of all disease, especially in families who "need" one.[57]

Another option is for the patient to be cared for by an interdisciplinary team, as exemplified by the Philadelphia Child Guidance Clinic/Pediatric Liaison model.[30] The team includes a pediatric gastroenterologist, nutritionist, nurse clinician, psychologist, and psychiatrist. The advantages of such team care are 1) the range and depth of expertise offered are more comprehensive than any individual clinician is capable of providing; and 2) mental health consultation is obligatory; those families who might have been disinclined towards psychosocial assessment may be less reluctant when it is presented as a requirement for receiving medical care. The possible disadvantages of team care are: 1) it is more cumbersome, requiring coordination of several busy clinicians; 2) the patient's motivation for forming a strong doctor-patient relationship may be weakened by the necessity for relating to several individuals instead of one principal physician; and 3) patients who are unwilling to accept assessment by mental health team members may reject the entire team and proceed with further doctor-shopping.

Another option is care by a psychologically trained pediatric gastroenterologist who is familiar with the psychotherapeutic aspects of clinical management[22] and able to recognize the myriad ways somatizing may contribute to a patient's illness. Rather than permit the patient's refusal of a mental health referral to be a roadblock, the physician uses the rapport developed during management of physical disorders to concurrently assess and manage psychosocial components of illness. He or she is enabled to do this by avoiding the dichotomy of physical versus mental disorders and instead takes a personal interest in the child and family as human beings. By avoiding psychologic jargon and other connotations of the mental health professional, the physician is able to approach mental health issues in patients who would have rejected such attention were it offered by a psychiatrist. Such a physician is capable of providing supportive psychologic care, while remaining alert to opportunities for lessening patients' resistance to formal mental health referral when needed.[22] At the same time, the physician continues being responsible for protecting the patient's health from chronic and/or intercurrent disease and ill-advised procedures,[52] and is capable of providing unfragmented care to somatizing patients.

MODELS OF ILLNESS

One model of illness casts the patient as "a vessel of disease" and dichotomizes disease as either in the mind or the body. Lask and Fosson[56] address the defects in the dichotomized model of illness by proposing that virtually all illnesses fall on a scale, one end of which represents illnesses that are psychosocial, the other end of which represents illnesses that are organic. The rest of the scale represents illnesses which are mixtures of psychosocial and organic components. Instead of these two aspects of illnesses being dichotomized, they are blended.

Where does the emotionally healthy child with RAP and no organic disease lie on this scale? The scale implies that both a pediatrician and a child psychiatrist might be required to treat patients whose illnesses are represented by intermediate points on the scale, but how does one serve the child and parents who may be unwilling to utilize psychiatric treatment? If the "organic" doctor has insufficient psychosocial skills, the child will fall into a gap created by the limitations of each kind of doctor.

Barr[58] offered a tripartite model for classifying recurrent abdominal pain that takes into account the child with RAP who has no organic or psychiatric disease. He classified abdominal pain as organic, dysfunctional, or psychogenic. Levine[59] criticized this as being an "either-or" classification which obscures the fact that any patient has the potential for having all three categories of pain simultaneously or at different times during his course.

Sorting Out Components of Illness

The following is offered as a tool for analyzing the components of the patient's illness and developing a plan of management.

Most factors contributing to illness fall into six categories: 1) organic disease, 2) mental disorders, 3) functional symptoms, 4) somatizing, 5) symptoms that accompany normal development processes, and 6) problems caused by a malfunctioning relationship between the individual and society. "Organic disease" requires no further definition. A "mental disorder" has been defined as a clinically significant behavioral or psychologic syndrome or pattern that is associated with distress or disability and does not result from a normal response to a particular event, such as the death of a loved one, but rather from dysfunction.[45] "Functional symptoms" are produced by organs free of organic disease. Somatizing is the use of bodily symptoms for psychologic purposes or personal advantage. This term is not related to bodily symptoms caused by emotional stress, eg, diarrhea before a final examination or tension headache associated with nerve-wracking work. Only if such symptoms are used to avoid obligations or the recognition of emotional distress can somatizing be applied to them. If they are not so used, such symptoms are functional.

Symptoms that accompany normal physical or psychologic development are sometimes mistaken for pathology, eg, premenarcheal vaginal discharge mistaken for a yeast infection, adolescent gynecomastia mistaken for a breast tumor, or crying at night in a 20-month-old with developmentally appropriate separation anxiety being mistaken for abdominal pain. Illness may be more severe and difficult to treat when the normally supportive relationship between the individual and society malfunctions. For example, patients who lack health insurance or are homeless have a component of illness that may override all other aspects of clinical importance.

Analyzing an illness enables the clinician to apply management strategies appropriate to each part. The young man with Crohn's disease in Case 1 had an organic disease (IBD), an emotional disturbance (acute anxiety), functional symptoms (acute diarrhea), and somatization (the unconscious use of his organic disease and functional symptoms to prevent awareness of his anxiety and its cause). The girl with more frequent sickle cell crises in Case 2 had an organic disease (sickle cell anemia), psychosocial problems (family dysfunction and resultant emotional distress), and somatizing (the largely unconscious use of her disease to bring comfort during stress). In Case 3, Donald had no organic disease, a psychiatric disorder (separation anxiety associated with family dysfunction), functional symptoms (RAP), and somatization (his use of RAP and other physical complaints to gain the comfort of his mother's presence and avoid recognition of his emotional pain).

Any patient can suffer any or all of the six possible components of illness at any time. Common diagnostic and management errors result when, for example, an emotionally disturbed child develops symptoms of organic disease that are mistakenly attributed to his psychiatric disorder. Or, a patient with a chronic organic disease may somatize and distort symptoms, misleading the physician into performing procedures that may be inappropriate.[15] Some of the most intractable somatizers also have some of the most severe organic diseases.

Therapeutic Approaches to Each Component of Illness

Many clinicians doubt their competence in managing the psychiatric components of illness. When they recognize emotional illness or family dysfunction in their patients, they feel they have no option but to refer the patient to a mental health professional, regardless of whether the patient will accept such a referral. Pediatricians and mental health professionals alike[60] often seem unaware that overcoming a patient's resistance to a mental health referral is a procedure that requires the utmost sensitivity and patience during a collaborative doctor-patient relationship.[49,52,61] In evaluating a family's readiness for a mental health referral, consider the following:

1. Are the parents able to recognize psychologic (rather than exclusively physical) distress in their child?

2. Does the child's psychologic distress cause enough concern in the parents for them to seek help for it? Some parents recognize their child's distress, but are able to dismiss their worry about it.

3. Do the parents view a mental health referral as potentially useful? Many, especially families prone to somatizing, do not.[15,46,57]

4. Is a mental health referral feasible in terms of cost and distance?

5. A successful referral for psychologic treatment should be viewed as the recruitment of an added care modality rather than the transfer of the patient to another caregiver. The referring physician should remain involved in the management of the child's abdominal pain and responsible for assessment of new symptoms of any etiology.[19,49,52]

These conditions are not met by many patients who need psychiatric care. The question remains: What is a nonpsychiatrist physician's competence with respect to psychiatric aspects of management? Hollis'[19] hierarchic classification of psychotherapeutic procedures serves as a guide to physicians whose patients are reluctant to receive psychiatric treatment. Its six levels, from elementary to complex, are: 1) sustaining procedures, ie, demonstrating an interest, a desire to help, understanding, and expressions of confidence or helpful reassurance; 2) procedures of direct influence, eg, suggestions and advice; 3) catharsis or ventilation, eg, encouraging the patient to pour out pent-up feelings to relieve tension; 4) reflective discussions about the patient's current situation, eg, helping the patient to consider the effects of his actions on others and himself or to look at relevant but withheld feelings, attitudes, and beliefs; 5) encouraging the patient to think about the emotional forces that cause response patterns, eg, thinking about feelings that cause unwanted behavior; and 6) reflective discussions on the origins of response patterns and tendencies.

Sustaining procedures and those of direct influence occur during most visits to a doctor. Catharsis or ventilation takes place whenever a physician gives a patient a sympathetic ear. Reflective discussion of a patient's predicament is a procedure that physicians perform if they take the time and avoid viewing it as "not really practicing medicine" or as a lapse in the efficient use of time.[22] The following vignette illustrates the procedure of encouraging the patient to think about emotional forces that cause response patterns.

Case 4. An 11-year-old girl was brought by her mother for evaluation of recurrent abdominal pain and excessive school absence.

It was obvious to the observer that the girl's incapacity was out of proportion to the severity of symptoms. The patient had a dour demeanor. Her mother was intensely concerned. When they went into the examining room, the patient was asked to undress except for her underwear, put on a gown, and sit up on the examining table. When the doctor returned a few minutes later, the patient had done most of what had been requested. Her mother was sitting in a chair facing her child. Noticing that the patient had not removed her shoes and socks, the physician asked her to take them off, too. The girl, without saying a word or changing her facial expression, extended one foot. Her mother leapt from her chair and began untying her daughter's shoe. The doctor intervened and said that he'd prefer the girl to take off her own shoes and socks. The girl shot her mother a look of annoyance. The mother then appeared embarrassed and flustered.

After the physical examination, the girl returned to the waiting room and the mother and doctor retired to the consultation room. The physician told the mother that her child's pains were due to RAP and explained the mechanism and safety of this common symptom. He then voiced his concern about how much invalidism and distress her daughter's mild, nondangerous symptoms had caused. He recalled her mentioning that her two older sons seldom missed an opportunity to berate their sister. The physician remembered that, in eliciting the history of the mother's childhood, she too had grown up as the only girl with older brothers. He asked her what it was like during her own childhood. She said her brothers had made her life miserable with taunting and denigration. The physician then mentioned that he had noticed how uncomfortable she seemed when he stopped her from taking off her daughter's shoe. "What were your thoughts at that moment?" he asked. "I felt as though I had to help her!" she said. She acknowledged feeling this need to provide assistance whenever her daughter appeared distressed or complained of abdominal pain. The physician then reflected on how hard her sons were on

their sister and how good it must make her daughter feel each time her mother responded to the girl's expression of pain or need. Perhaps the girl needed her pain complaints to get this special feeling. The physician wondered out loud about the effect the mother's devotion had on her daughter's ability to master adversity, compete successfully, and, in the process, develop self-esteem. The mother immediately recognized that she viewed her daughter as a child who suffered the same emotional abuse she had sustained during her own childhood. Her facial expression changed from sorrow to mild annoyance and her tone of voice in speaking to her daughter became more matter-of-fact. Stomachaches became less of a problem and the child's school attendance normalized.

Hollis' sixth and most complex category of psychotherapeutic procedures is elucidation of the origins of psychopathologic response patterns. This is the goal of analytic psychotherapy, in which the patient is helped to understand pathologic emotional forces as well as the defense mechanisms that obscure their recognition and prevent change. This level of intervention requires psychologic training and is generally beyond the scope of medical practitioners. Nevertheless, medical practitioners can and do incorporate a great deal of psychotherapy in their daily practice.

Hollis made an observation beneficial not only to her social work students, but to all clinicians:

> There is a tendency to think that there is something mysterious about the case work relationship, something that makes it fragile and untouchable except by the very expert. In fact, it is no more complicated than—but just as complicated as—any other relationship.[19]

The functional component of illness is treated with education, effective reassurance, and the offer of continuity and accessibility by the physician. Any symptomatic treatment that is effective and safe should be employed. However, when the physician and parents focus mainly on the pain and its treatment, as though it resulted from organic disease rather than a harmless event causing discomfort, the child is likely to move into the sick role, with all of its entitlements.

The child's complaints may become more intense as dependency needs are indulged. As soon as the functional nature of pain is established, the goal of management should dramatically shift to preventing the symptom from interfering with school attendance and other developmental pursuits. Everyone goes to school or work on days when he or she does not feel entirely well. Missing school only adds to the child's problems; the longer the absenteeism, the further behind the child becomes both academically and socially.

Efforts by the parents, physician, teacher, and school nurse must be coordinated, and all inappropriate "gains" eliminated.[48,62] If a child cannot go to school, the physician must be notified immediately. Such calls should be responded to as an emergency because the event acutely endangers successful management. When the physician senses that the parent (especially the single parent) may not have sufficient strength to effect the immediate return of the child to school, the physician may go with them. As Nader stated, a school visit can be exceedingly productive and is worth the physician's time.[49] It almost always convinces the child of his parents' and doctor's resolve. The physician speaks with the school nurse and/or principal with the child present, explaining the importance of not missing another day of school. Communication is established between the school nurse, parent, and physician so that the physician immediately participates in any decision about what should be done if and when the child becomes ill at school.

The management goals of the somatizing component of illness depend on its pervasiveness within the family. Families prone to somatizing are less able to recognize and stop somatizing in their child than families in which abnormal illness behavior is viewed as aberrant.[15,52,58,63] When the parents' preoccupation with their child's abdominal pain is so tenacious that all explanations, attempts at reassurance, and appeals to reason fail to change parental attitudes and behavior, the

management goal must shift towards ongoing supportive care and the relinquishment of a cure as the index of success. Successful management keeps the persistently somatizing patient from switching doctors and possibly encountering iatrogenic harm, while at the same time recognizing and treating intercurrent disease appropriately.[52]

It is a mistake to prejudge the complaints of patients who somatize. The more it appears that the patient is somatizing, the more important it is to be open-minded, take a careful history, and do a thorough physical examination. Invasive procedures should not be based on subjective complaints alone; objective findings must suggest organic disease. Avoid using psychiatric terms;[30] eg, "stress" may be a more acceptable term than "anxiety."[15] The functional symptoms they experience are best explained in terms of the mechanical events occurring in the organ from which symptoms originate. Allow patients to develop ideas about the meaning of their symptoms. Prescribe medications in small amounts with limited or no refills. Avoid, as much as possible, potentially addictive psychotropic drugs. Avoid the paternalistic role that patients often want the physician to assume. The more a patient views the doctor as omnipotent, the more he views his own role as passive and dependent on the physician, to whom he assigns responsibility for making him well.

Charles Ford, a liaison psychiatrist, wrote:

> Referral to a psychiatrist is frequently not well accepted and not necessarily of benefit...Despite the severity of the underlying psychopathology, these patients may do better with a primary care physician, with whom they can have a long-term relationship, than with a psychiatrist.[15]

He then summarized how the doctor-patient relationship can be used to treat somatization:

> As the doctor becomes better acquainted with the patient, there can be increased recognition of the patient's use of physical symptoms as a metaphor. Symptoms are often attempts to convey feelings of hurt, needs for affection, anger, and a wish for help in an

ongoing psychosocial crisis. The physician's ability to communicate that these feelings have been recognized, without ever directly confronting the patient concerning the symptom, may alleviate the need for the symptom. With receptive encouragement extending over time, the patient may gradually learn to express emotions and needs more directly, thereby making somatization unnecessary.[15]

Management of symptoms that accompany normal developmental processes requires little more than clarity, effective reassurance, and the offer of continuity and accessibility. Management of problems caused by malfunction in the relationship between the individual and society requires the doctor to be the patient's advocate. The assistance of colleagues in clinical social work is helpful, if not indispensable.

HOSPITALIZATION FOR INTRACTABLE RAP

Hospitalization on the pediatric ward is a valuable option in the management of children whose symptoms have created a crisis refractory to outpatient management.[40,64,65] Outpatient studies often fail to identify an organic cause of the child's symptoms and accumulate in number and cost.[38] Outpatient management may fail because the responsibility for gauging and interpreting the child's symptoms and administering remedies rests entirely on the parents. They may be stressed, prone to irrational guilt, inclined towards somatizing, and so enmeshed in their child's illness that objectivity is impossible. Health insurers may try to disallow hospitalization because they equate illness only with organic disease.

A 5- to 7-day hospitalization for RAP is different from hospitalization for acute pediatric illnesses. It has four purposes: 1) testing the premise that the child is in pain by observation and documentation of symptoms; 2) developing a data base regarding the child's somatic well-being; 3) exploring family life and the parents' life experiences to elucidate sources of distress that trouble the child and family; and 4) conducting pre-discharge conferences with the parents and child to review what has been learned and plan future management.[52]

Two caveats are needed before describing how these four purposes are accomplished:

1. There must be no prejudgments of the causes of the child's illness. If the parents feel that the physician and other hospital personnel are biased and view their child's symptoms as nonorganic, they may not collaborate. Remain open-minded and avoid an adversarial tone with the parents regarding who is "right" and what is best for the child.

2. Although individuals from several disciplines participate in assessment and management (nurses, house officers, social worker, play therapist, psychologist, and medical, surgical, or psychiatric consultants), there must be a principal physician who leads the effort, keeps all the participating colleagues accountable, and who in turn remains accountable and freely accessible to the child and parents during and following the hospital stay. A team effort without this kind of leadership is counterproductive.

Observation is at least as important as any diagnostic test. Parent-physician collaboration is strengthened by acknowledging that two kinds of expertise are necessary to arrive at a true picture of the child's symptoms: the parents, who know the child more intimately than any doctor or nurse can ever know him, but who, by virtue of their parental feelings, lack objectivity; and the principal physician, who knows a great deal about abdominal pain in children and can be objective.

Diagnostic tests scheduled over several days allow time for observation. The child's symptoms may change in surprising ways. Distortions and inconsistencies which become apparent allow parents and physicians to question their erroneous but firmly held preconceptions. The parent and physician speak to each other about their observations and thoughts during hospital visits, out of the child's presence.

Asking the child or parents for a subjective account of pain, however, does not provide an accurate estimate of its severity. Teaching them to report pain intensity on a scale of one to ten substitutes a numerical expression for a qualitative description, but adds nothing to the objectivity of their description. Second-hand descriptions of pain should not be used for assessment. Personal observations yield more useful, less distorted information.

Subjective feelings of extreme bodily distress may accompany anxiety attacks. Prompt administration of an anxiolytic agent with little or no analgesic properties, followed by close observation of its effect, may reveal that the cause of distress was acute anxiety.

Rarely, exacerbations may become so intense that analgesia is required. If analgesics are given for RAP, they should be ordered as a single dose and given only after a prompt clinical assessment. It is helpful to assess the hospitalized child in apparent acute distress by walking with him to the examining room, where a thorough physical examination can be performed. If his complaints are heavily influenced by anxiety, or if he is somatizing, the way he walks, gets on and off the examining table, and responds to a request to jump in place ten times may reveal more to the physician and observing parent than any blood test or x-ray. Should the child's performance during this out-of-bed procedure show surprisingly little impairment, in contrast to his pain behavior while in bed with parents and visitors present, it is imperative that the clinician *not* express satisfaction in proving that the child's pains were exaggerated. The parents may feel accused of misjudging their child and react by being less open-minded and more intent on proving the doctor wrong. A more useful response by the clinician is to reflect on how well the child performed and wonder out loud about what the discrepancy between his description of pain and his behavior could mean. This avoids damaging the collaborative relationship that will be needed in discussions concerning the nature of the real distress—the pain underneath the pain.

A data base of diagnostic studies should be developed for organic disease. A prudent but thorough series of tests should be based on the differential diagnoses of organic causes of the presenting symptoms and any other bodily symptoms that may appear during hospitalization. Physicians are often tempted to omit large portions of the work-up because the nonorganic nature of the patient's symptoms seems so apparent. These omissions become important deficiencies when the patient develops symptoms after discharge and the parents experience renewed doubts about their child's health and the integrity of the physician.[49] The diagnostic process succeeds if it identifies not only what is wrong with the child, but also affirms the extent of his health. In this regard, every test result that is negative for disease has therapeutic value.

The feelings and attitudes of the child can be explored through skillful interviews[34] and during therapeutic play in a child activity program. The parents' feelings and attitudes that enhance somatization in their child can be investigated during individual diagnostic interviews. If parents are willing to speak with a social worker, psychologist, or psychiatrist, arrange for them to do so. Forcing unwilling parents to talk with mental health colleagues, however, is likely to damage rapport and subsequent management.

The diagnostic interview supplements and deepens the clinician's knowledge of the parents' feelings and attitudes during their child's evaluation and treatment.[26,50] It is typically an hour-long, relatively unstructured discussion with an individual parent during which information is elicited concerning their values, the parenting they received during childhood, the stresses experienced during personal illnesses or those of significant figures, their marriage, and any other area that might be relevant to helping their child towards well-being.[33,66-72]

If hospitalization succeeds in helping the parents understand the sources of their child's distress and recognize somatizing, they are then ready to implement management strategies to prevent the child from staying out of school or using the illness to solve problems. Both parents need to collaborate.[49] The pre-discharge conference is the physician's opportunity to organize this effort. Issues regarding family dysfunction can be addressed and the options available for overcoming it discussed. A follow-up appointment is made. The physician calls the school principal so that the school is prepared for the patient's return. The parents may transport the child directly from the hospital to school.

CONCLUSION

The clinical process raises questions regarding the dynamics of the doctor-patient relationship, its diagnostic and therapeutic use, the nature of illness and disease, and the often difficult distinctions between what is therapeutic, nontherapeutic, and countertherapeutic. Nontechnologic, interpersonal procedures are just as worthy of study and support as pharmacologic, surgical, or physiologic procedures.[19] Clinical process theory,[13,17,22] communication skills,[54,73] and relevant psychiatric concepts[51] add a powerful dimension to our capacity for solving clinical problems.

The author thanks Paul E. Hyman, MD, whose encouragement and editorial assistance made this work possible; Giulio J. Barbero, MD, Edward J. Feldman, MD, Jane Fleisher, RN, Johnna Russell, MD, Dale Fitch, LCSW, Deb Gayer, RN, and Soraya Kashani, MD, for helpful discussion and criticism of the manuscript, and Shirley Haden for her unstinting efforts in its preparation.

REFERENCES

1. Berger HG, Honig PJ, Liebman R. Recurrent abdominal pain: gaining control of the symptom. *Am J Dis Child* 1977;131:1340-4.

2. Fleisher DR, Recurrent abdominal pain. In: Gellis SS, Kagan, BM, eds. *Current Pediatric Therapy.* Philadelphia, PA: WB Saunders, 1980;9:183-5.

3. Christensen, MF, Mortensen O. Long-term prognosis in children with recurrent abdominal pain. *Arch Dis Child* 1975;50:110-4.

4. Apley J, Hale B. Children with recurrent abdominal pain: how do they grow up? *Br Med J* 1973;3:7-9.

5. Olson A. Recurrent abdominal pain: an approach to diagnosis and management. *Pediatr Ann* 1987;16(10):834-42.

6. Sharrer VW, Ryan-Wenger NM. Measurements of stress and coping among school-aged children with and without recurrent abdominal pain. *J Sch Health* 1991;61(1):86-91.

7. Fiedorek SC, Casteel HB, Pumphrey CL, et al. The role of *Helicobacter pylori* in recurrent, functional abdominal pain in children. *Am J Gastroenterol* 1992;87(3):347-9.

8. Mavromichalis I, Zaramboukas T, Richman PI, et al. Recurrent abdominal pain of gastrointestinal origin. *Eur J Pediatr* 1992;151:560-3.

9. Engle GL. The need for a new medical model: a challenge for biomedicine. *Science* 1977;196:129-36.

10. Zeltzer LK, Barr RG, McGrath PA, et al. Pediatric pain: interacting behavioral and physical factors. *Pediatrics* 1992;90(5):816-21.

11. Waitzkin H. Doctor-patient communication: clinical implications of social scientific research. *JAMA* 1984;252:2441-6.

12. Engel GM. "The best and the brightest": the missing dimension in medical education. *Pharos* 1973;36(4):129-33.

13. Roter DL, Hall JA. *Doctors Talking with Patients, Patients Talking With Doctors: Improving Communication in Medical Visits.* Westport CT: Auburn House, 1992;21-37,174.

14. Carson RA. What are physicians for? *JAMA* 1977;238(10):1029-31.

15. Ford CV. *The Somatizing Disorders—Illness as a Way of Life.* New York, NY: Elsevier, 1983;1-10,36-48,70-87,243-54.

16. Szaz TS, Hollender MH. A contribution to the philosophy of medicine: the basic models of the doctor-patient relationship. In: Stoeckle JD, ed. *Encounters Between Patient and Doctors.* Cambridge, MA: MIT Press, 1987;Ch 3.

17. Billings JA, Stoeckle JD. *The Clinical Encounter.* Chicago, IL: Year Book Medical Publishers, 1989;165-99,277-85.

18. Lipkin M, Quill, TE, Hapodano RJ. The medi-

cal interview: a core curriculum for residencies in internal medicine. *Ann Intern Med* 1984;100:277-84.

19. Hollis F. *Casework - A Psychosocial Therapy*. New York, NY: Random House, 1966;12-13,71-5,108.

20. Parsons T. Social structure and dynamic process: the case of modern medical practice. In: *The Social System*. New York, NY: Free Press, 1951;4228-479.

21. Quill TE. Partnership in patient care: a contractual approach. *Ann Intern Med* 1983;98:228-34.

22. Prugh, DG. *The Psychosocial Aspects of Pediatrics*. Philadelphia, PA: Lea & Febiger, 1983;207-34.

23. Korsch BM, Aley, EF. Pediatric interviewing techniques. *Current Problems in Pediatrics* 1973;3(7):3-422.

24. Barr RG. Pain tolerance and developmental change in pain perception. In: Levine MD, Carey WB, Crocker AC, Gross RT, eds. *Developmental - Behavioral Pediatrics*. Philadelphia, PA: WB Saunders, 1983;505-511.

25. Dolgin MJ, Phipps S. Pediatric pain: the parents role. *Pediatrician* 1989;16:103-9.

26. Green M. Sources of pain. In: Levine MD, Carey WB, Crocker AC, Gross RT, eds. *Developmental-Behavioral Pediatrics*. Philadelphia, PA: WB Saunders, 1983:512-17.

27. Korsch B. Psychological reactions to physical illness in children. *J Med Assoc Ga* 1961;50:519-23.

28. Sigal J, Gagnon P. Effects of parents' and pediatricians' worry concerning severe gastroenteritis in early childhood on later disturbances in the child's behavior. *J Pediatr* 1975;87(5):809-14.

29. Green M, Solnit AJ. Reactions to the threatened loss of a child: a vulnerable child syndrome. *Pediatrics* 1964;34:58-66.

30. Wood B. Biopsychosocial care. In: Walker WA, Durie PR, Hamilton JR, Walker-Smith JA, Watkins J, eds. *Pediatric Gastrointestinal Disease*. Philadelphia, PA: Decker, 1991;1750-52.

31. Morgan WL, Engle GL. *The Clinical Approach to the Patient*. Philadelphia, PA: WB Saunders, 1969;27-30.

32. Stoeckle JD. *Encounters Between Patients and Doctors*. Cambridge, Mass: MIT Press 1987;10-16.

33. McGrath PJ, Feldman W. Clinical approach to recurrent abdominal pain in children. *J Dev Behav Pediatr* 1986;7(1):56-61.

34. Richtsmeier AJ. Individual interviews of children with unexplained symptoms. *Am J Dis Child* 1985;139:506-8.

35. Friedman R. Some characteristics of children with psychogenic pain. *Clin Pediatr* 1972;11:331-3.

36. Korsch BM, Gozzi EK, Francis V. Gaps in doctor-patient communication. *Pediatrics* 1968;42:855-71.

37. Zighelboim J, Talley NJ. What are functional bowel disorders? *Gastroenterology* 1993104:1196-1201.

38. Coleman J, Levine MD. Recurrent abdominal pain: the cost of the aches and the aches of the cost. *Pediatr Rev* 1986;8:143-51.

39. Stickler GB, Murphy DB. Recurrent abdominal pain. *Am J Dis Child* 1970;133:486-9.

40. Rosenberg AJ. Recurrent abdominal pain in children. *Drug Ther* July,1982;161-76.

41. Pearce J. Migraine: a psychosomatic disorder. *Headache* 1977;17:125-8.

42. Kolb LC. *Modern Clinical Psychiatry*, 9th ed. Philadelphia, PA: WB Saunders, 1977;549-50.

43. Lichstein J. Abdominal pain in children: how to know when it's psychogenic. *Consultant* July,1977;129-36.

44. McGrath PJ Goodman JT, Firestone R, et al. Recurrent abdominal pain—a psychogenic disorder? *Arch Dis Child* 1983;58:888-90.

45. Diagnostic and Statistical Manual of Mental Disorders—III-R. Washington, DC, American Psychiatric Association, 1987;38-65,255-68,257-259,315-20,360,401.

46. Rickles WH. Personality characteristics of psychosomatic patients. In: Rickles, Sandweiss, Jacobs, Grove, Criswell, eds. *Biofeedback and Fam-*

ily Practice Medicine. Plenum Publishing Corp. 1983;159-65.

47. Quill TE. Somatization disorder: one of medicine's blind spots. JAMA 1985;254(21):3075-9.

48. Schmitt B. School phobia: the great imitator—a pediatrician's viewpoint. Pediatrics 1971;48:433-41.

49. Nader PR, Bullock D, Caldwell B. School phobia. Pediatr Clin North Am 1975;22(3):605-17.

50. Green M. Interviewing. In: Green M, Haggerty RJ. Ambulatory Pediatrics II. Philadelphia, PA: WB Saunders, 1977;Ch 53.

51. Harris JC. Separation anxiety disorder. In: Oski, FA, De Angelis CD, Feigin RD, Warshaw JB, eds. Principles and Practice of Pediatrics. Philadelphia, PA: JB Lippincott, 1990;652-4.

52. Hughes MC, Zimin R. Children with psychogenic abdominal pain and their families: management during hospitalization. Clin Pediatr 1978;17(7):569-73.

53. Peabody FW. The care of the patient. JAMA 1927;88:877-82.

54. Wilmer AA. The doctor-patient relationship and the issues of pity, sympathy, and empathy. In: Stoeckle JD, ed. Encounters Between Patients and Doctors. Cambridge, MA: MIT Press, 1987;403-11.

55. Dickson DA, Hargie O, Morrow NC. Communication Skills Training for Health Professionals. London, England: Chapman & Hall, 1989;42.

56. Lask B, Fosson A. Childhood Illness: The Psychosomatic Approach. Chichester, England: J Wiley & Sons, 1989;85.

57. Gordon GH. Treating somatizing patients. West J Med 1987;147:88-91.

58. Barr RG. Recurrent abdominal pain. In: Levine MD, Carey WB, Crocker AC, Gross, RT, eds. Developmental-Behavioral Pediatrics. Philadelphia, PA: WB Saunders, 1983;524.

59. Levine MD, Rappaport LA. Recurrent abdominal pain in school children: the loneliness of the long-distance physician. Pediatr Clin North Am 1984;31(5):969-91.

60. Furman L. Letter to editor. J Pediatr 1990;117:322.

61. Fleisher DR, Morrison A. Authors' reply. J Pediatr 1990;117:322.

62. Mews CF, Sinatra FR. Abdominal pain. In: Wyllie R, Hyams JS, eds. Pediatric Gastrointestinal Disease. Philadelphia, PA: WB Saunders, 1993;183-4.

63. Shapiro EG, Rosenfeld AA. The Somatizing Child. New York, NY: Springer-Verlag, 1987;56-7.

64. Liebman WM. Recurrent abdominal pain in children. Clin Pediatr 1978;17:149-53.

65. Galdston R, Hughes MC. Pediatric hospitalization as crisis intervention. Am J Psychiatry 1972;129:721.

66. Barbero GJ. Children with recurrent hospitalizations: a problem of disabled children, parents, and physicians. J Dev Behav Pediatr 1984;5(6):319-24.

67. Buccini RV, Drossman DA. Chronic idiopathic abdominal pain. Current Concepts in Gastroenterology 1988;12(1):3-11.

68. Hodges K, Klein JJ, Barbero GJ, et al. Life events occurring in families of children with recurrent abdominal pain. J Psychosom Res 1984;28(3):185-8.

69. Robinson JO, Alverez JH, Dodge JA. Life events and family history in children with recurrent abdominal pain. J Psychosom Res 1990;34(2):171-81.

70. Waker LS, Greene JW. Negative life events and symptom resolution in pediatric abdominal pain patients. J Pediatr Psychol 1991;16(3):341-60.

71. Drossman DA, Leserman J, Nachman G, et al. Sexual and physical abuse in women with functional and organic gastrointestinal disorders. Ann Int Med 1990;113:828-33.

72. Garber J, Zeman J, Waker LS. Recurrent abdominal pain in children: psychiatric diagnoses and parental psychopathology. J Am Acad Child Adolesc Psychiatry 1990;29(4):648-56.

73. Coulehan JL, Block MR. The Medical Interview - A Primer for Students of the Art, 2nd ed. Philadelphia, PA: FA Davis, 1992.

Clinical Spectra of Chronic Enteric Neuromuscular Disorders

3

Diagnosis and Management of Children With Feeding Disorders

COLIN D. RUDOLPH

Feeding an infant is a rewarding experience for most parents. The infant is comforted and consoled by eating, and the parent achieves a sense of accomplishment by satisfying the infant's emotional and nutritional needs. This positive reciprocal interaction reinforces the bond between infant and parent. Feeding disorders disrupt this process and may prevent the infant from ingesting adequate nutrients for growth.[1,2] Understanding the underlying causes of feeding disorders allows appropriate intervention.

Feeding is a complex process which is easier to understand if it is separated into phases (Fig. 3.1). Successful feeding is initiated when an infant or child senses hunger and communicates a desire to eat. The parent responds by providing food in a manner appropriate to the child's abilities. For an infant, this requires bringing the breast or bottle to the infant's mouth. In an older child, only access to food need be provided since feeding is essentially independent. The second phase of feeding requires the formation of food into a bolus in the oral cavity. The bolus is transported safely through the pharynx into the esophagus, rather than being aspirated into the lungs. The third phase consists of food passing through the esophagus to the stomach, where it is digested and absorbed.

Abnormalities in any phase can interrupt successful feeding. For example, a child with a structural abnormality of the larynx may aspirate and choke during feeding, creating an aversive experience that the child attempts to avoid by refusing further meals. Often the parents' frustration with efforts to feed the child interferes with their coping abilities and parenting skills. A different clinical scenario may present with a similar parent/child relationship and food refusal. An overburdened or misinformed parent may force-feed an essentially normal child, or feed solids to an infant, which causes choking. This child will learn that feeding is unpleasant and will avoid eating. Thus, determining the primary cause of a feeding disorder requires the careful review of the potential for disorders in each phase. Treatment initially addresses any correctable underlying physical cause, then attempts to resolve secondary acquired adverse behaviors.

This chapter reviews the normal development of each phase of feeding. Subsequently, the diagnostic and therapeutic approaches to children with feeding disorders are discussed. The more common disorders that affect each phase of feeding are listed in Table 3.1.

APPETITE, FOOD-SEEKING, AND INGESTION

Appetite

Appetite is controlled by hunger and satiety centers in the hypothalamus that integrate a variety of sensory and central nervous system inputs in adult animals and humans. Sensory stimuli such as taste, smell, and vision provide environmental feedback. Visceral sensors relay information about gastric volume,[3] blood glucose concentrations, and intraluminal intestinal substrates[4]—all of which affect the appetite

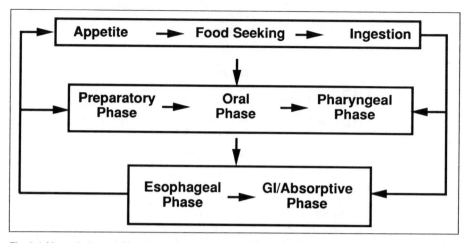

Fig. 3.1 Normal phases of feeding in infants and children. Complex interactions between each phase of feeding often obscure the diagnosis of the primary cause of a feeding disorder.

centers. Similarly, emotional states alter appetite via limbic and cortical inputs.[5] A variety of hormonal and neurochemical factors (eg, cholecystokinin,[6] endogenous opioids,[7] norepinephrine, and serotonin[8]) are involved in controlling appetite and feeding behavior, making appetite susceptible to pharmacologic interventions.[9-11]

Although appetite is difficult to assess in infants, it is clear that sensory inputs affect infant feeding behavior. Infants clearly prefer sweeter formulas.[12] Salt preference does not appear until after the age of 4 months.[13] Minor alterations in the composition of human breast milk—such as those induced by maternal ingestion of alcohol or garlic—can alter the infant's milk intake.[14,15] Physiologic visceral feedback also appears to be intact because infants and children receiving enteral tube feedings or parenteral nutrition have a reduced drive to eat. As in adults, mood or environment can also reduce food intake; infants who are not nurtured eat less.[16] The complex feeding relationship between the parent and infant is briefly reviewed in the discussion below on food-seeking behavior.

Reduced appetite is frequently observed in infants and children with chronic debilitating disease. Very specific food aversions, however, may be observed in healthy children and adults. If ingestion of a specific food is associated with a painful or uncomfortable experience, such as vomiting, a child may refuse to eat the food again. Understanding that a different stimulus, such as motion sickness or a viral illness, caused the discomfort often does not overcome the learned aversion to the specific food—even into adulthood.[17] The rapid and sustained acquisition of food aversions probably evolved to protect our ancestors from eating noxious substances repetitively.[18] The development of this type of specific feeding aversion has been observed in children with cancer. If the child is given a certain flavor of ice cream before chemotherapy, an aversion to that flavor is induced.[19] Similarly, children with metabolic diseases or allergies can experience nausea or discomfort after ingesting nutrients such as fructose or protein, leading to aversions to foods containing them.[20] Learned aversion to foods with fructose explains the low incidence of dental caries in children with hereditary fructose intolerance.[21]

It is easy to extend these observations to explain the development of more generalized feeding aversions if an infant has a negative experience, such as aspiration or choking, after most feeding experiences.[22-24] Infants that have required prolonged airway intubation or tube feeding often learn that any efforts by a caretaker to approach their mouth or face will result in discomfort from airway suctioning, tape removal, or tube

TABLE 3.1 Alterations in Normal Feeding and Their Causes

Appetite, Food-seeking Behavior, and Ingestion
Depression[35,5]
Deprivation[16]
CNS (diencephalic syndrome)[157]
Metabolic diseases
  hereditary fructose intolerance[21]
  urea cycle disorders[20]
  organic acidemias[20]
Sensory defects
  anosmia
  blindness[38,39]
Neuromuscular disease (see below)
Oral hypersensitivity or aversion
Conditioned dysphagia
  aspiration[22-24]
  oral inflammation (see below)
  GER[27]
  dumping syndrome or gastric bloating after gastric surgery[25,26]
Fatigue (heart disease, lung disease)[40,41]
Poverty[158,159]
Anorexia nervosa[160]

Oral, Pharyngeal, and Esophageal Swallowing
Anatomic abnormalities of the oropharynx
  cleft lip and/or palate[57]
  macroglossia[62-64]
  lingual ankyloglossia[161-164]
  Pierre-Robin malformation sequence[53,61]
  cleft larynx[165,166]
  retropharyngeal mass or abscess
Anatomic abnormalities of the esophagus
  tracheoesophageal fistula[167-170]
  congenital esophageal atresia[54,171-175]
  congenital esophageal stenosis due to tracheobronchial remnants[176,177]
  esophageal stricture, web, or ring[178-180]
  esophageal mass or tumor[181-183]
  foreign body[184]
  vascular rings and dysphagia lusorum[185-187]

Suck-swallow-breathing Coordination
Choanal atresia[53-55]
Bronchopulmonary dysplasia[51,52,188,189]
Cardiac disease[41,190-192]
Tachypnea (respiratory rates >60/min)[97,50]

Neuromuscular Coordination of Swallowing
Cerebral palsy[70,114,115,193-195]
Bulbar atresia or palsy[72]
Brain stem glioma[196]
Arnold-Chiari malformation[71,138,197,198]
Myelomeningocele[197,199]

Familial dysautonomia[68,69]
Tardive dyskinesia[85-87]
Nitrazepam-induced dysphagia[139]
Postdiphtheritic and polio paralysis[200,201]
Möbius syndrome (cranial nerve abnormalities)[202,203]
Myasthenia gravis[73,74]
Infant botulism[79,80]
Congenital myotonic dystrophy[75,76]
Oculopharyngeal dystrophy[77,78]
Muscular dystrophies and myopathies[204]
Cricopharyngeal achalasia[136,137]
Polymyositis/dermatomyositis[81-84]
Rheumatoid arthritis[91]

Esophageal Peristalsis
Achalasia[130-132]
Chagas disease[205,206]
Diffuse esophageal spasm[133,134]
Pseudo-obstruction[207,208]
Scleroderma[81,209]
Mixed connective tissue disease[210]
Systemic lupus erythematosus[211]
Polymyositis/dermatomyositis[81,82,83]
Rheumatoid arthritis[91]

Mucosal Infections and Inflammatory Disorders Causing Dysphagia
Candida pharyngitis or esophagitis[212]
Peptic esophagitis[27,213]
Herpes simplex esophagitis[214-216]
HIV[217]
Cytomegalovirus esophagitis[214-218]
Medication-induced esophagitis[219]
Crohn's disease[220,221]
Behcet's disease[222,81,223]
Chronic graft v host disease[224]

Feeding and Swallowing Difficulties
Xerostomia[81,88-90]
Hypothyroidism[67]
Neonatal hyperparathyroidism[225]
Trisomy 18 & 21[65,226,227]
Prader-Willi syndrome[66]
Allergies[228,229]
Lipid and lipoprotein metabolism disorders[230]
Neurofibromatosis[231]
Williams syndrome[232,227]
Coffin-Siris syndrome[233,234]
Opitz-G syndrome[235-237]
Cornelia de Lange syndrome[238]
Interstitial deletion (13)(q21.3q31)[239]
Globus pharyngeus[240-242]
Epidermolysis bullosa dystrophica[243]

manipulation. Therefore, they resist efforts to approach their face. When oral feeding can be initiated, this "oral aversion" must be gently extinguished. Similarly, older children with gastrointestinal motility disorders[25,26] or inflammation of the mouth or esophagus[27,28] can have dysphagia that results in decreased oral intake.

Food-seeking Behavior

Food-seeking behavior and ingestion are initiated by hunger. Infants and children must provide appropriate cues to a provider, indicating that they are hungry. Infants usually cry, toddlers may become irritable or sullen, and older children simply complain of hunger. Parents with marginal interactive skills often misinterpret or are unaware of these cues. Thus, the availability of appropriate food and the parent-child interaction determine the normal child's success in obtaining food.

Factors that affect the parent-child feeding interaction have been extensively studied because of the high incidence of failure to thrive (FTT) and possible long-term sequelae of infant undernutrition.[29] Emotional deprivation due to family dysfunction, chaos, or poverty has clearly been linked to FTT and poor feeding in infants.[30-32] This has led to a tendency of pediatricians to assume that in those infants with no obvious reason for poor oral intake, environmental factors are responsible for FTT. However, the primary role of emotional deprivation as a cause of inadequate food intake by infants has probably been overstated.

Infants with subtle feeding disorders may be less resilient in responding to environmental deprivation than normal infants.[33] A recent study[34] demonstrated that the reported incidence of an abnormal duration of feeding time, poor appetite, delayed tolerance of food textures, and difficulty in feeding in the first few months of life were similar in infants with nonorganic and organic FTT. Furthermore, the incidence of maternal affective and interactive behavior disorders was similar for infants with clear, organic causes of food refusal and those labelled with nonorganic FTT.[35] Even in in-ner-city children, where there is a high risk of family dysfunction, subtle abnormalities of oral motor function are identified in many children with FTT.[36] Thus, it is likely that many children with nonorganic FTT have subtle feeding impairments that prevent the intake of adequate calories. This impairment may require increased feeding time or other adjustments which are not achievable for a stressed caretaker in a dysfunctional family. Feeding difficulties frustrate even highly educated, experienced parents.[2]

Ingestion

Ingestion of food requires coordination of sensory apparatus as well as fine- and gross-motor skills to move the mouth toward a nipple or manipulate food with fingers or utensils. Ingram[37] observed that integrating the motor activities and reflexes for feeding is the most complicated challenge to the newborn infant nervous system. Feeding deficits therefore may provide the first indication that a child has an underlying neurologic deficit. Sensory defects such as anosmia or blindness[38,39] can also impair the ability to locate the nipple or bottle. Similarly, fatigue due to chronic lung disease or congestive heart disease may prevent coordination of normal feeding skills.[40,41]

ORAL AND PHARYNGEAL PHASES OF FEEDING

The oral and pharyngeal phases of feeding are conventionally separated into preparative, oral-transfer, and pharyngeal phases (Fig. 3.2A). Ingested food is first chewed and formed into a bolus in the anterior oral cavity. It is then transported into the pharynx and past the laryngeal inlet into the esophagus without being aspirated into the lungs. The anatomy of the oropharynx changes during development (Fig. 3.2), and the motor skills required for developmentally appropriate feeding evolve concurrently. The infant mouth and pharynx are adept at sucking, while the older child progresses to efficient biting and chewing. At each stage of development, successful feeding and swallowing requires split-second, coordinated,

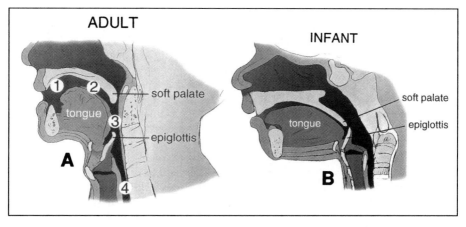

Fig. 3.2 **A,** Adult oropharynx. The phases of swallowing are: 1) preparatory phase, 2) oral phase, 3) pharyngeal phase, and 4) esophageal phase. **B,** Infant oropharynx. Note that the infant oral cavity is much smaller than that of the adult, providing little space for manipulating the food bolus. The larynx is elevated so that the epiglottis almost touches the soft palate. The tongue is entirely within the oral cavity, with no oral region of the pharynx.

sequential timing of tongue movements, pharyngeal and laryngeal muscles, as well as the appropriate cessation of breathing. In this section, the ontogeny of the oral and pharyngeal phases of swallowing will be reviewed and the causes of abnormal oropharyngeal swallowing discussed.

Oral Phase

The human oral cavity changes in shape and function during the first 2 years of life. The small size and shape of the infant oral cavity make it ideal for sucking. The buccal fat pads and palate stabilize the lateral and superior walls of the oral cavity. To suck, the lips close around the nipple and the tongue seals against the pharynx posteriorly,[42] forming a closed intraoral chamber. Depression of the tongue and mandible generates suction up to 150 mm Hg in the oral cavity.[43] The primary nonnutritive pattern of tongue movement is to extend and retract the tongue, allowing the nipple to be drawn into the mouth. As the infant matures, the oral cavity enlarges, allowing manipulation of a pureed or solid food bolus. Alveolar ridges and, subsequently, teeth develop to allow biting and mastication. The anatomic relationships then no longer favor sucking but rather promote cup and spoon feeding.

Mouthing and sucking movements have been observed in utero at 15 weeks' gestation.[44] Mouthing patterns persist until about 32 weeks' gestational age, when a disordered pattern of sucking bursts and pauses are observed. These are replaced with a stable pattern of rhythmic sucking and swallowing by 34 to 36 weeks' gestation.[45,46] After birth, swallowing is triggered when a certain volume of milk has been delivered. Since a brief cessation of breathing occurs during swallowing, significant reductions of ventilation and even hypoxia may occur during feeding in normal preterm and term infants, particularly during the initial phase of feeding when hungry infants can have a 1:1 correlation between suck and swallow.[47-49] Infants with tachypnea or borderline respiratory function may have profound difficulties coordinating feeding and breathing.[50-52] Similarly, lack of a nasal airway due to choanal atresia can prevent maintained sucking and feeding.[53-55]

Nipple shape, composition, and hole size determine the rate of milk flow. The usual volume of milk taken in during each suck is about 0.2 ml; 300 sucking and swallowing events are required to consume 60 ml, which the normal infant can ingest over 5 minutes.[56] More rapid milk delivery through nipples with larger holes increases the frequency of swallowing and therefore may decrease the time available for breathing. However, decreasing hole size increases the work of sucking, thereby increasing the time required for feeding. Term infants and, to a limited extent, preterm infants alter the strength of suck to control the volume of flow. Inadequate feedback control of flow rates can lead to either inadequate flow and increased work or overly rapid flow with respiratory compromise, particularly in infants with neurologic disorders. Thoughtful and careful alterations in nipple types and hole sizes provide a therapeutic strategy in many disorders of sucking and swallowing in infants.

Feeding an infant with a cleft palate is particularly challenging because the infant is unable to generate a negative pressure suck in the oral cavity. Feeding is usually most successful when a paced feeding is delivered by positive pressure into the oral cavity, allowing the infant to initiate swallows. With a consistent feeder, the infant can learn to coordinate the rate of formula delivery and swallows to allow successful oral feeding.[57] This accommodation to a severe anatomic abnormality demonstrates the adaptability of the neurologically normal child to variations in feeding approaches.

At approximately 3 to 4 months of age, the infant begins to develop tongue movements that allow bolus movement from the front of the mouth back towards the pharynx. Tongue extrusion becomes less dominant. By 6 months, infants use lip occlusion to remove soft foods from a spoon and tend to move food boluses to the midline for chewing.[58] Later, the development of increased tongue mobility allows lateralization of the solid food bolus for mastication. Mature patterns of mastication develop between 6 and 8 months of age.[59] Children may develop feeding problems if offered pureed or thickened feedings before they are developmentally ready (ie, approximately 5 to 7 months).

Limited feeding experience due to prolonged parenteral or enteral feeding during any phase of development can result in long-term disabilities in feeding skills. Illingworth[60] described "sensitive periods" for learning specific oral skills such as sucking or chewing. Infants that do not experience feeding during these critical periods of development have a far more difficult time mastering these skills later.

The development of a normal oral phase of swallowing requires normal anatomy (including dentition), intact sensory feedback from the mouth (via cranial nerves V_2, VII, IX, and X), as well as intact muscular strength and coordination of the orbicularis oris and buccal muscles (via cranial nerve VII and the ansa cervicales), muscles of mastication (cranial nerve V_3), and the tongue (cranial nerve XII). Anatomic defects, including cleft lip and palate[57] as well as micrognathia associated with the Pierre Robin malformation sequence,[53,61] can disrupt this phase of swallowing. Macroglossia as noted with Beckwith-Weidemann syndrome, glycogen storage diseases, and hypothyroidism[62-64] may also interfere with normal swallowing. A weak suck is often observed in infants with trisomy 18, trisomy 21,[65] Prader-Willi syndrome,[66] hypothyroidism,[67] familial dysautonomia[68,69] or neurologic abnormalities[70] including Möbius syndrome, Arnold-Chiari malformations,[71] bulbar atresia,[72] infantile myasthenia gravis,[73,74] congenital myotonic dystrophy, and myopathies.[75-78] Perinatal central nervous system (CNS) insults including infection, asphyxia, and hypoglycemia can also result in a weak suck reflex. Acquired disorders such as Guillain-Barré syndrome, infant botulism,[79,80] dermatopolymyositis,[81-84] and tardive dyskinesias due to treatment with phenothiazines or metoclopramide[85-87] may also perturb the oral phase of swallowing. Other overlooked causes of oral phase problems include xerostomia[81,88-90] and arthritis of the temporomandibular joints.[91]

Pharyngeal Phase

The pharynx provides a common passage for the respiratory, digestive, and vocal pathways (see Fig. 3.2A).[92] In the human infant and most adult mammals, the airway is relatively separate from the digestive pathway. During normal respiration, the larynx is situated fairly high in the neck at the level of cervical vertebrae C1-3, enabling the epiglottis to pass up behind the soft palate. At times the larynx almost opens directly into the nasopharynx, essentially creating separate respiratory and digestive tracts. The airway consists of a passage for air through the nares and nasopharynx directly into the larynx. Ingested liquids pass over the tongue, around the epiglottis into the isthmus faucium, through the piriform sinuses, and into the esophagus. The tongue lies entirely in the oral cavity. The elevated position of the larynx acts as a barrier between the airway and digestive pathway.

During the first 2 years of life, the human larynx remains relatively high in the neck. The major descent occurs between 2 and 3 years of age as the upper border of the larynx descends to the level of cervical vertebra C-3 and the lower border of the larynx descends to C-5 (see Fig. 3.2B). The descent of the larynx prevents the epiglottis from approximating the soft palate. Thus, in the mature human, even during maximum laryngeal elevation a region of oropharynx is always located above the laryngeal inlet and the airway and digestive pathways cannot be entirely separated. Among mammals, this anatomic arrangement is unique to the adult human, probably evolving to allow the use of the larger tongue surface to form a broader range of sounds for communication. Unfortunately, the sophisticated neuromuscular protective mechanisms which evolved to prevent aspiration are less robust than the simpler mechanical protection provided by anatomic positioning of the larynx above the digestive pathway. Minor anatomic or neuromuscular disorders that are not problematic in an infant can compromise protective mechanisms when the larynx descends because the separation of air and digestive pathways becomes more challenging.

Pharyngeal swallows are initiated in an ordered, sequential pattern in response to stimulation by food or secretions in the pharynx.[93,94] Tactile receptors in the pharynx provide sensory stimulation to the medullary swallowing center (ie, nucleus tractus solitarius and ventromedial reticular formation) via cranial nerves V, IX, and X.[95] The medullary swallowing center initiates a swallow by stimulating the ambiguous nucleus and dorsomedial vagal nucleus. In the older child or adult, the upper pharynx and the soft palate close against the posterior pharynx as the food bolus is propelled by the tongue into the pharynx, sealing the nasal cavity. The bolus is pushed through the oropharynx by the contraction of the pharyngeal muscles against the tongue, which forms the anterior wall of the oropharynx. Proprioceptive feedback adjusts the peristaltic activity appropriately for different food bolus sizes and consistencies. Simultaneously, respiration ceases and the larynx is pulled superiorly and anteriorly by the mylohoid, geniohyoid, and thyrohyoid muscles, moving the laryngeal inlet out of the path of the bolus. When the larynx closes, the epiglottis flips over the top of the larynx and the false and true vocal cords close to further protect the laryngeal inlet. The upper esophageal sphincter opens and peristaltic contractions of the pharyngeal constrictor muscles drive the bolus through the pharynx, past the displaced, closed larynx, into the esophagus.

Coordination of the oral and pharyngeal phases of swallowing is essential for preventing aspiration.[96] Early overflow of the food bolus into the pharynx before respiration ceases and the swallow is initiated may allow food to be aspirated during inspiration. An unrelaxed upper esophageal sphincter results in pooling of food in the piriform sinus. This food overflows into the airway when the larynx descends after a swallow sequence and inspiration begins.

Anatomic abnormalities, including laryngeal clefts and other laryngeal deformities, can result in dysphagia and aspiration. Rigid laryngoscopy may be required to ensure that there are no anatomic abnormalities. Myopathies, CNS abnormalities, tumor masses or foreign bodies, esophageal peristaltic disorders or inflammatory disorders all can disrupt the pharyngeal phase of swallowing (see Table 3.1). As noted above, infants or children with tachypnea (respiratory rates >60) often have difficulty disassociating swallowing from inspiration, making feeding difficult.[50,97]

ESOPHAGEAL SWALLOWING AND THE GASTROINTESTINAL ABSORPTIVE PHASE

The esophagus is a conduit between the pharynx and the stomach, with the muscular upper and lower esophageal sphincters at either end. The upper esophageal sphincter relaxes during swallowing to allow the food bolus to enter the esophagus. Peristaltic contractions propel the bolus down into the stomach. The lower esophageal sphincter relaxes to allow bolus passage into the stomach. Propagation of the peristaltic wave depends on the intrinsic myenteric plexus and on vagal afferents (see Chapters 1 and 11 for details on normal esophageal physiology and disorders of esophageal motility). Abnormal peristalsis, inflammation, or mechanical obstruction due to esophageal atresia or esophageal narrowing as a result of congenital stenosis, strictures, webs, vascular rings, tumor, or foreign body may all result in dysphagia in infants and children (see Table 3.1).

Successful acquisition of food, ingestion, and swallowing ensures that feedings enter the stomach. Normally, when food enters the stomach and relieves hunger, future feeding behavior is reinforced. In fact, visceral receptors may influence further feeding behavior. In rats, food preferences can be altered by the infusion of glucose into the portal vein—but not a peripheral vein—suggesting that some hepatic receptors modify behavioral responses.[98] Problems such as gastroparesis, dumping syndrome (postfundoplication),[26,99,100] peptic disease, pancreatitis, and cholelithiasis all can cause postprandial pain or discomfort, limiting food intake.

EVALUATION OF FEEDING DISORDERS

Symptoms of feeding disorders can include the refusal to eat or drink, failure to gain weight, aversion to specific food types or textures, and recurrent pneumonias. Because of the complexity of the behavioral and physiologic components of those disorders, the evaluation of an infant or child is most readily achieved by a multidisciplinary team approach. Usually, a careful developmental, medical, feeding, and dietary history in addition to a physical examination provides clues to the diagnosis. Observation of a feeding session where the child is fed by his or her usual primary feeder is often enlightening. Subsequent diagnostic evaluation varies depending on suspected pathology.

Observation of Feeding

Observation of a feeding session by experienced occupational therapists, speech pathologists, psychologists, and nurses often provides tremendous insight into the underlying problem. Positive interactions between the child and parent (eg, shared eye contact, reciprocal vocalizations, praise, and touch) or negative interactions (eg, lack of conversation, eye contact, or touch as well as forced feeding, threats, bribes, and inconsistency) are noted. These observations highlight primary or secondary behavioral problems, which allows future structuring of appropriate interventions.[101] The child's responses to offered foods—including disruptive behaviors such as turning the head away from or throwing food—are also noted.

Attention to the child's position and posture, as well as the mechanics of feeding skills during the ingestion of various textures, also provides clues regarding any underlying anatomic or physiologic problems. Observations of the ability to handle oral secretions, pace of feeding, escape of food from the mouth, tongue and jaw movements, number of swallows to clear a bolus, noisy airway sounds after swallowing, coordinaton of suck and/or swallow, laryngeal elevation and gagging, coughing, or emesis associated with feedings can indicate that there may be an underlying neurologic or structural problem. Attention to articulation and voice quality also may provide useful information since the structures used for the oropharyngeal phases of feeding are also used for speech production. Systematic evaluation of infant sucking that focuses on jaw and tongue movements as well as rhythm, may allow more reliable assessment of patient progress and treatment success.[102] A complete review of the clinical assessment of suck and swallowing function is beyond the scope of this chapter, but is extensively reviewed in several texts.[103-105] Unfortunately, despite careful observation, it is often difficult to ascertain the cause of a feeding disorder or the safety of feeding using only clinical observations.[106-109]

Diagnostic Tests

Careful examination of oral, pharyngeal, laryngeal, and esophageal anatomy and function are important during the evaluation of children with feeding disorders. Three basic approaches are utilized: radiographic studies, direct visualization of structures with fiberoptic endoscopes, and manometry to assess patterns of change in intraluminal pressure. Each approach provides different, useful information.

Radiographic studies have two separate goals. First, anatomic or structural abnormalities such as strictures, fistulae, or masses need to be excluded. Second, images of the coordination of movement of a bolus through the oropharynx and esophagus can be studied. Standard upper gastrointestinal contrast studies using barium suspensions are required for careful anatomic studies. Children with feeding disorders frequently will not ingest an adequate amount of barium for successful completion of these studies; a nasogastric feeding tube is required for a thorough study. Because this unpleasant experience usually prevents further cooperation, children frequently require a different session for evaluation of the functional aspects of swallowing.

Functional studies of swallowing are usually best performed by a speech pathologist or occupational therapist in cooperation with a radiologist. The details of normal videofluoroscopic observations of swallowing have been described in adults[110] and infants.[111] Videofluoroscopic swallowing studies (VSS)[112-115] are performed in patients with feeding disorders after a careful history is obtained so that the study can be initiated using the most readily acceptable foods, textures, and position. Maximizing the like-

lihood of successful swallows at the beginning of the study ensures that some observations are obtained before the patient experiences discomfort and refuses further efforts at evaluation. Subsequently, other textures are examined and the therapeutic efficacy of modifications in bolus volume, nipple or utensil types, and body posture all may be explored.[106,116,117] VSS allows the relatively noninvasive assessment of the oral stage of swallowing and can help determine the consistencies and conditions for safe swallowing. A large, accumulated experience in the interpretation of VSS makes this test the "gold standard" for evaluating children with swallowing disorders. Unfortunately, radiation exposure limits the use of fluoroscopy for teaching therapeutic maneuvers. In addition, patients must be transported to a facility with expensive fluoroscopic equipment.

Ultrasound provides an attractive alternative for evaluating the oral phase of swallowing and allows observation of the coordination of laryngeal elevation during swallows.[118-120] Unfortunately, ultrasound lacks sensitivity in visualizing pharyngeal motion and determining if aspiration has occurred. Therefore it cannot reliably determine swallowing safety. Ultrasound also allows the study of infant swallowing mechanisms,[49,121] especially tongue movements. Ultrasound may be a useful tool for biofeedback training in compensatory maneuvers because it allows visual feedback on tongue and laryngeal movements, with no discomfort or risk to the patient.

Fiberoptic endoscopic examinations of swallowing (FEES) is a recently described approach to the evaluation of swallowing, performed by passing a flexible laryngoscope into the oropharynx after anesthetizing the nares and nasopharynx.[122] In experienced hands, this test can be performed in adults with minimal discomfort. Initially, pharyngeal anatomy and movement of pharyngeal and laryngeal structures can be evaluated during speech. The management of secretions is examined by placing a small amount of green food coloring on the tongue. Accumulation of secretions in the valleculae or piriform sinus, or aspiration of secretions may be directly observed. Finally, swallows of varying volumes and textures are administered by mouth and the coordination of swallowing and efficiency of pharyngeal clearance are assessed. FEES does not provide information regarding the oral phase of swallowing but compares favorably with VSS for the evaluation of the pharyngeal phase of swallowing.[123-125] FEES is particularly valuable for evaluating swallowing safety in children who refuse to ingest adequate amounts of barium for VSS. In such cases, studying the anatomy and evaluating the patient's ability to handle the oral secretions provides useful information. In addition, FEES may prove useful for teaching compensatory maneuvers to prevent aspiration because it provides easily recognized visual feedback.[126] Fiberendoscopic evaluation of the esophagus, stomach, and duodenum is easily achieved with standard upper endoscopy in children of all ages.[127]

Manometry is useful for evaluating esophageal peristalsis, as discussed in Chapter 11, and more recently has been utilized for evaluating pharyngeal and upper esophageal sphincter function.[128,129] Esophageal manometry can identify disorders of esophageal motility, including achalasia[130-132] and diffuse esophageal spasm.[133,134] The function of the normal upper esophageal sphincter has been well studied in children,[135] but only isolated cases of primary cricopharyngeal achalasia[136,137] and abnormalities in the coordination of upper esophageal sphincter function in children with Arnold-Chiari malformations[138] and nitrazepam-induced dysphagia[139] have been reported. The role of manometry in the evaluation of pharyngeal swallowing in adults and children requires further investigation.

TREATMENT

Careful evaluation of children with feeding disorders should demonstrate treatable anatomic or inflammatory lesions. A child may refuse to eat even after an underlying anatomic abnormality has been corrected because of a learned aversion to feeding. Behavior therapy often can overcome this type of conditioned food refusal. Unfortu-nately, many children with feeding disorders have noncorrectable neurologic or anatomic abnormalities which make oral feeding difficult or impossible. Behavioral therapy and various therapeutic approaches may improve the efficiency and safety of feeding.

The emotional rewards and convenience of oral feeding must be balanced with the potential risks of aspiration and chronic lung disease. The amount of aspiration that is safe depends on the patient's ability to clear the airway with cough and ciliary flow. Society and health professionals often impose a value system on families and patients that stresses the importance of providing oral nutrition. Some patients, though, are at risk for aspiration. In others, providing oral nutrition consumes the parents' and child's lives, leaving little time for other nurturing activities. Thus, supplying some nutrition by nasogastric or gastrostomy feedings may be beneficial. Families may need counseling to help them realize that alternate approaches may be better for the child's overall well-being than persisting in efforts to provide nutrition only by mouth. The timing for aggressive behavioral intervention or for initiating oral feeding must be decided in the context of the child's overall development and well-being. Because anatomic relationships of the larynx change during development and disease progression may alter swallowing, episodic reevaluation of the safety or approach to feeding is essential.

Behavioral Therapy

Behavioral feeding disorders and the approach to their management has recently been comprehensively reviewed.[140] Normal preschool children can be induced to change their dietary selections by using a combination of social praise and a program that makes the consumption of preferred foods contingent upon eating disliked foods.[141] This type of contingency management has been combined with other therapeutic approaches to treat more serious feeding disorders, including food refusal in children with FTT,[142] cerebral palsy,[143,144] cystic fibrosis,[145] metabolic disorders,[20] and after long-term gastrostomy feedings[146] or other chronic disorders that prevent oral feeding.[147] Treatment strategies include "shaping" by rewarding successive approximations of targeted behaviors, "positively reinforcing" by rewarding with praise, access to favored toys, music, clapping, stickers, and/or socialization if a desired behavior is completed, and "ignoring" or inattention when the child engages in inappropriate behaviors.[145] The slow, hierarchical advancement of rewarded goals eventually leads to full oral feeding. Successful implementation usually requires a structured inpatient management program.

Children with real or perceived feeding disorders are at increased risk of long-term psychosocial problems.[148] Therefore, in cases of nonorganic FTT, a multidisciplinary intervention that includes provisions to ensure access to food, parental training in compensatory approaches to feeding, and efforts to improve family support systems provides the most promise for successful intervention.[149] In children with underlying physiologic disorders, many parents suffer tremendous emotional distress, which also needs to be acknowledged and addressed.[2] Assuaging parental feelings of inadequacy and guilt resulting from their previous unsuccessful efforts at feeding is likely to be therapeutic. Family support services, respite care, and financial assistance programs need to be integrated with the child's chronic care medical needs.[150,151]

Therapeutic Maneuvers for Swallowing Disorders

Combining the clinical history, examination, and videofluoroscopic swallowing study or fiberoptic examination of swallowing allows the therapist to determine the best bolus volume and texture, pace of administration, and use of nipples or utensils for oral feeding.

Changes in body and head position may also protect the airway or allow more efficient passage of a bolus through the oropharynx. For example, tilting the head forward widens the vallecular space, thereby diverting food away from the laryngeal inlet. General strategies which may alter the safety of swallowing in patients with a variety of

disorders have been reviewed in several texts[103-105,152] and recent publications.[153,154]

Prosthodontic approaches to swallowing disorders may be effective in specific cases, particularly when there are major anatomic abnormalities.[155] Use of a palatal prosthesis that increases pharyngeal mechanical stimulation during swallowing has been reported to be effective for treating infants with delayed initiation of the pharyngeal phase of swallowing.[156]

Even if full oral feeding cannot be achieved, providing some feedings of sterile water may be possible and desirable. This experience will facilitate the possible later introduction of oral feeds and is usually rewarding for the parents. Also, continuing oral stimulation will prevent the development of aversion to oral touch, allowing good dental care. It is essential to remember that the nutritional requirements of every patient must be met by either an oral or alternate route. Similarly, the development of social skills and interactions achieved during mealtimes must be incorporated into patients' lives, despite their lack of oral intake.

REFERENCES

1. Galler JR, Ricciuti HN, Crawford MA, Kucharski LT. The role of the mother-infant interaction in nutritional disorders. In: Galler, ed. *Nutrition and Behavior.* New York, NY: Plenum Press, 1984.

2. Budd KS, McGraw TE, Farbisz R, et al. Psychosocial concomitants of children's feeding disorders. *J Pediatr Psychol* 1992;17:81-94.

3. Mook DG. On the organization of appetite. *Appetite* 1988;12:27-39.

4. Welch I, Saunders K, Read NW. Effect of ileal and intravenous infusions of fat emulsions on feeding and satiety in human volunteers. *Gastroenterology* 1985;89:1293-7.

5. Fernstrom M. Depression, antidepressants, and body weight change. *Ann NY Acad Sci* 1989;575:31-40.

6. Cheng CA, Geoghegan JG, Lawson C, Berlang-

ieri SU, Akwari O, Pappas TN. Central and peripheral effects of CCK receptor antagonists on satiety in dogs. *Am J Physiol* 1993;265:G219-23.

7. Fantino M, Hosotte J, Apfelbaum M. An opioid antagonist, naltrexone, reduces preference for sucrose in humans. *Am J Physiol* 1986;251:R91-6.

8. Blundell JE. Serotonin and appetite. *Neuropharmacology* 1984;23:1537-51.

9. Bruera E. Clinical management of anorexia and cachexia in patients with advanced cancer. *Oncology* 1992;49(suppl 2):35-42.

10. Loprinzi C, Goldberg R, Burnham N. Cancer-associated anorexia and cachexia: implications for drug therapy. *Drugs* 1992;43:499-506.

11. Sullivan A, Nauss-Karol C, Hogan S, Triscari J. Pharmacologic modification of appetite. *Curr Concepts Nutr* 1988;16:79-90.

12. Lipsitt LP, Behl G. Taste-mediated differences in sucking behavior of human newborns. In: Capaldi, Powley, eds. *Taste Experience and Feeding.* New York, NY: American Psychiatric Association, 1990.

13. Beauchamp GK, Cowart BJ, Moran M. Developmental changes in salt acceptability in human infants. *Dev Psychobiol* 1986;19:17-25.

14. Mennella JA, Beauchamp GK. The transfer of alcohol to human milk. *N Engl J Med* 1991;325:981-5.

15. Mennella J, Beauchamp G. The effects of repeated exposure to garlic-flavored milk on the nursling's behavior. *Pediatr Res* 1993;34:805-8.

16. Gagan RJ, Cupoli JM, Watkins AH. The families of children who fail to thrive: preliminary investigations of parental deprivation among organic and non-organic cases. *Child Abuse Negl* 1984;8:93-103.

17. Garb JL, Stunkard AJ. Taste aversions in man. *Am J Psychiatry* 1974;131:1204-7.

18. Garcia J, Hankins WG, Rusiniak KW. Behavioral regulation of the milieu interne in man and rat. *Science* 1974;185:824.

19. Bernstein, IL. Learned taste aversions in children receiving chemotherapy. *Science* 1978;200:1302-3.

20. Hyman SL, Porter CA, Page TJ, Iwata BA, Kissel R, Batshaw ML. Behavior management of feeding disturbances in urea cycle and organic acid disorders. *J Pediatr* 1987;111:558-62.

21. Baerlocher K, Gitzelmann R, Steinmann B, Gitzelmann-Cumarasamy N. Hereditary fructose intolerance in early childhood: a major diagnostic challenge: survey of 20 symptomatic cases. *Helv Paediatr Acta* 1978;33:465-7.

22. Vogel, S. Oral motor and feeding problems in the tube fed infant: suggested treatment strategies for occupational therapists. In: Cromwell, ed. *Occupational Therapy for People with Eating Dysfunctions.* New York, NY: Haworth Press, 1986.

23. DiScipio W, Kaslon K, Ruben R. Traumatically acquired conditioned dysphagia in children. *Ann Otol* 1978;87:509-14.

24. Di Scipio W, Kaslon K. Conditioned dysphagia in cleft palate children after pharyngeal flap surgery. *Psychosom Med* 1982;44:247-57.

25. Borowitz S, Borowitz K. Oral dysfunction following Nissen fundoplication. *Dysphagia* 1992;7:234-7.

26. Hirsig J, Baals H, Tuchschmid P, Spitz L, Stauffer U. Dumping syndrome following Nissen's fundoplication: a cause for refusal to feed. *J Pediatr Surg* 1984;19:155-7.

27. Catto-Smith AG, Machida H, Butzner JD, Gall DG, Scott RB. The role of gastroesophageal reflux in pediatric dysphagia. *J Pediatr Gastroenterol Nutr* 1991;12:159-65.

28. Dellert SF, Hyams JS, Treem WR, Geertsma MA. Feeding resistance and gastroesophageal reflux in infancy. *J Pediatr Gastroenterol Nutr* 1993;17:66-71.

29. Black M, Dubowitz H. Failure to thrive: lessons from animal models and developing countries. *Dev Behav Pediatr* 1991;12:259-67.

30. Kerr MAD, Bogues JL, Kerr DS. Psychosocial functioning of mothers of malnourished children. *Pediatrics* 1978;62:778-84.

31. Cravioto, J. and DeLicardie E. Microenviron-

mental factors in severe protein-calorie malnutrition. In: Scrimshaw, Behar, eds. *Nutrition and Agricultural Development*. New York, NY: Plenum, 1976.

32. Altemeier W, O'Connor S, Sherrod K, et al. Prospective study of antecedents for nonorganic failure to thrive. *J Pediatr* 1985;106:360-5.

33. Accardo P. Growth and development: an interactional context for failure to thrive. In: Accardo, ed. *Failure to Thrive in Infancy and Early Childhood: a Multidisciplinary Team Approach*. Baltimore, MD: University Park Press, 1982.

34. Ramsay M, Gisel EG, and Boutry M. Non-organic failure to thrive: Growth failure secondary to feeding-skills disorder. *Dev Med Child Neurol* 1993;35:285-97.

35. Singer LT, Song LY, Hill BP, Jaffe AC. Stress and depression in mothers of failure to thrive children. *J Pediatr Psychology* 1990;15:711-20.

36. Mathisen B, Skuse D, Wolke D, Reilly S. Oral-motor dysfunction and failure to thrive among inner-city infants. *Dev Med Child Neurol* 1989;31:293-302.

37. Ingram TTS. Clinical significance of the infantile feeding reflexes. *Dev Med Child Neurol* 1962;4:159-69.

38. Troster H, Brambrin M, and Beelmann A. Prevalence and situational causes of stereotyped behaviors in blind infants and preschoolers. *J Abnorm Child Psychol* 1991;19:569-90.

39. Thommessen M, Trygg K, Riis G, and Kase B. Nutrition and growth retardation in 10 children with congenital deaf-blindness. *J Am Diet Assoc* 1989;89:69-73.

40. Lobo M. Parent-infant interaction during feeding when the infant has congenital heart disease. *J Pediatr Nurs* 1992;7:97-105.

41. Thommessen M, Heiberg A, Kase B. Feeding problems in children with congenital heart disease: the impact on energy intake and growth outcome. *Eur J Clin Nutr* 1992;46:457-64.

42. Mathew OP. Science of bottle feeding. *J Pediatr* 1991;119:511-9.

43. Brenman HS, Pierce L, Mackowiak R, Friedman MHF. Multisensor nipple recording of oral variables. *J Appl Physiol* 1969;26:494-6.

44. Ianniruberto A, Tejani E. Ultrasound study of fetal movements. *Semin Perinatol* 1981;5:175-81.

45. Hack M, Estabrook MM. Development of sucking rhythm in preterm infants. *Early Hum Dev* 1985;11:133-40.

46. Meier P, Anderson G. Responses of small preterm infants to bottle and breast feeding. *MCN* 1987;12:84-92.

47. Mathew OP, Bhatia J. Sucking and breathing patterns during breast and bottle-feeding in term neonates: effects of nutrient delivery and composition. *Am J Dis Child* 1989;143:588-92.

48. Mathew OP. Respiratory control during nipple feeding in preterm infants. *Pediatr Pulmonol* 1988;5:220-4.

49. BuLock F, Woolridge M, Baum J. Development of coordination of sucking, swallowing, and breathing: ultrasound study of term and preterm infants. *Dev Med Child Neurol* 1990;32:669-78.

50. Timms B, DiFiore J, Martin R, Miller M. Increased respiratory drive as an inhibitor of oral feeding of preterm infants. *J Pediatr* 1993;123:127-31.

51. Kurzner S, Garg M, Bautista D, Sargent C, Bowman M, and Keens T. Growth failure in bronchopulmonary dysplasia; elevated metabolic rates and pulmonary mechanics. *J Pediatr* 1988;112:73-80.

52. Singer L, Martin R, Hawkins S, Benson-Szekely L, Yamashita T, Carlo W. Oxygen desaturation complicates feeding in infants with bronchopulmonary dysplasia after discharge. *Pediatrics* 1992;30:380-4.

53. Cozzi F, Pierro A. Glossoptosis-apnea syndrome in infancy. *Pediatrics* 1985;75:836-43.

54. Cozzi F, Myers N, Madonna L, Drago S, Fiocca G, Piacenti S, Pierro A. Esophageal atresia, choanal atresia and dysautonomia. *J Pediatr Surg* 1991;26:548-52.

55. Pagon R, Graham J Jr, Zonana J, Yong S. Coloboma, congenital heart disease and choanal atresia with multiple anomalies: CHARGE association. *J Pediatr* 1981;99:223-7.

56. Selley W, Ellis R, Flack F, Brooks W. Coordination of sucking, swallowing and breathing in the newborn: its relationship to infant feeding and normal development. *Br J Disord Commun* 1990;25:311-27.

57. Kaufman F. Managing the cleft lip and palate patient. *Pediatr Clin North Am* 1991;38:1127-47.

58. Stolovitz P, Gisel E. Circumoral movements in response to three different food textures in children 6 months to 2 years of age. *Dysphagia* 1991;6:17-25.

59. Sheppard JJ, Mysak ED. Ontogeny of infantile oral reflexes and emerging chewing. *Child Devel* 1984;55:831-43.

60. Illingworth RS, and Lister JL. The critical or sensitive period, with special reference to certain feeding problems in infants and children. *J Pediatr* 1964;65:839-48.

61. Singer L, Sidoti E. Pediatric management of Robin sequence. *Cleft Palate Craniofac J* 1992;29:220-3.

62. Rizer F, Schechter G, Richardson M. Macroglossia: etiologic considerations and management techniques. *Int J Ped Otorhinol* 1985;8:225-36.

63. Salman R. Oral manifestations of Beckwith-Wiedemann syndrome. *Spec Care Dentist* 1988;8:23-4.

64. Rice J, Carson S. A case report of lingual lymphangioma presenting as recurrent massive tongue enlargement. *Clin Pediatr* 1985;24:47-50.

65. Cullen S, Cronk C, Pueschel S, Schnell R, Reed R. Social development and feeding milestones of young Down syndrome children. *Am J Ment Defic* 1981;85:410-5.

66. Holm VA, Cassidy SB, Butler MG, et al. Prader-Willi syndrome: consensus diagnostic criteria. *Pediatrics* 1993;91:398-402.

67. Grant D, Smith I, Fuggle P, Tokar S, Chapple J. Congenital hypothyroidism detected by neonatal screening: relationship between biochemical severity and early clinical features. *Arch Dis Child* 1992;67:87-90.

68. Axelrod F, Porges R, Sein M. Neonatal recognition of familial dysautonomia. *J Pediatr* 1987;110:946-8.

69. Margulies S, Brunt P, Donner M, and Silbiger M. Familial dysautonomia: a cineradiographic study of swallowing mechanisms. *Radiology* 1968;90:107-16.

70. McBride M, Danner S. Sucking disorders in neurologically impaired infants: assessment and facilitation of breastfeeding. *Clin Perinatol* 1987;14:109-30.

71. Pollack I, Pang D, Kocoshis S, Putnam P. Neurogenic dysphagia resulting from Chiari malformations. *Neurosurgery* 1992;30:709-19.

72. Grundy D, McSweeney T, Jones H. Cranial nerve palsies in cervical injuries. *Spine* 1984;9:339-43.

73. Papzian O. Transient neonatal myasthenia gravis. *J Child Neurol* 1992;7:135-41.

74. Fenichel G. Myasthenia gravis in children. *Int Pediatr* 1989;4:151-4.

75. Wesstrom T, Bensch J, Schollin J. Congenital myotonic dystrophy. *Acta Paediatr Scand* 1986;75:849-54.

76. Hageman A, Gabreels F, Liem K, Renkawek K, Boon J. Congenital myotonic dystrophy: a report on thirteen cases and a review of the literature. *J Neurol Sci* 1993;115:95-101.

77. Lacomis D, Kupsky W, Kuban K, Specht L. Childhood onset oculopharyngeal muscular dystrophy. *Pediatr Neurol* 1991;7:382-4.

78. Duranceau A, Beauchamp G, Jamieson G, Barbeau A. Oropharyngeal dysphagia and oculopharyngeal muscular dystrophy. *Surg Clin North Am* 1983;63:825-32.

79. Gay C, Marks W, Riley HJ, Bodensteiner J, Hamza M, Noorani P, Bobele G. Infantile botulism. *South Med J* 1988;81:457-60.

80. Thilo E, Townsend S, Deacon J. Infant botulism at 1 week of age: report of two cases. *Pediatrics* 1993;92:151-3.

81. Bubl R, Schon B. Dysphagia in dermatologic disease. *Dysphagia* 1993;8:85-90.

82. Vencovsky J, Rehak F, Pafko P, et al. Acute

cricopharyngeal obstruction in dermatomyositis. *J Rheumatol* 1988;15:1016-8.

83. Horowitz M, McNeil J, Maddern G, Collins P, Shearman D. Abnormalities of gastric and esophageal emptying in polymyositis and dermatomyositis. *Gastroenterology* 1986;90:434-9.

84. Metheny, J. Dermatomyositis. A vocal and swallowing disease entity. *Laryngoscope* 1978;88:147-61.

85. Putnam P, Orenstein S, Wessel H, Stowe R. Tardive dyskinesia associated with use of metoclopramide in a child. *J Pediatr* 1992;121:983-5.

86. Craig T, Richardson M, Bark N, Klevanov R. Impairment of swallowing, tardive dyskinesia and anticholinergic drug use. *Psychopharmacol Bull* 1982;18:83-6.

87. Bazemore P, Tonkonogy J, Ananth R. Dysphagia in psychiatric patients: clinical and video fluoroscopic study. *Dysphagia* 1991;6:2-5.

88. Stoschus B, Allescher H. Drug induced dysphagia. *Dysphagia* 1993;8:154-9.

89. Fox P, vander Ven P, Sonies B, Weiffenbach J, Baum B. Xerostomia: evaluation of a symptom with increasing significance. *J Am Dent Assoc* 1985;100:519-25.

90. Caruso A, Sonies B, Atkinson J, Fox P. Objective measures of swallowing in patients with primary Sjogren's syndrome. *Dysphagia* 1989;4:101-5.

91. Ekberg O, Redlund-Johnell I, and Sjoblom K. Pharyngeal function in patients with rheumatoid arthritis of the cervical spine and temporomandibular joint. *Acta Radiol* 1987;28:35-39.

92. Laitman JT, Reidenberg JS. Specialization of the human upper respiratory and upper digestive systems as seen through comparative and developmental anatomy. *Dysphagia* 1993;8:318-25.

93. Dodds W. The physiology of swallowing. *Dysphagia* 1989;3:171- 8.

94. Kahrilas P. Pharyngeal structure and function. *Dysphagia* 1993;8:303-7.

95. Miller A. The search for the central swallowing pathway: the quest for clarity. *Dysphagia* 1993;8:185-94.

96. Logemann J. Treatment for aspiration related to dysphagia: an overview. *Dysphagia* 1986;1:34-8.

97. Peiper A. Neurology of food intake. In: *Cerebral Function in Infancy and Childhood.* New York, NY: Publishing Consultants Bureau, 1963.

98. Tordoff M, Friedman M. Hepatic portal glucose infusions decrease food intake and increase food preference. *Am J Physiol* 1986;251:R192-6.

99. Caulfield M, Wyllie R, Firor H, Michener W. Dumping syndrome in children. *J Pediatr* 1987;110:212-5.

100. Meyer S, Deckelbaum R, Lax E, Schiller M. Infant dumping syndrome after gastroesophageal reflux surgery. *J Pediatr* 1981;99:235-7.

101. Padgett D. Behavior management of feeding problems. *Nutr Focus* 1992;7:1-6.

102. Palmer M, Crawley K, Blanco I. Neonatal oral-motor assessment scale: a reliability study. *J Perinatol* 1993;13:28-35.

103. Wolf L, Glass R. *Feeding and Swallowing Disorders in Infancy.* Tucson, AZ: Therapy Skill Builders, 1992.

104. Logemann J. *Evaluation and Treatment of Swallowing Disorders.* Sandiego, CA: College-Hill Press, 1983.

105. Morris S, Klein M. *Pre-feeding Skills.* Tucson, AZ: Therapy Skill Builders, 1987.

106. Zerilli K, Stefans V, DiPietro M. Protocol for the use of videofluoroscopy in pediatric swallowing dysfunction. *Am J Occup Ther* 1989;44:441-6.

107. Linden P, Siebens A. Dysphagia: Predicting laryngeal penetration. *Arch Phys Med Rehab* 1983;64:281-4.

108. Splaingard M, Hutchins B, Sultan L, Chaudhuri G. Aspiration in rehabilitation patients: a blinded study of videofluoroscopy versus bedside clinical assessment. *Arch Phys Med Rehab* 1986;67:622-3.

109. Linden P, Kuhlemeier K, Patterson C. The probability of correctly predicting subglottic penetration from clinical observations. *Dysphagia* 1993;8:170-9.

110. Dodds W, Stewart E, Logemann J. Physiology and radiology of the normal oral and pharyngeal phases of swallowing. *AJR* 1990;154:953-63.

111. Newman L, Cleveland R, Blickman J, Hillman R, Jaramillo D. Videofluoroscopic analysis of the infant swallow. *Invest Radiol* 1991;26:870-3.

112. Dodds W, Logemann J, Stewart E. Radiologic assessment of abnormal oral and pharyngeal phases of swallowing. *AJR* 1990;154:965-74.

113. Kramer S. Radiologic examination of the swallowing-impaired child. *Dysphagia* 1989;3:117-25.

114. Griggs C, Jones P, Lee R. Videofluoroscopic investigation of feeding disorders of children with multiple handicaps. *Dev Med Child Neurol* 1989;31:303-8.

115. Morton R, Bonas R, Fourie B, Minford J. Videofluoroscopy in the assessment of feeding disorders of children with neurological problems. *Dev Med Child Neurol* 1993;35:388-95.

116. Palmer J, Kkuhlemeier K, Tippett D, Lynch C. A protocol for the videofluorographic swallowing study. *Dysphagia* 1993;8: 209-14.

117. Linden P. Videofluoroscopy in the rehabilitation of swallowing dysfunction. *Dysphagia* 1989;3:189-91.

118. Shawker T, Sonies B, Hall T, Baum B. Ultrasound analysis of tongue, hyoid, and larynx activity during swallowing. *Invest Radiol* 1984;19:82-6.

119. Maniere-Ezvan A, Duval J, Darnault P. Ultrasonic assessment of the anatomy and function of the tongue. *Surg Radiol Anat* 1993;15:55-61.

120. Wein B, Bockler R, Klajman S. Temporal reconstruction of sonographic imaging of disturbed tongue movements. *Dysphagia* 1991;6:135-9.

121. Bosma J, Hepburn L, Josell S, Baker K. Ultrasound demonstration of tongue motions during suckle feeding. *Dev Med Child Neurol* 1990;32:223-9.

122. Langmore S, Schatz K, Olsen N. Fiberoptic endoscopic examination of swallowing safety: a new procedure. *Dysphagia* 1988;2:216-9.

123. Bastian R. Videoendoscopic evaluation of patients with dysphagia: an adjunct to the modified barium swallow. *Otolaryngol Head Neck Surg* 1991;104:339-50.

124. Langmore S, Schatz K, Olson N. Endoscopic and videofluoroscopic evaluations of swallowing and aspiration. *Ann Otol Rhinol Laryngol* 1991;100:678-81.

125. Bastian R. The videoendoscopic swallowing study: an alternative and partner to the videofluoroscopic swallowing study. *Dysphagia* 1993;8:359-67.

126. Yamaoka M, Matsuya T, Miyazaki T, Nishio J, Ibuki K. Visual training for velopharyngeal closure in cleft palate patients: a fibrescopic procedure (preliminary report). *J Max-fac Surg* 1983;11:191-3.

127. Ament M, Berquist W, Vargas J, Perisic V. Fiberoptic upper intestinal endoscopy in infants and children. *Pediatr Clin North Am* 1988;35:141-55.

128. Cook I. Cricopharyngeal function and dysfunction. *Dysphagia* 1993;8:244-251.

129. Castell J, Castell D. Modern solid state computerized manometry of the pharyngoesophageal segment. *Dysphagia* 1993;8:270-5.

130. Moore P, Couch R, Perry Y, et al. Allgrove syndrome: an autosomal recessive syndrome of ACTH insensitivity, achalasia, and alacrima. *Clin Endocrinol* 1991;34:107-14.

131. Rapeport K, Bremner C. Marfan's syndrome presenting with achalasia of the oesophagus: a case report. *S Afr Med J* 1981;59:766-8.

132. Azizkhan RG, Tapper D, Eraklis A. Achalasia in childhood: a 20-year experience. *J Pediatr Surg* 1980;15:452-6.

133. Wyllie E, Wyllie R, Rothner D, Morris H. Diffuse esophageal spasm: a cause of paroxysmal posturing and irritability in infants and mentally retarded children. *J Pediatr* 1989;15:261- 3.

134. Milov D, Cynamon H, Andres J. Chest pain and dysphagia in adolescents caused by diffuse esophageal spasm. *J Pediatr Gastroenterol Nutr* 1989;9:450-3.

135. Davidson G, Dent J, Willing J. Monitoring of upper oesophageal sphincter pressure in children. *Gut* 1991;32:607-11.

136. Skinner M, Shorter N. Primary neonatal cricopharyngeal achalasia: a case report and review of the literature. *J Pediatr Surg* 1992;27:1509-11.

137. Mihailovic T, Perisic V. Balloon dilatation of cricopharyngeal achalasia. *Pediatr Radiol* 1992;22:522-4.

138. Putnam P, Orenstein S, Pang D, Pollack I, Proujansky R, Kocoshis S. Cricopharyngeal dysfunction associated with Chiari malformations. *Pediatrics* 1992;89:871-6.

139. Wyllie E, Wyllie R, Cruse R, et al. The mechanism of nitrazepam-induced drooling and aspiration. *N Engl J Med* 1986;314:35-8.

140. Babbitt R, Hoch T, Coe D. Behavioral feeding disorders. In: Tuchman, Walter, eds. *Disorders of Feeding and Swallowing in Infants and Children: Pathophysiology, Diagnosis and Treatment*. San Diego, CA: Singular Publishing Group, 1994.

141. Madsen C, Madsen C, Thompson F. Increasing rural Head Start children's consumption of middle class meals. *J Appl Behav Analysis* 1974;7:257-62.

142. Larson K, Ayllon T, Barnett Q. A behavioral feeding program for failure to thrive infants. *Behav Res Ther* 1985;25: 39-47.

143. Riordan M, Iwata B, Finney J, Wohl M, Stanley A. Behavioral assessment and treatment of chronic food refusal in handicapped children. *J Appl Behav Anal* 1984;17:327-41.

144. Riordan M, Iwata B, Wohl M, and Finney J. Behavioral treatment of food refusal and selectivity in developmentally disabled children. *Appl Res Mental Retard* 1980;1:95-112.

145. Singer L, Nofer J, Benson-Szekely L, Brooks L. Behavioral assessment and management of food refusal in children with cystic fibrosis. *Dev Behav Pediatr* 1991;12:115-20.

146. Blackman J, Nelson C. Reinstituting oral feedings in children fed by gastrostomy tube. *Clin Pediatr* 1985;24:434-8.

147. Handen B, Mandell F, Russo D. Feeding induction in children who refuse to eat. *Am J Dis Child* 1986;140:52-4.

148. Rutter M. The long-term effects of early experience. *Dev Med Child Neurol* 1980;22:800-15.

149. Drotar D. The family context of nonorganic failure to thrive. *Am J Othopsychiatry* 1991;61:23-33.

150. Chamberlin J, Henry M, Roberts J, Sapsford A, Courtney S. An infant and toddler feeding group program. *Am J Occup Ther* 1991;45:907-11.

151. Gallageher J, Vietze PM. *Families of Handicapped Persons: Current Research, Programs, and Policy Issues*. Baltimore, MD: Paul Brookes, 1993:115-27.

152. Tuchman D, Walter R. Disorders of feeding and swallowing in infants and children: pathophysiology, diagnosis and treatment. 1994.

153. Bartolome G, Neumann S. Swallowing therapy in patients with neurological disorders causing cricopharyngeal dysfunction. *Dysphagia* 1993;8:146-9.

154. Neumann S. Swallowing therapy with neurologic patients: results of direct and indirect therapy methods in 66 patients suffering from neurological disorders. *Dysphagia* 1993;8:150-3.

155. Davis J. Prosthodontic management of swallowing disorders. *Dysphagia* 1989;3:199-205.

156. Selley W, Boxall J. A new way to treat sucking and swallowing difficulties in babies. *Lancet* 1986;1:1182-4.

157. Lavery M, ONeill J, Chu F, Martyn L. Acquired nystagmus in early childhood: a presenting sign of intracranial tumor. *Ophthalmology* 1984;91:425-53.

158. Mayer J. Hunger and undernutrition in the United States. *J Nutr* 1990;120:919-23.

159. Field J. Famine: a perspective for the nutrition community. *Nutr Rev* 1991;49:144-52.

160. Milanese A. Eating disorders and obesity. In: Willie, Hyams, eds. *Pediatric Gastrointestinal Disease: Pathophysiology, Diagnosis, Management*. Philadelphia, PA: WB Saunders, 1993.

161. Nicholson W. Tongue-tie (ankyloglossia) associated with breastfeeding problems. *J Hum Lact* 1991;7:82-4.

162. Fleiss P, Burger M, Ramkumar H, Carrington

P. Ankyloglossia: a cause of breastfeeding problems? *J Hum Lact* 1990;6:128-9.

163. Conway A. Ankyloglossia—to snip or not to snip: is that the question? *J Hum Lact* 1990;6:101-2.

164. Williams W, Waldron C. Assessment of lingual function when ankyloglossia (tongue-tie) is suspected. *J Am Dent Assoc* 1985;110:353-6.

165. Cotton R, Schreiber J. Management of laryngotracheo-esophageal cleft. *Ann Otol Rhinol Laryngol* 1981;90:401-5.

166. Ericksen C, Zwillenberg D, Robinson N. Diagnosis and management of cleft larynx: literature review and case report. *Ann Otol Rhinol Laryngol* 1990;99:703-8.

167. Curci M, Dibbins A. Problems associated with a Nissen fundoplicaton following tracheoesophageal fistual and esophageal atresia repair. *Arch Surg* 1988;123:618-20.

168. Milligan D, Levison H. Lung function in children following repair of tracheoesophageal fistula. *J Pediatr* 1979;95:24-7.

169. Desjardins J, Stephens C, Moses C. Results of surgical treatment of congenital tracheo-esophageal fistula with a note on cine-fluorographic findings. *Am Surg* 1964;160:141.

170. Laks H, Wildinson R, Schuster S. Long-term results following correction of esophageal atresia with tracheoesophageal fistula: a clinical and cine-fluorographic study. *J Pediatr Surg* 1972;7:591.

171. Anderson K, Noblett H, Belsey R, Randolph J. Long-term follow-up of children with colon and gastric tube interposition for esophageal atresia. *Surgery* 1992;111:131-6.

172. Orringer M, Kirsch M, Sloan H. Long-term esophageal function following repair of esophageal atresia. *Ann Surg* 1977;186:436-43.

173. Romeo G, Zuccarello B, Proietto F, et al. Disorders of the esophageal motor activity in atresia of the esophagus. *J Pediatr Surg* 1987;22:120-4.

174. Ashcraft K, Goodwin C, Amoury R, Holder T. Early recognition and aggressive treatment of gastroesophageal reflux following repair of esophageal atresia. *J Pediatr Surg* 1977;12:317-21.

175. Chetcuti P, Phelan P. Gastrointestinal morbidity and growth after repair of oesophageal atresia and tracheo-oesophageal fistula. *Arch Dis Child* 1993;68:163-6.

176. Yeung C, Spitz L, Brereton R, Kiely E, Leake J. Congenital esophageal stenosis due to tracheobronchial remnants: a rare but important association with esophageal atresia. *J Pediatr Surg* 1992;27:852-5.

177. Shoshany G, Bar-Maor J. Congenital stenosis of the esophagus due to tracheobronchial remnants: a missed diagnosis. *J Pediatr Gastroenterol Nutr* 1986;5:977-9.

178. Newman S, Caplan D. Lower esophageal ring in childhood. *Am J Gastroenterol* 1980;73:165-7.

179. Waldenstrom J, Kjelberg S. The roentgenological diagnosis of sideropenic dysphagia (Plummer-Vinson's syndrome). *Acta Radiol* 1939;20:618-38.

180. Puntis J, Chapman S, Proops D, Sartori P. Dysphagia due to oesophageal web. *Arch Dis Child* 1989;64:141-3.

181. Everett C, Volberg F, Ulshen M, Murray G. Intramural esophageal hamartoma: a report of two cases and review of the literature. *Gastrointest Radiol* 1980;5:317-9.

182. Taal B, Van Heerde P, Somers R. Isolated primary oesophageal involvement by lymphoma: a rare cause of dysphagia—two case histories and a review of other published data. *Gut* 1993;34:994-8.

183. Wolf Y, Katz S, Lax E. Okon E, Schiller M. Dysphagia in a child with aggressive fibromatosis of the esophagus. *J Pediatr Surg* 1989;24:1137-9.

184. Vos G, Heymans H, Urbanus N. Inspiratory stridor and dysphagia because of prolonged oesophageal foreign body. *Eur J Pediatr* 1987;146:86-7.

185. Orenstein S. Manometric demonstration of aberrant right subclavian artery associated with dysphagia. *J Pediatr Gastroenterol Nutr* 1984;3:634-6.

186. Martin G, Rudolph C, Hillemeier C, Heyman MB. Dysphagia lusorum in children. *AJDC* 1986;140:815-6.

187. van Son J, Vincent J, van Oort A, Lacquet L. Translocation of aberrant right subclavian artery in dysphagia lusoria in children through a right thoracotomy. *Thorac Cardiovasc Surg* 1988;37:52-4.

188. Sindel B, Maisels J, Ballantine T. Gastroesophageal reflux to the proximal esophagus in infants with bronchopulmonary dysplasia. *AJDC* 1989;143:1103-6.

189. Pridham K, Sondel S, Chang A, Green C. Nipple feeding for preterm infants with bronchopulmonary dysplasia. *J Obstet Gynecol Neonatal Nurs* 1993;22:147-55.

190. Ehlers K. Growth failure in association with congenital heart disease. *Pediatr Ann* 1978;7:750-9.

191. Yahav J, Avigad S, Frand M, Shem-Tov A, Barzilay Z, Linn S, Jonas A. Assessment of intestinal and cardiorespiratory function in children with congenital heart disease on high-caloric formulas. *J Pediatr Gastroenterol Nutr* 1985;4:778-85.

192. Combs V, Marino B. A comparison of growth patterns in breast and bottle-fed infants with congenital heart disease. *Pediatr Nurs* 1993;19:175-9.

193. Gisel E, Patrick J. Identification of children with cerebral palsy unable to maintain a normal nutritional state. *Lancet* 1988;1:283-5.

194. Rogers B, Arvedson J, Msall M, Demerath R. Hypoxemia during oral feeding of children with severe cerebral palsy. *Dev Med Child Neurol* 1993;35:3-10.

195. Waterman E, Koltai P, Downey J, Cacace A. Swallowing disorders in a population of children with cerebral palsy. *Int J Pediatr Otolaryn* 1992;24:63-71.

196. Frank Y, Schwartz S, Epstein N, Beresford H. Chronic dysphagia, vomiting, and gastroesophageal reflux as manifestations of a brain stem glioma: a case report. *Pediatr Neurosci* 1989;15:265-8.

197. Vandertop W, Asai A, Hoffman H, Drake J, Humphreys R, Rutka J, Becker L. Surgical decompression for symptomatic Chiari II malformation in neonates with myelomeningocele. *J Neurosurg* 1992;77:541-4.

198. Wolpert S, Scott R, Platenberg C, Runge V. The clinical significance of hindbrain herniation and deformity as shown on MR images of patients with Chiari II malformation. *AJNR* 1988;9:1075-8.

199. Fernbach S, McLone D. Derangement of swallowing in children with myelomeningocele. *Pediatr Radiol* 1985;15:311-4.

200. Coelho C, Ferranti R. Incidence and nature of dysphagia in polio survivors. *Arch Phys Med Rehabil* 1991;72:1071-5.

201. Sonies B, Dalakas M. Dysphagia in patients with the post-polio syndrome. *N Engl J Med* 1991;3234:1162-7.

202. Sudarshan A, Goldie W. The spectrum of congenital facial diplegia (Moebius syndrome). *Pediatr Neurol* 1985;1:180-4.

203. Kumar D. Moebius syndrome. *J Med Genet* 1990;27:122-6.

204. Jaffe K, McDonald C, Ingman E, Haas J. Symptoms of upper gastrointestinal dysfunction in Duchenne muscular dystrophy: case-control study. *Arch Phys Med Rehabil* 1990;71:742-4.

205. Tanowitz H, Kirchhoff L, Simon D, Morris S, Weiss L, Wittner M. Chagas' disease. *Clin Microbiol Rev* 1992;5:400-19.

206. Bittencourt A, Vieira G, Tavares H, Mota E, and Maguire J. Esophageal involvement in congenital Chagas' disease: report of a case with megaesophagus. *Am J Trop Med* 1984;33:30-3.

207. Glassman M, Spivak W, Mininberg D, Madara J. Chronic idiopathic intestinal pseudoobstruction: a commonly misdiagnosed disease in infants and children. *Pediatrics* 1989;83:603-8.

208. Schuffler M, Pope C. Esophageal motor dysfunction in idiopathic intestinal pseudoobstruction. *Gastroenterology* 1976;70:677-82.

209. Cohen S, Fisher R, Lipshutz W, Turner R, Myers A, et al. The pathogenesis of esophageal dysfunction in scleroderma and Raynaud's disease. *J Clin Invest* 1972;51:2663-8.

210. Marshall J, Kretschmar J, Gerhardt D, Winship D, Winn D, Treadwell E, Sharp G. Gastrointestinal manifestations of mixed connective tissue disease. *Gastroenterology* 1990;98:1232-8.

211. Ramirez-Mata M, Reyes P, Alarcon-Segovia

D, Garza R. Esophageal motility in systemic lupus erythematosus. *Am J Dig Dis* 1974;19:132-6.

212. Kodsi B, Wickremesinghe P, Kozinn P, Iswara K, Goldberg P. Candida esophagitis: a prospective study of 27 cases. *Gastroenterology* 1976;71:715-9.

213. Cucchiara S, Staiano A, Di Lorenzo C, D'Ambrosio R, Andreotti M, Prato M, DeFillipo P, Auricchio S. Esophageal motor abnormalities in children with gastroesophageal reflux and peptic esophagitis. *Pediatrics* 1986;108:907-10.

214. Moore D, Davidson G, Binns G. Herpes simplex oesophagitis in young children. *Med J Aust* 1986;144:716-7.

215. Nash G, Ross J. Herpetic esophagitis: a common cause of esophageal ulceration. *Hum Pathol* 1974;5:339-45.

216. McBane R, Gross JJ. Herpes esophagitis-clinical syndrome, endoscopic appearance and diagnosis in 23 patients. *Gastrointest Endosc* 1991;37:600-3.

217. Rabeneck L, Popovic M, Gartner S, McLean D, McLeod W, Read, E, Wong K, Boyko W. Acute HIV infection presenting with painful swallowing and esophageal ulcers. *JAMA* 1990;263:2318-22.

218. Balthazar E, Megibow A, Hulnik D, Cho K, Beranbaum E. Cytomegalovirus esophagitis in AIDS: radiographic features in 16 patients. *AJR* 1987;149:919-23.

219. Kikendall J, Friedman A, Oyewole M, Fleischer D, Johnson L. Pill-induced esophageal injury: case reports and review of the medical literature. *Dig Dis Sci* 1983;28:174-82.

220. Lenaerts C, Roy C, Vaillancourt M, Weber A, Morin C, Seidman E. High incidence of upper gastrointestinal tract involvement in children with Crohn's disease. *Pediatrics* 1989;83:777-81.

221. Gelfand M, Krone C. Dysphagia and esophageal ulceration in Crohn's disease. *Gastrointest Radiol* 1968;7:199-203.

222. Bottomley W, Dakkak M, Walton S, Bennett J. Esophageal involvement in Behcet's disease: is endoscopy necessary? *Dig Dis Sci* 1992;37:594-7.

223. Lebwohl O, Forder K, Berdon M, Morrison S, Challop R. Ulcerative esophagitis and colitis in a pediatric patient with Behcet's syndrome. *Am J Gastroenterol* 1977;68:550-5.

224. McDonald G, Sullivan K, Schuffler M, Shulmann H, Thomas E. Esophageal abnormalities in chronic graft versus host disease in humans. *Gastroenterology* 1981;80:914-21.

225. Cole D, Forsythe C, Dooley J, Grantmyre E, Salisbury S. Primary neonatal hyperparthyroidisms: a devastating neurodevelopmental disorder if left untreated. *J Craniofac Genet Devel Biol* 1990;10:205-14.

226. Gisel E, Lange L, Niman C. Chewing cycles in 4- and 5-year-old Down's syndrome children: a comparison of eating efficacy with normals. *Am J Occup Ther* 1984;38:666-70.

227. Trauner D, Bellugi U, Chase C. Neurologic features of Williams and Down syndromes. *Pediatr Neurol* 1989;5:166-8.

228. Crowe S, Perdue M. Gastrointestinal food hypersensitivity: basic mechanisms of pathophysiology. *Gastroenterology* 1992;103: 1075-95.

229. Bock S, Atkins F. Patterns of food hypersensitivity during sixteen years of double-blind placebo-controlled food challenges. *J Pediatr* 1990;117:561-7.

230. Brady R. Disorders of lipid metabolism. In: Berg, ed. *Neurologic Manifestations of Pediatric Diseases.* Stoneham, MA: Butterworth, 1990.

231. Tees D, Lofchy N, Rutka J. Deafness, dysphagia, and a middle ear mass in a patient with neurofibromatosis type 2. *J Otolaryngol* 1992;21:227-9.

232. Morris C, Demsey S, Leonard C, Dilts C, Blackburn B. Natural history of Williams syndrome: physical characteristics. *J Pediatr* 1988;113:318-26.

233. Quazi, OH, Heckman LS, Markouizos D, Verma RS. The Coffin-Siris syndrome. *J Med Genet* 1990;27:333-6.

234. Lucaya J, Garcia-Conesa J, Bosch-Banyeras J, Pons-Peradejordi G. The Coffin-Siris syndrome: a report of four cases and review of the literature. *Pediatr Radiol* 1981;11:35-8.

235. Einfeld S, Fairley M, Green B, Opitz J. Brief clinical report: sudden death in childhood in a case of the G syndrome. *Am J Med Genet* 1987;28:293-6.

236. Patton M, Baraitser M, Nickolaides K, Rodeck C, Gamsu H. Prenatal treatment of fetal hydrops associated with hypertelorism-dysphagia syndrome (Opitz-G syndrome). *Prenatal Diag* 1986;6:109-15.

237. Wilson G, Oliver W. Further delineation of the G syndrome: a manageable genetic cause of infantile dysphagia. *J Med Genet* 1989;25:157-63.

238. Cates M, Billmire B, Bull M, Grosfeld J. Gastroesophageal dysfunction in Cornelia de Lange syndrome. *J Pediatr Surg* 1989;24:248-50.

239. Peet P, Rodrigues Pereira R, Van Hemel J, Hoogeboom A. Interstitial del(13)(q21.3q31) associated with psychomotor retardation, eczema, and absent suck and swallowing reflex. *J Med Genet* 1987;24:786-8.

240. Batch A. Globus pharyngeus. *J Laryngol Otol* 1988;102:152-8, 227-30.

241. Ossakow S, Elta G, Colturi T, Bogdasarian R, Nostrant T. Esophageal reflux and dysmotility as the basis for persistent cervical symptoms. *Ann Otol Rhinol Laryngol* 1987;96:387-92.

242. Timon C, O'Dwyer T, Cagney D, Walsh M. Globus pharyngeus: long-term follow-up and prognostic factors. *Ann Otol Rhinol Laryngol* 1991;100:351-4.

243. Kern I, Esenberg M, Willis S. Management of esophageal stenosis in epidermolysis bullosa dystrophica. *Arch Dis Child* 1989;64:551-6.

CHAPTER
4
Gastroesophageal Reflux

SUSAN R. ORENSTEIN

Gastroesophageal reflux disease (GERD) is one of the most common motility disorders. Indeed, it is one of the most common pediatric disorders of any sort. During the last few decades, a great deal of progress has been made in understanding its pathophysiology and in defining optimal evaluation and treatment. This progress, however, has also illuminated the complexity of the disease, as well as the limitations of current therapy. This chapter will describe our current understanding of the pathophysiology of GERD, delineate what is known about its epidemiology, elaborate its multiple clinical presentations, and discuss diagnostic and treatment strategies. It will focus particularly on difficult management issues.

ESOPHAGEAL SPHINCTER PHYSIOLOGY

At rest (ie, in the absence of peristalsis) esophageal pressure is raised only at the upper and lower esophageal sphincters (UES and LES). Lower esophageal sphincter pressure normally varies depending on the characteristics of the manometry equipment (see Chapter 12), but most reports suggest a normal pressure of about 20 mm Hg. Values below 10 mm Hg are usually considered abnormal. The LES pressure is fairly static, but it does rise during gastric contractions in phase 3 of the migrating motor complex.[1] Experimentally, the human LES pressure was increased by cholinergic stimuli (eg, bethanechol, cisapride), metoclopramide, gastrin, and gastric alkalinization.[2,3] It was decreased by anesthesia, morphine, diazepam, intraduodenal fat, β-adrenergic agents

(eg, epinephrine, isoproterenol, salbutamol), dopamine, secretin, cholecystokinin, glucagon, vasoactive inhibitory peptide, progesterone, estrogen, nitrites, nifedipine, theophylline, ethanol, and nicotine.[2,4-7] Some of these effects hint at the physiologic controls of the LES: myogenic tone that is reduced by inhibitory effects of vasoactive inhibitory peptide and nitric oxide. Neuromuscular factors affecting the LES are shown in Figure 4.1.

Upper esophageal sphincter pressure is usually higher and more variable than that of the LES. Upper esophageal sphincter pressure decreases during deep sleep until it is virtually absent,[8] and increases markedly during emotional stress and straining.[9-11] It also increases during experimental esophageal balloon distention and fluid perfusion, especially with acidic fluids.[12,13]

Relaxation of the LES and UES occurs during swallowing as well as in other situations. Secondary peristalsis that originates in the esophagus rather than in the oropharynx includes a relaxation of the LES, which allows esophageal material to be propelled into the stomach. Inflating an esophageal balloon induces a similar relaxation of the LES. The LES and UES both relax to retrogradely vent the stomach and then the esophagus during belching or vomiting. The relaxation of the LES during belching[14] is similar to inappropriate transient lower esophageal sphincter relaxation (TLESR). It is considered inappropriate because it is not associated with swallowing. Although other mechanisms have been proposed,[15] normal individuals apparently increase the rate of TLESRs postprandially[16-18] due to gastric

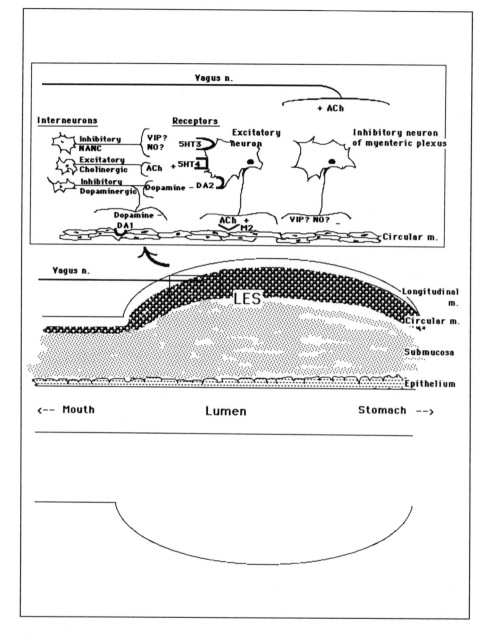

Fig. 4.1 Some of the probable modulators of lower esophageal sphincter (LES) function. The detail shows the circular muscle of the LES and its neural controls. Basic LES tone is myogenic, but the sphincter's pressure can be augmented by the direct, stimulatory effects of excitatory cholingeric neurons releasing acetylcholine on M_2 muscarinic receptors on the muscle. Bethanechol's main site for raising LES pressure is probably also at this receptor. Metoclopramide, a dopamine antagonist, may function by blocking dopamine's inhibition of the excitatory neuron at DA_2 receptors, or by a direct action on DA_1 dopamine receptors on myocytes. Cisapride directly potentiates acetylcholine release at the neuromuscular junction. LES relaxation, whether due to vagal input initiated by a swallow or occurring spontaneously, is mediated by inhibitory neurons releasing vasoactive inhibitory peptide (VIP) or nitric oxide (NO). Current therapy for reflux does not address the primary pathophysiology—inappropriate relaxations of the LES.

distention, particularly in the lesser curvature.[19,20] These LES relaxations are accompanied by relaxation of the crural diaphragm,[21] which abolishes the pressure at the gastroesophageal junction. Transient lower esophageal sphincter relaxations are eliminated by anesthesia, vagal blockade, and lesions of the dorsal motor nucleus of the vagus in animals, thus suggesting central as well as reflexive controls.[22-24] They are suppressed in the supine position, as compared with the seated position.[25,26] This suppression inhibits sphincter relaxation when fluid, rather than air, is likely to be at the gastroesophageal junction. These relaxations are also reduced in frequency by cold stress[27] and reduced in amplitude by somatostatin.[28] Nifedipine and ingestion of raw onion[29] cause an increase in frequency. Transient lower esophageal sphincter relaxations are probably mediated by the actions of vasoactive inhibitory peptide and/or nitric oxide.

As noted above, relaxations of the UES occur during swallowing and belching. They have also been induced experimentally by the rapid insufflation of air into the esophagus.[13] The exquisite controls of esophageal function are evident in the differential responses of the UES to esophageal balloon distention (analogous to a food bolus), and esophageal air insufflation (analogous to a belch).

THE PATHOPHYSIOLOGY OF REFLUX

Several issues have hindered attempts to understand gastroesophageal reflux. Reflux, regurgitation, and vomiting are ambiguous terms that are sometimes confused. Reflux is generally characterized as effortless, in contrast to rumination and vomiting.[30] The presence of abdominal wall muscle contraction in association with regurgitant reflux episodes,[31,32] however, clouds the distinction, particularly with rumination. Rumination involves some voluntary effort.[33-38] Vomiting involves much more effort, often including powerful retching and retrograde duodenogastric contractions.

Another issue that confuses our understanding of gastroesophageal reflux is that reflux is a normal phenomenon, occurring in virtually everyone. Thus there is a continuum between normals and those with severe and obvious GERD. Reflux disease is present when the reflux has produced harm: disability, discomfort, or impairment of function. This often occurs when physiologic reflux episodes are increased in frequency or duration, but reflux disease may be produced by subtler changes, including increased noxiousness of the refluxate itself, decreased defenses against harmful effects of reflux, or hazardous responses to reflux.

The determination of cause and effect is also difficult, since there are many aspects of reflux disease where cause-and-effect relationships are cyclical. Reflux causes esophagitis, which causes dysmotility, which causes further reflux. Reflux causes respiratory disease, which leads to abnormal thoracoabdominal pressure relationships and occasions provocative therapies and medications, all of which result in further reflux. The original factor initiating the cycle is usually impossible to determine.

Frequency

When the barriers to reflux are compromised or the provocations of reflux are augmented, reflux frequency increases. Many of the contributors to increased frequency have been illustrated in children as well as in adults.

LES pressure. When the antireflux mechanism is inadequate, reflux frequency increases. The primary part of the antireflux mechanism is the LES itself. Early discussions of the pathophysiology of reflux disease centered on low tonic LES pressure; esophagitis, for example, was found more often in those with low pressure. This issue is now, of course, more complex than it seemed initially, since severe esophagitis may be a cause of low LES pressure as well as the result of it. Low LES pressure is rarely the primary cause of reflux disease, although it may be an important perpetuating factor.

It has been suggested that pressures above 3 mm Hg are sufficient to maintain LES competence.[39] Relaxations below this value are now believed responsible for most reflux episodes.

Crural diaphragm. The LES tone is augmented by the crural diaphragm, which bolsters the LES during inspiration,[40] straining (eg, leg raising), and whenever the sphincter's competence is threatened. This function of the diaphragm explains why individuals with significant hiatal hernias have increased incidence of reflux disease; the hernia prevents the crura from bolstering the LES during abdominal straining and increased intra-abdominal pressure.[41] Even in the absence of a hiatal hernia, the crura's protection is reflexively inhibited when TLESRs mediate reflux episodes.[21,42]

It is important to recognize that in the past, particularly in Europe, there was a low threshold for identifying "hiatal hernia" on barium fluoroscopy. Stress manuevers were sometimes used for demonstration and in some centers "hiatal hernia" was virtually synonymous with gastroesophageal reflux disease.[43-47] The manometric rarity of these small, sliding hiatal hernias and the frequency with which they were seen fluoroscopically calls into question their physiologic significance.

TLESRs. While tonic LES pressure is important, TLESRs were identified as the most crucial mediators of reflux episodes once development[48] of the Dent sleeve allowed their detection. The study of TLESRs is still in its infancy, and they have been little studied in children.[49-51] Adult studies have suggested that TLESRs are more frequent in those with reflux disease than in normal controls, at least postprandially.[20,52] Nitric oxide and vasoactive inhibitory peptide may have a role in relaxing the LES, but whether dysfunctions of these inhibitory agents underlie TLESRs is unclear.[53]

Other. Other physiologic disturbances may worsen reflux frequency. Increased gastric contents due to larger meal size,[54] increased gastric secretion,[55-57] delayed gastric emptying, or duodenogastric reflux makes more potential refluxate available in the stomach

for a longer time. Infants with refractory or severe reflux, associated either with pulmonary disease or with failure to thrive, have significantly delayed gastric emptying.[58-62] Studies contesting this association are flawed by unphysiologic, clear-liquid feedings or apparently milder reflux disease.[63-65] Older children with esophagitis and low LES pressure also have been found to experience delayed gastric emptying.[66]

Greater gastric pressure due to obesity,[67,68] pregnancy,[69,70] peritoneal dialysis,[71] coughing, sneezing, straining,[72] or perhaps, reflux-associated fundic contractions,[73,74] increases the likelihood of reflux, particularly in the presence of a hiatal hernia or a concurrent TLESR. Sudden pressure increases may also change the character of reflux from nonregurgitant to regurgitant.[75]

Duration

When esophageal clearance mechanisms are impaired, the reflux episodes last longer. Gravity, peristalsis, and saliva are components of the esophageal clearance mechanism.[76-78] Deficiencies in all three components are responsible for the marked delay in clearance of reflux that occurs during sleep.[79]

Gravity. Gravity promotes bulk esophageal clearance, particularly of liquids, in the upright, seated, or standing postures. Although gravity contributes little in the presence of normal peristalsis, it may play an important role when peristalsis is defective, which often occurs with severe esophagitis.[76]

Peristaltic bulk clearance. Peristalsis is responsible for clearing the bulk of refluxate from the esophagus. Primary peristalsis, originating with a swallow, is stimulated by esophageal acidification or heartburn. Secondary peristalsis, originating in the esophagus, is stimulated by the volume of fluid in the esophagus.[80,81] A single, normal peristaltic wave clears the entire esophagus of refluxate.[82] Peristaltic amplitude of 30 mm Hg is necessary for effective volume clearance.[82] Incomplete or low-pressure waves permit retrograde escape of refluxate; these abnormalities occur frequently in patients with esophagitis. Even infants and children with severe reflux disease manifest these abnormalities,[62,83-86] although they were not found in children with mild esophagitis.[87]

The role of hiatal hernia in impairing bulk clearance from the esophagus has also been noted.[88-91]

Salivary neutralization. The outflow of bicarbonate-rich saliva (ie, waterbrash) that occurs during esophageal acidification[92,93] contributes in two ways to esophageal clearance. The most obvious of these is the stepwise neutralization of residual esophageal acid during swallows that follow the initial bulk-clearing swallow. The second contribution of reflux-stimulated salivation is to provoke further primary peristaltic waves, carrying the saliva into the esophagus and clearing residual bulk if necessary.

The bicarbonate in saliva is supplemented by esophageal bicarbonate secretion,[94] probably originating in submucosal glands.

Reflux Noxiousness

When the refluxate contains more acid, pepsin, or damaging duodenal components, reflux noxiousness increases and esophagitis is worsened.

Acid. Hydrochloric acid has long been understood as an important harmful component of refluxate. The degree of esophagitis has been associated with the degree of acid exposure, expressed as the "area under the curve" of pH probe studies.[95] Greater damage occurs with lower pH and with intermittent, rather than continuous, acid exposure if the total exposure time is constant.[96,97] Even newborn term infants secrete acid effectively, although less than adults. In very young prematures, the secretion may not be enough to support peptic activity.[98-101]

Pepsin. The contribution of pepsin has been relatively ignored. An experimental study suggested that hydrochloric acid without pepsin produces comparatively few changes, at least in the rabbit epithelium.[102] Much of the damaging effect of increased gastric acid exposure is probably due to the accompanying increased gastric peptic activity, which promotes cell shedding. Pepsinogen is secreted by newborns, but not by very premature infants.[103]

Bile acids and trypsin. The contribution of duodenal contents—particularly bile acids and trypsin—to esophagitis has been controversial. These materials can cause esophagitis in the absence of gastric acid or pepsin, as is evident from the occurrence of esophagitis in patients with achlorhydria or postgastrectomy.[104-106] Experimental models have confirmed the ability of bile acids and trypsin to damage the esophagus severely. Bile acids disrupt cell membranes and cause cell shedding. Trypsin causes morphologic changes and hemorrhage.[107-110] These materials may be particularly important in the development of complicated esophagitis such as Barrett's esophagus or stricture.[111] They are even present in reduced concentrations in the newborn's duodenal contents.[112] Recent studies of infants and children have described pH-probe parameters of such alkaline (presumably duodenogastric) reflux, and have related them to esophagitis.[113-114] The controversial aspect is the possible confusion of alkaline saliva with alkaline duodenal contents when using an esophageal pH probe to document duodenogastroesophageal reflux. Recently, it was estimated that gastric juice would need to be more than 80% duodenal juice by volume in order to elevate the pH of the fluid above 7 (T.R. DeMeester, MD, unpublished data, OESO meeting, Paris, 1993).

Reflux Defenses

Once gastroesophageal reflux has occurred, the factors that protect the esophageal mucosa from refluxate and those that prevent the refluxate from escaping the esophagus before being returned to the stomach can be considered the defenses against reflux.

Mucosal defense. The study of esophageal mucosal defenses is still a new field. Possible components of mucosal defense include esophageal mucus, the "mucosal barrier" to ion influx, mucosal blood flow that brings bicarbonate as well as other factors, prostaglandins, and epithelial growth factor from the capillary epithelium, platelets, or possibly saliva.[115,116]

"Escape" defense. When the refluxate finds its way to a hazardous location, the noxiousness of reflux is increased. The most common of these "escapes" from the esophagus is regurgitation, which causes failure to thrive in many infants. Other problematic destinations for escaped refluxate are the airway and the nasopharynx. Refluxate in the airway is designated aspiration, and is one cause of upper and lower airway disease. The most proximal portion of the airway has recently been identified as extremely susceptible to damage by refluxate,[117,118] so that minimal contact can produce serious symptoms (see Clinical Presentations, later this chapter). Pharyngonasal reflux has not been well examined, although parents of some infants describe frequent nasal regurgitation. Pharyngonasal reflux during swallowing results from velopalatal insufficiency; the mechanisms of pharyngonasal reflux associated with gastroesophageal reflux are unclear, as is the issue of whether it contributes to sinusitis or otitis.[119] The UES may play a role in preventing these phenomena, which affect infants more frequently than older children, but this role is not yet clear. Similarly, the defensive roles of the soft palate, epiglottis, and larynx during reflux are incompletely defined.

Hazardous Responses to Reflux

When an individual becomes more susceptible to the effects of refluxate, reflux noxiousness may rise without any change in the reflux parameters themselves. Examples of these hazardous responses to reflux include reflux-induced bronchospasm (eg, asthma or wheezing) and laryngospasm (eg, obstructive apnea), both of which seem to occur in some children on a reflexive basis, as well as during actual aspiration. Other possible reflexes are central apnea and bradycardia. All of these responses are probably vagally mediated. They

will be discussed in more detail under Clinical Presentations.

EPIDEMIOLOGY

The incidence and prevalence of reflux disease are difficult to determine because it is a loosely defined condition that cannot be reliably identified noninvasively. The many recently recognized manifestations of reflux are thus often difficult to link to reflux in individual instances. This section will describe the age-related normal ranges of reflux episode frequency, differentiate physiologic from pathologic reflux, contrast the infantile and adult forms of reflux disease, estimate the frequency of disease in infants and older children, and discuss some groups that have been identified as being particularly susceptible to reflux disease.

Reflux in Normals

Regurgitant reflux. Regurgitation was the earliest form of reflux identified, and it is still the most commonly used marker of reflux disease in infants. Regurgitant reflux represents only the tip of the iceberg of reflux episodes; it may even result from different mechanisms than nonregurgitant reflux.[32] Parents report that approximately 70% of infants referred for evaluation of reflux disease (and a similar proportion of those who are subsequently shown to have reflux disease) will have regurgitation as a problem,[120] in contrast to about 20% of infants seen in a well-baby clinic (unpublished data). Specifically, 80% of the infants with reflux are reported to regurgitate at least once a day at greater than 5 ml per average episode, whereas only 40% of well infants do so. There is clearly considerably more regurgitation in infants with reflux disease, but there is also a great deal of overlap between them and normal infants. After 1 year of age, regurgitation is as infrequent in children with reflux disease as it is in normals.

Fluoroscopic reflux. Fluoroscopic barium gastroesophagography, without provocative maneuvers, shows reflux episodes occurring more often and reaching higher in the esophagus in children with reflux disease than in those without symptoms of reflux disease. Again, normals and reflux patients overlap. The reflux episodes also decrease in frequency and height in the esophagus with age in normals. A retrospective study of 470 children delineated the upper range of normal for the number of episodes seen in 5 minutes of fluoroscopy. Those younger than 6 weeks had three episodes; children from 7 weeks to 1 year had two episodes; those between 1 and 6 years had one episode; and those over 6 years had fewer than one episode.[121] This study also crudely quantified the volume of refluxate by distinguishing reflux that reached the level of the clavicles from reflux that did not. Of the reflux episodes in each age group of asymptomatic children, the proportion which reached the

clavicles decreased with age: 86% of episodes in normal infants younger than 6 weeks reached the clavicles, whereas only 20% of the episodes in the normal teenagers did.

pH probe reflux. The pH probe can detect acid reflux frequency, duration, and acidity throughout prolonged periods of monitoring—typically 24 hours. Using this method, investigators have characterized the range of normal for total duration of esophageal acidification (pH <4) and for frequency of acid reflux episodes related to age during infancy, childhood, and adulthood (Fig. 4.2).[122-124] However, since most reflux episodes occur postprandially, the pH probe often cannot detect reflux because of the buffering of gastric contents by the meal, an effect that is particularly evident in infants. These nor-

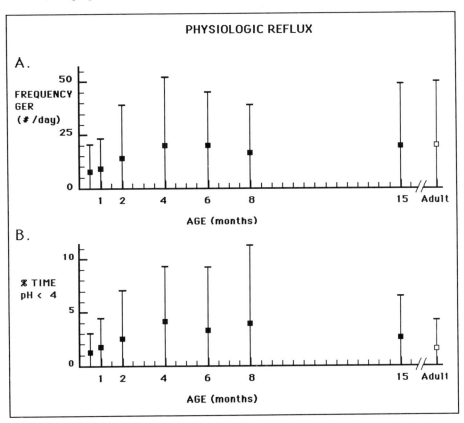

Fig. 4.2 Physiologic reflux: range of normal values during development. Graphic representation of normal ranges (mean ± 2 SD) for reflux in children of various ages (n = 285) and in adults (n = 15). **A,** Frequency of reflux episodes. **B,** Total duration of esophageal acidification throughout the day, during normal activities and diet. (Reprinted with permission from Orenstein SR, 1991[244])

mal values therefore significantly underestimate the frequency and duration of total reflux—acid and nonacid combined.

Physiologic and Pathologic Reflux

Since reflux is present in normal individuals, a continuum from normal to diseased exists with respect to gastroesophageal reflux. We should not define reflux disease simply by the deviation from normal values of frequency or duration; we should demand that symptoms, harm, or disability must be produced to meet our definition of disease. This may be difficult to determine, however. Does the patient who has pain induced by acidification, but who does not have histologic esophagitis or esophageal dysmotility, have reflux disease? If so, it may often be missed. Does the patient who has normal reflux frequency, but who occasionally aspirates refluxate, have reflux disease? Certainly, but this course of events is often extremely difficult to document.

Infantile and "Adult" Reflux

Clinically, pediatric gastroesophageal reflux takes two forms: infantile reflux and "adult" reflux. The former becomes symptomatic during the first months of life and resolves clinically by 12 to 24 months of age in at least 80% of afflicted babies.[125,126] The latter form may develop with a background of infantile reflux in some children, but often appears anew in children beyond infancy. This form, like reflux in adults, tends to persist, waxing and waning symptomatically. As many as 50% of affected older children, like adults, will not obtain permanent relief of symptoms, and will require chronic or intermittent therapy.[127,128] In addition to the difference in the course of the disease for the infantile and adult forms, there are some differences in clinical presentation. These will be described in detail in Clinical Presentations, but can be summarized as being due to older childrens' developmental maturation, longer chronicity, and verbal abilities. Developmental maturation results in the virtual disappearance of regurgitation, apnea, and stridor as manifestations of reflux, but asthma increases. The

almost exclusive confinement of Barrett's epithelium and strictures to older individuals is due to the longer chronicity of reflux. Because infants cannot speak, complaints of heartburn or other descriptions of pain do not occur, although intractable crying may be an analogous symptom.[129,130]

Mildly Symptomatic Reflux and GERD

The prevalence, incidence, and disappearance of GERD is unknown for infants, older children, and even for adults. The diversity of symptoms which may represent GERD has contributed to this informational vacuum.

Adults. Using only the most obvious symptoms—heartburn and/or acid regurgitation more than once a week in adults—a population-based study from Olmsted County, Minnesota (Mayo Clinic), found a 15% incidence of these symptoms.[131] Nearly 50% of these adults lost their symptoms within the next year or so, but were replaced by a similar number with new onset of symptoms. A similar survey found 36% of adults to have heartburn at least monthly, and 7% to have it daily.[132] These studies probably overestimate actual disease, in the sense that once-weekly heartburn may be insignificant, but underestimate it in the sense that other symptoms of reflux disease (eg, respiratory symptoms) were not assessed, and that the patients with asymptomatic esophagitis and Barrett's esophagus were ignored. A review of the epidemiology of reflux suggests that the prevalence of reflux disease is approximately 5%, and for reflux esophagitis it is approximately 2%.[133] Another study indicated that the yearly incidence of endoscopically proven esophagitis is 0.12%, with complicated cases (strictures and Barrett's) making up 12% of the diagnoses.[134] This latter study contrasts with one which found only 1.2% of esophagitis cases to have strictures.[135] It has also been suggested that 5% to 10% of patients referred to hospital for investigation require surgery.[136]

Infants. As noted above, 20% of parents of

well infants describe regurgitation as a problem. This figure may correspond to the 15% of adults in the Mayo study with obvious but relatively benign symptoms. (Both groups are likely to respond well to conservative treatment measures, as will be discussed.) A description of the estimated incidence of infantile reflux of any severity is also 20%.[137] This source estimates that 33% (6.7% of all infants) come to medical attention, of whom 80% (5.4% of all infants) are resolved with minimal therapy and no investigation. Of the other 1.3% who are investigated, the large majority are successfully treated medically, but 0.4% of all infants require antireflux surgery (>25% of those investigated). These incidence estimates seem fairly reasonable, but confirmatory data are needed. The legitimacy of the estimates is suggested by the yearly rate of approximately 200 discharge diagnoses of reflux disease in infants younger than 12 months at the 200-bed Children's Hospital of Pittsburgh. The affiliated referral maternity hospital has a delivery rate of about 10,000 per year, producing an estimated 2% incidence of reflux severe enough to be investigated in hospital in the first year of life, which is very similar to the 1.3% figure cited above. The incidence of symptomatic GERD in very low birthweight infants is higher; 3%[138] to 10%[139] of such infants have symptoms of reflux-associated apnea, bradycardia, or exacerbated bronchopulmonary dysplasia. Prolongation of reflux episodes is common in these tiny infants, suggesting impaired esophageal acid clearance as an important mechanism.

Older children. Reflux was diagnosed annually in about 300 children older than 1 year of age admitted to Children's Hospital of Pittsburgh. This rate suggests an average yearly incidence of investigated reflux of 18 in each 1-year age group, in comparison to the 200 per year in the first year of life, or not more than 0.2% yearly incidence of investigated reflux after 1 year of age. If there were no repeat admissions, which is not the case, 5% of individuals would have a hospitalization with a diagnosis of reflux disease at some time during their childhood. The actual number is probably less. A study of 126

infants and children with reflux disease cited 17% as presenting after the first year of life;[126] combined with our figures, this would correspond to 0.4% of all children developing reflux disease beyond infancy, and 2.4% of all children—including infants—developing reflux disease.

Sex Ratio

Many studies suggest a slight preponderance of males with GERD in infancy (eg, 1.27:1), as well as in older patients, but this may not be statistically or clinically significant.[126,140] Barrett's esophagus, a complication of severe reflux, is more prevalent in males.[141,142] If there is a male preponderance, the cause in children is unknown. In adults, the differences could be genetic, hormonal, or related to socioenvironmental factors such as nicotine and ethanol exposure.

Groups With Increased Incidence of GERD

Some groups have been noted to have more reflux disease than the general population.

Neurologic disease. Neurologic disease is associated with a high prevalence of GERD, which often persists beyond infancy. As many as 15% of institutionalized, severely retarded children have recurrent vomiting, mostly attributed to reflux.[143] An unknown further proportion may have nonregurgitant reflux responsible for esophagitis or respiratory symptoms. Neurologic disease associated with hypertonia and spasticity may provoke reflux episodes by increasing abdominal pressure. Since children with spasticity have a high incidence of hiatal hernia, this rise in abdominal pressure often occurs without a protective increase in crural support of the LES. One study suggests that extensor spasm, air swallowing, and kyphoscoliosis play roles in the development of the hiatal hernias found in these children.[144]

Hypotonia may be present in other children with severe neurologic disease. Hypotonia leads to supine or slumped postures, which are also provocative for reflux episodes.

Although Down syndrome occurs in 1 out of 660 newborns, 2% to 10% of infants undergoing fundoplication in various series have had this diagnosis.[145] These children may be somewhat hypotonic, but esophageal manometry also showed a high frequency of simultaneous esophageal contractions in five children studied in detail.[145] The contrasting normalcy of the LES pressure suggests the possibility that the motility changes may have been primary, rather than secondary to esophagitis.

Myopathy, dysautonomia, systemic sclerosis.

Children with myopathy[146] or systemic sclerosis[147] may also be predisposed to reflux disease because their reflux episodes are poorly cleared. A high prevalence of reflux disease is reported in familial dysautonomia,[148] although it could be argued that the episodes of nausea, retching, and actual vomiting that these patients exhibit differs from what is commonly understood as gastroesophageal reflux. The autonomic nervous system plays a role in reflux, however, so that abnormalities in autonomic functioning could promote reflux. Although the mechanisms underlying vomiting in familial dysautonomia are incompletely understood, the vomiting often results in esophagitis, thereby promoting cycles of further dysmotility and reflux.

Chronic respiratory disease.

Bronchopulmonary dysplasia, cystic fibrosis, and asthma are associated with a high prevalence of GERD in children. Increased abdominal pressure during wheezing or coughing, decreased thoracic pressure during stridor, provocative medications, and positioning during ventilation or physiotherapy all may exacerbate physiologic reflux to pathologic proportions in these children.

As many as 20% of premature infants with bronchopulmonary dysplasia have abnormal quantities of reflux, as compared with 1% to 2% of prematures without bronchopulmonary dysplasia.[138]

Children with cystic fibrosis experience increased reflux by several measures. Report of any heartburn in approximately 25%[149,150] and heartburn more than once weekly in 9%[150] is similar to the rate in normal adults, although perhaps more than

in normal children. However, regurgitation occurs more than once weekly in 3% of children with cystic fibrosis who are older than 5 years of age.[151] This is certainly an abnormal frequency, and may represent posttussive emesis. Similarly, complications of reflux such as esophageal erosions (occurring in up to 50%[149]), hematemesis (up to 6%[149-151]), and strictures (up to 2%[150,151]) are increased in cystic fibrosis. The provocative effect of the degree of respiratory disease is suggested by increased frequency of esophagitis (76% v 25%) in those with severe respiratory disease compared to those with mild cases.[149]

Children with asthma also experience increased frequency of reflux. Prevalence of abnormal reflux is reported to range from 45% to 78% in these children,[152-157] which is similar to the high prevalence in adult asthmatics.[158,159]

Congenital esophageal anomalies.

Esophageal atresia is associated with a high incidence of symptomatic GERD, which complicates the management of the accompanying respiratory disease and the frequent anastomotic strictures.[160] The reflux seems to be a product of intrinsic esophageal dysmotility, LES dysfunction related to postoperative traction on the lower esophageal segment, and possibly delayed gastric emptying due to operative vagal damage.[150,161-166] The disparity between studies showing no evidence of symptomatic reflux[163] and those showing up to two thirds with symptomatic reflux[166] may be due to preoperative differences, such as the length of the gap between the ends of the esophagus.

Increased abdominal pressure.

Particularly if the LES is not bolstered by the crural diaphragm, as occurs in hiatal hernia, increased abdominal pressure facilitates reflux. Abdominal pressure is increased in situations other than the hypertonic, neurologically devastated children discussed above. Chronically increased abdominal pressure occurs in obesity, and explains the reported 73% prevalence of heartburn in 55 unselected massively obese adults.[67] The 29% prevalence of hiatal hernia in the same unselected adults, and a 100% prevalence of hiatal hernia in a smaller study[68] provides evidence for the pathophysiology. Although low LES pressure and deranged esophageal clearance were also reported in many of these patients, these abnormalities may be secondary to the esophagitis. Less research has been performed on obese children, but they probably experience similar problems.

During pregnancy, not only does chronic abdominal distention increase abdominal pressure and predispose to hiatal hernia, but other changes occur.[69,70] The normal nausea and vomiting of morning sickness early in pregnancy may cause esophagitis and thus lead to esophageal dysmotility. Delayed gastric emptying has been reported, perhaps simply due to the crowded intra-abdominal conditions. Hormonal changes, such as the rise in progesterone, mediate LES relaxation. Twenty-five percent of pregnant women—both adults and adolescents—have reported daily heartburn, and up to 80% have reported some heartburn during pregnancy.[69,132]

Gastrostomy feedings induce GERD in initially nonrefluxing children after treatment with a percutaneous endoscopic gastrostomy[167] (60%) or after treatment with an operative Stamm gastrostomy (25%).[168] The postulated mechanisms by which gastrostomies induce GERD include changing the gastroesophageal angle[169] and decreasing the LES pressure or length,[170] but clinical experience suggests that the most important factor may be the rapid bolus feedings often given to these children after gastrostomy. The resulting abrupt increase in intragastric pressure may overwhelm the rate of gastric receptive relaxation and provoke LES relaxation.[171]

Peritoneal dialysis may delay gastric emptying,[71] but increased reflux in these patients with chronic renal failure may also be due to a changed hormonal environment and foregut motor function independent of the mechanical effects on the abdomen.[172]

Exercise is occasionally cited as a cause of symptomatic gastroesophageal reflux in children as well as adults.[173-175] The effects of exercise on gastroesophageal motility are complex, and depend on type (eg, bicycle, treadmill, etc), intensity (measured as % of maximal), and duration of exercise. This complexity explains some of the diversity of reported study results: gastric emptying, for example, is accelerated by moderate exercise, but delayed by severe exercise.[176,177] Gastric acid secretion is inhibited by strenuous exercise at greater than 70% of maximal.[177-179] Esophageal contraction amplitude and duration are decreased by increasing intensity of exercise,[180] as is LES pressure.[181] Finally, abdominothoracic pressure relationships are likely to be affected by the strenuous breathing associated with heavy exertion.

Postural effects. Disorders leading to hypotonia and chronic supine or semisupine postures[182,183] promote reflux. Premature infants may have increased reflux on this basis.

Hormonal effects. The reflux associated with pregnancy[69] or chronic renal failure[172] may be promoted by hormonal effects on the LES, specifically progesterone and gastrin.

Vagal dysfunction or injury. Reflux associated with familial dysautonomia, repaired esophageal atresia, and mediastinal or hiatal surgery may have vagal dysfunction in common.[148,184,185]

Genetic predisposition. A case report on a series of twins with reflux disease postulated a genetic influence on the incidence of reflux.[186] However, a small number of case reports in twins or even triplets is clearly insufficient evidence for a genetic influence on a disease with a childhood incidence over 2%. Furthermore, even if an increased incidence within families were shown, environmental factors would still need to be seriously considered.

CLINICAL PRESENTATIONS

In this section the myriad clinical presentations currently associated with reflux will be reviewed. Salient diagnostic and therapeutic aspects particular to each type of presentation will be outlined. A more comprehensive discussion of the particulars of the diagnostic and therapeutic armamentarium will be developed in Diagnostic Evaluation and Treatment.

Regurgitation

Infantile regurgitation is the most common presentation of GERD. As discussed above, 20% of normal infants have enough regurgitation that their parents consider it a problem, although less than 2% of infants require investigation. Considering GERD as the cause of this system is no challenge; the challenges lie in avoiding inappropriate investigation and in not missing other causes of vomiting in children.

Happy spitters. Babies whose parents' main complaint is the mess they make require no investigation of therapy, other than conservative measures (see Treatment). Thickening of milk formula with rice cereal, for example, is usually enough to reduce the spitting and the mess.

Regurgitation with weight loss. The infant with regurgitation and weight loss should be evaluated for anatomic abnormalities with barium fluoroscopy. To avoid a lethal midgut volvulus, particular attention should be paid to whether intestinal rotation is normal. Antral and duodenal webs may also present with regurgitation, and may be difficult to demonstrate radiographically if the webs are not perpendicular to the plane of the image. Consideration of allergic disease (eg, formula protein intolerance) in these infants is often fruitful, particularly in the context of a family history of allergies. This is most simply evaluated by an empiric therapeutic trial of 2 to 3 weeks of a protein hydrolysate formula, remembering that symptoms of food allergy may take that long to improve after dietary modification. The use of soy formula in this context is common, but only adds confusion, because of the large proportion of infants with allergy to both cow's milk and soy. Although the pH probe is commonly used to evaluate the infant whose presenting symptom is regurgitation, it contributes little to the evaluation and should be avoided.

Regurgitation with irritability. The infant with regurgitation and irritability should be considered for evaluation or treatment for esophagitis (see below), but irritability may also be a sign of metabolic disease, central nervous system disease, or partial obstruction. These diagnoses should be seriously considered in irritable regurgitating infants.

Regurgitation with ill appearance. The infant with regurgitation who appears ill, manifests developmental delay, neurologic abnormalities, or seizures, etc., requires more evaluation, and GERD is the least ominous of the possible diagnoses. One should not automatically diagnose these infants as having "the reflux that often accompanies neurologic deficits" without seriously considering metabolic disease as the cause for both the neurologic problems and the regurgitation.

Rumination. Infantile rumination and regurgitant reflux share some characteristics, and there may be a continuum between their pathophysiologies and therapies.[33,34,38] Evidence of a disturbed parent-infant relationship, self-gagging, or apparently pleasurable regurgitation and reswallowing suggest rumination. However, rumination may also produce esophagitis, thus causing dysmotility and self-perpetuating reflux. Several infants who were sticking their fingers in their throats have been successfully treated with therapy for reflux. Thus, even the infant with apparent classical rumination may benefit from consideration for therapy of reflux disease in combination with any modification of their psychosocial situation.

Regurgitation in older children. Regurgitation in older children and adults is far less common than it is in infants. Even material which escapes from the esophagus to the mouth is often reswallowed. A history of acid coming up into the mouth effortlessly or during frequent burping is a useful symptom. Usually this symptom alone will not bring an older child to medical attention, and heartburn or similar symptoms are often the presenting complaint. Toddlers who have actual regurgitation persisting from infancy may require investigation and treatment if this manifestation of reflux has not resolved as their posture has become upright and their diet has become largely solids.

Adult-type rumination. As with infantile rumination, "adult-type" rumination shares some characteristics with regurgitant reflux.[35,37,38] These patients, like those with bulimia and anorexia nervosa, deserve consideration of esophagitis therapy in combination with behavioral- or psychotherapy.

Esophagitis

Symptoms of esophagitis are the most common manifestations of GERD that bring older children and adults to medical attention.

Chest pain. Pain in the chest, designated "heartburn" because of the difficulty distinguishing it from ischemic heart pain in adults, is the most common symptom of esophagitis in verbal children. The pain of heartburn parallels both the duration and the concentration of acid exposure in experimental protocols. Similarly, the endoscopic and histologic findings of esophagitis bear a relationship to the area under the curve—the pH probe representation of the duration and concentration of esophageal acid exposure.[95,97,187] In children, the difficulty of distinguishing cardiac pain is far less an issue than it is in adults, in whom the Bernstein test gained favor because of its diagnostic utility for this discrimination. In children with typical complaints of heartburn, as in adults, a 2-month course of empiric pharmacotherapy combined with conservative therapy is a rational diagnostic strategy. Endoscopic evaluation is reserved for persistent or recurrent symptoms. Chest pain in children may indicate the presence of a primary motility disorder.[188]

Abdominal pain. Epigastric abdominal pain may also represent esophagitis. If the characteristics of the pain suggest either typical peptic ulcer disease or esophagitis, antisecretory therapy may be employed for the 2-month empiric trial of therapy before proceeding to further diagnostic evaluation. If such evaluation is needed, endoscopy is the optimal initial procedure.

Infantile irritability. Chronic crying in infants was mentioned above as a manifestation of esophagitis. The suction biopsy technique[189-191] can be used as a rapid, minimally invasive test to evaluate for esophagitis in these babies. Because this symptom is less specific than heartburn, 2 months of empiric therapy is less desirable in this setting. The alternative diagnostic evaluations—pH probe or endoscopy with biopsy—are significantly more invasive and expensive, so that optimal evaluation of such irritable infants is difficult if suction biopsies are unavailable. The immediate response to a dose of a liquid antacid may be diagnostically helpful. It is crucial in any case to keep in mind the nonspecific nature of this symptom, and the tremendous range of possible diagnoses, from benign "colic" to life-threatening diseases.

Feeding resistance. Refusal to eat while appearing hungry is another manifestation of infantile esophagitis. It often coexists with meal-associated irritability. We have seen several infants with severe failure to thrive due to refusal to drink formula, in whom dramatic esophagitis was evident on esophageal biopsies, and in whom aggressive nonsurgical therapy for reflux esophagitis produced resolution of their feeding refusal and subsequent rapid weight gain. Others have reported similar cases.[192] When confronted with an infant with feeding refusal, other diagnostic considerations to keep in mind are an acquired distaste for the formula due to an association of the taste with symptoms from allergy, or metabolic disease such as hereditary fructose intolerance or even galactosemia (depending on the formula). A switch to a casein-hydrolysate formula without sucrose (ie, Pregestamil) will treat all of these possibilities concurrently, if a rapid improvement of the failure to thrive is desired. The possibilities of these diagnoses should not be forgotten, however, when considering resumption of formula containing cow's milk, soy, lactose, sucrose, or fructose.

Hematemesis. Bleeding is far less common than pain as a symptom of peptic esophagitis, particularly in children. Evidence for bleeding due to esophagitis are hematemesis or, more subtly, anemia. Hematemesis usually demands endoscopic evaluation, which will distinguish esophagitis from other causes such as varices, gastroduodenal erosions or ulceration, or arteriovenous malformations. Other causes of hematemesis to be kept in mind are swallowed maternal blood (in newborns or nursing infants), nosebleeds, oropharyngeal lesions, or hemoptysis. The evaluation may need to be directed toward these entities if the history is suggestive or the endoscopy is normal.

Anemia. Anemia is rarely a presentation of otherwise asymptomatic esophagitis. Any child presenting with significant anemia requires hemoccult testing of stool as part of the initial physical examination. Those with hemoccult-positive stool but without hematochezia should usually have upper endoscopy, which will disclose esophagitis if it is present. Even in the absence of hemoccult-positive stool, if the anemia remains unexplained evaluation for esophagitis may be warranted.

Dysphagia. Difficulty swallowing may be a manifestation of esophagitis in two ways. The esophagitis-associated dysmotility mentioned earlier may cause dysphagia. As is typical with dysphagia due to dysmotility, it affects swallowing of liquids as much as or even more than swallowing of solids. In contrast, esophagitis which has progressed to esophageal stricture presents as dysphagia, which affects swallowing of solids earlier and more severely than swallowing of liquids.

Evaluation of dysphagia should begin with barium fluoroscopy. If a stricture is demonstrated, endoscopy for histology and therapeutic dilation is the next step. If there is no stricture and no classic evidence for a primary motility disorder, but the history otherwise suggests esophagitis, a 2-month trial of empiric therapy for esophagitis is reasonable. If there is ambiguity about the likelihood of esophagitis, endoscopy should be performed; if esophagitis is present it should be treated for several months before reevaluating for the presence of dysphagia. If no esophagitis is found, esophageal manometry should be performed to evaluate for a primary motility disorder.

Clinically-silent esophagitis. Barrett's esophagus is usually unsuspected before endoscopy discloses the pinker columnar epithelium extending into and replacing the normal pale squamous epithelium.[142,193] Barrett's esophagus is important both because it is associated with other complications (eg, esophageal ulcers and strictures) and because it is a premalignant lesion. Recent evidence suggests that this form of complicated esophagitis, in particular, is linked with reflux of duodenal contents. In addition, the complexity of distinguishing hiatal hernias from Barrett's epithelium with a propensity for dysplasia has been simplified recently by the suggestion that only intestinal metaplasia carries the increased risk of dysplasia and carcinoma. The development of Barrett's esophagus seems to depend on the chronicity of reflux disease. Thus it occurs infrequently in young children. However, because it has been seen as early as 5 years of age, and esophageal adenocarcinoma appears as early as 11 years of age,[193] vigilance for this complication is needed, and histologic evaluation of the esophagus in GERD assumes even greater importance.

Respiratory Presentations

Respiratory presentations of GERD were unsuspected until the past 10 to 20 years. The range of such manifestations is gradually being clarified, but in many cases the pathophysiology remains ambiguous. That reflux may cause these respiratory manifestations is compounded by the fact that many respiratory symptoms or treatments may, in turn, provoke reflux. Coughing, wheezing, stridor, chest physiotherapy, medications (eg, theophylline, β-adrenergic bronchodilators, caffeine), and mechanical ventilation may all contribute to reflux.

This vicious cycle explains the epidemiologic data, discussed above, that show an increased rate of GERD in children with respiratory disease. In settings such as cystic fibrosis, bronchopulmonary dysplasia, repaired esophageal atresia, and asthma, treatment of reflux-associated respiratory disease can be facilitated by minimizing β-adrenergic or theophylline bronchodilators, avoiding supine mechanical ventilation, and performing chest physiotherapy prior to (rather than following) meals.

Pneumonia. Rarely, aspiration of refluxate causes pneumonia in children. It can be suspected in neurologically abnormal children, whose airway protective mechanisms are often defective. However, in these children it may be difficult to distinguish aspiration during reflux from aspiration during swallowing. Barium fluoroscopy can identify defects in the swallowing mechanism, and rarely may show aspiration during reflux. Scintigraphy is slightly more sensitive for reflux-associated aspiration because it documents small volumes of aspiration that occur during 6 hours (the half-life of technetium 99m) or more, rather than only during the few minutes of a barium study. (Theoretically, children could be also be fluoroscoped for several hours after barium ingestion, but aspirated barium must be distinguished from many other faint radiopacities in the chest, whereas the technetium radionuclide must only be distinguished from background activity and radionuclide spilled on the exterior of the patient.) Other techniques to diagnose aspiration include bronchoscopic evaluation of the laryngeal and tracheal epithelium as well as staining tracheobronchial macrophages for milk-derived lipid. In the child with a tracheostomy, the use of dyes such as methylene blue in several feedings will easily disclose any aspirated material in substances suctioned from the trachea. In children who are fed intragastrically, finding the material in the trachea is diagnostic of aspiration of refluxate.

Children who aspirate refluxate recurrently also often aspirate during swallowing. Optimal therapy frequently includes gastrostomy, which can be accompanied either by surgical fundoplication or gastrojejunal tube placement for feeding,[194] thus protecting against reflux. Even if aspiration during oral feedings is not certain, many of these neurologically devastated patients take so long to feed that other means of enteral nutrition are desirable. The same surgical options can be considered.

Children who are not candidates for gastrostomy and who receive nutrition orally may benefit from thickened liquid feedings, which minimize regurgitation and improve dysfunctional swallowing.[119]

Wheezing and asthma. These symptoms are caused by reflux in several different ways (Fig. 4.3). Aspirated material, inflammatory changes of the bronchial mucosa, and spasms of the bronchial musculature all may contribute to reflux-associated wheezing.

The challenge in wheezing patients is to determine who should be evaluated for reflux. Patients whose symptoms are clearly associated with allergens, upper respiratory illnesses, or exercise, and who respond well to standard therapy for such asthma do not require evaluation for reflux. Patients with unexplained exacerbations, nocturnal symptoms, or intractability to standard nonsteroidal therapy should be considered for evaluation. Wheezing patients with heartburn should be evaluated endoscopically. In contrast, those with heartburn alone should not be treated empirically because therapy for reflux-associated asthma is likely to be more prolonged than that of simple heartburn. The endpoint of therapy is also less clear, and the use of concurrent medications further complicates the issue. Wheezing patients without heartburn can be evaluated with endoscopy, with a Bernstein test, or with a pH probe test, in that order.

Pharmacologic therapy for reflux-associated wheezing is similar to that of esoph-

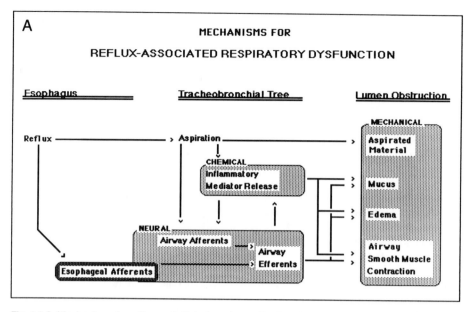

Fig. 4.3 **A,** Mechanisms for reflux-associated respiratory dysfunction. Reflux may produce respiratory disease directly, by mechanical occlusion of the lumen with aspirated material, or indirectly. Reflux narrows the airway indirectly via neural or chemical induction of mucus secretion, edema, or muscle contraction. The neural mechanism can have local (airway) or distal (esophageal) afferents. **B,** Four potential components of bronchial obstruction. Concentric loci of airway obstruction are the lumen, which can be narrowed by material from extra- or intrapulmonary sources; the lamina propria, which can be expanded at the expense of the lumen by edema; and the bronchial musculature, which can narrow the lumen by contracting. (Reprinted with permission from Putnam PE, et al, 1991[245])

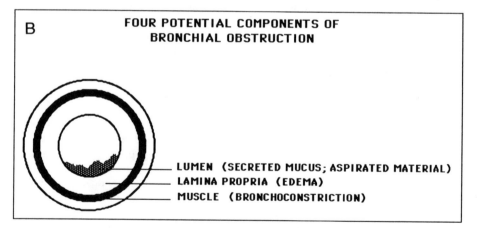

agitis. The relatively slow response of respiratory symptoms, as compared with that of heartburn, mandates continuing therapy for several months even if respiratory symptoms do not initially respond. A hydrogen pump blockade for optimal acid suppression (eg, omeprazole) may also be warranted, particularly as initial therapy while the diagnostic accuracy is being judged. Occasionally, patients with intractable or chronic disease will benefit from fundoplication.

Apnea. Apnea, stridor, and croup may be the ends of a continuum of reflux-associated upper-airway symptoms in infants or very young children. Apnea may be due to reflux-mediated vagal reflexes, with the stimulus in the esophagus or larynx, or it may be caused by microaspiration. (Exacerbated aspiration would be more likely to present as pneumonia.) This manifestation occurs only in infants, who are predisposed by neurologic immaturity to apnea as a response to various stimuli. The main difficulty in understanding pathophysiology is the conflicting clinical and experimental data. Clinical evidence suggests that such apnea is usually obstructive (due to laryngospasm) occurring in the awake infant postprandially.[195,196] Experimental evidence, however, demonstrates that reflexive laryngospasm requires acid refluxate as the stimulus;[197] this acid reflux does not occur postprandially after an infant formula feeding.[198,199]

Sleep apnea and central apnea seem much less likely to be due to reflux. In contrast, many single episodes of gagging, choking, and turning blue during regurgitation are so clearly related to reflux that further evaluation is not necessary, and pharmacotherapy can be instituted on that basis. For recurrent apnea with an ambiguous cause, a pneumogram can be helpful in distinguishing central from obstructive apnea, if a nasal thermistor or end-tidal Co_2 measurement is incorporated. If reflux is a possible cause and esophageal pH probe output can be included as one of the lines of analog data, the temporal association between reflux episodes and any apneas which occur can be assessed. In addition, even if no apneas occur, a markedly abnormal pH probe record can justify pharmacotherapy for reflux, particularly if the evaluation identifies no other cause of apnea. Reflux-associated infantile apnea rarely necessitates fundoplication.

Stridor and croup. These audible signs of upper-airway narrowing may be due to laryngospasm, insufficient stiffness of the upper-airway structures (ie, laryngotracheomalacia), or to inflammatory narrowing of the upper airway (ie, epiglottitis or reflux laryngitis). These signs of airway narrowing predominate in infants and younger children because the upper airway enlarges and stiffens with age. Both laryngospasm (see Apnea, above) and laryngeal inflammation (see Hoarseness, below) are sequellae of reflux. Children with chronic or intermittent stridor or croup should be evaluated for reflux.

When designing the evaluation, it should be remembered that only 1 minute of subglottic exposure every other day for a few days is sufficient to produce considerable airway narrowing, at least when superimposed on a mucosal lesion.[117] This exquisite susceptibility to acid injury contrasts with the response of the esophageal epithelium, which is protected by clearance mechanisms such as frequent peristalsis and lavage with salivary bicarbonate. This susceptibility is the reason why children without esophagitis or abnormal esophageal acid exposure nonetheless manifest laryngeal abnormalities. While a positive esophageal biopsy may be able to indicate a pathologic reflux that requires therapy, a normal biopsy is useless in this setting. Similarly, if the respiratory symptom is both intermittent and frequent, a pH probe may document that the symptom follows esophageal acidification predictably,[200] but a normal pH probe does not prove that the respiratory symptom is unrelated to reflux. Dual-level esophageal pH monitoring should be avoided, both for the above reasons and because the upper and lower esophagus are functionally a single space, separated only by gravity in the upright position. In contrast, fiberoptic laryngoscopic evaluation is important because it can disclose isolated laryngomalacia (which would mediate against reflux as a cause) or posterior laryngeal inflammation (which would mediate for reflux as a cause). Straight laryngoscopic evaluations, however, may be falsely negative for laryngomalacia. Fiberoptic laryngoscopy can also document unusual anatomic abnormalities responsible for the symptom, such as the epiglottic cyst that produced intermittent stridor in one child. Intermittent stridor due to reflux may be optimally diagnosed using a modified Bernstein test.[201]

Reflux-induced laryngeal symptoms are treated similarly to those of reflux-associated bronchospasm. They may be even more resistant to therapy, however, given the minimal laryngeal acid exposure that can produce symptoms. Episodic life-threatening laryngeal obstruction justifies fundoplication, if it is clearly due to reflux.

Hoarseness. Laryngitis is manifested by hoarseness in verbal children, or by a hoarse cry in nonverbal children.[202,203] The pathophysiology, diagnostic, and therapeutic strategies are similar to those discussed for laryngeal inflammation and croup, above.

Otitis and sinusitis. These otolaryngologic symptoms may occasionally be due to refluxate causing inflammation and subsequent obstruction of the openings of the eustachian tubes or the sinuses, although there is little literature to support this connection.[119] Regurgitation—particularly nasal regurgitation—suggests this association in infants and young children with intractable otitis or sinusitis.

Neurobehavioral Presentations

Sandifer's syndrome. This very odd, dystonic posturing is caused by reflux.[204] An interesting case report suggested a therapeutic benefit from this posturing, which seemed to improve esophageal motility and clearance.[205] Dystonic posturing due to metoclopramide or other drugs that cause extrapyramidal side effects should be considered in the differential diagnosis as should other primary neurologic causes. Endoscopy for esophagitis, pH probe to document temporal association of the behavior with reflux episodes (if the posturing occurs more often than daily), or a modified Bernstein test may all be helpful in determining whether the posturing is due to reflux. Detailed neurologic evaluation is particularly useful in the differential diagnosis.

Infantile arching. This subtler, more common posturing is also clinically associated with reflux. As with Sandifer syndrome, it may represent attempts to improve clearance of refluxed acid, or may be a nonspecific response to esophageal discomfort. It is rarely a presenting complaint, but its presence in the history adds support to the possibility of abnormal reflux and esophagitis.

DIAGNOSTIC EVALUATION
History

The diagnostic evaluation begins with a complete history. Inquiring about the reflux-associated symptoms discussed under Clinical Presentations is useful, even if they were not part of the presenting complaint. Due to the breadth of the differential diagnostic considerations, however, the history must be complete, rather than simply reflux-related. A questionnaire related to infantile reflux[120] can be developed and validated to streamline the history and keep it consistent.

Physical Examination

In many—perhaps most—patients with reflux disease, the physical examination is normal. As with the history, however, a complete physical examination is crucial to focusing the differential diagnosis.

pH Probe

The pH probe study is discussed in detail in Chapter 15 so only a few salient issues will be mentioned here.

The pH probe test is unnecessary in the regurgitating patient, or in the patient already diagnosed for uncomplicated esophagitis. In patients with intermittent symptoms that might be related to reflux, the probe can show an association only if the symptoms occur frequently enough to be demonstrated during the 24-hour test and their occurrence is recorded reliably enough for exact temporal linkage to the pH probe events. Simply showing a statistically abnormal quantity of reflux is a poor substitute for temporal linkage. The relative costs and benefits of endoscopy, or suction biopsy in infants, versus pH probe should be considered when evaluating which procedure is better in a particular clinical setting. If the pH probe requires a day of admission for reliable recording, and if it will only produce suggestive rather than diagnostic information, the endoscopy may have the favorable cost-benefit ratio. The probe may be most useful in settings where direct linking of symptoms to reflux episodes is possible, or where evaluation of the effect of a treatment on reflux parameters is desired. The pH probe does not detect reflux in the postprandial period after neutral pH feedings, particularly in infants.[198,199]

When pH probe studies are scored for reflux quantity, rather than used simply to document a temporal association between reflux episodes and a particular symptom, several scoring systems have been described. Mathematically-derived pH probe scores designed to select obscure patients with reflux disease[206,207] may provide suggestive information, but they also obscure the primary data.[208,209]

In contrast, several simpler scores have been shown to correlate with different manifestations of reflux disease. The "reflux index" (the percentage of the day with esophageal pH <4) is greater in those with esophagitis than in those without esophagitis, with a threshold of 7% to 10% in both children and adults.[152,210,211] Prolonged (>3 or 4 min) "mean duration of reflux during sleep" predicted reflux-associated respiratory disease.[212-214]

Manometry

Manometry is discussed in detail in Chapter 11. Although it plays an investigational role in determining the pathophysiology and optimal therapy of reflux disease, it has little value in the evaluation of a patient with suspected GERD. One exception is when dysphagia is a presenting complaint; a suggested diagnostic approach is outlined under Dysphagia, in the Clinical Presentations section of this chapter.

Barium Fluoroscopy

Barium fluoroscopy should not be used to diagnose reflux, despite the normal ranges of the number and height of reflux episodes defined in a fairly large study. In numerically quantifying radiographic reflux, it is often difficult to be certain that comparable techniques were used. Furthermore, regurgitation by an agitated, trussed, frantic child may have little to do with the physiologic situation. Provocative manuevers such as artifically increasing abdominal pressure have also fallen out of favor because they are unacceptably unphysiologic.

Barium upper gastrointestinal study (not simply an esophagram) should be performed in the regurgitating child, however, to evaluate the anatomy and eliminate structural disorders in the differential diagnosis. When present, the serendipitous findings on fluoroscopy of copious free-flowing reflux, a large hiatal hernia, reflux with aspiration, or radiographic esophagitis provide evidence for reflux disease.

Technetium Scintigraphy

Technetium 99m sulfur colloid gastroesophageal scintigraphy is most often used to document pulmonary aspiration but, like other tests for this purpose, its sensitivity is mediocre. Scintigraphy can also characterize the frequency and duration of postprandial reflux after a physiologic meal, but attention must be paid to specific technical aspects.[215] Furthermore, it can define gastric emptying. The characteristics of the meal used to define normal values of gastric emptying should be comparable and physiologic, and the possibility of artefact from superimposition of the stomach and ligament of Treitz must be remembered.

Endoscopy

Endoscopy is the most useful procedure in older children who are evaluated for reflux esophagitis. Esophageal erosions, ulcerations, strictures, and Barrett's epithelium can be visualized and many disorders in the differential diagnosis of the symptoms can be assessed. The endoscope can even be tipped anteriorly as it is withdrawn into the pharynx, to visualize the larynx and look for posterior laryngeal inflammation associated with some of the upper-airway manifestations of reflux disease. During endoscopy, esophageal histology should always be evaluated with multiple biopsies to provide a screen for infectious causes of esophagitis, and a means of identifying Barrett's epithelium reliably. The findings indicative of reflux esophagitis itself are most reliably evaluated on large-suction biopsies (see below). Others, particularly the inflammatory cell infiltrates, can also be seen on endoscopic grasp biopsies. Endoscopic findings have been scored by Savary's classification and subsequent variations.[216] In general, these systems grade esophageal findings as grade I (single linear erosion), grade II (multiple erosions), grade III (confluent circumferential erosions), grade IV (strictures or ulcers), and grade V (Barrett's epithelium). It has been shown in children that endoscopic findings short of erosions are unreliable manifestations of reflux esophagitis, although these patients often have histologic evidence of the disorder.[217]

Esophageal Histology and Suction Biopsies

The histology of reflux esophagitis is seen most clearly on large-suction biopsies, which can be oriented easily for optimal quantification of papillary height and basal-cell thickness. The latter is the most sensitive measure of reflux esophagitis.[189-191,218] In addition, inflammatory markers of reflux esophagitis are identifiable and quantifiable: eosinophils, lymphocytes ("squiggle cells"), and polymorphonuclear leukocytes. Other findings probably associated with reflux include papillary telangiectasias. Table 4.1 shows the upper limit of normal as derived from autopsy material from infants who died suddenly of nonreflux causes.

Suction biopsies are particularly useful for evaluating reflux esophagitis in infants because the differential diagnosis does not usually require endoscopy. Endoscopy is more difficult to perform safely without general anesthesia in infants than in older children because the grasp specimens obtained through the small-infant endoscopes are inadequate for evaluation of the sensitive morphometric parameters of esophagitis. The high grades of esophagitis reliable for diagnosing reflux esophagitis endoscopically are uncommon in infants. The Quinton-Rubin instrument has been used successfully to obtain these biopsies in over 1000 patients at Children's Hospital of Pittsburgh without any complications that required treatment. It is to be hoped that the demonstrated utility and safety of the technique will prompt resumption of its manufacture.

Bernstein Test

The Bernstein test, which alternates esophageal infusion of acid and saline to determine if the acid produces heartburn, was initially developed to distinguish ischemic cardiac disease from the "heartburn" of reflux disease. It has been modified since then to determine in particular patients whether esophageal acidification produces bronchospasm, stridor, or other symptoms.[201,219] To determine clearly that these symptoms are due to reflux alone, rather than to aspiration of the infused acid, a pH probe located in the esophagus but high above the infusion point is useful. The Bernstein test is a relatively efficient and reliable way of associating intermittent symptoms with esophageal acidification. Its advantages over the pH probe, which is useful in similar situations, are that rigorous observations can be made efficiently at a defined time of esophageal acidification, and that esophageal acidification can be more clearly shown to be the cause of the symptom, rather than an effect or accompaniment.

TREATMENT

Therapy for GERD has many components, directed at different aspects of its pathophysiology. Unfortunately, no therapy exists that can be specifically directed at the most important component of the pathophysiology—the TLESR.

GERD can be treated conservatively, pharmacologically, or surgically. Conservative therapy is applicable to virtually anyone with symptoms suggestive of reflux. Pharmacologic therapy is used for children shown to have reflux disease, or it may be used empirically for a limited time in some specific instances. Surgery is reserved for those with reflux disease that is intractable to medical therapy, those with symptoms too hazardous to evaluate for intractability, or, sometimes, in those whose symptoms respond well to medical therapy but who face a lifetime of such therapy because of recurrent relapses when medications are withdrawn.

Conservative Therapy

Conservative therapies are accompanied by little or no risk, and sometimes consider-

(Reprinted with permission from Black DO, et al, 1990[189])

TABLE 4.1 Upper Limits of Normal: Morphometric Criteria for Esophagitis in Infants

Criterion	Upper Limit of Normal	Sensitivity
Basal layer thickness	25%	.89
Papillary height	53%	.30
Epithelial eosinophils	0/mm muscularis mucosae	.26
Epithelial neutrophils	0/mm muscularis mucosae	.15
Lamina propria eosinophils	0.8/mm muscularis mucosae	.41

able benefit. Thus there is little reason not to use them in anyone with symptoms suspected to be due to reflux. These therapies are also continued when pharmacologic therapy is added.

Dietary measures. Reflux is minimized by measures that decrease the volume of meals while maintaining adequate daily caloric intake (ie, small-volume feedings, noncarbonated drinks, thickened infant feedings), improve gastric emptying (eg, avoiding high-fat meals), minimize the noxiousness of gastric contents (eg, nonacid, noncaffeine drinks), and avoid impairment of LES function (eg, abstaining from nicotine).

Thickened infant feedings are the most clinically useful of these measures.[220-222] Adding a tablespoon (15 ml) of dry rice cereal to each ounce of formula provides equicaloric intake at two thirds the volume and markedly reduces the number of regurgitative episodes. It is excellent therapy for infants with regurgitation as the presenting symptom, and is often sufficient even for infants with regurgitation and failure to thrive. It is particularly ideal for infants who have loose stools prior to therapy, since it causes constipation in many infants. There are several methods of treating such constipation if it occurs. A magnesium-containing antacid has the dual benefits of acid neutralization and constipation treatment. The use of a less-constipating nonrice cereal also may have similar benefits for reflux; this has not been tested, however, and rice has the

advantage of hypoallergenicity. A few parents have found that adding a bottle of apple juice thickened with rice cereal to each day's feedings improves the stooling without adverse effects on regurgitation, despite the low pH (4) of apple juice and its tendency to increase regurgitation when given alone. Postprandial coughing sometimes increases after rice-thickening;[223] the possible pathophysiology and clinical significance of this reaction is being explored.

Positioning measures. Positioning is difficult to manipulate in older children, but avoidance of slumped or supine postures, especially postprandially, is ideal. Infants should also avoid supine and seated positions.[182] They should be prone when they are not held directly upright. There seems to be no additional benefit when the head of the bed is elevated.[224] The benefit of lateral positions—particularly the right lateral position, which speeds gastric emptying—is ambiguous. An avoidable provocative maneuver a few young parents use is "the postprandial jiggle;" counselling against this activity has considerable therapeutic effect.

Other. Some conservative measures useful in older children are the avoidance of obesity, tight clothing, and bedtime snacking. In some situations the use of antacids as needed for symptoms can be considered "conservative" therapy, but in children antacid use should not be protracted without a definite diagnosis.

Pharmacologic Therapy

Pharmacotherapy is utilized when reflux disease has been diagnosed. Whether it also should be used empirically in children is debatable, but a 2-month course of therapy for classical symptoms is reasonable. Empiric use should not continue longer than 2 months without diagnostic evaluation.

A prokinetic agent can be used in virtually all children with reflux disease, adding an acid-secretion inhibitor in those with esophagitis. An acid-secretion inhibitor should not usually be used alone, particularly in complicated reflux disease (ie, respiratory disease, esophageal ulceration, strictures, Barrett's esophagus) because of the roles of gastric emptying and duodenogastric reflux in these patients.

Prokinetic agents. Prokinetic medications are discussed in Chapter 25. They are useful in children with reflux disease, whether or not they have esophagitis.

Bethanechol was the first prokinetic drug widely used for reflux. Its cholinergic mechanism increases LES pressure and peristaltic amplitude and velocity,[225] but does not change gastric emptying. Stimulation of salivation may also improve clearance parameters. Overall, however, its beneficial effects on reflux are ambiguous[226] and appear to be confined to improvement of esophageal clearance.[227] Bethanechol is disadvantageous for patients with respiratory symptoms because it causes bronchospasm. While no longer a first-line drug for reflux disease, it may be useful in the occasional child who does not respond well to cisapride or metoclopramide.

Metoclopramide, an antidopaminergic agent, increases the LES pressure, improves peristaltic function, and also improves gastric emptying.[228,229] It appears to have more clinical efficacy than bethanechol in reflux disease,[230-232] but its narrow therapeutic margin[228,233] results in a considerable number of infants being irritable or somnolent while taking a relatively low dose (0.1 mg/kg qid). Most of these infants improve when the dose is reduced by 50%; however, some clinical effect seems to persist. The terrible permanent extrapyramidal effects (eg, tardive dys-

kinesia) are far more common in the elderly and almost never occur in children[233] but are a salient reason for avoiding high doses and prolonged usage. Even in older children, a dose higher than 0.1 mg/kg four times daily should not be given.

Cisapride's recent availability in the United States may make the negative aspects of bethanechol and metoclopramide largely irrelevant. While not a cholinergic agent itself, it promotes the release of acetylcholine from postganglionic nerve endings in the myenteric plexus. Its clinical efficacy seems to be greater than the two previously mentioned drugs, and its safety record is excellent. Currently it is the first-line prokinetic for reflux disease. The suggested dosage in children ranges from 0.1 to 0.3 mg/kg, up to four times daily.[234]

Anti-acid agents. These medications are the foundation of treatment of esophagitis in adults, in whom they are often used alone. They do nothing for the motility abnormalities that are the basis for reflux disease, but they nonetheless heal esophagitis, highlighting the role of acid and acid-activated pepsin as chief noxious agents.

Antacids are used empirically, prior to diagnosis, to neutralize gastric acid. They are also used as needed for symptoms that "break through" the more powerful agents discussed below. It is useful to choose antacids based on pretreatment stool characteristics: patients with constipation will benefit from the magnesium-containing products, such as Mylanta or Maalox, whereas those with loose stools require products higher in aluminum (the "gel" antacids), including Basalgel, Amphogel, and Alternagel). A dosage of 1 cc/kg is usually appropriate.[235] Side effects from overdosage rarely occur, but indicate that even these benign medications are not completely risk free.[236] Although these medications were found in one study to be comparable to H_2-receptor blockade,[235] the dosage frequency was prohibitive for routine clinical use and the costs would probably not be less than that of the H_2-receptor antagonists.

H_2-receptor antagonists are currently

the basis of standard antisecretory therapy. The fundic parietal cell, which is responsible for gastric acid secretion, is stimulated to secrete by occupation of several different receptors. The vagus nerve provides acetylcholine for the cholinergic receptor, the antral G-cell provides gastrin for the gastrin receptor, and histamine-secreting mast cells provide histamine for the H_2-receptor.[237]

H_2-receptor antagonists differ in frequency of administration. Ranitidine, with its twice-daily dosing, is commonly used in acid-peptic diseases, but parents using a four-times-daily prokinetic agent often find a four-times-daily antisecretory agent (eg, cimetidine) simplest to administer. The monthly cost of the latter may be lower as well.

Hydrogen pump inhibitors suppress gastric acid secretion more completely than H_2-receptor blockade alone, by irreversibly inhibiting H^+/K^+-ATPase ("the hydrogen pump") in the parietal cell. Omeprazole blocks acid secretion in this way. True to its mechanism, it has been shown to be a powerful antisecretory agent. There is even less experience with this drug in children than in adults. Concerns about the negative effects of such complete acid suppression, such as bacterial overgrowth and hypergastrinemia, have been raised. For many reasons, in children it is best to reserve this powerful medication for very resistant esophagitis and special situations, starting with a daily dose of 0.7 mg/kg.[238] It is debatable that antireflux surgery may provide a less expensive and more permanent solution to refractory reflux disease in children.

Surgical Therapy

Nissen fundoplication. Fundoplication, which is the wrapping of the fundus around the LES, produces a dramatic reduction of reflux when successfully performed. Most children treated with fundoplication manifest less reflux than normal individuals. Fundoplication is most commonly performed by the Nissen method, a 360° wrap that completely prevents reflux episodes. Other types of fundoplication prevent reflux less completely, but may have a lower incidence of negative side effects such as dysphagia, bloating, and inability to vomit when ill. Fundoplication can be combined with a gastrostomy in neurologically abnormal children who need it for feeding, and in young infants, in whom a temporary gastrostomy for venting prevents postoperative difficulties.

Most esophagitis can be healed with optimal prokinetic and antisecretory medication superimposed on careful conservative treatment. Some patients, however, benefit from surgical treatment of their reflux disease. Reported fundoplication rates of 18% to 30% of all children investigated for reflux disease[126,137] seem high. Whether this figure was due to a high threshold for investigation or a low threshold for surgery is unclear. If the benefits of fundoplication persist over many decades, the optimal rate of fundoplication may be higher in children than in adults, because of the costs and risks of a lifetime of medication use. Continuing improvements in pharmacotherapy, however, may modulate enthusiasm for surgery. Such decisions between long-term pharmacotherapy and fundoplication are necessarily a gamble, particularly in children.

Children with peptic esophageal strictures (irregular mid- to lower-esophageal strictures with histologic esophagitis in the epithelium below the stricture) and children with Barrett's intestinal metaplasia should have fundoplication. Preparing the child for surgery with aggressive pharmacologic therapy, and dilations if there is a stricture, is potentially beneficial but there is little rationale for attempting protracted medical therapy. Because of the combined roles of acid and duodenogastric reflux, such therapy would require two potent drugs for many decades. The cost-benefit analysis clearly favors surgery in these children, whose risks are considerable if reflux continues.

The uncommon older child with persistent esophagitis despite 6 to 12 months of cisapride up to 0.3mg/kg qid and omeprazole up to 2.0 mg/kg qid should have fundoplication to prevent the more serious sequelae of stricture or Barrett's.

Less clear-cut cases involve children whose relapsing esophagitis is healed by aggressive pharmacotherapy, but who relapse whenever drugs are withdrawn. If this pattern persists, surgery is an option, but different families may come to different decisions given this difficult choice.

Children with severe chronic respiratory disease also may benefit from the complete resolution of reflux that fundoplication provides. In considering children with repaired esophageal atresia for fundoplication, the primary esophageal motility abnormalities will mandate a looser wrap to prevent postoperative dysphagia.

Children with severe neurologic disability and reflux often have dysphagia that necessitates enteral feedings; fundoplication and gastrostomy is often the most efficient solution to these problems. The procedure must be performed with care to try to minimize its complications in this difficult group of children.[239]

Infants with reflux-associated apnea were often treated surgically in the past, but it has become clear that most of these infants can safely outgrow both their reflux and their propensity for apnea during the first year of life. Careful medical management of these infants thus has a potentially great benefit.

Some have argued that the child who requires a gastrostomy should have a fundoplication in all cases but this may not be the best approach.[240] A child being prepared for a percutaneous endoscopic gastrostomy (PEG) usually benefits from an upper gastrointestinal barium study to document a normal upper gastrointestinal tract. If there is no evidence for severe reflux or other abnormalities on that study, the child is taken to the operating room for the PEG, which can be performed under general anesthesia in conjunction with pediatric surgeons. In the rare instance when unexpected endoscopic esophagitis is seen during the initial insertion of the endoscope, the procedure is changed to fundoplication with gastrostomy. The parents are advised of that possibility preoperatively, and sign consents for both procedures. Postoperative gastrostomy feedings should be given slowly, to approx-imate a normal meal time of at least 15 minutes, and allow gastric receptive relaxation. In the rare child in whom GERD develops subsequently, a secondary fundoplication can be performed at that time. This approach has received more support.[241-243]

GASTROJEJUNAL TUBE FEEDING

Gastrostomy combined with gastrojejunal tube feedings has been proposed as an alternative to gastrostomy with fundoplication. The relative risks and benefits have been studied.[194] A higher initial cost of the fundoplication may be offset by higher recurrent costs due to displacement of the enteral tube.

REFERENCES

1. Dent J, Dodds WJ, Sekiguchi T, Hogan WJ, Arndorfer RC. Interdigestive phasic contractions of the human lower esophageal sphincter. *Gastroenterology* 1983;84:453-60.

2. Goyal RK. The lower esophageal sphincter. *Viewpoints on Digestive Diseases* 1976;8:1-4.

3. Lipshutz W, Gaskins R, Lukash WML, et al. Pathogenesis of lower-esophageal-sphincter incompetence. *N Engl J Med* 1973;289:182-4.

4. Cotton BR, Smith G. The lower oesophageal sphincter and anesthesia. *Br J Anaesth* 1984;56:37-46.

5. Hall A, Moossa A, Clark J, Cooley G, Skinner D. The effects of premedication drugs on the lower oesophageal high-pressure zone and reflux status of Rhesus monkeys and man. *Gut* 1975;16:347-52.

6. Mittal R, Frank E, Lange R, McCallum R. Effects of morphine and naloxone on esophageal motility and gastric emptying in man. *Dig Dis Sci* 1986;31:936-42.

7. Holloway R, Lyrenas E, Dent J, Tippett M. Effect of intraduodenal fat on lower esophageal sphincter function and gastroesophageal reflux. *Gastroenterology* 1989;96:A215.

8. Kahrilas P, Dodds W, Dent J, Haeberle B, Hogan W, Arndorfer R. Effect of sleep, spontaneous gastroesophageal reflux, and a meal on upper esophageal sphincter pressure in normal human volun-

teers. *Gastroenterology* 1987;92:466-71.

9. Cook IJ, Dent J, Shannon S, Collins SM. Measurement of upper esophageal sphincter pressure: effect of acute emotional stress. *Gastroenterology* 1987;93:526-32.

10. Davidson GP, Dent J, Willing J. Monitoring of upper oesophageal sphincter pressure in children. *Gut* 1991;32:607-11.

11. Davidson GP, Willing J, Furukawa Y, Dent J. Strain-induced augmentation of upper oesophageal sphincter pressure in children. *J Paediatr Child Health* 1992;28:

12. Gerhardt DC, Shuck TJ, Bordeaux RA, Winship DH. Human upper esophageal sphincter: response to volume, osmotic, and acid stimuli. *Gastroenterology* 1978;75:268-74.

13. Kahrilas P, Dodds W, Dent J, Wyman J, Hogan W, Arndorfer R. Upper esophageal sphincter function during belching. *Gastroenterology* 1986;91:133-40.

14. McNally E, Kelly J, Ingelfinger F. Mechanism of belching: effects of gastric distension with air. *Gastroenterology* 1964;46:254-9.

15. Mittal R, McCallum R. Characteristics of transient lower esophageal sphincter relaxation in humans. *Am J Physiol* 1987;252:G636-41.

16. Holloway RH, Kocyan P, Dent J. Meals provoke gastroesophageal reflux by increasing the rate of transient lower esophageal sphincter relaxation. *Gastroenterology* 1989;96:A214.

17. Freidin N, Ren J, Sluss J, McCallum RW. The effect of large meal on the frequency and quality of transient LES relaxations (TLESR). *Gastroenterology* 1989;96:A159.

18. Sivri B, Freidin N, McCallum R. The effect of large meals on the characteristics of transient lower esophageal sphincter relaxation (TLESR). *Am J Gastroenterol* 1990;85:1226.

19. Holloway R, Hongo M, Berger K, McCallum R. Gastric distension: A mechanism for post-prandial gastroesophageal reflux. *Gastroenterology* 1984;1115.

20. Franzi S, Martin C, Cox M, Dent J. Response of canine lower esophageal sphincter to gastric dis-

tension. *Am J Physiol* 1990;259:G380.

21. Mittal R, Fisher M. Electrical and mechanical inhibition of the crural diaphragm during transient relaxation of the lower esophageal sphincter. *Gastroenterology* 1990;99:1265-8.

22. Martin C, Patrikios J, Dent J. Abolition of gas reflux and transient lower esophageal sphincter relaxation by vagal blockade in the dog. *Gastroenterology* 1986;91:890-6.

23. Cox MR, Martin CJ, Dent J, Westmore M. Effect of general anaesthesia on transient lower oesophageal sphincter relaxations in the dog. *Aust N Z J Surg* 1988;58:825-30.

24. Nguyen C, Rossiter C, Benjamin S, Gillis R. Blockade of gastric distention-induced lower esophageal sphincter (LES) relaxations by lesioning the caudal portion of the dorsal motor nucleus (DMV) of the vagus in cats. *Gastroenterology* 1991;100:A476.

25. Ireland A, Dent J, Holloway R. Preservation of postural suppression of belching in patients with refluxesophagitis. *Gastroenterology* 1992; 102:A87.

26. Wyman J, Dent J, Heddle R, et al. Control of belching by the lower oesophageal sphincter. *Gut* 1990;31:639-46.

27. Penagini R, Bartesaghi B, Blanchi PA. Effect of cold stress on postprandial lower esophageal sphincter competence and gastroesophageal reflux in healthy subjects. *Dig Dis Sci* 1992;37:1200-5.

28. Branch MS, Gessner FM, Smith JW, Brazer SP. Somatostatin analogue (octreotide) inhibits lower esophageal sphincter relaxation. *Gastroenterology* 1991;100:A425.

29. Allen M, DiMarino A, Robinson M. The effect of raw onions on inappropriate transient lower esophageal sphincter relaxations (TLESR) and gastroesophageal reflux (GER). *Am J Gastroenterol* 1991;87:1242.

30. Lang I, Sarna S. Motor and myoelectric activity associated with vomiting, regurgitation, and nausea. In: Wood J, ed. *Motility and Circulation.* Bethesda, MD: American Physiological Society, 1989;1193.

31. Menon AP, Schefft GL, Thach BT. Airway

protective and abdominal expulsive mechanisms in infantile regurgitation. *J Appl Physiol* 1985;59:716-21.

32. Orenstein SR, Deneault LG, Lutz JW, Wessel HB, Dent J. Regurgitant reflux, in contrast to non-regurgitant reflux, is associated with rectus abdominus contraction in infants. *Gastroenterology* 1991;100:A135.

33. Fleisher DR. Infant rumination syndrome: report of a case and review of the literature. *Am J Dis Child* 1979;133:266-9.

34. Whitehead WE, Drescher VM, Morrill CE, Cataldo MF. Rumination syndrome in children treated by increased holding. *J Pediatr Gastroenterol Nutr* 1985;4:650-6.

35. Amarnath RP, Abell TL, Malagelada J-R. The rumination syndrome in adults. *Ann Intern Med* 1986;105:513-8.

36. Amarnath RP, Perrault JF. Rumination in normal children: diagnosis and clinical considerations. *Gastroenterology* 1991;100A25. Abstract.

37. Shay S, Johnson L, Wong R, et al. Rumination, heartburn, and daytime gastroesophageal reflux: a case study with mechanisms defined and successfully treated with biofeedback therapy. *J Clin Gastroenterol* 1986;8:115-26.

38. Smout A, Breumelhof R. Voluntary induction of transient lower esophageal sphincter relaxation in an adult patient with the rumination syndrome. *Am J Gastroenterol* 1990;85:1621-5.

39. Dent J, Dodds WJ, Hogan WJ, Toculi J. Factors that influence induction of gastroesophageal reflux in normal human subjects. *Dig Dis Sci* 1988;33:270-5.

40. Marino W, Jain N, Pitchumoni C. Induction of lower esophageal sphincter (LES) dysfunction during use of the negative pressure body ventilator. *Am J Gastroenterol* 1988;83:1376-80.

41. Sloan S, Rademaker AW, Kahrilas PJ. Determinants of gastroesophageal junction incompetence: hiatal hernia, lower esophageal sphincter, or both. *Ann Int Med* 1992;117:977-82.

42. Martin CJ, Dodds WJ, Liem HH, Dantas RO, Layman RD, Dent J. Diaphragmatic contribution to gastroesophageal competence and reflux in dogs. *Am J Physiol* 1992;263:G551-7.

43. Friedland GW, Dodds WJ, Sunshine P, Zboraiske FF. Apparent disparity in incidence of hiatal hernia in infants and children in Britain and the United States. *Am J Roentgenol Radium Ther Nucl Med* 1974;120:305-14.

44. Darling DB, Fisher JH, Gellis SS. Hiatal hernia and gastroesophageal reflux in infants and children: analysis of the incidence in North American children. *Pediatrics* 1974;54:450-5.

45. Carre IJ, Astley R, Smellie JM. Minor degrees of partial thoracic stomach in childhood: review of 112 cases. *Lancet* 1952;2:1150-3.

46. Carre IJ. Familial incidence of the partial thoracic stomach ("hiatus hernia") in children. *International Congress of Pediatrics, 11th,* Tokyo, University of Tokyo Press. 1965;566-7.

47. Jewett TC Jr, Siegel M. Hiatal hernia and gastroesophageal reflux. *J Pediatr Gastroenterol Nutr* 1984;3:340-5.

48. Dent J. A new technique for continuous sphincter pressure measurement. *Gastroenterology* 1976;71:263-7.

49. Dent J, Davidson GP, Barnes BE, Freeman JK, Kirubakaran C. The mechanism of gastro-oesophageal reflux in children. *Aust Paediatr J* 1981;17:125.

50. Werlin SL, Dodds WJ, Hogan WJ, Glicklich M, Arndorfer R. Esophageal function in esophageal atresia. *Dig Dis Sci* 1981;26:796-800.

51. Cucchiara S, Staiano A, Di Lorenzo C, DeLuca G, dellaRocca A, Auricchio S. Pathophysiology of gastroesophageal reflux and distal esophageal motility in children with gastroesophageal reflux disease. *J Pediatr Gastroenterol Nutr* 1988;7:830-6.

52. Holloway RH, Kocyan P, Dent J. Provocation of transient lower esophageal sphincter relaxations by meals in patients with symptomatic gastroesophageal reflux. *Dig Dis Sci* 1991;36:1034-9.

53. Mittal RK, Smith TK. Is nitric oxide the noncholinergic, nonadrenergic neurotransmitter responsible for lower esophageal sphincter relaxation? *Gastroenterology* 1993;104:656-8.

54. Sutphen JL, Dillard VL. Effect of feeding volume on early postcibal gastroesophageal reflux in infants. *J Pediatr Gastroenterol Nutr*

1988;7:185-8.

55. Agha FP. Esophageal involvement in Zollinger-Ellison syndrome. *AJR* 1985;144:721-5.

56. Collen MJ, Lewis JH, Benjamin SB. Gastric acid hypersecretion in refractory gastroesophageal reflux disease. *Gastroenterology* 1990;98:654-61.

57. Sutphen JL, Dillard VL. Effects of maturation and gastric acidity on gastroesophageal reflux in infants. *Am J Dis Child* 1986;140:1062-4.

58. Hillemeier AC, Lange R, McCallum R, Seashore J, Gryboski J. Delayed gastric emptying in infants with gastroesophageal reflux. *J Pediatr* 1981;98:190-3.

59. Lin C-H, Tolia V, Kuhns L, Dubois R. Role of gastric emptying in infants with complicated gastroesophageal reflux. *Pediatr Res* 1989;25:118A.

60. Carroccio A, Iacono G, Li Voti G, et al. Gastric emptying in infants with gastroesophageal reflux: ultrasound evaluation before and after cisapride administration. *Scand J Gastroenterol* 1992;27:799-804.

61. Cucchiara S, Bortolotti M, Minella R, Pagano A. Study of antro-duodeno-jejunal (A-D-J) motility in children with refractory gastro-oesoghageal reflux (GOR) disease. *J Pediatr Gastroenterol Nutr* 1991;13:325.

62. Hillemeier AC, Grill BB, McCallum R, Gryboski J. Esophageal and gastric motor abnormalities in gastroesophageal reflux during infancy. *Gastroenterology* 1983;84:741-6.

63. Euler AR, Byrne WJ. Gastric emptying times of water in infants and children: comparison of those with and without gastroesophageal reflux. *J Pediatr Gastroenterol Nutr* 1983;2:595-8.

64. Jackson PT, Glasgow JF, Thomas PS, Carre IJ. Children with gastroesophageal reflux with or without partial thoracic stomach (hiatal hernia) have normal gastric emptying. *J Pediatr Gastroenterol Nutr* 1989;8:37-40.

65. Jolley SG, Leonard JC, Tunell WP. Gastric emptying in children with gastroesophageal reflux: an estimate of effective gastric emptying. *J Pediatr Surg* 1987;22:923-6.

66. Di Lorenzo C, Piepsz A, Ham H, Cadranel S.

Gastric emptying with gastro-oesophageal reflux. *Arch Dis Child* 1987;62:449-53.

67. Hagen J, Deitel M, Khanna RK, Ilves R. Gastroesophageal reflux in the massively obese. *Int Surg* 1987;72:1-3.

68. Beauchamp G. Gastroesophageal reflux and obesity. *Surg Clin North Am* 1983;63:869-76.

69. Singer A, Brandt L. Pathophysiology of the gastrointestinal tract during pregnancy. *Am J Gastroenterol* 1991;86:1695-1712.

70. Galmiche J, Denis P. Reflux gastro-oesophagien et grossesse: une enigme physiopathologique non-resoluel. *Gastroenterol Clin Biol* 1982;6:421-3.

71. Brown-Cartwright D, Smith H, Feldman M. Gastric emptying of an indigestible solid in patients with end-stage renal disease on continuous ambulatory peritoneal dialysis. *Gastroenterology* 1988;95:49-51.

72. Barham C, Gotley D, Miller R, Mills A, Alderson D. Pressure events surrounding oesophageal acid reflux episodes and acid clearance in ambulant healthy volunteers. *Gut* 1993;34:444-9.

73. Sarna S, Gleysteen J, Ryan R. Fundic motor activity and its role in gastroesophageal reflux. *Gastroenterology* 1986;90 (5 parts):1615. Abstract.

74. Muller-Lissner S, Blum A. Fundic pressure rise lowers lower esophageal sphincter pressure in man. *Hepatogastroenterology* 1982;29:151-2.

75. Orenstein SR, Deneault LG, Lutz JW, Wessel HB, Dent J. Regurgitant reflux, in contrast to non-regurgitant reflux, is associated with rectus abdominus contraction in infants. *Gastroenterology* 1991;100:A135.

76. Helm JF, Dodds WJ, Riedel DR. Determinants of esophageal acid clearance in normal subjects. *Gastroenterology* 1983;85:607-12.

77. Helm JF, Dodds WJ, Pelc LR. Effect of esophageal emptying and saliva on clearance of acid from the esophagus. *N Engl J Med* 1984;310:284-8.

78. Allen ML, Orr WC, Woodruff DM, et al. The effects of swallowing frequency and transdermal scopolamine on esophageal acid clearance. *Am J Gastroenterol* 1985;80:669-72.

79. Sondheimer JM. Clearance of spontaneous gastroesophageal reflux in awake and sleeping infants. *Gastroenterology* 1989;97:821-6.

80. Madsen T, Wallin L, Boesby S, Larsen V. Oesophageal peristalsis in normal subjects. *Scand J Gastroenterol* 1983;18:513-18.

81. Carron DA, Massey BT, Dodds WJ, et al. Heartburn, but not esophageal acidification, per se, increases the rate of spontaneous swallowing. *Gastroenterology* 1989;96:A74.

82. Kahrilas P, Dodds W, Hogan W. Effect of peristaltic dysfunction on esophageal volume clearance. *Gastroenterology* 1988;94:73-80.

83. Cucchiara S, Staiano A, Di Lorenzo C, De-Luca G, dellaRocca A, Auricchio S. Pathophysiology of gastroesophageal reflux and distal esophageal motility in children with gastroesophageal reflux disease. *J Pediatr Gastroenterol Nutr* 1988;7:830-6.

84. Cucchiara S, Staiano A, Di Lorenzo C, et al. Esophageal motor abnormalities in children with gastroesophageal reflux and peptic esophagitis. *J Pediatr* 1986;108:907-10.

85. Mahony M, Migliavacca M, Spitz L, Milla P. Motor disorders of the oesophagus in gastrooesophageal reflux. *Arch Dis Child* 1988;63:1333-8.

86. Arana J, Tovar JA. Motor efficiency of the refluxing esophagus in basal conditions and after acid challenge. *J Pediatr Surg* 1989;24:1049-54.

87. Berezin S, Halata MS, Newman LJ, Glassman MS, Medow MS. Esophageal manometry in children with esophagitis. *Am J Gastroenterol* 1993;88:680-2.

88. Stewart R, Johnston B, Boston V, Dodge J. Role of hiatal hernia in delaying acid clearance. *Arch Dis Child* 1993;68:662-4.

89. Petersen H, Johannessen T, Sandvik A, et al. Relationship between endoscopic hiatus hernia and gastroesophageal reflux symptoms. *Scand J Gastroenterol* 1991;26:921-6.

90. Mittal R, Lange R, McCallum R. Identification and mechanism of delayed esophageal clearance in subjects with hiatus hernia. *Gastroenterology* 1987;92:130-5.

91. Sloan S, Kahrilas P. Impairment of esophageal emptying with hiatal hernia. *Gastroenterology* 1991;100:596-605.

92. Helm JF, Dodds WJ, Hogan WJ. Salivary response to esophageal acid in normal subjects and patients with reflux esophagitis. *Gastroenterology* 1987;93:1393-7.

93. Dutta SK, Matossian HB, Melrowitz RF, Vaeth J. Modulation of salivary secretion by acid infusion in the distal esophagus in humans. *Gastroenterology* 1992;103:1833-41.

94. Meyers R, Orlando R. In vivo bicarbonate secretion by human esophagus. *Gastroenterology* 1991;103:1174-8.

95. Vandenplas Y, Franckx GA, Pipeleers MM, Derde MP, Sacre SL. Area under pH 4: advantages of a new parameter in the interpretation of esophageal pH monitoring data in infants. *J Pediatr Gastroenterol Nutr* 1989;9:34-9.

96. Cassidy KT, Geisinger KR, Kraus BB, Castell DO. Continuous versus intermittent acid exposure in production of esophagitis in feline model. *Dig Dis Sci* 1992;37:1206-11.

97. Bremner RM, Crookes PF, DeMeester TR, Peters JH, Stein HJ. Concentration of refluxed acid and esophageal mucosal injury. *Am J Surg* 1992;164:522-7.

98. Hyman PE, Clarke DD, Everett SL, et al. Gastric acid secretory function in preterm infants. *J Pediatr* 1985;106:467-70.

99. Harada T, Hyman PE, Everett S, Ament ME. Meal-stimulated gastric acid secretion in infants. *J Pediatr* 1984;104:534-8.

100. Sondheimer J, Clark D, Gervaise E. Continuous gastric pH measurement in young and older healthy preterm infants receiving formula and clear liquid feedings. *J Pediatr Gastroenterol Nutr* 1985;4:352-5.

101. DiPalma J, Kirk CL, Hamosh M, Colon AR, Benjamin SB, Hamosh P. Lipase and pepsin activity in the gastric mucosa of infants, children, and adults. *Gastroenterology* 1991;101:116-21.

102. Salo J, Lehto V-P, Kivilaakso E. Morphological alterations in experimental esophagitis: light microscopic and scanning and transmission electron microscopic study. *Dig Dis Sci* 1983;28:440-8.

103. Weisselberg B, Yahav J, Reichman B, Jonas A. Basal and meal-stimulated pepsinogen secretion in preterm infants: a longitudinal study. *J Pediatr Gastroenterol Nutr* 1992;15:58-62.

104. Orlando R, Bozymski E. Heartburn in pernicious anemia—a consequence of bile reflux. *N Engl J Med* 1973;289:522-3.

105. Morrow D, Passaro E. Alkaline reflux esophagitis after total gastrectomy. *Am J Surg* 1976;132:287-91.

106. Palmer E. Subacute erosive ("peptic") esophagitis associated with achlorhydria. *N Engl J Med* 1960;262:927-9.

107. Lillemoe K, Johnson L, Harmon J. Alkaline esophagitis: a comparison of the ability of components of gastroduodenal contents to injure the rabbit esophagus. *Gastroenterology* 1983;85:621-8.

108. Salo J, Lehto V-P, Kivilaakso E. Morphological alterations in experimental esophagitis: light microscopic and scanning and transmission electron microscopic study. *Dig Dis Sci* 1983;28:440-8.

109. Salo J, Kivilaakso E. Contribution of trypsin and cholate to the pathogenesis of experimental alkaline reflux esophagitis. *Scand J Gastroenterol* 1984;19:875-81.

110. Evander A, Little AG, Riddell RH, et al. Composition of the refluxed material determines the degree of reflux esophagitis in the dog. *Gastroenterology* 1987;93:280-6.

111. Stein HJ, Barlow AP, DeMeester TR, Hinder RA. Complications of gastroesophageal reflux disease: role of the lower esophageal sphincter, esophageal acid and acid/alkaline exposure, and duodenogastric reflux. *Ann Surg* 1992;216:35-43.

112. Lebenthal E, Lee P. Development of functional response in human exocrine pancreas. *Pediatrics* 1980;66:556-60.

113. Vandenplas Y, Loeb H. Alkaline gastro-esophageal reflux in infancy. *J Pediatr Gastroenterol Nutr* 1991;12:448-52.

114. Malthaner R, Newman K, Parry R, Duffy L, Randolph J. Alkaline gastroeophageal reflux in infants and children. *J Pediatr Surg* 1991;26:986-91.

115. Orlando R. Esophageal epithelial resistance.

In: Castell DO, Wu WC, Ott DJ, eds. *Gastro-Esophageal Reflux Disease*. Mount Kisco, NY: Futura Publishing, 1985;55-79.

116. Orlando R, Lacy E, Tobey N, Cowart K. Barriers to paracellular permeability in rabbit esophageal epithelium. *Gastroenterology* 1992;102:910-23.

117. Little F, Kohut R, Koufman J, Marshall R. Effect of gastric acid on the pathogenesis of subglottic stenosis. *Ann Otol Rhinol Laryngol* 1985;94:516-9.

118. Richter J. Hoarseness and gastroesophageal reflux: what is the relationship (selected summary). *Gastroenterology* 1990;98:1717-9.

119. Oestreich A, Dunbar J. Pharyngonasal reflux: spectrum and significance in early childhood. *AJR* 1984;141:923-5.

120. Orenstein SR, Cohn JF, Shalaby TM, Kartan R. Reliability and validity of an infant gastroesophageal reflux questionnaire. *Clin Pediatr* 1993;32:472-84.

121. Cleveland RH, Kushner DC, Schwartz AN. Gastroesophageal reflux in children: results of a standardized fluoroscopic approach. *AJR* 1983;141:53-6.

122. Vandenplas Y, Sacre-Smits L. Continuous 24-hour eosphageal pH monitoring in 285 asymptomatic infants 0-15 months old. *J Pediatr Gastroenterol Nutr* 1987;6:220-4.

123. Vandenplas Y, Goyvaerts H, Helven R, Sacre L. Gastroesophageal reflux, as measured by 24-hour pH monitoring, in 509 healthy infants screened for risk of sudden infant death syndrome. *Pediatrics* 1991;88:834-40.

124. Johnson L, DeMeester T. Twenty-four-hour pH monitoring of the distal esophagus: a quantitative measure of gastroesophageal reflux. *Am J Gastroenterol* 1974;62:325-32.

125. Carre IJ. A historical review of the clinical consequences of hiatal hernia (partial thoracic stomach) and gastroesophageal reflux. In: Gellis S. *Gastroesophageal Reflux: Report of the 76th Ross Conference on Pediatric Research*. Columbus, OH: Ross Laboratories, 1979;1-12.

126. Shepherd RW, Wren J, Evans S, Lander M, Ong TH. Gastroesophageal reflux in children: clinical profile, course, and outcome with active thera-

py in 126 cases. *Clin Pediatr (Phila)* 1987;26:55-60.

127. Treem W, Davis P, Hyams J. Gastroesophageal reflux in the older child: presentation, response to treatment and long-term follow-up. *Clin Pediatr* 1991;30:435-40.

128. Schindlbeck N, Klauser A, Berghammer G, Londong W, Muller-Lissner S. Three year follow up of patients with gastroesophageal reflux disease. *Gut* 1992;33:1016-9.

129. Ryan P, Lander M, Ong TH, Shepherd R. When does reflux oesophagitis occur with gastro-oesophageal reflux in infants? A clinical and endoscopic study, and correlation with outcome. *Aust Paediatr J* 1983;19:90-3.

130. Flores AF, Katz AJ. The crying baby syndrome: the role of gastroesophageal reflux. *Pediatr Res* 1984;18:195A.

131. Talley N, Zinsmeister A, Schleck C, Melton L. Natural history of gastroesophageal reflux: a population-based study. *Gastroenterology* 1992;102-28.

132. Nebel O, Fornes M, Castell D. Symptomatic gastroesophageal reflux: incidence and precipitating factors. *Am J Dig Dis* 1976;21:953-6.

133. Wienbeck M, Barnert J. Epidemiology of reflux disease and reflux esophagitis. *Scand J Gastroenterol* 1989;24:7-13.

134. Loof L, Gotell P, Eifberg B. The incidence of reflux oesophagitis: a study of endoscopy reports from a defined catchment area in Sweden. *Scand J Gastroenterol* 1993;28:113-8.

135. Ben Rajeb M, Bouche O, Zeitoun P. Study of 47 consecutive patients with peptic esophageal stricture compared with 3880 cases of reflux esophagitis. *Dig Dis Sci* 1992;37:733-6.

136. Heading R. Epidemiology of oesophageal reflux disease. *Scand J Gastroenterol* 1989;24:33-7.

137. Aronow E. Silverberg M. Normal and abnormal GI motility. In: Silverberg M. ed. *Pediatric Gastroenterology*. New York, NY: Medical Examination Publishing, 1983;214.

138. Hrabovsky EE, Mullett MD. Gastroesophageal reflux and the premature infant. *J Pediatr Surg* 1986;21:583-7.

139. Campfield J, Shah B, Angelides A, Hirsch B. Incidence of gastroesophageal reflux (GER) in VLBW. *Pediatr Res* 1992;31:106A.

140. Peeters S, Vandenplas Y. Sex ratio of gastroesophageal reflux in infancy. *J Pediatr Gastroenterol Nutr* 1991;13:314.

141. Skinner D. Controversies about Barrett's esophagus. *Ann Thorac Surg* 1990;49:523-4.

142. Hassall E, Weinstein WM, Ament ME. Barrett's esophagus in childhood. *Gastroenterology* 1985;89:1331-7.

143. Sondheimer JM, Morris BA. Gastroesophageal reflux among severely retarded children. *J Pediatr* 1979;94:710-4.

144. Abrahams P, Burkitt BF. Hiatus hernia and gastro-oesophageal reflux in children and adolescents with cerebral palsy. *Aust Paediatr J* 1970;6:41-6.

145. Hillemeier C, Buchin PJ, Gryboski J. Esophageal dysfunction in Down's syndrome. *J Pediatr Gastroenterol Nutr* 1982;1:101-4.

146. Berezin S, Newman LJ, Schwarz SM, Spiro AJ. Gastroesophageal reflux associated with nemaline myopathy of infancy. *Pediatrics* 1988;81:111-5.

147. Murphy JR, McNally P, Peller P, Shay SS. Prolonged clearance is the primary abnormal reflux parameter in patients with progressive systemic sclerosis and esophagitis. *Dig Dis Sci* 1992;37:833-41.

148. Axelrod FB, Gouge TH, Ginsburg HB, Bangaru BS, Hazzi C. Fundoplication and gastrostomy in familial dysautonomia. *J Pediatr* 1991;118:388-94.

149. Feigelson J, Girault F, Pecau Y. Gastro-oesophageal reflux and esophagitis in cystic fibrosis. *Acta Paediatr Scand* 1987;76:989-90.

150. Scott RB, OLoughlin EV, Gall DG. Gastroesophageal reflux in patients with cystic fibrosis. *J Pediatr* 1985;106:223-7.

151. Bendig DW, Seilheimer DK, Wagner ML, Ferry GD, Barrison GM. Complications of gastroesophageal reflux in patients with cystic fibrosis. *J Pediatr* 1982;100:536-40.

152. Baer M, Maki M, Nurminen J, Turjanmaa V,

Pukander J, Vesikarl T. Esophagitis and findings of long-term esophageal pH recording in children with repeated lower respiratory tract symptoms. *J Pediatr Gastroenterol Nutr* 1986;5:187-90.

153. Shapiro GG, Christie DL. Gastroesophageal reflux in steroid-dependent asthmatic youths. *Pediatrics* 1979;63:207-12.

154. Gustafsson PM, Kjellman NIM, Tibbling L. Bronchial asthma and acid reflux into the distal and proximal oesophagus. *Arch Dis Child* 1990;65:1255-8.

155. Gustafsson PM, Kjellman NIM, Tibbling L. Oesophageal function and symptoms in moderate and severe asthma. *Acta Paediatr Scand* 1986;75:729-36.

156. Martin ME, Grunstein MM, Larsen GL. The relationship of gastroesophageal reflux to nocturnal wheezing in children with asthma. *Ann Allergy* 1982;49:318-22.

157. Hoyoux C, Forget P, Lambrechts L, Geubelle F. Chronic bronchopulmonary disease and gastroesophageal reflux in children. *Pediatr Pulmonol* 1985;1:149-53.

158. Sontag S, O'Connell S, Khandeiwal S, et al. Most asthmatics have gastroesophageal reflux with or without bronchodilator therapy. *Gastroenterology* 1990;99:613-20.

159. Ducolone A, Vandevenne A, Joulin H, et al. Gastroesophageal reflux in patients with asthma and chronic bronchitis. *Am Rev Respir Dis* 1987;135:327-32.

160. Ashcraft KW, Goodwin C, Amoury RA, Holder TM. Early recognition and aggressive treatment of gastroesophageal reflux following repair of esophageal atresia. *J Pediatr Surg* 1977;12:317-21.

161. Nakazato Y, Landing BH, Wells TR. Abnormal Auerbach plexus in the esophagus and stomach of patients with esophageal atresia and tracheoesophageal fistula. *J Pediatr Surg* 1986;21:831-7.

162. Whitington PF, Shermeta DW, Seto DS, Jones L, Hendrix TR. Role of lower esophageal sphincter incompetence in recurrent pneumonia after repair of esophageal atresia. *J Pediatr* 1977;91:550-4.

163. Putnam T, Lawrence R, Wood B, et al. Esophageal function after repair of esophageal atresia. *Surg Gynecol Obstet* 1984;158:344-8.

164. Parker AF, Christie DL, Cahill JL. Incidence and significance of gastroesophageal reflux following repair of esophageal atresia and tracheoesophageal fistula and the need for anti-reflux procedures. *J Pediatr Surg* 1979;14:5-8.

165. Lind J, Bianchard R, Guyda H. Esophageal motility in tracheoesophageal fistula and esophageal atresia. *Surg Gynecol Obstet* 1966;123:557-64.

166. Jolley SG, Johnson DG, Roberts CC, et al. Patterns of gastroesophageal reflux in children following repair of esophageal atresia and distal tracheoesophageal fistula. *J Pediatr Surg* 1980;15:857-62.

167. Grunow JE, Al-Hafidh A-S. Gastroesophageal reflux following percutaneous endoscopic gastrostomy in children. *J Pediatr Surg* 1989;24:42-5.

168. Mollitt DL, Golladay ES, Selbert JJ. Symptomatic gastro-esophageal reflux following gastrostomy in neurologically impaired patients. *Pediatrics* 1985;75:1124-6.

169. Papaila JG, Vane DW, Colville C, et al. The effect of various types of gastrostomy on the lower esophageal sphincter. *J Pediatr Surg* 1987;22:1198-202.

170. Jolley SG, Tunell WP, Hoelzer DJ, Thomas S, Smith El. Lower esophageal pressure changes with tube gastrostomy: a causative factor of gastroesophageal reflux in children? *J Pediatr Surg* 1986;21:624-7.

171. Coben R, Weintraub A, DiMarino A, Cohen S. Bolus PEG feeding decreases lower esophageal sphincter pressure. *Gastroenterology* 1991;100:A45.

172. Ravelli A, Ledermann S, Bisset W, Trompeter R, Barratt T, Milla F. Foregut motor function in chronic renal failure. *Arch Dis Child* 1992;67:1343-7.

173. Motil KJ, Ostendorf J, Bricker JT, Klish WJ. Exercise-induced gastroesophageal reflux in an athletic child. *J Pediatr Gastroenterol Nutr* 1987;6:989-91.

174. Kraus B, Sinclair J, Castell D. Gastroesophageal reflux in runners: characteristics and treatment. *Ann Int Med* 1990;112:429-33.

175. Schofield P, Bennett D, Whorwell P, et al. Exertional gastro-oesophageal reflux: a mechanism for symptoms in patients with angina pectoris and normal coronary angiograms. *BMJ* 1987;294:1459-61.

176. Cammack J, Read NW, Cann PA, Greenwood B, Holgate AM. Effect of prolonged exercise on the passage of a solid meal through the stomach and small intestine. *Gut* 1982;23:957-61.

177. Ramsbottom N, Hunt J. Effect of exercise on gastric emptying and gastric secretion. *Digestion* 1974;10:1-8.

178. Feldman M, Nixon JV. Effect of exercise on postprandial gastric secretion and emptying in humans. *J Appl Physiol* 1982;53:851-4.

179. Costill DL, Saltin B. Factors limiting gastric emptying during rest and exercise. *J Appl Physiol* 1974;37:679-83.

180. Soffer E, Merchant R, Deuthman G, Launspach J, Gisolfi C. The effect of graded exercise on esophageal motility and gastro-esophageal reflux in trained athletes. *Gastroenterology* 1991;100:A497.

181. Hamois D, Tighe D, Georgeson S, Castell D, Kastenberg D. Lower esophageal sphincter (LES) pressure decreases following exercise. *Am J Gastroenterol* 1993;88:1488. Abstract.

182. Orenstein SR, Whitington PF, Orenstein DM. The infant seat as treatment for gastroesophageal reflux. *N Engl J Med* 1983;309:760-3.

183. Torres A, Serra-Batlles J, Ros E, et al. Pulmonary aspiration of gastric contents in patients receiving mechanical ventilation: the effect of body position. *Ann Int Med* 1992;116:540-3.

184. Reid K, McKenzie F, Menkis A. Importance of chronic aspiration in recipients of heart-lung transplants. *Lancet* 1990;336:206-8.

185. Udassin R, Seror D, Vinograd I, et al. Nissen fundoplication in the treatment of children with familial dysautonomia. *Am J Surg* 1992;164:332-6.

186. Iacono G, Carroccio A, Montalto G, Cavataio F, Balsamo V. Gastroesophageal reflux: clinical presentation in two pairs of twins. *J Pediatr Gastroenterol Nutr* 1992;14:460-2.

187. Fiorucci S, Santucci L, Chiucchiu S, Morelli A. Gastric acidity and gastroesophageal reflux patterns in patients with esophagitis. *Gastroenterology* 1992;103:855-61.

188. Glassman MS, Medow MS, Berezin S, Newman LJ. Spectrum of esophageal disorders in children with chest pain. *Dig Dis Sci* 1992;37:663-6.

189. Black DD, Haggitt RC, Orenstein SR, Whitington PF. Esophagitis in infants: morphometric histologic diagnosis and correlation with measures of gastroesophageal reflux. *Gastroenterology* 1990;98:1408-14.

190. Putnam PE, Orenstein SR. Blind esophageal suction biopsy in children less than 2 years of age. *Gastroenterology* 1992;102:A149.

191. Whitington PF, Orenstein SR. Manometric guidance in suction biopsy of the esophagus in children. *J Pediatr Gastroenterol Nutr* 1984;3:535-8.

192. Dellert S, Hyams J, Treem W, Geertsma M. Feeding resistance and gastroesophageal reflux in infancy. *J Pediatr Gastroenterol Nutr* 1993;17:66-71.

193. Hassall E. Barrett's esophagus: new definitions and approaches in children [invited review]. *J Pediatr Gastroenterol Nutr* 1993;16:345-64.

194. Albanese C, Towbin R, Ulman I, Lewis J, Smith S. Percutaneous gastrojejunostomy versus Nissen fundoplication for enteral feeding of the neurologically impaired child with gastroesophageal reflux. *J Pediatr* 1993;123:371-5

195. Newman LJ, Russe J, Glassman MS, et al. Patterns of gastroesophageal reflux (GER) in patients with apparent life-threatening events. *J Pediatr Gastroenterol Nutr* 1989;8:157-60.

196. Spitzer AR, Boyle JT, Tuchman DN, Fox WW. Awake apnea associated with gastroesophageal reflux: a specific clinical syndrome. *J Pediatr* 1984;104:200-5.

197. Herbst JJ, Minton SD, Book LS. Gastroesophageal reflux causing respiratory distrass and apnea in newborn infants. *J Pediatr* 1979;95:763-8.

198. Tolia V, Kauffman RE. Comparison of evaluation of gastro-esophageal reflux in infants using different feedings during intraesophageal pH

monitoring. *J Pediatr Gastroenterol Nutr* 1990;10:426-9.

199. Sutphen J, Dillard V. pH-adjusted formula and gastroesophageal reflux. *J Pediatr Gastroenterol Nutr* 1991;12:48-51.

200. Orenstein SR, Orenstein DM, Whitington PF. Gastroesophageal reflux causing stridor. *Chest* 1983;84:301-2.

201. Orenstein SR, Kocoshis SA, Orenstein DM, Proujansky R. Stridor and gastroesophageal reflux: diagnostic use of intraluminal esophageal acid perfusion (Bernstein test). *Pediatr Pulmonol* 1987;3:420-4.

202. Putnam PE, Orenstein SR: Hoarseness in a child with gastro-esophageal reflux. *Acta Pediatr Scand* 1992;81:635-6.

203. Buts JP, Barudi C, Moulin D, Cornu G, Otte JB. Prevalence and treatment of silent gastro-oesophageal reflux in children with recurrent respiratory disorders. *Eur J Pediatr* 1986;145:396-400.

204. Kinsbourne M. Hiatus hernia with contortions of the neck. *Lancet* 1964;1:1058-61.

205. Puntis J, Smith H, Buick R. Booth I. Effect of dystonic movements on oesophageal peristalsis in Sandifer's syndrome. *Arch Dis Child* 1989;64:1311-3.

206. Jolley S, Johnson D, Herbst J, Pena A, Garnier R. An assessment of gastroesophageal reflux in children by extended monitoring of the distal esophagus. *Surgery* 1978;84:16-22.

207. Euler AR, Byrne WJ. Twenty-four-hour esophageal intraluminal pH probe testing: a comparative analysis. *Gastroenterology* 1981;80:957-61.

208. Grill BB. Twenty-four-hour esophageal pH monitoring: what's the score? *J Pediatr Gastroenterol Nutr* 1992;14:249-51.

209. Friesen CA, Hayes R, Hodge C, Roberts CC. Comparison of methods of assessing 24-hour intraesophageal pH recordings in children. *J Pediatr Gastroenterol Nutr* 1992;14:252-5.

210. Schiesinger P, Donahue P, Schmid B, Layden T. Limitations of 24-hour intraesophageal pH monitoring in the hospital setting. *Gastroenterology* 1985;89:797-804.

211. Schindlbeck N, Heinrich C, Konig A, Dendorfer A, Pace F, Muller-Lissner S. Optimal thresholds, sensitivity, and specificity of long-term pH-metry for the detection of gastroesophageal reflux disease. *Gastroenterology* 1987;93:85-90.

212. Jolley S, Herbst J, Johnson D, Matlak M, Book L. Esophageal pH monitoring during sleep identifies children with respiratory symptoms from gastroesophageal reflux. *Gastroenterology* 1981;80:1501-6.

213. Halpern LM, Jolley SG, Tunnell WP, Johnson DG, Sterling CE. The mean duration of gastroesophageal reflux during sleep as an indicator of respiratory symptoms from gastroesophageal reflux in children. *J Pediatr Surg* 1991;26:686-90.

214. Eizaguirre I, Tovar JA. Predicting preoperatively the outcome of respiratory symptoms of gastroesophageal reflux. *J Pediatr Surg* 1992;27:848-51.

215. Orenstein SR, Klein HA, Rosenthal MS. Scintigraphic images for quantifying pediatric gastroesophageal reflux: a study of simultaneous scintigraphy and pH probe using multiplexed data and acid feedings. *J Nucl Med* 1993;34:1228-34.

216. Miller L. Endoscopy of the esophagus. In: Hennessy T, Cuschieri A, eds. *Surgery of the Oesophagus.* Oxford, England: Butterworth, Heinemann, 1992;89-142.

217. Biller JA, Winter HS, Grand RJ, Allred EN. Are endoscopic changes predictive of histologic esophagitis in children. *J Pediatr* 1983;103:215-8.

218. Orenstein SR, DiGiorgio CJ, Putnam PE, Kelsey SF, Shalaby TM, Becich MJ. Histology of infantile reflux esophagitis: evaluation of an objective, quantitative, analytic technique. *Gastroenterology* 1993;104 (4 parts):A166.

219. Berezin S, Medow MS, Glassman MS, Newman LJ. Esophageal chest pain in children with asthma. *J Pediatr Gastroenterol Nutr* 1991;12:52-5.

220. Orenstein SR, Magill HL, Brooks P. Thickening of infant feedings for therapy of gastroesophageal reflux. *J Pediatr* 1987;110:181-6.

221. Vandenplas Y, Sacre L. Milk-thickening agents as a treatment for gastroesophageal reflux [published erratum appears in *Clin Pediatr (Phila)* 1987 Mar;26(3):148]. *Clin Pediatr (Phila)* 1987;26:66-8.

222. Ramenofsky ML, Leape LL. Continuous upper esophageal pH monitoring in infants and children with gastroesophageal reflux, pneumonia, and apneic spells. *J Pediatr Surg* 1981;16:374-8.

223. Orenstein SR, Shalaby TM, Putnam PE: Thickened feedings as a cause of increased coughing when used as therapy for gastroesophageal reflux in infants. *J Pediatr* 1992;121:913-5.

224. Orenstein SR. Prone positioning in infant gastroesophageal reflux: is elevation of the head worth the trouble? *J Pediatr* 1990;117:184-7.

225. Sondheimer JM, Arnold GL. Early effects of bethanechol on the esophageal motor function of infants with gastroesophageal reflux. *J Pediatr Gastroenterol Nutr* 1986;5:47-51.

226. Orenstein SR, Lofton SW, Orenstein DM. Bethanechol for pediatric gastroesophageal reflux. a prospective, blind, controlled study. *J Pediatr Gastroenterol Nutr* 1986;5:549-55.

227. Sondheimer JM, Mintz HL, Michaels M. Bethanechol treatment of gastroesophageal reflux in infants: effect on continuous esophageal pH records. *J Pediatr* 1984;104:128-31.

228. Machida H, Forbes D, Gall D, Scott R. Metoclopramide in gastroesophageal reflux of infancy. *J Pediatr* 1988;112:483-7.

229. Hyman PE, Abrams CE, Dubois A. Gastric emptying in infants: response to metoclopramide depends on the underlying condition. *J Pediatr Gastroenterol Nutr* 1988;7:181-4.

230. Leung A, Lai P. Use of metoclopramide for the treatment of gastroesophageal reflux in infants and children. *Curr Ther Res* 1984;36:911-5.

231. Tolia V, Calhoun J, Kuhns L, Kauffman RE. Randomized, prospective double-blind trial of metoclopramide and placebo for gastroesophageal reflux in infants. *J Pediatr* 1989;115:141-5.

232. Hyams JS, Leichtner AM, Zamett LO, Walters JK. Effects of metoclopramide on prolonged intraesophageal pH testing in infants with gastroesophageal reflux. *J Pediatr Gastroenterol Nutr* 1986;5:716-20.

233. Putnam PE, Orenstein SR, Wessel HB, Stowe RM. Tardive dyskinesia associated with metoclopramide use in a child. *J Pediatr* 1992;121:983-5.

234. Cucchiara S, Staiano A, Capozzi C, Di Lorenzo C, Boccierl A, Auricchio S. Cisapride for gastro-oesophageal reflux and peptic oesophagitis. *Arch Dis Child* 1987;62:454-7.

235. Cucchiara S, Staiano A, Romaniello G, Capobianco S, Auricchio S. Antacids and cimetidine treatment for gastro-oesophageal reflux and peptic oesophagitis. *Arch Dis Child* 1984;59:842-7.

236. Brand JM, Greer FR. Hypermagnesemia and intestinal perforation following antacid administration in a premature infant. *Pediatrics* 1990;85:121-4.

237. Black J. Reflections on the analytical pharmacology of histamine H_2-receptor antagonists. *Gastroenterology* 1993;105:963-8.

238. Gunasekaran T, Hassall E. Efficacy and safety of omeprazole for severe gastroesophageal reflux in children. *J Pediatr* 1993;123:148-54.

239. Rice H, Seashore J, Toulouklan R. Evaluation of Nissen fundoplication in neurologically impaired children. *J Pediatr Surg* 1991;26:697-701.

240. Jolley S, Smith E, Tunell W. Protective antireflux operation with feeding gastrostomy. *Ann Surg* 1985;201:736-40.

241. Duffy L, Kerzner B, Newman K, Taylor G, Majd M, Randolph J: Gastrostomy tube (GT) placement: relationship to gastroesophageal reflux (GER). *Pediatr Res* 1989;25:111A.

242. Berezin S, Schwartz SM, Halata MS, Newman LJ. Gastroesophageal reflux secondary to gastrostomy tube placement. *Am J Dis Child* 1986;140:699-701.

243. Gauderer MW. Feeding gastrostomy or feeding gastrostomy plus antireflux procedure? *J Pediatr Gastroenterol Nutr* 1988;7:795-6.

244. Orenstein SR. Gastroesophageal reflux. In: Stockman JA II, Winter RJ, eds. *Current Problems in Pediatrics.* Chicago, IL: Year Book Medical Publishers, 1991;21(5):202.

245. Putnam PE, Ricker DH, Orenstein SR. Gastroesophageal reflux. In: Beckerman R, Brouilette R, Hunt C, eds. *Respiratory Control Disorders in Infants and Children.* Baltimore, MD: Williams & Wilkins; 1991:324-5.

5

Cyclic Vomiting

DAVID R. FLEISHER

Samuel Gee's powers of clinical observation are exemplified by his description of cyclic vomiting. Although published more than a century ago, it is still accurate and useful:

These cases seem to be all of the same kind, their characteristic being fits of vomiting, which recur after intervals of uncertain length. The intervals themselves are free from sign of disease. The vomiting continues for a few hours or a few days. When it had been severe, the patients are left much exhausted. The patients are children: the oldest...being about 9 years old. In 4 cases at least, the disorder began in babyhood. Pain, in the upper part of the belly or around the navel, often accompanies the vomiting. Sometimes the pain is so severe as to throw the vomiting into the shade. The state of the bowels during the attack is uncertain: they are costive, or loose, or unaffected...The conditions under which the vomiting occurs is not constant. They are: 1) exhaustion after traveling, or excitement of any kind. 2) indigestible food; by no means a common condition. 3) exposure to cold. But, in some cases, the closest observation fails to discover anything which can be called a cause.[1]

The characteristic that distinguishes cyclic vomiting from recurrent vomiting caused by peptic ulcer, giardiasis, or other diseases of the upper gastrointestinal mucosa is its episodic pattern. In cyclic vomiting, there is intense nausea, vomiting, and retching many times per day or hour, for hours or days at a time; the episodes are separated by symp-tom-free intervals of days or months. In other vomiting disorders, vomiting is typically less intense, occurring once or several times on a more or less daily basis.[2]

Cyclic vomiting is uncommon,[3] and little has been written about it during the past 60 years.[2,4-7] Relatively few physicians have encountered it, felt able to diagnose it with confidence, or experienced success in treating it. Cyclic vomiting is noted for an absence of pathognomonic historical features, physical signs, or pathologic, radiologic, or encephalographic markers. Recurrent vomiting has a large differential diagnosis, including many serious and life-threatening diseases.[3] There is no standard management for this disorder. These factors hinder clinicians in making an unequivocal diagnosis of cyclic vomiting. This in turn creates feelings of distress and isolation in parents, who fear that they are powerless in coping with an ailment that is unique to their child and baffling to their physicians.

FEATURES OF CYCLIC VOMITING

The prevalence of cyclic vomiting is unknown. However, reports from early in the century to the present—from England, New York City, the Midwest, and Los Angeles—suggest the disorder is diagnosed three to six times a year in tertiary pediatric centers.[2-5,8] Cyclic vomiting was more common in Germany following World War II, where it was diagnosed 20 to 30 times a year in two large pediatric clinics.[9,10] Boys and girls are affected in equal numbers.

Figure 5.1 depicts the age of onset of the disorder in three series of patients.[3-5] Al-

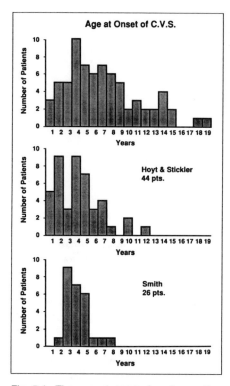

Fig. 5.1 The age at onset of cyclic vomiting syndrome (CVS) in patients. (Reprinted with permission from Fleisher DR, Matar M, 1993[3]; Hoyt C, Stickler G, 1960[5]; Smith C, 1937[4])

though cyclic vomiting commonly begins in preschool and early school-age children, onset may occur any time from infancy to late adolescence, and adult-onset cases have been reported as well.[11]

Cyclic vomiting episodes tend to be similar in duration and symptoms over months or years. In one series, 85% of those affected had attacks of fairly uniform length and 15% had attacks of variable length (Fig. 5.2).[3] Over the course of the disorder, episodes may worsen or improve in frequency and severity before recurrences cease.

The frequency of episodes ranges from 1 to 70 per year, averaging 12 per year.[3] The term "cyclic" implies regular, rhythmic recurrences. Episodes of vomiting are fairly regular in only about 50% of patients. Other patients' episodes occur at intervals that have no temporal predictability. Figure 5.3 shows the pattern of recurrences in four patients.

Vomiting begins at characteristic times of the day or night in 76% of patients (Fig. 5.4).[3] The most common times of onset are the middle of the night and/or on arising in the morning.

Many episodes are accompanied by characteristic symptoms and signs in addition to

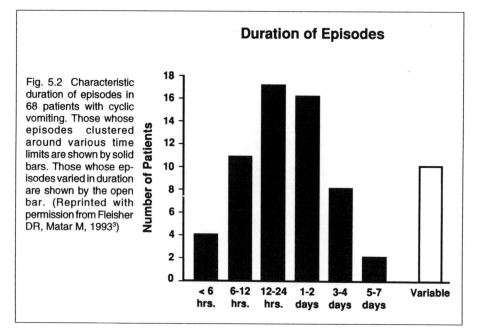

Fig. 5.2 Characteristic duration of episodes in 68 patients with cyclic vomiting. Those whose episodes clustered around various time limits are shown by solid bars. Those whose episodes varied in duration are shown by the open bar. (Reprinted with permission from Fleisher DR, Matar M, 1993[3])

vomiting. Most patients complain of abdominal pain located in the periumbilical and/or epigastric regions. Children often refer to nausea as "pain," making it difficult to differentiate these two kinds of distress. Nevertheless, some children writhe and groan while complaining of pain, behavior indicative of more than nausea alone. Intense nausea sometimes prompts children to spit out, rather than swallow, their saliva; they may carry a pan or towel in which to expectorate. Others are prevented from speaking by a mouthful of saliva they are unwilling to swallow.

Loose stools near the onset or during cyclic vomiting episodes have been reported by 30% of patients.[3] Headache accompanied

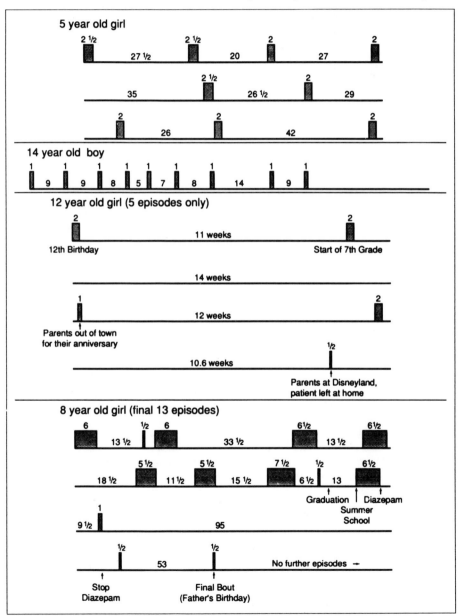

Fig. 5.3 The duration of and intervals between episodes in four representative patients with cyclic vomiting. The numbers above and between bars signify days, unless otherwise indicated.

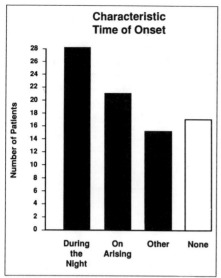

Characteristic Time of Onset

Number of Patients

28, 26, 24, 22, 20, 18, 16, 14, 12, 10, 8, 6, 4, 2, 0

During the Night | On Arising | Other | None

Fig. 5.4 Seventy-six percent of patients had one or two characteristic times of onset of episodes. Twenty-four percent had no characteristic time of onset. Vomiting began most commonly during the night and on arising in the morning.

nausea and vomiting in 27%. Fever, usually 100° to 102°, occurs in 23% of patients during episodes.[3] Other phenomena indicative of autonomic dysfunction during attacks include hypertension and tachycardia,[3,12] which may be present throughout episodes, even while the patient appears to be asleep. These abnormal vital signs remit when episodes end. Inappropriate secretion of antidiuretic hormone may accompany prolonged nausea.[13] Transient leukocytosis is sometimes found during attacks, even in the absence of infection.[14]

Cyclic vomiting attacks cause reflux esophagitis, which is manifested by retrosternal pain and hematemesis. Esophagitis is thought to be secondary to the vomiting rather than its cause, although severe esophagitis may prolong episodes by contributing to nausea. Some patients seem driven to drink water even though they vomit as soon as they swallow it. Compulsive water drinking by intravenously well-hydrated patients seemed puzzling until the following patient's letter was read: "I drink the water because sometimes vomiting helps to relieve the nausea and, as I know I'm going to vomit anyway, it is far less unpleasant to bring up a dilute solution than to vomit concentrated hydrochloric acid which causes the agonizing pain of severe heartburn."

Patients are uncommunicative and withdrawn during cyclic vomiting episodes and may seem "psychotically depressed."[12] The literature on cyclic vomiting lacks descriptions of the subjective experience of an attack. The following, written by patients, contributes to the clinician's understanding of patient behavior during attacks.

A 13-year-old girl wrote, "I start to get a headache, feel sick, unable to swallow, [feel a] stomachache, dizziness and just general nausea. Then, often I will suddenly vomit and start salivating...When I'm having an attack, I am in a semicomatose state. I am not aware of any goings on around. All I feel like doing is sleeping. I sometimes hear Mom or Dad or Sam saying something where they need an answer. Although I am asleep, I hear them and my mind knows the answer, but it's trapped so I can't tell them."

Another young woman wrote of her attacks, "They would usually hit me the minute I woke up in the morning, or sometimes in the middle of the night. Never did I have any warning; I would rarely make it to the bathroom before getting sick upon waking. The telling symptom for me is extreme nausea, which is worsened by the slightest movement or faintest odor. The nausea is an extremely controlling, dominating force. Oddly enough, it's almost as if the vomiting is my body's reaction to the nausea or is meant to relieve it, because the vomiting would quell the nausea wave and allow me to sleep, if only for a while. The intervals between vomiting episodes always lessened as the day wore on, and [I] inevitably would end up vomiting every 15 minutes. I would alternate between sleep and vomiting... I felt possessed during the episodes. Even though there was nothing in me, my body just had to vomit, and I would vomit bile and blood. During these episodes, I am also extremely lethargic and have a difficult time talking, as the nausea consumes every ounce of strength. It is an extremely difficult experience to articulate, sick or well."

Another patient wrote, "At the onset of an attack, when I have vomited once, I know I am going to go through hell before I recover. At this stage, I do not feel too bad physically, because vomiting relieves the nausea. But, as the attack progresses, the nausea becomes constant. Nothing will relieve it...I am utterly exhausted, and all I want to do is sleep...I am not aware of the nausea and the pain while sleeping. But, as soon as I lie down to try and sleep, the nausea intensifies and I have to sit up again...I end up falling asleep while sitting up, not exactly a comfortable position. If I wake up during the night, I'm always confused. I am aware of incredible discomfort and pain... I don't understand what's happening to me."

Seventy-seven percent of patients identify specific conditions or events that seem to trigger episodes.[3] Noxious emotional stress, such as parental conflict, is mentioned most as a precipitating factor.[15] Almost as frequently, nonnoxious excitement, such as birthdays or vacations, seem to precipitate episodes.[16] Infections, such as colds, influenza, or sinusitis, are the third most common cause of vomiting episodes. Active infections during episodes probably interfere with the efficacy of antiemetic agents. Other triggers reported by patients include physical exhaustion, hot weather, motion sickness, overeating, eating at bedtime, specific foods, menstruation, and asthma attacks.

CHARACTERISTICS OF PATIENTS AND THEIR FAMILIES

The review of systems in cyclic vomiting patients[3] reveals that, between vomiting episodes, 67% have symptoms of irritable bowel syndrome (IBS), such as pellet stools, diarrhea induced by stress or fatty meals, or recurrent abdominal pain.[17] This is two to six times the prevalence of IBS in the general population.[18-21]

Eleven percent of patients have migraine headaches,[3] almost twice the prevalence of migraine in unselected children.[22-24] Susceptibility to motion sickness is reported by 46% of patients.[3] This figure is similar to the susceptibility to motion sickness in 45% of

migrainous children, and significantly greater than the 5% to 7% susceptibility to motion sickness in two groups of nonmigrainous children.[25]

When parents were asked to characterize their child's personality, 76% viewed their children as having one or more of the following traits: competitive, perfectionistic, high-achieving, aggressive, strong-willed, moralistic, caring, and enthusiastic.[3]

Four of 71 patients (5.6%) had epilepsy.[3] This is ten times the prevalence of epilepsy in unselected children.[26] Anticonvulsants are effective for controlling seizures, but do not control cyclic vomiting episodes.

Family histories reveal that first- and/or second-degree relatives have IBS in 62% of cases and recurrent headaches in 58%, including 40% whose headaches are migrainous.[3] Three of 71 patients had a parent with a history of cyclic vomiting.[3]

The features of cyclic vomiting are summarized in Table 5.1.[3]

THE COURSE OF ILLNESS

Figure 5.5 depicts the natural history of cyclic vomiting in 29 patients.[3] Sixteen had been symptom-free for more than a year at the time of follow-up. In some, the disorder continued (with one or more episodes per year) for decades; in others, the illness lasted a year or less. Although its course defines it as a self-limited disorder, it is impossible to predict when it will end. The statement that cyclic vomiting usually terminates before puberty[5,27] is questionable, since the disorder may persist well beyond puberty or begin years after.[3]

ETIOLOGY AND PATHOGENESIS

There appears to be a relationship between cyclic vomiting, migraine, IBS, and personality.[3] The theory that cyclic vomiting is a migraine variant or equivalent[28,29] is based on features shared by both disorders,[2,4,5,16,30,31] ie, both are episodic.[1-5] The episodes in these disorders tend to be stereotypic for individual patients,[1,3-5] are frequently precipitated by stress or excitement,[3,16] and often begin during the night or morn-

TABLE 5.1 Clinical Features of Cyclic Vomiting

Recurrent, self-limited episodes of nausea, vomiting and pallor	100%
Intervals between episodes are symptom-free	100%
The duration and symptomatology of episodes are stereotyped and characteristic for each patient over time	85%
Episodes are triggered by heightened emotional states and/or physical stress	77%
Patients have typical personality features	76%
Episodes may be accompanied by headache and/or loose stooling, and/or mild pyrexia, and/or mild hypertension, and tachycardia	67%
Episodes begin during the night and/or on arising in the morning	65%
Family history of irritable bowel syndrome	62%
Patients are prone to motion sickness	46%
Family history of migraine headaches	40%
Patients expectorate saliva or hold it in their mouths without swallowing for extended periods	13%

(Reprinted with permission from Fleisher DR, Matar M, 1993[3])

ing.[3,4,14,16,32] Migraine is familial[29] and the impression exists that it is more common in the families of patients with cyclic vomiting, although this remains to be proved by prospective study.[4,16]

Increased susceptibility to motion sickness and IBS are more frequent in both disorders.[3,4,15] The prevalence of irritable bowel symptoms between attacks in cyclic vomiting patients is more than that of the general population.[33,34] Children with recurrent abdominal pain are more likely to experience frequent headaches and cyclic vomiting.[35-38] Considering that the pathogenesis of migraine is unclear[39] and agents which ameliorate migraine headaches are generally ineffective during cyclic vomiting episodes, equating cyclic vomiting with migraine does not advance understanding or management of the disorder.

Although cyclic vomiting is considered by some to be a seizure disorder,[35] its relationship with epilepsy remains unclear. Cyclic vomiting episodes of brief duration, associated with other features of seizures (eg, olfactory hallucinations, epileptiform EEG, postictal sleep) are well documented.[40] One published series describes five patients with abnormal EEGs, whose periodic episodes of vomiting lasted several days.[14] Two of the cases appeared to be indistinguishable from cyclic vomiting. The unexpectedly high prevalence of epilepsy in patients with cyclic vomiting[3] might support the hypothesis that cyclic vomiting is a seizure disorder. However, in patients referred to a pediatric neurology clinic, cyclic vomiting was almost seven times more frequent in migrainous children than in epileptics.[35] It is likely that cyclic vomiting, migraine, and epilepsy originate in the central nervous system, and that stress or excitement are important precipitants to symptom production. The precise pathogenesis for these three paroxysmal disorders remains unknown; the categorical distinctions between them are based on clinical appearances and responses to empiric therapies. Moreover, cyclic vomiting and epilepsy are not mutually exclusive. It is quite possible for both disorders to coexist in the same patient.

Cyclic vomiting, migraine, and epilepsy are clinically distinct entities, even though some patients present with overlapping symptomatology. Of the three, cyclic vomiting seems the least prevalent. It has also re-

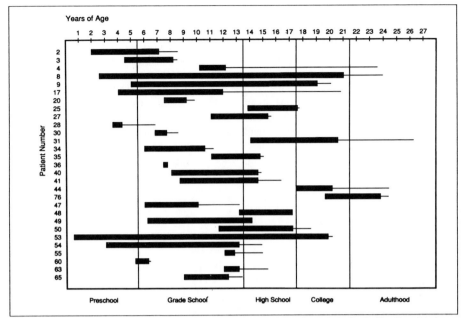

Fig. 5.5 The age at onset and duration of cyclic vomiting in 29 patients is indicated by the wide bars. Narrow, horizontal lines indicate the duration of follow-up, during which patients were free of symptoms. (Reprinted with permission from Fleisher DR, Matar M, 1993[3])

ceived the least scrutiny and analysis.

DIFFERENTIAL DIAGNOSIS

The differential diagnosis of cyclic vomiting includes diseases that present with similar symptoms during at least part of their course.

Brain Stem Glioma

Brain stem glioma may mimic cyclic vomiting. One case history concerned an infant whose frequent vomiting became cyclic by 3 years of age, at which point the diagnosis of cyclic vomiting was made.[5] At 6 years, she presented with papilledema and later died of an astrocytoma arising from the floor of the fourth ventricle. The emesis of cyclic vomiting resembles that of increased intracranial pressure, in that both tend to occur in the morning and are unrelated to food intake.[41] Vomiting as a symptom of brain tumor is readily diagnosed when there are signs of increased intracranial pressure. Brain stem glioma, however, may infiltrate the medulla without obstructing the flow of cerebrospinal fluid. This may cause vomit-

ing by direct encroachment on the medullary vomiting centers and the cranial nerve nuclei that control gastrointestinal motility.[42,43] Therefore, a high index of suspicion is necessary for brain stem lesions in a vomiting child without increased intracranial pressure.[44,45] Although most children with brain stem gliomas die within 18 months of the diagnosis,[46] and treatment is at best palliative, there are atypical cases of brain stem gliomas that grow slowly and may be amenable to surgery.[47] The prognosis in patients with such tumors would be seriously compromised by misdiagnosis.

Obstructive Uropathy

Obstructive uropathy is a relatively common cause of vomiting in children. The following patients exhibited a pattern of symptoms that, by history, was indistinguishable from cyclic vomiting.

Case 1. A 3½-year-old girl had been well until 11 months previously, when she experienced the first of 13 discrete episodes of vomiting. These episodes were similar in duration and self-limited, but had become progressively more frequent. They usually began with anorexia at dinner. She went to bed at the usual time only to be awakened after midnight by abdominal pain and vomiting of clear or bilious material. She then vomited a few or many times until about 5 a.m., when she resumed sleeping. She usually awoke at 7 a.m., ate breakfast, and felt well until the next episode. Physical examination showed a healthy-appearing, well-nourished girl (BP = 116/60). There was subtle convexity of her left flank and a soft, nontender left upper-quadrant mass whose lower edge was palpable 5 cm below the left costal margin. There were no other physical abnormalities. Urinalysis was negative. Ultrasonography and excretory urography showed left hydronephrosis with obstruction of the ureteropelvic junction. She had no vomiting episodes after decompression by percutaneous nephrostomy followed by pyeloplasty.

Case 2. At 18 months of age, a 7½-year-old boy began having episodes of vomiting that lasted 12 to 24 hours. He then suffered 8 to 13 episodes per year, each beginning with abdominal pain at 5 p.m., followed by the onset of vomiting at 8 p.m. The vomiting recurred every hour until 2:30 a.m., when it increased in frequency to every 15 minutes, and continued throughout the night until tapering off by morning. Lethargy and anorexia gradually subsided during the following 3 days, after which he was well until the next episode. Most episodes had similar symptoms, although a few were of shorter duration. During these briefer episodes he vomited once or twice daily for a day or two and was not incapacitated with pain or nausea between emeses.

His temperature rose as high as 100° during episodes. There was no headache or diarrhea. He sometimes held saliva in his mouth to avoid swallowing. Although he never complained of retrosternal pain, he vomited "coffee-grounds" material during some attacks. The patient's mother, father, and paternal grandmother were subject to migraine headaches. His mother had IBS. The patient had been treated with cyprohep-

tadine for 3 months, during which he had no bouts. Breakthrough systems prompted 6 months of oral lorazepam every day followed by 3 months of carbamazepine, neither of which seemed to help. Physical examination revealed a blood pressure of 146/78 at the start of the visit and 130/80 at the end. While supine, the silhouette of the left side of the abdomen was slightly less concave than the right when the patient was viewed from the foot of the examining table. On palpation, the left upper quadrant felt fuller than the right, although no discrete mass was definable. There was slight tenderness without guarding below the left costal margin as compared with the right. Urinalysis showed 1 + protein; the sediment contained 10 red blood cells and 4 white blood cells per high-power field and no evidence of infection. Abdominal ultrasound showed left hydronephrosis. The patient underwent surgery for left ureteropelvic junction obstruction.

Comment: Dietl's crisis[48] is a plausible explanation for the periodicity of vomiting in these two cases. The partially obstructed renal pelvis may not cause symptoms until periods of increased urine production cause acute exacerbation of hydronephrosis. The symptoms subside as soon as the renal pelvis drains sufficiently,[49,50] and recur with the next diuresis. Although many children with unilateral ureteropelvic junction obstruction localize the pain that accompanies vomiting ipsilateral through their hydronephrosis, others localize their pain to the midabdomen.[51] Their midabdominal pain might therefore be confused with the midabdominal or midepigastric pain that is typical for cyclic vomiting.

Children lose weight during episodes of cyclic vomiting and the weight loss in children having 5- to 10-day episodes can be dramatic.[4] Nevertheless, weight is regained rapidly after the end of each attack and their overall pattern of weight gain is normal.[5] Growth lag suggests the presence of chronic disease.[52]

Transient leukocytosis without apparent infection may accompany some attacks[14] and, together with abdominal pain, vomit-

TABLE 5.2 **Diagnosis of Cyclic Vomiting**

Gastrointestinal
  Peptic ulcer disease[54]
  Pancreatitis[55]
  Pancreatic pseudocyst[56]
  Intestinal parasitism[57]
  Intermittent small-bowel obstruction[58]
  Recurrent subacute appendicitis[59,60]
  Chronic idiopathic intestinal pseudo-
    obstruction[61]
  Bochdalek's hernia[62]
Central Nervous System
  Brain tumors causing increased
    intracranial pressure
  Brain stem tumors, with or without
    increased intracranial pressure[43,44]
  Subdural hematoma or effusions[63,64]
  Abdominal epilepsy[40]
  Hydrocephalus—slit ventricle
    syndrome[65,66]
Autonomic Nervous System
  Familial dysautonomia[52,67]
Urinary Tract
  Obstructive uropathies[48,49]
Endocrine
  Pheochromocytoma[68,69]
  Adrenal insufficiency[70]
  Diabetes mellitus[71]
Metabolic
  Ornithine transcarbamylase deficiency[72]
  Medium-chain acyl coenzyme A
    dehydrogenase deficiency[73]
  Propionic acidemia[74]
  Isovaleric acidemia
    (chronic intermittent form)[75]
  Porphyria[76]

(Reprinted with permission from Fleisher DR, Matar M 1993[3])

ing, and hypoactive bowel sounds, may prompt a misdiagnosis of appendicitis.[4,5]

A progressive disease may cause vomiting that is intermittent, even periodic. The patient's well-being between vomiting episodes does not guarantee the absence of ongoing organic disease. Furthermore, vomiting caused by any organic disease may be triggered or intensified by emotional stress or excitement. Therefore, the view that nausea and vomiting is *either* organic *or* functional is an oversimplification that may result in inadequate or excessive diagnostic testing and treatment.[53]

Table 5.2 contains diseases to be considered in the differential diagnosis of cyclic vomiting. Table 5.3 contains studies to be considered in the diagnostic process.

MANAGEMENT

Children with cyclic vomiting suffer alarming symptoms. The diagnosis is often delayed or unrecognized because cyclic vomiting is seldom encountered in general medical practice. As a result, the parents' feelings of not knowing what is wrong or what to do about it can cause despair, anger, and a loss of all sense of well-being. As one parent put it, "You wonder when you wake up—is this another bad day? And then I hold my breath each morning until she appears. We are so thankful to learn of other people with cyclic vomiting. For many years we thought it was just a strange thing with our child. Now we know it's a 'real disease' with a 'real name.' "

A single diagnostic consultation with a knowledgeable clinician whom the family likes and respects may result in an immediate sense of improvement and a decrease in the frequency and/or severity of attacks. Figure 5.6 depicts the recurrence rates of cyclic vomiting before and after the initial diagnostic consultation. Undoubtedly, the trend towards resolution shown by most patients is partly due to the natural history of the disorder. However, if feelings of dread and powerlessness potentiate nausea,[77] then the diagnostic clarity, hopeful prognosis, and therapeutic alliance established between the physician, child, and parents will probably have a beneficial effect on symptoms.[78]

Nevertheless, the disruptions caused by episodes may overwhelm the family by depriving the parents of sleep, draining their financial resources, and causing them to miss work. A plan should be developed for each child that maximizes convenience for the family, while minimizing frustrating waits in emergency rooms, hospitalizations, and exposure to care givers who are unfamiliar with the patient and the disorder.

Management of cyclic vomiting involves the relief of nausea and vomiting, treatment of its acute complications, and prophylaxis. It is logical to assume that the sooner antiemetic treatment is instituted, the easier it is to affect a remission. Therefore, it is recommended that treatment begin within an hour of the onset of an attack. Waiting it out—

hoping for early subsidence without intervention—merely prolongs the child's suffering and increases the dehydration and other complications of an attack. No controlled studies have been published concerning antiemetics in cyclic vomiting. The following statements regarding use and efficacy are based on personal experience and anecdotal reports.

Ondansetron is an antiemetic agent used extensively in oncology patients to lessen or abolish the nausea and vomiting associated with chemotherapy. It blocks serotonin receptors of the 5-HT$_3$ type located in the chemoreceptor trigger zone, as well as in the vomiting centers of the medulla and on vagal nerve terminals.[79,80] Limited personal experience in the use of ondansetron during cyclic vomiting episodes has thus far provided no evidence contradictory to its manufacturer's claims that it is safe, nonsedating, unlikely to cause extrapyramidal or other serious side effects, and does not interact with benzodiazepines. An initial dose of 0.3 to 0.4 mg/kg administered intravenously over 15 to 30 minutes is recommended. Resolution of nausea often occurs during this infusion. If nausea continues, or if it temporarily subsides but then recurs, a course of 1 mg/h intravenously for 12 hours up to a total dose of 0.8 mg/kg every 24 hours, or a maximum of 12 mg subsequent to the initial dose of 0.3 to 0.4 mg/kg is suggested.

Induction of sleep has long been considered beneficial in controlling attacks.[4] Lorazepam, a benzodiazepine with antiemetic, anxiolytic, and sedative properties,[81] has been used to suppress or shorten bouts of cyclic vomiting.[82] An intravenous injection of lorazepam 0.05 to 0.2 mg/kg, administered over a few minutes, often produces sedation and diminishes nausea within a short time. The patient should then be allowed to sleep. If the patient awakens after several hours with renewed nausea, the dose should be repeated every 6 hours for no more than four doses,

---

TABLE 5.3 Diagnostic Studies in the Differential Diagnosis of Cyclic Vomiting

Blood Studies
   CBC with differential and RBC morphology
   Electrolytes, blood urea nitrogen, creatinine, glucose
   Tests of hepatic function (AST, ALT, alkaline phosphatase, bilirubin, serum protein, and albumin)
   Blood ammonia
   Lactate and pyruvate
   Amylase and lipase
   Blood lead
   Pregnancy test

Urine Studies
   Urinalysis with microscopic examination of sediment
   Urine culture
   Urine for amino acids, organic acids, catecholamines, porphobilinogen, aminolevulinic acid, uroporphyrin and coproporphyrin

Stool Studies
   Occult blood
   Stool leukocytes
   Ova parasites

Radiologic Studies
   Ultrasonography of liver, biliary tract, pancreas, kidneys, and adrenal glands
   Chest roentgenograms
   Abdominal roentgenograms
   Barium study of upper GI tract and small bowel
   Contrast enema study
   MRI of brain

Other Studies
   EEG

(Reprinted with permission from Fleisher DR, Matar M, 1993[3])

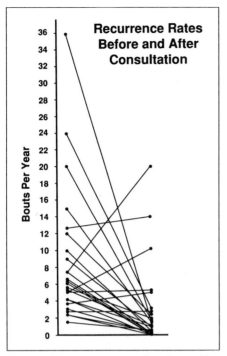

Recurrence Rates Before and After Consultation

Bouts Per Year

Fig. 5.6 Recurrence rates of cyclic vomiting before and after the initial diagnostic consultation.

until he or she awakens without nausea. Side effects include somnolence, unsteady gait, and sometimes transient hallucinosis. The above dosages of lorazepam are similar to those used in status epilepticus.[83,84] This use of lorazepam resembles the use of diazepam for the vomiting crises of familial dysautonomia.[85] Lorazepam has been used in addition to ondansetron when the latter proved ineffective. The immediate, oral use of a benzodiazepine at the perceived approach of a vomiting attack has been effective for some children and adolescents whose bouts are triggered by acute anxiety.

Phenothiazines (eg, chlorpromazine), butyrophenones (eg, droperidol), and benzamides (eg, metoclopramide or trimethobenzamide) seem less effective and entail the risk of extrapyramidal reactions.

Prior to administration of antiemetics, every child with cyclic vomiting should be assessed clinically for infection or some other cause of acute vomiting. "Over-the-phone" treatment of episodes, or treatment by home-infusion service personnel who are unable to provide competent clinical assessment, is hazardous.

At least three kinds of problems should be looked for whenever antiemetic therapy seems ineffective: 1) supervening disorder that causes vomiting, eg, meningitis, pregnancy, or intestinal obstruction; 2) sleep deprivation caused by noise, light, or commotion in the room, or by overly conscientious nursing observations and procedures; and 3) complications of prolonged vomiting, which, in themselves, cause nausea.

Complications of prolonged nausea and vomiting include peptic esophagitis and depletion of extracellular and intracellular electrolytes. Bloody or "coffee grounds" vomitus and heartburn indicate the presence of peptic esophagitis, which should be treated promptly and vigorously by administration of intravenous H_2-histamine receptor antagonists to raise the pH of the vomitus above 4. Potassium losses may be profound, even when serum potassium levels are in the low to normal range. The patient may be receiving "maintenance" potassium input while losing much more in expectorated saliva and vomited gastric juice. Magnesium may also be required in above-maintenance amounts.[86]

Patients who are fearful of venipunctures or have difficult venous access may benefit from the use of a topical anesthetic (Emla cream, Astra Pharmaceuticals, Westborough, MD) to lessen the stress of intravenous procedures.

Finding an antiemetic regimen that is effective and readily available seems, in itself, to lessen the frequency of attacks in many patients, perhaps because it restores a sense of control and lessens the dread of future attacks. In those patients who continue to have frequent, prolonged attacks, long-term propranolol,[32] amitriptyline, or erythromycin[87] may be effective in the prophylaxis of recurrences.

Many patients are intensely hungry at the end of vomiting episodes. Some are able to resume an unrestricted diet, while others suffer recurrence of symptoms after eating their first postepisodic meal. An unknown number of patients with cyclic nausea and vomiting have abnormal gastric myoelectrical function, even when asymptomatic.[11] Patients with gastric dysrhythmias tolerate liquids better than solid foods.[88] Therefore, it is advisable to limit oral intake to isotonic or hypotonic nutrient liquids for a day or so in children who have had recurrences of nausea after eating solid food.

Psychiatric Aspects of Management

Cyclic vomiting is best viewed as functional, ie, a disorder caused by an organ dysfunction rather than an underlying organic or mental disease. Parents of children with cyclic vomiting may fear for their child's life. Their unallayed fears may cause them to view their child as excessively vulnerable and fragile.[89] The child's and family's psychopathology may also be utilized for somatizing, the process by which patients consciously or unconsciously use bodily symptoms for psychologic purposes or personal advantage.[90] For example, domestic strife may precipitate an episode of vomiting, which then shifts the parent's attention away from conflict and towards caring for the sick child. Cyclic vomiting, as the child's defense against the anxiety caused by the parents' hostility towards each other, may thereby be unwittingly reinforced and perpetuated.

However, the presence of family dysfunction is not, in itself, sufficient cause for referral to a mental health professional. Parents must be willing and able to view such a referral as potentially useful. Otherwise, the referral may hinder rather than help the therapeutic program.

Although cyclic vomiting may be a reaction to psychologic stress and attention to psychologic factors is imperative,[91] it should not be labeled psychosomatic, ie, due to a primary neurotic illness.[92] The implication that bodily symptoms with no discernible organic cause are the result of a psychologic disorder may offend the patient, damage doctor-patient rapport, and reduce the clinician's efficacy. By viewing the etiology of cyclic vomiting nonspecifically—as functional rather than psychiatric—that implication is avoided and patients who are, in fact, emotionally well are not offended. Those patients who have significant psychologic and family pathology, but are unable to utilize formal mental health resources, need the support of an undamaged doctor-patient relationship. If the clinician avoids setting up the "psychosomatic" barrier from the start, mental health issues (including resistance to a mental health referral) can be dealt with during management of the child's functional disorder.[93]

The author is grateful to Giulio Barbero, MD, Larry Puls, MD, Edward Feldman, MD, and Harry Cynamon, MD, for seminal ideas and observations; to Marla Matar, MD, and William Altemeier, MD, for help with writing and editing; to Fiona McRonald, Lucy Ryall, and Jennifer Parsons for their contributions towards the understanding of cyclic vomiting; and to Mrs. Kathleen Adams, President of the Cyclic Vomiting Association of America. The author also thanks Mrs. Shirley Haden for preparation of the manuscript.

REFERENCES

1. Gee S. On fitful or recurrent vomiting. *Saint Bartholomew's Hospital Reports.* 1882;18(1)1-6.

2. Pfau BT, Li B UK, Murray RD, et al. Cyclic vomiting in children: a migraine equivalent? *Gastroenterology* 1992;102:A23.

3. Fleisher DR, Matar M. The cyclic vomiting syndrome: a report of 71 cases and literature review. *J Pediatr Gastroenterol Nutr* 1993;17(4):361-9.

4. Smith C. Recurrent vomiting in children. *J Pediatr* 1937; 10(6)719-42.

5. Hoyt C, Stickler G. A study of 44 children with the syndrome of recurrent (cyclic) vomiting. *Pediatrics* 1960;25:775-80.

6. Reinhart J, Evans S, McFadden D. Cyclic vomiting in children: seen through the psychiatrist's eye. *Pediatrics* 1977;59(3):371-7.

7. Li B UK. Cyclic vomiting syndrome: a pediatric Rorschach test. *J Pediatr Gastroenterol Nutr* 1993;17(4)351-3.

8. Hammond J. The late sequellae of recurrent

vomiting of childhood. *Dev Med Child Neurol* 1974;16:15-22.

9. Lorber J. Causes of cyclical vomiting. *Develop Med Child Neurol* 1963;5:645.

10. Lang K. On the importance of central nervous damage in periodic vomiting in childhood. (German) *Mschr Kinderheilk* 1963;111(5):161-7.

11. Abell T, Chung H, Malagelada J. Idiopathic cyclic nausea and vomiting—a disorder of gastrointestinal motility? *Mayo Clin Proc* 1988;63:1169-75.

12. Sato T, Igarashi N, Minami S, et al. Recurrent attacks of vomiting, hypertension, and psychotic depression: a syndrome of periodic catecholamine and prostaglandin discharge. *Acta Endocrinol (Copenh)* 1988;117:189-97.

13. Rowe J, Shelton R, Helderman H, et al. Influence of the emetic reflex on vasopressin release in man. *Kidney Int* 1979;16:729-35.

14. Millichap J, Lombroso C, Lennox W. Cyclic vomiting as a form of epilepsy in children. *Pediatrics* 1955;15:705-14.

15. Hammond J. The prognosis for severe cyclical vomiting in childhood. In: Cumings J, ed. *Background to Migraine*. New York, NY: Springer-Verlag; 1973:chap 14.

16. Farquhar HG. Abdominal migraine in children. *Br Med J* 5-12-56; 1082-5.

17. Thompson W. The irritable bowel: one disease, or several, or none? In: Read N, ed. *Irritable Bowel Syndrome*. London: Gruen & Stratton, 1985:3-14.

18. Fleisher DR, Hyman PE. *Recurrent Abdominal Pain in Children: Seminars in GI Diseases*. Chicago, IL: WB Saunders. (In press)

19. Apley J. *The Child with Abdominal Pains*, Oxford: Blackwell Scientific Publications, 2nd ed., 1975:23-5.

20. Thompson W, Heaton K. Functional bowel disorders in apparently healthy people. *Gastroenterology* 1980;79:283-8.

21. Schuster MM. Irritable bowel syndrome. In: Sleisenger MH, Fordtran JS, eds. *Gastrointestinal Disease*, Philadelphia, PA: WB Saunders, 1993:930.

22. Sillanpac M. Changes in the prevalence of migraine and other headaches during the first seven school years. *Headache* 1982; 23:15-9.

23. Bille B. Migraine in school children. *Acta Paediatr* 1962; Suppl. 136:1-151.

24. Oster J. Recurrent abdominal pain, headache, and limb pains in children and adolescents. *Pediatrics* 1972;50:429-36.

25. Barabas G, Matthews W, Ferrari M. Childhood migraine and motion sickness. *Pediatrics* 1983;72:188-90.

26. Huttenlocher PR. Idiopathic epilepsy. In: Behrman RE, Vaughn VC, eds. *Nelson Textbook of Pediatrics*. Philadelphia, PA: WB Saunders; 1987:1288.

27. Thompson W. *The Irritable Gut*. Baltimore, MD: University Park Press; 1979:203.

28. Hockaday J. Migraine and its equivalents in childhood. *Dev Med Child Neurol* 1987;29:258-70.

29. Prensky A. Migraine and migrainous variants in pediatric patients. *Pediatr Clin North Am* 1976;23(3):461-71.

30. Jernigan S, Ware L. Reversible quantitative EEG changes in a case of cyclic vomiting: evidence for migraine equivalent. *Dev Med Child Neurol* 1991;33:80-5.

31. Mortimer M. The VER as a diagnostic marker for childhood abdominal migraine. *Headache* 1990;30:642-5.

32. Symon D, Russell G. Abdominal migraine: a childhood syndrome defined. *Cephalalgia* 1986;6:223-8.

33. Thompson W, Heaton K. Functional bowel disorders in apparently healthy people. *Gastroenterology* 1980;79:283-8.

34. Apley J, Naish N. Recurrent abdominal pain: a field survey of 1000 school children. *Arch Dis Child* 1958;33:165-70.

35. Lanzi G, Balottin U, Ottolini F, et al. Cyclic vomiting and recurrent abdominal pains as migraine or epileptic equivalents. *Cephalalgia* 1983;3:115-8.

36. Lanz G, Ballotin U, Fazzi E, et al. The periodic

syndrome in pediatric migraine sufferers. *Cephalalgia* 1983;(Suppl 1):91-3.

37. Lundberg P. Abdominal migraine. *Headache* July 1975:122-5.

38. Apley J. *The Child with Abdominal Pains.* Oxford, England: Blackwell Scientific Publications, 2nd ed. 1975;16-17.

39. Welch K. Migraine—a biobehavioral disorder. *Arch Neurol* 1987;44:323-7.

40. Mitchell W, Greenwood R, Messenheimer J. Abdominal epilepsy: Cyclic vomiting as a major symptom of simple partial seizures. *Arch Neurol* 1983;40:251-2.

41. Menkes J. *Textbook of Child Neurology,* 3rd ed. Philadelphia, PA: Lea & Febiger; 1985:534.

42. Mahony M, Kennedy J, Leaf D, et al. Brain stem glioma presenting as gastro-esophageal reflux. *Arch Dis Child* 1987;62:731-3.

43. Frank Y, Schwartz S, Epstein N, et al. Chronic dysphagia, vomiting, and gastroesophageal reflux as manifestations of a brain stem glioma. *Pediatr Neurosci* 1989;15:265-8.

44. Sarkari N, Bickerstaff E. Relapses and remissions in brain stem tumors. *Br Med J* 1969;2:21-3.

45. Bray P, Corter S, Taveras T. Brain stem tumors in children. *Neurology* 1958;8(1)1-7.

46. Huttenlocher P. Glioma of the brain stem. In: Berman RE, Vaughn VC, eds. *Nelson Textbook of Pediatrics,* 13th ed. Philadelphia, PA: WB Saunders; 1987:1320.

47. Lassiter K, Eben A, Davis C, et al. Surgical treatment of brain stem gliomas. *J Neurosurg* 1971;34:719-25.

48. Elder J, Duckett J. Dietl's crisis. In: Gillenwater J, Grayhack J, Howards S, et al, eds. *Adult and Pediatric Urology.* Chicago, IL: Year Book Medical Publishers; 1987:1555.

49. Koff S, Hayden L, Cirulli C, et al. Pathophysiology of ureteropelvic junction obstruction. *J Urol* 1986;136:336-8.

50. Homsy Y, Mehta P, Hout D, et al. Intermittent hydronephrosis: a diagnostic challenge. *J Urol* 1988;140:1222-6.

51. Kelalis P, King L, Belman A. *Clinical Pediatric Urology,* 2nd ed. Philadelphia, PA: WB Saunders; 1985:445.

52. Axelrod F. Familial dysautonomia. In: Gellis S, Kagan B, eds. *Current Pediatric Therapy,* 13th ed. Philadelphia, PA: WB Saunders, 1990:94.

53. Gonzalez-Heydrich J, Kerner J, Steiner H. Testing the psychogenic vomiting diagnosis. *Am J Dis Child* 1991:145:913-6.

54. Gryboski J, Walker W. *Gastrointestinal Problems in the Infant, 2nd* ed. Philadelphia, PA: WB Saunders; 1983:237.

55. Hendren W, Greep J, Patton A. Pancreatitis in childhood. *Arch Dis Child* 1965;40:1322-45.

56. Silverman A, Roy C. *Pediatric Clinical Gastroenterology,* 3rd ed. St. Louis, MO: CV Mosby Co, 1983:851.

57. Green M. *Pediatric Diagnosis,* 4th ed. Philadelphia, PA: *WB Saunders,* 1986:217-19.

58. Jahin Y, Stone A, Wise L. Mesenteric hernia. *Surg Gynecol Obstet* 1980;150:747-54.

59. Lee A, Bell R, Griffen W, et al. Recurrent appendiceal colic. *Surg Gynecol Obstet* 1985;161:21-4.

60. Silverman A, Roy C. *Pediatric Clinical Gastroenterology,* 3rd ed. St. Louis, MO: CV Mosby, 1983:851.

61. Anuras S, Anuras J. Clinical manifestations of severe gastrointestinal motility disturbance. *J Intensive Care Med* 1988;3:99-108.

62. Hight D, Hixson S, Reed J, et al. Intermittent diaphragmatic hernia of Bochdalek. *Pediatrics* 1982;69(5):601-4.

63. Til K. Subdural haematoma and effusion in infancy. *Br Med J* 1968;3:400-2.

64. Weil M. Infections of the nervous system. In: Menkes J, ed. *Textbook of Child Neurology,* 3rd ed. Philadelphia, PA: Lea & Ferbiger, 1985:322-3.

65. Coker S. Cyclic vomiting and the slit ventricle syndrome. *Pediatr Neurol* 1987;3:297-9.

66. Nowak T, James H. Migraine headaches in hydrocephalic children. *Child's Nerv Syst* 1989;5:310-4.

67. Linde L, Westover J. Esophageal and gastric abnormalities in dysautonomia. *Pediatrics* 1962;29:303.

68. Stackpole R, Melicow M, Uson A. Pheochromocytoma in children. *J Pediatr* 1963;63(2):315-30.

69. DiGeorge A. Pheochromocytoma. In: Behrman R, Vaughn V, eds. *Nelson Textbook of Pediatrics,* 13th ed. Philadelphia, PA: WB Saunders, 1987:1227.

70. Valenzuela G, Smalley W, Schain D, et al. Reversibility of gastric dysmotility in cortisol deficiency. *Am J Gastroenterol* 1987;82(10):1066-8.

71. Feldman M. Nausea and vomiting. In: Sleisenger M, Fordtran J. *Gastrointestinal Disease,* 4th ed. Philadelphia, PA: WB Saunders, 1989:227.

72. Berry G. Disorders of amino acid metabolism. In: Walker W, Durie P, Hamilton J, et al. *Pediatric Gastrointestinal Disease.* Philadelphia, PA: BC Decker, 1991;948-50.

73. Coates P, Hale D, Stanley C, et al. Genetic deficiency of medium-chain acyl coenzyme A dehydrogenase. *Pediatr Res* 1985;19(7):627-76.

74. Rezvani I, Auerbach V. Propionic acidemia. In: Behrman R, Vaughn V, eds. *Nelson Textbook of Pediatrics,* 13th ed. Philadelphia, PA: WB Saunders, 1987:292-3.

75. Sweetman L. Branched chain organic acidurias. In: Scriver C, Beaudet A, Siy W, et al, eds. *The Metabolic Basis of Inherited Disease,* 6th ed. New York, NY: McGraw Hill, 1989:795.

76. Stein J, Tschudy D. Acute intermittent porphyria. *Medicine* 1970;49:1-16.

77. Stacher G. Physiology of brain-gut interactions. In: Tache Y, Wingate D. *Brain-Gut Interactions,* Boca Raton, FL: CRC Press, 1991:281-3.

78. Ford CV. *The Somatizing Disorders.* New York, NY: Elsevier, 1983:232-231.

79. Richardson B, Engel G, Donatch P, et al. Identification of serotonin m-receptor subtypes and their specific blockade by a new class of drugs. *Nature* 1985;316:126-31.

80. Ireland SJ, Tyers MB. Pharmacological characterization of 5-hydroxytryptamine-induced deplorization of the rat isolated vagus nerve. *Br J Pharmacol* 1987;90:229-38.

81. *AMA Drug Evaluations,* 6th ed. New York, NY: J Wiley & Sons, 1986:272.

82. Puls L. A recurrent vomiting syndrome in children. *Contemp Pediatr;* Sept 1990:8-11.

83. Leppik I, Derivan A, Homan R, et al. Double-blind study of lorazepam and diazepam in status epilepticus. *JAMA* 1983; 249(11):1452-4.

84. Holmes G. Seizure disorders. In: Gellis S, Kagan B, eds. *Current Pediatric Therapy,* 13th ed. Philadelphia, PA: WB Saunders, 1990:75-6.

85. Axelrod F. Familial dysautonomia. In: Gellis S, Kagan B. *Current Pediatric Therapy,* 13th ed. Philadelphia, PA: WB Saunders, 1990:94.

86. Harris I, Wilkinson A. Magnesium depletion in children. *Lancet* 1971:735-6.

87. Vanderhoof JA, Young R, Kaufman SS, Ernst L. Treatment of cyclic vomiting in childhood with erythromycin. *J Pediatr Gastroenterol Nutr* 1993;17:387-91

88. McCallum R. Motor functions of the stomach in health and disease. In: Sleisenger M, Fordtran J. *Gastrointestinal Disease,* 4th ed. Philadelphia, PA: WB Saunders, 1989:675-713.

89. Waters W. Migraine and symptoms in childhood: bilious attacks, travel sickness and eczema. *Headache* 1972:55-61.

90. Ford CV. *The Somatizing Disorders.* New York, NY: Elsevier, 1983:1-2.

91. Reinhart J, Evans S, McFadden D. Cyclic vomiting in children: seen through the psychiatrist's eye. *Pediatrics* 1977;59(3):371-7.

92. Pearce J. Migraine: psychosomatic disorder. *Headache* 1977;17:125-8.

93. Ford CV. *The Somatizing Disorders.* New York, NY: Elsevier, 1983:256.

6

Functional Abdominal Pain
As Etiology of Recurrent Abdominal Pain

J. TIMOTHY BOYLE

Recurrent abdominal pain (RAP) is a popular descriptor that has evolved from the seminal definition by Apley of intermittent abdominal pain in children between the ages of 4 to 16 years which persists for longer than 3 months and affects normal activity.[1] Although the focal point of the disorder is abdominal pain, patients exhibit a broad range of symptoms. No standard diagnostic criteria have evolved from Apley's original description. Most physicians continue to dichotomize RAP etiologies into "organic" and "nonorganic." This approach is clearly inadequate, especially since the term nonorganic may imply a psychologic etiology. RAP etiologies are better classified into five broad categories: anatomic, infectious, noninfectious inflammatory, biochemical, or functional. Expression of pain from all causes of RAP may be influenced by both physical and psychosocial factors.

Functional abdominal pain (FAP) comprises a group of disorders that includes paroxysmal periumbilical abdominal pain, nonulcer dyspepsia, and irritable bowel syndrome (IBS). Although it is usually possible to classify a patient into a specific group, it is unclear whether the symptoms in the distinct groups have different underlying pathophysiologic mechanisms. Since the exact etiology and pathogenesis of the pain are unknown, and no specific diagnostic markers exist for any group, FAP is too often perceived as a diagnosis of exclusion.

The purpose of this chapter is to provide a practical approach to children with FAP by discussing epidemiology, possible etiologies and pathogenesis, clinical presentation, diagnostic approach, and management.

INCIDENCE

Recurrent abdominal pain that affects normal activity has been reported to occur in 10% to 15% of school-aged children between 4 and 14 years.[2-5] Another 15% of school-aged children may have paroxysmal abdominal pain lasting in excess of 3 months which either does not affect activity, or is not brought to the attention of a physician.[5] There may be a slight predominance towards girls in children with RAP, but data are sparse.

Prevalence figures for FAP are unknown. Functional abdominal pain is by far the most common etiology of RAP in children.

PATHOPHYSIOLOGY

It is not clear whether the different clinical presentations of FAP result from a heterogeneous group of disorders, or represent variable expressions of the same disorder. The frequent occurrence of upper- and lower-bowel symptoms in the same patient (particularly nonulcer dyspepsia and IBS in adolescents) suggest that the latter may be the case.[6,7] It is generally agreed that patients in all subgroups experience real visceral pain. There is no evidence that the pain is imagined, represents social modeling of parental pain, or is a means of avoiding unwanted experiences (eg, school phobia or malingering).

The prevailing viewpoint is that the pathogenesis of the pain and associated symptoms involves disordered gastrointestinal motility, or visceral hypersensitivity.[8] Motility disturbances have been described using manometric evaluation, measurements of intestinal transit, and surface electrophysiologic recordings. No characteristic motility disturbance has yet been identified for any of the subgroups of FAP. Studies in adults with functional bowel disease have described clusters of jejunal pressure activity and ileal propulsive waves that coincided with pain,[9] accelerated small- and large-bowel transit times in patients with diarrhea,[10] delayed small-bowel and whole-gut transit in patients with constipation,[10] and gastric dysarrythmia as well as delayed gastric emptying in patients with nausea and vomiting.[6] A few poorly controlled pediatric studies have described delayed intestinal transit,[11] exaggerated colonic motor response to pharmacologic stimulation,[12] and high-amplitude duodenal contractions[13] in patients with RAP. Only the latter study described a temporal association between abdominal pain and the motility disturbance.

Visceral hypersensitivity in patients with functional bowel disease is suggested by reports of enhanced awareness of balloon distention in all segments of the GI tract from the esophagus to the rectum.[8] There may be an increased awareness of normal motor activity in some adults with IBS because they describe abdominal pain during antroduodenal phase-3 activity of the migrating motor complex.[14] Although altered visceral distention thresholds may reflect a more generalized phenomenon of lowered tolerance for any kind of uncomfortable somatic stimulus, adults and pediatric patients do not differ in their tolerance to hand-immersion in ice water.[15,16] An altered threshold of gut-wall receptors, an altered modulation in the conduction of the sensory input, or a decreased threshold for pain perception at the central level may all contribute to visceral hypersensitivity.

Altered motor response or altered visceral sensation to gut distention caused by substances such as lactose, fructose, sorbitol, fatty acids, and bile acids may explain why some patients enjoy a qualitative improvement in pain symptoms when given stringent dietary restrictions.[10,17,18]

The fact that a wide variety of physical and psychosocial stress factors external to the gastrointestinal tract may trigger abdominal symptoms suggests that dysfunction of the extrinsic innervation of the gut may also contribute to the pathogenesis of the condition.[8] Dysfunction of the extrinsic innervation could originate within the motor pathways of the vagus, or within the central nervous system. Following cold stress, for instance, pupillary responses for FAP patients differ from those of controls, providing indirect evidence for such dysfunction.[19]

Nonspecific histologic inflammatory changes occur at all levels of the gastrointestinal tract in patients with functional abdominal pain.[6,7] Mild inflammatory changes may be the cause or the effect of altered intestinal motility. Immune responses change neural and endocrinal function. In turn, neural and endocrinal activity modifies immunologic function.[20] Activated immunocompetent cells such as monocytes, lymphocytes, and macrophages that take up residence in the intestinal tract may secrete a variety of cytokines and inflammatory mediators, which can lead to profound changes in enteric neural function. The possibility that some aspect of personality, behavior, coping style, or emotional state influences immune responses may also have implications.[20] The enteric or central nervous systems may modulate intestinal immune responses. Activation of the sympathetic nervous system causes leukocytosis, sequestration of lymphocytes, and inhibition of natural killer-cell activity.[21] Sensory neurons contain a variety of neurotransmitters and neuropeptides that can affect lymphocyte function, including substance P, vasoactive intestinal polypeptide, angiotensin II, calcitonin gene-related peptide, and somatostatin.[22]

Finally, the higher incidence of functional disorders in the parents of these children suggests a genetic predisposition.[1] The natural history of the disorder, however, suggests that development may also be a factor in the pathophysiology.[23,24]

CLINICAL PRESENTATIONS

A well structured medical history and physical examination usually indicates that functional abdominal pain is the likely diagnosis in a child presenting with RAP. The pain must be chronic with a duration in excess of 3 months. The logic behind this time requirement is the poorly documented belief that self-limiting motility disturbances follow a number of acute gastrointestinal inflammatory conditions, particularly viral gastritis and gastroenteritis. Children with FAP tend to exhibit one of three clinical presentations: 1) paroxysmal abdominal pain, 2) abdominal pain associated with symptoms of dyspepsia, and 3) abdominal pain associated with symptoms of IBS. The frequency of the various presentations in the pediatric population has not been well defined.

Chronic Paroxysmal Abdominal Pain

Isolated paroxysmal abdominal pain tends to occur in children less than 10 years of age. The pain varies in severity. Its onset is usually gradual. Pain episodes last less than 1 hour in 50% of patients, and less than 3 hours in the vast majority. Continuous pain has been described in less than 10% of patients. The patient may look well while vocalizing the presence of pain. During severe attacks, the child may exhibit behaviors such as doubling over, grimacing, crying, and clenching or pushing on the abdomen. Parents describe the child as miserable and appearing pale or listless during these episodes.

The child is usually unable to describe the nature of the pain (eg, stabbing, burning, dull). Even when asked to locate the point of maximal pain with one finger, the child will usually move his or her whole hand around the periumbilical area. Pain radiating to the back, chest, or legs is rare. The parent or young child is usually unable to describe a temporal relationship to meals, activity, stress, or bowel movements. The pain rarely awakens the child from sleep, but it is not uncommon for pain to occur in the evening, affecting the ability of the child to fall asleep.

Chronic Abdominal Pain Associated With Dyspepsia

The symptoms of dyspepsia in association with chronic abdominal pain suggest upper gastrointestinal tract dysfunction. Abdominal pain is often localized to the epigastrium, in the right or left upper quadrants. In younger children, however, pain is more likely to be periumbilical. There is often a temporal relationship between meal ingestion and symptoms. In some cases, the rhythmicity between food ingestion and symptoms may be delayed, resembling that of classical ulcer disease. In others, the pain develops immediately or shortly after eating and persists for 3 to 4 hours, stimulating gallbladder or pancreatic dysfunction. Nausea, heartburn (ie, a substernal burning discomfort which radiates cephalad), oral regurgitation, early satiety, postprandial abdominal bloating and/or distention, and excess gas with or without increased belching or flatulence are common associated problems. A history of occasional vomiting is not uncommon, but vomiting is not an important component of the clinical presentation.

Chronic Abdominal Pain Associated With Signs of IBS

The symptoms of IBS in association with chronic abdominal pain suggest colonic dysfunction. Abdominal pain is relieved by defecation, or associated with an irregular pattern of defecation including change in frequency or consistency of stool, straining or urgency, feeling of incomplete evacuation, passage of mucus, or a feeling of bloating or abdominal distention. Abdominal distention is a common associated symptom.

All three clinical presentations of FAP may include nongastrointestinal symptoms such as headache, pallor, dizziness, fatigability, urologic dysfunction, and gynecologic problems. Parents may report "fever" between 99° and 100° F.

In addition to the clinical features of the pain and associated symptoms, RAP is characterized by a constellation of historical features that facilitate recognition of the syndrome:

1. Concurrent physical or psychosocial stress factors. Examples of physical stress include viral infection, lactose intolerance, or menses. Psychosocial stresses can include death or separation of a family member,

physical illness or chronic handicap in parents or siblings, school problems, poverty, financial problems, or recent geographical move.

2. A positive family history for IBS, peptic ulcer, previous appendectomy, or migraine headaches.

3. A characteristic reinforcement response to the pain behavior by parents, school, and primary physician. Reinforcement responses include social attention, rest periods during pain episodes, missed school, medication, escalating diagnostic tests, and hospitalization. Parents characteristically respond to a report of pain by requesting that the child lie down on a couch or bed. Toys, TV, books, drinks, or food are provided for distraction. The parent will usually administer some type of symptomatic therapy—either tactile (eg, massaging the abdomen or using a heating pad) or medical (eg, acetaminophen, ibuprofen, or an anticholinergic agent).

DIAGNOSIS

The optimal diagnostic evaluation of the patient who presents with RAP remains controversial. Since most patients will have functional pain, optimal care is facilitated by approaching the diagnosis positively. Rather than a shotgun approach to rule out all potential infectious, inflammatory, structural, and biochemical causes, diagnostic evaluation should be driven by an index of suspicion based on pertinent red flags in the history and physical examination.

Chronic Isolated Paroxysmal Abdominal Pain

Table 6.1 lists the major differentials of chronic paroxysmal abdominal pain in children. The indicators in the history in patients with this presentation include pain localized away from the umbilicus, pain that interferes with normal sleep patterns, discrete episodes of pain of acute onset, pain precipitated by eating, weight loss, associated neurologic symptoms, and extraintestinal symptoms such as fever, rash, and joint pains. Physical findings such as abdominal mass, hepatosplenomegaly, joint swelling, lymphadenopathy, jaundice, ascites, costoverte-

TABLE 6.1 **Differential Diagnoses for Chronic Isolated Paroxysmal Abdominal Pain**

Crohn's Disease
Recurrent Partial Small-bowel
  Obstruction
    malrotation w/wo volvulus
    intussusception caused by
    Meckel's adhesions
Appendical Colic
  (Inspissated casts of fecal
  material within the appendix)
Neoplasia
Lymphoma
Carcinoma
Gynecologic Disorders
  Endometriosis
  Chronic pelvic pain following
    pelvic inflammatory disease
  Cystic teratoma of ovary
Musculoskeletal Pain
Renal Disorders
  Chronic pyelonephritis
  Ureteropelvic junction
    obstruction
Psychiatric Disorders
  Depression
  Somatization
  Anxiety
  Panic disorders
  Conversion reaction

bral angle tenderness, patulous anal tone, capacious stool-filled rectum, positive fecal occult-blood test, and perianal fistula, fissure, or ulceration are incompatible with a diagnosis of FAP, and require further evaluation.

Criteria for a positive diagnosis of FAP in patients who present with recurrent paroxysmal abdominal pain include a characteristic history, negative physical examination (except for abdominal pressure tenderness), and negative results of laboratory studies, including a complete blood count, an erythrocyte sedimentation rate, and urinalysis to screen for inflammatory bowel disease and urinary tract infection. A stool O&P (giardia, blastocystis hominis, or dientamoeba fragilis) and lactose hydrogen breath test should also be obtained. Lactose intolerance, parasitic colonization, and FAP are all common and may coexist. Lactose intolerance and parasitic infection should not be viewed as primary causes of paroxysmal abdominal pain in the absence of an altered bowel pattern, but rather as a physical trigger of pain symptoms. Often the primary physician will recommend elimination of dairy products from the diet to see if pain symptoms are affected. Parents may be over-diligent, however, subjecting their children to prolonged dietary restrictions even though no therapeutic benefit is perceived.

Endoscopy, barium contrast studies, ultrasonography, and CT scanning have no role in the diagnostic evaluation of the pediatric patient with isolated paroxysmal abdominal pain who fulfills diagnostic criteria for FAP. The most valuable diagnostic test in a patient with historical red flags is an upper-gastrointestinal series and small-bowel follow through. The x-ray request should specifically ask the radiologist to rule out peptic ulcer, malrotation, and Crohn's disease. Rare conditions such as lymphoma or pseudo-obstruction will also be picked up by an upper gastrointestinal series. Barium enema should be considered to evaluate the appendix in patients with chronic right lower quadrant pain. Filling defects, focal globular or diffuse distention of the appendix, or retained barium in the appendix 72 hours after contrast study should raise the possibility of appendical colic. Meckel's diverticulum should not be included in the differential diagnosis of chronic abdominal pain unless there are signs of obstruction or gastrointestinal bleeding. Abdominal ultrasound has a low diagnostic yield, but may pick up rare cases of uteropelvic obstruction, chronic fibrosing pancreatitis, hereditary pancreatitis, and cystic teratoma of the ovary. Benign ovarian cysts in adolescent females do not cause RAP.

Chronic Abdominal Pain With Vomiting and/or Dyspepsia

The presence of vomiting and/or dyspepsia in patients with chronic abdominal pain

TABLE 6.2 **Possible Diagnoses in Patients With Chronic Abdominal Pain and Dyspepsia**

Functional Dyspepsia
Gastroesophageal Reflux Disease
Peptic Ulcer
NSAID Ulcer
Helicobacter pylori Gastritis
Eosinophilic Gastroenteritis
Parasitic Infection
   Giardia
   Blastocystis hominis
   Dientamoeba fragilis
Bacterial Overgrowth
Crohn's Disease
Malrotation w/wo Volvulus
Lymphoma, Carcinoma
Chronic Pancreatitis
Chronic Hepatitis
Ureteropelvic Junction Obstruction
Idiopathic Gastroparesis
Biliary Dyskinesia
Intestinal Pseudo-obstruction
Psychiatric Disorders
   Depression
   Somatization
   Anxiety
   Panic disorders
   Conversion reaction

expands the differential to include diagnoses listed in Table 6.2. Unlike isolated paroxysmal abdominal pain, symptoms and physical examination do not distinguish functional dyspepsia from upper-gastrointestinal inflammatory, structural, or motility disorders. Thus, symptoms of dyspepsia generate a more extensive evaluation. A reasonable initial laboratory evaluation of this clinical presentation includes a complete blood count, measurement of the erythrocyte sedimentation rate, chemistry profile, stool O&P, urinalysis, and serologic evaluation of *Helicobacter pylori*. This will screen for eosinophilic gastroenteritis, inflammatory bowel disease, chronic hepatitis, chronic renal disease, parasitic disease, and *H pylori* gastritis. An upper-gastrointestinal series with small-bowel follow through is indicated in those patients with recurrent vomiting to rule out gastric outlet disorder, malrotation, and inflammatory bowel disease. Serum amylase, lipase, and ultrasonography are indicated where the history reveals discrete acute episodes of pain, triggered by a meal, or localized to the right or left upper quadrants. Ultrasonography will screen for gallstones, pancreatic edema/pseudocyst, hydronephroses secondary to ureteropelvic junction obstruction, and retroperitoneal mass.

The cornerstone of the diagnostic evaluation of chronic abdominal pain associated with vomiting and/or dyspepsia is upper endoscopy. By gross examination of the upper gastrointestinal mucosa, as well as selective histology and culture, upper endoscopy allows the consultant to rule out erosive esophagitis, peptic ulcer, *H pylori* gastritis, and bacterial overgrowth. The diagnostic value of identifying microscopic inflammation in the duodenum, stomach, or esophagus in the context of grossly normal-appearing upper gastrointestinal mucosa is less clear. Microscopic upper gastrointestinal inflammation is very common in pediatric patients with chronic abdominal pain and dyspepsia, probably approaching the 30% to 50% incidence described in adults with non-ulcer dyspepsia.[6] If the same therapeutic principles applied to patients with gross esophagitis or peptic ulcer are applied to patients with functional dyspepsia with microscopic inflammation, an empiric trial of H_2-receptor antagonists should be made for all patients prior to endoscopy. However, the diagnostic value of microscopic upper gastrointestinal inflammation is unknown. Such nonspecific findings have been described in asymptomatic adults as well as patients with IBS. A visually normal upper endoscopy, together with an appropriate negative screening evaluation, should allow a positive diagnosis of functional dyspepsia, thus facilitating long-term management. The consistent presence of central nervous system symptoms associated with RAP justifies neurologic consultation for evaluation of migraine, and urine porphyrin determination. The yield of such evaluation is low, however, in the absence of vomiting.

Criteria for a positive diagnosis of functional dyspepsia in patients with RAP and dyspepsia include a characteristic history, negative physical examination (except for abdominal pressure tenderness), a laboratory evaluation which includes a normal complete blood count, erythrocyte sedimentation rate, stool O&P, serology for *H pylori* (if available), and an upper endoscopy which reveals no gross evidence of peptic ulceration or *H pylori* (antral nodularity), or microscopic evidence of Crohn's disease, *H pylori* eosinophilic gastroenteritis, or reflux esophatitis. Mild histologic gastritis or duodenitis in the absence of chronic ingestion of nonsteroidal anti-inflammatory drugs (NSAIDS), gross peptic ulceration, and *H pylori* are considered nonspecific findings, and consistent with a diagnosis of functional dyspepsia.

Further evaluation of motility disorders such as idiopathic gastroparesis, biliary dyskinesia, enterogastric reflux, and pseudo-obstruction is only indicated in patients who do not respond to management strategies for functional dyspepsia.

Chronic Abdominal Pain With Altered Bowel Pattern

Table 6.3 lists the major differential of chronic abdominal pain associated with altered bowel pattern. The major red flags in the history include pain localized away from the umbilicus, pain that interferes with normal sleep patterns, diarrhea that awakens the patient from sleep, visible or occult blood in the stool, weight loss, and extraintestinal symptoms such as fever, rash, and joint pain. Red flags on physical examination include abdominal mass, joint swelling, positive fecal occult-blood test, or perianal fistula, fissure, or ulceration.

Criteria for a positive diagnosis of functional irritable bowel in patients with RAP and altered bowel function include a characteristic history, negative physical examination (except for abdominal pressure tenderness), a laboratory evaluation which includes a normal complete blood count, erythrocyte sedimentation rate, stool O&P x 3, *Clostrid-*

TABLE 6.3 Differential Diagnoses for Chronic Abdominal Pain and Symptoms Suggesting IBS

Inflammatory Bowel Disease
  Ulcerative colitis
  Crohn's disease
Intestinal Parasites
  Giardia
  Blastocystis hominis
  Dientamoeba fragilis
Lactose Intolerance
Complication of Constipation
  Megacolon
  Encopresis
  Intermittent sigmoid volvulus
Drug-induced Diarrhea, Constipation
Pseudomembranous Enterocolitis
Bacterial Overgrowth
Celiac Disease
Gynecologic Disorders
  Endometriosis
  Chronic pelvic pain following
    pelvic inflammatory disease
  Cystic teratoma of ovary
Neoplasia
  Lymphoma
  Carcinoma
Psychiatric Disorders
  Depression
  Somatization
  Anxiety
  Panic disorders
  Conversion reaction

ium difficile toxin (if chronic diarrhea and history of chronic antibiotic ingestion are present), and lactose hydrogen breath test.

Flexible sigmoidoscopy or colonoscopy is indicated for patients with historical or physical red flags to exclude inflammatory bowel disease, microscopic (lymphocytic) colitis, and collagenous colitis.[7]

MANAGEMENT

Functional abdominal pain can be considered an illness that refers to the subjective state of the child who is aware of not being well. The management objective of FAP is to prevent the illness from leading to social dysfunction. The management goal cannot be total freedom from pain and associated symptoms, but maintaining good physical health and normal activity for age. Consultants may be needed in selected cases to confirm the diagnosis, recommend or reinforce treatment strategies, or address suspected significant psychosocial disturbances.

Management begins with a positive diagnosis, education, and establishment of realistic expectations and consistent limits. Thus, for patients who positively fulfill the symptom-based diagnostic criteria described above, a diagnostic label can be provided with confidence. This is reassuring to the child, family, and physician, and can make extensive, fruitless searches for other diseases unnecessary. Explaining to patients and parents the suspected mechanisms for symptoms can also help them take control of their disease. It is important to emphasize that the pain is real, and is most likely caused by an increased intensity of intestinal motor activity in response to a wide variety of stressful psychophysiologic stimuli. The concept of visceral hypersensitivity can be used to explain why some children may experience pain even with normal amounts of stress. The potential genetic vulnerability in those families with a strong history of pain should be stated. The expected excellent long-term prognosis in terms of life-expectancy and major morbidity must be explained. The family should understand that the chronic nature of the illness requires long-term follow-up with the primary care physician.

The initial therapy for FAP is directed towards environmental and dietary modifications. The first goal is to identify, clarify, and reverse stresses that may trigger pain. Equally important is to reverse environmental reinforcement of the pain behavior. Parents and school must support the child rather than the pain. Lifestyle must be normalized regardless of pain. Regular school attendance is essential. School officials must be encouraged to be responsive to the pain behavior, but not to let it disrupt attendance, class activity, or performance expectations. At home, parents need to foster the child's independence in dealing with the pain.

Dietary modifications that may lessen symptoms include restriction of dairy products or lactase supplementation in children with documented lactose intolerance, or restriction of gas-forming foods such as legumes. Because of its safety, a trial of fiber is reasonable in all patients with FAP, although efficacy has not been proved. Synthetic fiber supplements such as methylcellulose, psyllium, and polycarbophil may cause less bloating than natural fiber supplements because of improved solubility, but long-term compliance is always a problem. Because other dietary carbohydrates may be malabsorbed and act as provocative stimuli of pain, restriction of excessive intakes of carbonated beverages (fructose), dietary starches (corn, potato, wheat, oats), or products containing sorbitol (eg, oral medication, gum or candy, toothpaste, gelatin capsules) is reasonable.

Drug therapy of FAP is controversial since there is no convincing evidence that any one of the three symptom complexes can be effectively treated. However, an individual patient may benefit from treatment directed at alleviating the predominant symptom. Oral anticholinergic agents (eg, dicyclomine or hyoscyamine) often provide effective pain relief, particularly if used on a prn basis in conjunction with dietary fiber. Since many patients are hypersensitive to anticholinergics, it's very important to start out with a small dose, and titrate up to an adequate dose. A therapeutic dose of the drug will cause dryness of the mouth. If anticholinergic medication is used for treating severe exacerbations of pain, a sublingual administration should be considered to provide more rapid relief. Patients with predictable postprandial abdominal pain may be helped by anticholinergic agents taken 30 minutes before meals so that maximal effect occurs when symptoms are expected.

For patients with irritable bowel whose predominant symptom is diarrhea, an antidiarrheal agent (eg, loperamide) or the bile-salt binding agent, cholestyramine, may be helpful.

Uncertainty exists about the efficacy of short-term therapy with H_2-receptor antagonists for mild nonspecific gastritis or duodenitis in patients with functional dyspepsia. Similarly, there are no data to support the use of drugs which enhance gastroduodenal motility (eg, metoclopromide or cisapride).[25]

Future therapeutic approaches should include agents that modulate intestinal activity by blocking visceral afferent pathway transmission evoked by several peptides and hormones. Theoretically, receptor sites located in the enteric nervous system, afferent nerves, or central nervous system could be blocked using cholecystokinin antagonists, serotonin antagonists, somatostatin, selected antimuscarinics, and opioid antagonists.[8]

Alternative therapies that may be beneficial include psychotherapy, hypnotherapy, and biofeedback. Consultation with a child psychiatrist or psychologist is indicated if there is extreme internalizing behavior (eg, anxiety, depression, or low self-esteem), modeling or imitation of family pain behavior, maladaptive family coping mechanisms, or failure of initial attempts at environmental modification to return to a normal life-style.

PROGNOSIS

There are no prospective studies of the outcome of FAP in children. Once FAP is diagnosed, subsequent follow-up rarely identifies an occult organic disorder. Interestingly, pain resolves completely in 30% to 50% of patients within 2 to 6 weeks after diagnosis.[23,24] This high incidence of early resolution suggests that in most instances child and parent accept reassurance that the pain is not organic and that environmental modification is effective. More long-term studies, however, suggest that 30% to 50% of children with FAP in childhood experience pain as adults, although in 70% the pain does not limit normal activity. Christensen and Mortensen[23] and Apley and Hale[24] report that the clinical symptoms in adults are more consistent with IBS. Thirty percent of patients with FAP develop other chronic complaints as adults, including headaches, backaches, and menstrual irregularities.[24] Based on a small number of patients, Apley and

TABLE 6.4 **Factors That Affect Long-term Resolution of Functional Abdominal Pain**		
Factor	**Prognosis Better**	**Prognosis Worse**
Family	Normal	"Painful family"
Sex	Female	Male
Age of onset	>6 y	<6 y
Period before treatment	<6 mo	>6 mo

(Reproduced with permission from Apley J, Hale B, 1973[24])

Hale have described several factors that influence prognosis for a lasting resolution of pain symptoms during childhood (Table 6.4).[24]

CONCLUSION

There are three distinct clinical presentations of FAP in children and adolescents: primary periumbilical paroxysmal abdominal pain, functional dyspepsia, and IBS. Adequate data support the view that medical history, physical examination, and selected laboratory or endoscopic evaluation allows a positive diagnosis of each type of functional disorder. Therapy, however, remains largely empiric, directed equally towards relief of symptoms and maintenance of normal activity for age.

REFERENCES

1. Apley J. *The Child With Abdominal Pains.* London, England: Blackwell Scientific Publications, 1975.

2. Apley J, Naish N. Recurrent abdominal pains: a field survey of 1000 school children. *Arch Dis Child* 1958;33:165-70.

3. Oster J. Recurrent abdominal pain, headache, and limb pains in children and adolescents. *Pediatrics* 1972;50:429-36.

4. Pringle MLK, Butler NR, Davie R. *11,000 Seven Year Olds.* London, England: Longmans, 1966.

5. Faull C, Nicol AR. Abdominal pain in six-year-olds: an epidemiological study in a new town. *J Child Psychol Psychiatry* 1986;27:251-60.

6. Talley NJ, Phillips SF. Non-ulcer dyspepsia: potential causes and pathophysiology. *Ann Intern Med* 1988;108:865-79.

7. Lynn RB, Friedman LS. Irritable bowel syndrome. *N Eng J Med* 1993;329:1940-5.

8. Zighelboim J, Talley NJ. What are functional disorders? *Gastroenterology* 1993;104:1196-201.

9. Kellow JE, Phillips SF. Altered small bowel motility in irritable bowel syndrome is correlated with symptoms. *Gastroenterology* 1987;92:1885-93.

10. Phillips SF, Talley NJ, Camilleri M. The irritable bowel syndrome. In: Anuras S, ed. *Motility Disorders of the Gastrointestinal Tract.* New York NY: Raven Press, 1992;299-326.

11. Dimson SB. Transit time related to clinical findings in children with recurrent abdominal pain. *Pediatrics* 1972;47:666-74.

12. Kopel FB, Kim IC, Barbero GJ. Comparison of rectosigmoid motility in normal children, children with RAP, and children with ulcerative colitis. *Pediatrics* 1967;39:539-44.

13. Pineiro-Carrero VM, Andres JM, Davis RH, Mathias JR. Abnormal gastroduodenal motility in children and adolescents with recurrent functional abdominal pain. *J Pediatr* 1988;113:820-5.

14. Kellow JE, Eckerly GM, Jones MP. Enhanced perception of physiological intestinal motility in the irritable bowel syndrome. *Gastroenterology* 1991;101:1621-7.

15. Whitehead WE, Holotkotter B, Enck P, et al. Tolerance for rectosigmoid distention in irritable bowel syndrome. *Gastroenterology* 1990;98:1187-92.

16. Feuerstein M, Barr RG, Francoeur TE, Houle M, Rafman S. Potential biobehavioral mechanisms of recurrent abdominal pain in children. *Pain* 1982;13:287-98.

17. Barr RG, Levine MD, Watkins J. Recurrent abdominal pain in children due to lactose intolerance: a prospective study. *N Engl J Med* 1979;300:1449-52.

18. Hyams JS. Chronic abdominal pain caused by sorbitol malabsorption. *J Pediatr* 1982;100:772-3.

19. Rubin LS, Barbero GJ, Sibinga MS. Pupillary reactivity in children with recurrent abdominal pain. *Psychosom Med* 1967;29:111-20.

20. Reichlin S. Neuro-endocrine-immune reactions. *N Engl J Med* 1993;329:1246-53.

21. Kiecolt-Glaser JK, Glaser R. Stress and immune function in humans. In: Ader R, Felton DL, Cohen N, eds. *Psychoneuroimmunology,* 2nd ed. San Diego, CA: Academic Press, 1991:849-67.

22. Carr DJ. Neuroendocrine peptide receptors on cells of the system. In: Blalock JE, ed. *Neuroimmunoendocrinology,* 2nd ed. Basel, Switzerland: Karger, 1992:84-105.

23. Christensen MF, Mortenson O. Long-term prognosis in children with recurrent abdominal pain. *Arch Dis Child* 1975;50:110-4.

24. Apley J, Hale B. Children with recurrent abdominal pain: how do they grow up? *Br Med J* 1973;3:7-9.

25. Talley NJ. Non-ulcer dyspepsia: myths and realities. *Aliment Pharmacol Ther* 1991;5:145-62.

CHAPTER 7

Chronic Intestinal Pseudo-obstruction

PAUL E. HYMAN

Chronic intestinal pseudo-obstruction (CIP) is a clinical diagnosis that is based on signs and symptoms of intestinal obstruction in the absence of a lumen-blocking lesion. CIP is composed of a heterogeneous group of enteric neuromuscular disorders, differing in genetics, pathophysiology, histopathology, extent and severity of symptoms, associated illness, and response to therapy. CIP is the most severe form of enteric neuromuscular disease. Mild CIP falls on a continuum of symptomatic and pathophysiologic abnormalities. Other enteric neuromuscular disorders, such as recurrent abdominal pain of childhood, functional dyspepsia, irritable bowel syndrome, and cyclic vomiting, are less severe but more common. To differentiate CIP from less severe enteric neuromus-

cular disorders, CIP can be operationally defined as enteric neuromuscular disease of sufficient severity to require special nutritional support (ie, tube feeding or parenteral nutrition) to maintain nutritional sufficiency at some time during its course. The most common signs are abdominal distention and failure to thrive. The most common symptoms are abdominal pain, vomiting, and constipation or diarrhea. The term "chronic idiopathic intestinal pseudo-obstruction" was first used to organize an approach to the care of children with this group of unexplained symptoms.[1] More recently, chronic intestinal pseudo-obstruction has been understood to represent conditions that vary widely in cause, severity, course, and response to therapy (Table 7.1). Examples of genetic het-

---

TABLE 7.1 **Heterogeneity of Chronic Intestinal Pseudo-obstruction in Pediatric Patients**

Onset	**Symptoms**
in utero	constant or intermittent
neonatal	vary in intensity and character
infantile	cyclic
acquired	
	Areas of Gastrointestinal Involvement
Presentation	entire GI tract
acute bowel obstruction	segmental
gastroesophageal reflux	megaduodenum
constipation	small bowel
chronic abdominal pain	colon
chronic abdominal distention	
	Pathology
Systems	myopathy
gastrointestinal disease only	neuropathy
hollow viscera (bowel & bladder)	absent neurons
GI involvement in generalized	immature neurons
autonomic neuropathy	degenerating neurons
associated with systemic disease	no microscopic abnormality

(Adapted with permission from Hyman PE, Di Lorenzo C, 1993[57])

erogeneity in pseudo-obstruction include a wide spectrum of abnormal gastric, small intestinal, and colonic myoelectric activity and contractions, as well as nerve and muscle abnormalities. In some ways, chronic intestinal pseudo-obstruction is an obsolete term because it is now possible to employ pathologic and physiologic techniques to differentiate the many disorders that cause the symptoms.

Although these diseases have distinctive pathophysiologic characteristics, they are considered together because their clinical features are similar. There is sometimes disagreement and confusion among physicians concerning precisely what constitutes a diagnosis of CIP. For individual communications, it may be better to provide a description of the patient and the clinical course, but grouping may help increase awareness of these rare conditions.

ETIOLOGY

Pseudo-obstruction may occur as a primary disease, or as a secondary manifestation of other conditions that may transiently (eg, hypothyroidism or opiate ingestion) or permanently (eg, scleroderma or amyloidosis) alter bowel motility (Table 7.2).

The majority of congenital forms of neuropathic and myopathic pseudo-obstruction are sporadic. That is, there is no family history of pseudo-obstruction, no associated syndrome, and no evidence of predisposing factors such as toxins, infections, ischemia, or autoimmune disease.

In a minority of cases, CIP may result from a familial inherited disease. There are reports of autosomal dominant[2,3] and recessive[4-6] neuropathic, as well as dominant[7-9] and recessive[10-11] myopathic patterns of inheritance. In the autosomal dominant diseases, expressivity and penetrance vary; some of those affected die in childhood, but those who are less handicapped are able to reproduce.

Pseudo-obstruction may result from exposure to toxins in utero. A few children with fetal alcohol syndrome and a few with narcotic-abusing mothers have neuropathic forms of pseudo-obstruction. Presumably, any substance that alters neuronal migration

or maturation might affect myenteric plexus development and cause pseudo-obstruction.

Children with chromosomal abnormalities or syndromes may suffer from pseudo-obstruction. Children with Down syndrome may have abnormal esophageal motility,[12] neuronal dysplasia in the myenteric plexus, and a higher incidence of absent submucous plexus (Hirschsprung's disease) than the general population. A few children with Down syndrome have a myenteric plexus neuropathy that is so generalized and severe that they

---

TABLE 7.2 Causes of Chronic Pseudo-obstruction in Children

Primary Pseudo-obstruction
Visceral myopathies
   sporadic
   familial
Visceral neuropathies
   sporadic
   familial

Secondary Pseudo-obstruction (related to or associated with recognized causes)
Muscular dystrophies
Scleroderma and other connective-tissue diseases
Postischemic neuropathy
Postviral neuropathy
Generalized dysautonomia
Hypothyroidism
Diabetic autonomic neuropathy
Drugs—anticholinergics, opiates, Ca^{+2} channel blockers
Severe inflammatory bowel disease
After organ transplantation
Amyloidosis
Chagas disease
Fetal alcohol syndrome
Chromosome abnormalities
Multiple endocrine neoplasia, type 3
Radiation enteritis
Munchausen's syndrome-by-proxy

(Adapted with permission from Hyman PE, Di Lorenzo C, 1993[57])

require special nutritional support. Children with neurofibromatosis, multiple endocrine neoplasia type 3, Russell-Silver syndrome, and other chromosomal aberrations and autonomic neuropathies may suffer from severe neuropathic constipation. Children with Duchenne muscular dystrophy sometimes develop pseudo-obstruction,[13] especially in the terminal stages of life. Esophageal manometry[14] and gastric emptying[15] are abnormal in Duchenne dystrophy, suggesting that the myopathy includes gastrointestinal smooth muscle, even in asymptomatic children.

Acquired pseudo-obstruction may be a rare complication of viral acute gastroenteritis, presumably resulting from viral injury to the myenteric plexus.[16] Cytomegalovirus infection of the myenteric plexus is associated with pseudo-obstruction.[17] Preliminary observations implicate E-B virus[18] and rotavirus[19,20] in the pathogenesis of CIP.

Very premature infants often have prolonged feeding difficulties, which may be related in part to immature motility patterns or to ischemia induced by a failure to meet the increased need for gastrointestinal blood flow after feeding. Some infants with bronchopulmonary dysplasia appear to have severe gastrointestinal motility abnormalities. Their preterm birth and stormy courses, including chronic hypoxemia and ischemia, are consistent with the development of pseudo-obstruction due to myenteric plexus injury or maturational arrest. Children may develop pseudo-obstruction after necrotizing enterocolitis[21] or gastroschisis, presumably for similar reasons (ie, local ischemia and neuronal injury or maturational arrest).

Abnormalities in immune function may have a role in the pathogenesis of pseudo-obstruction in some cases. Many affected infants and toddlers have food allergies. A few older children have pseudo-obstruction associated with autoimmune features such as persistently positive antinuclear antibody (ANA) or systemic rhabdomyolysis.

PATHOLOGY

Histologic abnormalities may exist in the muscle or nerve, or (rarely) both.[22,23] Normal histology is found in about 10% of appropriately studied cases. In such cases, there is perhaps an abnormality in some biochemical aspect of stimulus-contraction coupling.

When laparotomy is imminent for a child with pseudo-obstruction, timely communication between the surgeon and the pathologist is essential. Laparotomy is not indicated for biopsy alone[24] because a pathologic diagnosis usually does not alter management. When elective surgery is indicated (eg, for cholecystectomy or creation of a feeding jejunostomy), the plan should include full-thickness bowel biopsy, at least 2 x 2 cm in diameter. The tissues should be processed for histology, histochemistry for selected peptides and enzymes, electron microscopy, and silver stains of the myenteric plexus.[25] The histopathology of enteric neuromuscular disease is described in Chapter 22.

CLINICAL FEATURES

More than 75% of affected children develop symptoms by the end of their first year, and the remainder present sporadically through their first 2 decades. The number and intensity of signs and symptoms vary in individual patients, but it may be useful to note the relative frequencies within this population. Abdominal distention and vomiting are the most common features, with complaints in approximately 75% of patients. Constipation, abdominal pain, and poor weight gain are features in about 60%. Diarrhea is a complaint in one third. Urinary tract smooth muscle is affected in a few with visceral neuropathy, but in nearly all with visceral myopathy (about 20% of all pseudo-obstruction patients).

In Utero

Children with a visceral myopathy or neuropathy involving urinary bladder as well as gastrointestinal smooth muscle may be diagnosed by fetal ultrasound examination during the second trimester.[26] The urinary bladder is distended, but rather than oligohydramnios as expected for renal disease alone, the in utero intestinal obstruction is associated with polyhydramnios.

Neonatal

Approximately two thirds of infants with congenital pseudo-obstruction are born prematurely. Occasionally, a massively distended bladder draws immediate attention because the abdominal distention impinges on the diaphragmatic excursion and prevents effective respiration. In the megacystis microcolon hypoperistalsis syndrome, the bladder may be catheterized, or a vesicotomy may be created. Once the bladder is decompressed and the child is stabilized, the gastrointestinal component of the illness becomes apparent. As attempts are made to initiate feeding, there is vomiting, gastroparesis, and abdominal distention. Radiographs show dilated bowel loops and little or no transit, but no evidence of ischemic disease. In the first days, a contrast enema shows microcolon. The microcolon resolves and the colon may dilate as time passes and the luminal contents stretch the diseased bowel wall. Intestinal malrotation is common, and will frequently be the indication for exploratory laparotomy. Intestinal malrotation is found in both neuropathic and myopathic congenital forms of pseudo-obstruction. Of children presenting at birth, about 40% have a malrotation. In CIP, correcting the malrotation does not alter the symptoms, and prolonged postoperative ileus will result.[27] After weeks of unsuccessful attempts to initiate enteral feeding, a central venous catheter is tunneled to provide total parenteral nutrition (TPN). After months, TPN-associated liver disease, sepsis, and other acute intercurrent illness may threaten the lives of these children. About half die in the first year, usually from TPN-associated complications.

Preterm infants with prolonged respiratory distress or neonatal necrotizing enterocolitis often have subsequent feeding difficulties. Preterm infants are born with immature patterns of gastrointestinal motility, which would be characterized as neuropathy in adults, because nonpropagating clusters dominate after 28 weeks, and the migrating motor complex does not appear until approximately 34 weeks postconception. The feeding difficulties encountered by the recovering preterm infant may arise from aversion to oral stimulation related to prolonged orotracheal intubation, or to gastroparesis and gastroesophageal reflux related to immaturity of gastrointestinal motility.[28] Speculation about the origins of the "maturational arrest" of the myenteric plexus in the sick preterm infant include local ischemia and hypoxemia secondary to lung and heart disease that leads to neuronal injury, or nutritional insufficiency during a critical period of neuronal maturation. In infants recovering from neonatal necrotizing enterocolitis, or gastroschisis, there may be a postinflammatory fibrosis in the intestinal wall with consequent impaired contractility, leading to bowel dilatation proximal to the fibrotic segment.

Infantile

Infants with less severe, less apparent problems may be characterized as colicky, poor feeders, or spitters in the nursery, but are well enough to be discharged home. The mothers of affected infants become frustrated and anxious as their children fail to gain weight. Such infants repeatedly regurgitate, cry distressingly through the day as if hungry, but spit out the breast or refuse the nipple after just a few sips. Often, bowel movements are infrequent, and progressive abdominal distention is relieved by passage of large, hard feces. Sleep is fitful and rarely lasts more than a few hours. Their mothers become frustrated and fatigued as earnest attempts to nurture are foiled by the infant. Visits to the pediatrician are frequent, with repeated, futile diet changes. Viral upper respiratory illness or gastroenteritis often results in hospitalization for dehydration. Parent-child interaction problems are part of the differential diagnosis, but exclusive attention to family psychodynamics sometimes delays appropriate diagnostic procedures.

When evaluated by pediatric gastroenterologists, no distinctive diagnostic signs or symptoms are apparent. Contrast studies rarely show a dilated bowel at this stage. Upper endoscopy is normal, or may show esophagitis, a consequence of pathologic gastroesophageal reflux that is only part of a more extensive gastrointestinal disorder. Similarly, esophageal pH monitoring may demonstrate that reflux episodes correlate with emesis. Characteristically, gastric emptying of a complex liquid meal is delayed. Testing for giardiasis, metabolic, central nervous system, and urologic disease is appropriate because their symptoms may mimic enteric neuromuscular disease.

No distinctive clinical features differentiate the pathophysiology or predict the prognosis. However, antroduodenal manometry has been used to define postprandial duodenal hypomotility,[29] one discrete entity that occurs in infancy but spontaneously resolves within a few years. In infants with a pseudo-obstruction, the features of postprandial duodenal hypomotility are: 1) few antral or duodenal contractions for an hour following a complex liquid meal, 2) normal fasting antroduodenal motility, 3) symptoms worsen following fundoplication, 4) symptoms and manometric disorder resolve with cisapride, and 5) resolution occurs within the first decade. In 90% of children, the presence of the migrating motor complex (MMC) is associated with successful enteral feeding, while 90% of those without MMC require parenteral nutrition. When the manometric result does not correlate with the clinical presentation, it is prudent to consider a coexistent behavioral disorder in the child or family.

Munchausen's syndrome-by-proxy is a psychiatric disorder in which a parent—almost always the mother—overreports or produces illness in her child. The fabrication of the helpless child's illness is exclusively for psychologic reasons and never for external incentives. Munchausen's syndrome-by-proxy presents as a group of signs and symptoms that are not explainable by examinations and standard medical tests, and so may present as CIP—a rare clinical diagnosis without a specific diagnostic test. A number of case reports document factitious illness due to chronic poisoning with laxatives or emetics initially diagnosed as CIP.[30,31]

Although the characteristics and behavior of the mothers whose children have pseudo-obstruction or Munchausen's syndrome-by-proxy superficially appear similar (Table 7.3), several clues can help separate the two. In Munchausen's syndrome-by-proxy, the parent is focused on technical medical information, and sometimes seems more connected to the medical team than to the child. In most children, symptoms of pseudo-obstruction are present from birth. Late onset of symptoms unassociated with some documented acute illness (eg, rotovirus gastroparesis, meningitis) is uncommon, even within the spectrum of pseudo-obstruction. Pseudo-obstruction is usually associated with vomiting and constipation. Although diarrhea may be a consequence of either active secretion or bacterial overgrowth in pseudo-obstruction, it may also suggest emetine poisoning. Multiple central venous catheter infections with enteric organisms in the absence of a dilated bowel (which may predispose to bacterial transmigration) should suggest a factitious disorder.[32,33]

Munchausen's syndrome-by-proxy may

TABLE 7.3 **Similarities in Patient Histories in Pseudo-obstruction and Munchausen's Syndrome-by-proxy**

- Unexplained persistent or recurrent illness
- Very rare disorder as the primary diagnosis
- Experienced physicians state that they "...have never seen a case like it!"
- Investigations at variance with the health of the child
- Overattentive mother who will not leave the child
- Treatments not tolerated (IV lines get infected, drugs are vomited)
- Mother complains that too little is being done to help the child

(Adapted with permission from Reece RM, 1990[58])

be suspected when symptoms given by history are not confirmed with direct observation, or when the degree of disability is not consistent with the observed symptoms. Sometimes normal antroduodenal or colonic manometry is inconsistent with the history of disability. However, abnormal manometry does not exclude Munchausen's syndrome-by-proxy for several reasons. First, drugs given by the abuser to the child may induce abnormal motility patterns. Second, the presence of an intestinal neuromuscular disorder does not preclude a coexistent factitious disorder. For example, an older sibling may have Hirschsprung's disease and the younger may have symptoms due to Munchausen's syndrome-by-proxy. Although difficult to arrange, hospitalizing the child for observation in the enforced absence of the mother (or with continuous video camera monitoring) is usually required to confirm Munchausen's syndrome-by-proxy. It is unusual to document poisoning, either by direct observation or by toxicology of the child's body fluids. Documentation of overreporting and fabrication by the parent, together with a continuous period of health for the child following separation is diagnostic for Munchausen's syndrome-by-proxy.

Acquired

A gastroparesis associated with rotovirus is common.[20] Rarely, persistent postviral gastroparesis and pseudo-obstruction is found. It is not clear whether such illness continues as a result of persistent viral infection within the myenteric plexus, from antibodies to the virus cross-reacting with enteric neurons, or from some other pathophysiology. Adolescents may develop acutely psychiatric symptoms, pseudo-obstruction, and genitourinary problems simultaneously, with no apparent cause. Esophageal, antroduodenal, and colonic manometry are consistent with loss of inhibitory neural tone. Toddlers may develop prolonged gastroparesis after neurologically devastating bacterial meningitis.

Colonic

Hirschsprung's disease, the absence of neuronal cell bodies in the submucous plexus, is the most common cause of pseudo-obstruction, occurring in 1 of 6000 births.[34] Much less common are neuropathies in which the colonic neurons are present in the submucous and myenteric plexi, but are abnormal in morphology and function. Affected children develop chronic constipation in infancy, but upper gastrointestinal symptoms are minor or absent. In contrast to the signs and symptoms in functional fecal retention, stools are soft, extrarectal fecal masses are common, and encopresis is unusual. There is no effort to retain stools, but the abdomen may become distended.

Colonic neuropathy should be considered after a trial of mineral oil and behavioral modification fails to improve the symptoms, suggesting that functional fecal retention is not the cause. A diagnosis can be established with colonic manometry[35] or full-thickness colonic biopsies (examined by standard H & E and Smith's silver stains of the myenteric plexus) unless the areas studied are irreversibly dilated. It is possible that dilated fibrotic bowel will demonstrate no contractions, and histopathology may be altered as a consequence of cathartic use and voluntary fecal retention, perhaps in the absence of a primary motility disorder.

Colonic lavage may be useful to evacuate the stools and decompress the distended colon. Often, the colon becomes refractory to all medical management, and colectomy is considered. Unfortunately, in about 50% of cases the neuronal abnormality does not recognize anatomic boundaries, but extends some distance proximal to the ileocecal valve. In such cases, the ileostomy functions poorly after colectomy. Pseudo-obstruction may persist, and abdominal pain may become a dominant symptom. Repeated explorations for "adhesions" and further bowel resections increase the morbidity of this condition.

At present, there is no way to assess ileal motility in children, so that successful surgery cannot be predicted by preoperative testing. Silver stains of the myenteric plexus cannot be performed emergently, which means that an intraoperative decision cannot be made, as is done in Hirschsprung's disease. When considering surgery, the possibility of a cure must be weighed against the possibility that several surgeries will be required.

CLINICAL COURSE

During childhood, the majority of children with CIP experience a clinical course that is characterized by relative remissions and exacerbations. Many can identify factors that precipitate deteriorations, including intercurrent infections, general anesthesia and laparotomy, psychologic stress, and poor nutritional status.

The radiographic signs are those of intestinal obstruction, with dilated small intestine in one third of children, and microcolon in those who were studied because of neonatal obstruction.[36] Stasis of contrast material placed into the affected bowel may be prolonged; it is prudent to plan a means to evacuate the contrast fluid, or to use a nontoxic, isotonic, water-soluble contrast that will avoid the problem of barium solidifying and presenting a true anatomic obstruction. Children may feel well but still show radiographic evidence of bowel obstruction. A problem arises when children develop an acute deterioration. X-rays may demonstrate the same patterns of bowel obstruction that are seen when the child feels well. In children who had previous surgery, discriminating between physical obstruction related to adhesions and an episodic increase in the symptoms of pseudo-obstruction can be difficult.

DIAGNOSIS

Pseudo-obstruction is a commonly misdiagnosed disease in infants and children.[37] Despite its early and dramatic clinical presentation in many children, the time between onset and diagnosis has averaged about 3 years, because physicians mistakenly attribute the symptoms to more common conditions.

Special diagnostic testing provides information about the nature and severity of the pathophysiology. Manometric studies are more sensitive than radiographic tests when evaluating the strength and coordination of contraction and relaxation in the esophagus,

gastric antrum, small intestine, colon, and anorectal area.

Gastric emptying of a solid nutrient meal is the best test for gastroparesis. In severely affected children, gastric emptying of solids or liquids may be very delayed, and intestinal contents may reflux into the stomach.

Esophageal abnormalities are found with manometry in about 50% of those affected by pseudo-obstruction. In children with myopathy, contractions are low amplitude but are coordinated in the distal two thirds of the esophagus. Lower esophageal sphincter pressure is low, and sphincter relaxation is complete. When the esophagus is affected by neuropathy, contraction amplitude in the esophageal body may be high, normal, low, or absent. Contractions may be simultaneous, spontaneous, or repetitive, and relaxation of the lower esophageal sphincter may be incomplete.

Antroduodenal manometry is always abnormal in intestinal pseudo-obstruction that involves the upper gastrointestinal tract. However, manometry is often abnormal in partial or complete small-bowel obstruction. Although the manometric patterns of true obstruction may differ from those of pseudo-obstruction in adults,[38,39] such a distinction was not clear in children we have studied. Antroduodenal manometry should not be used as a test to differentiate true bowel obstruction from pseudo-obstruction. Contrast radiography and—as a last resort—exploratory laparotomy, are best for differentiating true obstruction from pseudo-obstruction. Once a diagnosis of pseudo-obstruction is established, manometry can determine the physiologic correlates for the symptoms, assess drug responses, and establish the prognosis.

Increases in intraluminal pressure are inversely proportional to the bowel diameter (LaPlace's law). Therefore, no contractions are recorded in dilated bowel, and manometry is not useful. The normal and abnormal features of antroduodenal manometry are illustrated in Chapter 12.

In most cases, the manometric disorganization correlates with the clinical severity and the anatomic lesion. For example, children with total aganglionosis have contractions of normal amplitude that are never organized into MMCs, fed patterns, or even bursts or clusters of contractions, but are simply a monotonous pattern of random events. Children with such a pattern are TPN-dependent. In contrast, there are children with normal MMCs and a normal phase 2-like pattern after meals who have abnormal nonpropagating bursts of contractions. These children usually eat by mouth, although they complain of bloating, pain, vomiting, and constipation.

Colonic manometry is abnormal in colonic pseudo-obstruction. Patients with neuropathic disease have no postprandial gastrocolonic response.[40] That is, contractions are normal in amplitude, but the expected postprandial increase in the motility index is absent. In those with myopathy, there are usually no colonic contractions.[35] The transit of luminal contents is often decreased.

Anorectal manometry is normal in chronic intestinal pseudo-obstruction. The rectoinhibitory reflex is absent only in Hirschsprung's disease.

Electrogastrography (EGG) is in its formative stages, but may prove to be a useful, noninvasive diagnostic tool for evaluating both children with pseudo-obstruction and their families.[41] Skin electrodes are placed over the stomach, just as surface electrodes are placed over the heart to perform electrocardiography. The electrical slow-wave rhythms of the gastric body and antrum are recorded. Gastric slow waves are normally within a range of 2.4 to 3.8 per minute. Gastric neuropathies are characterized by decreases (bradygastria) or increases (tachygastria) in the dominant slow-wave frequency (see Chapter 19).

Intestinal sensory neurons link pain to motility.[42] Pain and stress alter motility,[43] just as abnormal motility may cause pain. Further investigations into this area may provide insight into the pathophysiology of pseudo-obstruction in some affected children.

TREATMENT
Nutritional Support

The goal of nutritional support is to promote normal growth and development with the fewest possible complications and greatest patient comfort. In children with pseudo-obstruction, motility improves as nutritional deficiencies resolve, and worsen as malnutrition recurs. Failure-to-thrive is a consistent feature in children with serious untreated enteric neuromuscular disease.

Approximately 50% of affected children require enteral tube feedings. Bolus intragastric feedings may be useful for infants and toddlers who will not suck or drink, or for administering unpalatable nutritional supplements for older children. If gastric bolus feedings are associated with vomiting and pain, then continuous drip feedings may be more successful. If anorexia and early satiety do not improve after several months of optimal nutritional support, then a percutaneous endoscopic or surgical gastrostomy offers the advantages of easing nutrient administration and avoiding the need for repeated nasogastric intubations.

Most children with visceral myopathy and a few with neuropathy have a flaccid stomach and almost no gastric emptying. When oral feedings fail because of gastroparesis, feedings into the small bowel will be successful in some cases. If there is generalized bowel dilatation, jejunal tube feedings are not likely to succeed. Dilatation results in ineffective contractions, which prolong transit and lead to bacterial overgrowth. Using antroduodenal or jejunal manometry, the presence of the migrating motor complex in the small bowel predicts success of jejunal tube feedings.[44] Even in the absence of the migrating motor complex but no bowel dilatation, jejunal feeding is sometimes successful. Children with gastroparesis vomit frequently, and catheters placed through the stomach into the duodenum are often retched out of place. Catheter placements through the pylorus are difficult in dilated atonic stomachs. Therefore, a surgical procedure to create a jejunostomy 30 cm distal to the ligament of Treitz can be recommended for long-term use.

In approximately 50% of children with CIP, parenteral nutrition is required to achieve optimal nutritional support. Ninety percent of the deaths in children with CIP are caused by TPN-associated complications. In the absence of enteral nutrients, the gastrointestinal tract does not grow or mature normally.[45] In the absence of the postprandial rise in trophic and stimulant gastrointestinal hormones, there is bile stasis and liver disease.[46] TPN-associated cholelithiasis[47] and progressive liver disease are important causes of morbidity and mortality in children with pseudo-obstruction. The minimal volume, composition, and route of enteral support required to reverse or prevent the progression of gastrointestinal complications has not been determined. It seems likely that a complex liquid formula containing protein and fat, contributing 10% to 25% of the total caloric requirement is sufficient to stimulate postprandial increases in splanchnic blood flow and the secretion of trophic factors. Every effort should be extended to maximize enteral nutritional support in parenteral nutrition-dependent children. As children live through their first years, their rate of growth slows and caloric requirements decrease, so that some children eventually can be weaned from parenteral nutrition.

Drugs

Cisapride has helped a minority of children with pseudo-obstruction. Cisapride's mechanism of action is to facilitate the release of acetylcholine from the myenteric plexus motor neurons. Cisapride increases the number and strength of contractions in the duodenum of children with pseudo-obstruction, but does not initiate phase 3 of the migrating motor complex in patients without it, or inhibit discrete abnormalities.[48] Cisapride is the first drug to demonstrate consistent efficacy in some patients with CIP. Factors that predict improved symptoms with cisapride in children include the presence of the migrating motor complex and the absence of bowel dilatation.[49] Cisapride, which is not appreciably absorbed in the stomach, may be given through a jejunal tube with good absorption. Rectal absorption with suppositories is erratic. Doses for children range from 0.15 to 0.3 mg/kg/dose three or four times daily. Increasing the dose above this range

has not had greater effect.

A trial of cisapride is appropriate for most children with pseudo-obstruction. For children on TPN, the trial should be initiated when there is no acute illness and no malnutrition, and should be coincident with the initiation of enteral feedings three or four times daily. Side effects include gastrointestinal complaints and irritability, which are observed in about 5% of children. Uraticarial rash or urinary incontinence occur rarely.

Erythromycin, a motilin receptor agonist, appears to facilitate gastric emptying in those with neuropathic gastroparesis by stimulating high-amplitude 3 per minute antral contractions, relaxing the pylorus, and inducing antral phase 3 episodes at low, non-antibiotic doses of 1 to 3 mg/kg IV or 3 to 5 mg orally. Erythromycin does not appear to be effective for more generalized motility disorders.

Metoclopramide, domperidone, somatostatin, misoprostil, leuprolide, and acetylcholinesterase inhibitors have no proven efficacy in childhood forms of pseudo-obstruction.

Antibiotics are used for bacterial overgrowth, which is associated with steatorrhea, fat-soluble vitamin malabsorption, and malabsorption of the intrinsic factor-vitamin B_{12} complex. It is possible that bacterial overgrowth contributes to bacteremias and frequent episodes of central venous catheter-related sepsis, and to TPN-associated liver disease. Further, bacterial overgrowth, mucosal injury, malabsorption, fluid secretion, and gas production may contribute to chronic dilatation of the intestine. Chronic use of antibiotics may result in the emergence of resistant strains of bacteria, or overgrowth with fungi. Thus, the advisability of treating bacterial overgrowth cannot be generalized, but should be considered on an individual basis.

Approximately one third of children with neuropathic pseudo-obstruction have evidence of gastric acid hypersecretion or peptic disease. However, excessive gastrostomy drainage may result from retrograde flow of intestinal contents into the stomach, and not from gastric acid hypersecretion. Gastric secretory function or gastric pH should be tested before beginning antisecretory drugs. Histamine H_2 receptor antagonists may be used to suppress gastric acid hypersecretion. Tolerance develops after a few months of intravenous use,[50] so the drug should be given enterally when possible. If the drug is added to TPN, gastric pH should be assessed at regular intervals to monitor efficacy. Inducing achlorhydria is inadvisable because it will permit bacterial overgrowth in the stomach.

Constipation is treated with mineral oil, suppositories, and/or enemas. An enteral lavage solution works well in those with disease confined to the colon, but will cause massive distention in children with more proximal disease.

Pain Management

Chronic abdominal pain is a symptom in more than 50% of affected children.[51] The management of chronic visceral pain is facilitated by a multidisciplinary approach, with input from anesthesiologists and psychologists interested in pain management. Chronic visceral pain may emanate from areas of tissue damage, from peripheral nerves that have been sensitized by repeated stimulation or from central nervous system hypersensitivity (see Chapter 10). Therapy may be aimed at one or more of these causes of pain. For example, a gastrostomy for decompression may ease pain from distention, epidural anesthesia may alleviate the pain of visceral hyperalgesia, and hypnosis or guided imagery may minimize centrally mediated pain. Tricyclic antidepressants and clonidine seem to be useful adjuncts in some patients with visceral hyperalgesia. In children who cannot eat, amitriptyline may be given intravenously, and clonidine is administered via skin patch. A bedtime dose of amitriptyline can improve the acceptability of nighttime drip enteral feedings in many cases, perhaps by acting as a sedative and decreasing visceral hyperalgesia.

Opiates are not useful in the management of chronic visceral pain. Visceral hyperalgesia and central nervous system hypersensitivity are not affected by opiates. Opiates have unfavorable effects on intestinal motility, and narcotic withdrawal may simulate the visceral pain of pseudo-obstruction.

Surgery

One of the management challenges in pseudo-obstruction is the evaluation and re-evaluation of acute obstructive episodes. Although most episodes are pseudo-obstruction, it is important to recognize and to intervene when there is a true bowel obstruction, appendicitis, cholecystitis, or other surgical condition. Children with episodes of pseudo-obstruction undergo repeated exploratory laparotomies. It is especially important to avoid unnecessary abdominal surgery in children with pseudo-obstruction for several reasons: 1) they often suffer from very prolonged postoperative ileus; 2) adhesions develop, creating a diagnostic problem each time a new obstructive episode occurs; and 3) adhesions following laparotomy may distort normal tissue planes, increasing the risk for bleeding and organ perforation during future surgeries. After several laparotomies with no evidence of mechanical obstruction, the surgeon may choose a more conservative management plan for subsequent episodes, including pain management, nutritional support, and abdominal decompression.

Gastrostomy is the only procedure that reduces the number of hospitalizations in adults with pseudo-obstruction[52] and the experience with children seems to be similar. Gastrostomy provides a quick and comfortable means for evacuating gastric contents, and for relieving nausea, vomiting, and pain related to gastric and bowel distention. Continued "venting" may decompress more distal regions of the small bowel, eliminating the need for nasogastric intubation and analgesics. Decompression may be useful not only for symptom relief, but also for preventing irreversible luminal distention. Gastrostomy is used for enteral feeding and the administration of enteral medication. Gastrostomy placement should be considered for those receiving parenteral nutrition and for children who will need tube feedings for longer than 2 months. In many patients, endoscopic gastrostomy placement is ideal. In those with contraindications to endoscopic placement, surgical placement is appropriate. Care must be taken to place the ostomy in a suitable position, above the gastric antrum in the midbody. Gastrostomy may be used for continuous drip feedings in children who have anorexia, early satiety, or symptoms arising from bolus, but not drip, feedings.

Fundoplication is rarely indicated in pseudo-obstruction. After fundoplication, symptoms may change from vomiting to repeated retching due to outlet obstruction at the lower esophageal sphincter.[53] Repeated retching is usually a more distressing and incapacitating symptom than vomiting. In children with pseudo-obstruction, vomiting is reduced by venting the gastrostomy. Acid reflux is controlled with gastric antisecretory medication.

Results of pyloroplasty or Roux-en-y gastrojejunostomy to improve gastric emptying in pseudo-obstruction have been poor; gastric emptying remains delayed. Altering the anatomy rarely improves the function of the dilated fundus and body.

Small-bowel resections or tapering operations may provide relief for months or even years. However, if the pathophysiologic condition was present in other areas of the bowel, then these areas gradually dilate and the symptoms recur.

Colectomy is sometimes necessary in congenital pseudo-obstruction to decompress an abdomen that is so distended it impairs respiration. In children with diffuse enteric neuromuscular disease, ileostomies and colostomies are seldom useful for decompression. Colectomy is preferable to diverting colostomy because the likelihood for improving colonic function or medical treatment is negligible, and there is a risk of pain, bleeding, and malaise from diversion colitis.[54] Diversion colitis develops after a year or two of diversion of the fecal stream, and may cause symptoms of abdominal pain and tenesmus, signs of hematochezia, and predispose to transmural bacteremia.

Colectomy may be curative in children with neuropathic pseudo-obstruction that is confined to the colon. These children are unable to defecate spontaneously due to colonic inertia. Their pathology may show neu-

ronal dysplasia or maturational arrest, and their colon manometry is abnormal, with an absence of a postprandial increase in the motility index. Before surgery, antroduodenal and esophageal manometry should be performed to determine if the upper gastrointestinal tract is involved. Abnormal antroduodenal manometry is a relative contraindication to colectomy, because symptoms of upper gastrointestinal involvement—usually with a pain component—often follow colon resection. Sometimes antroduodenal manometry is normal when a neuropathy is present in the distal small bowel. This possibility complicates management decisions, because there is no test for evaluating ileal motility alone. In patients with ileocolonic neuropathy who undergo colectomy without symptom resolution, a second surgery may be required to resect the involved ileum.

An ileostomy or cecostomy may be placed for regular infusion of an enteral lavage solution. The infusion ostomy using a small "button" ostomy appliance has not yet been thoroughly evaluated. It may be an option for patients with colonic pseudo-obstruction who do not choose colonic resection.

Failing medical management may signal a need for total enterectomy. Rarely, a mucosal secretory disorder complicates the management of pseudo-obstruction. Several liters of intestinal secretions drain from orifices each day. When secretions cannot be controlled with opiates, anticholinergics, antibiotics, steroids, or somatostatin analog, it may be necessary to resect the entire bowel to avoid life-threatening electrolyte abnormalities and nutritional disturbances caused by the large volume losses. Enterectomy may be used to treat repeated life-threatening central venous catheter infections due to bacterial transmigration across stagnant dilated bowel loops. Total bowel resection should be considered alone or in combination with small-bowel transplantation.

Intestinal Transplantation

Successful intestinal transplantation holds the promise of lifesaving cure for children with TPN-dependent chronic intestinal pseudo-obstruction. In 1987, an intestinal graft functioned for more than 6 months in a recipient treated with cyclosporine, prednisone, and OKT3.[55] With increasing availability of the immunosuppressant FK506, more patients will undergo successful intestinal or combined intestinal and liver transplantation.[56] Some problems distinct from those of transplantation immunology will complicate postoperative management for some children with pseudo-obstruction. The gastroparesis present in all affected children means that oral or gastrostomy tube feedings will not succeed after intestinal transplantation. Venous access may be limited due to years of total parenteral nutrition. The liver may be cirrhotic, and a multiple-organ transplantation may be necessary. In fact, the timing of transplantation will be related to the onset of liver failure in many children with pseudo-obstruction. In those whose liver is functioning well, gallbladder and duct involvement with enteric neuromuscular disease may predispose to biliary tract complications. Urinary bladder function is abnormal in most of those with myopathy and a few with neuropathy.

CONCLUSIONS

Pseudo-obstruction is a rare condition. Appropriate evaluations and lifesaving treatments require extraordinary resources. Care for children with pseudo-obstruction should probably be limited to a few centers with personnel who have the time, interest, and expertise to coordinate optimal care for these children.

REFERENCES

1. Byrne W, Cipel L, Euler A, et al. Chronic idiopathic intestinal pseudo-obstruction syndrome in children: clinical characteristics and prognosis. *J Pediatr* 1977;90:585-9.

2. Roy AD, Bharucha H, Nevin NC, et al. Idiopathic intestinal pseudo-obstruction: a familial visceral neuropathy. *Clin Genet* 1980;18:291-7.

3. Mayer EA, Schuffler MD, Rotter JI, et al. Familial visceral neuropathy with autosomal dominant transmission. *Gastroenterology* 1986;91:1528-35.

4. Schuffler MD, Bird TD, Sumi SM, et al. A familial neuronal disease presenting as intestinal pseudo-obstruction. *Gastroenterology* 1978;75:889-98.

5. Haltia M, Somer H, Palo J, et al. Neuronal intranuclear inclusion disease in identical twins. *Ann Neurol* 1984;15:316-21.

6. Patel H, Norman MG, Perry TL, et al. Multiple system atrophy with neuronal intranuclear hyaline inclusions: report of a case and review of the literature. *J Neurol Sci* 1985;67:57-65.

7. Faulk DL, Anuras S, Gardner D. A familial visceral myopathy. *Ann Intern Med* 1987;89:600-6.

8. Schuffler MD, Pope CE. Studies of idiopathic intestinal pseudo-obstruction: hereditary hollow visceral myopathy—family studies. *Gastroenterology* 1977;73:339-44.

9. Schuffler MD, Lowe MC, Bill AH. Studies of idiopathic intestinal pseudo-obstruction: hereditary hollow visceral myopathy—clinical and pathological studies. *Gastroenterology* 1977;73:327-8.

10. Anuras S, Mitros FA, Nowak TV, et al. A familial visceral myopathy with external ophthalmoplegia and autosomal recessive transmission. *Gastroenterology* 1983;84:346-53.

11. Ionasescu V, Thompson SH, Ionasescu R, et al. Inherited ophthalmoplegia with intestinal pseudo-obstruction. *J Neurol Sci* 1983;59:215-28.

12. Hillemeier C, Buchin PJ, Gryboski J. Esophageal dysfunction in Down syndrome. *J Ped Gastro Nutr* 1982;1:101-4.

13. Leon SH, Schuffler MD, Kettler M, Rohrmann CA. Chronic intestinal pseudo-obstruction as a complication of Duchenne's muscular dystrophy. *Gastroenterology* 1986;90:455-9.

14. Staiano A, DelGiudice E, Romano A, et al. Upper gastrointestinal tract motility in children with progressive muscular dystrophy. *J Pediatr* 1992;121:720-4.

15. Barohn RJ, Levine EJ, Olson JO, Mendell JR. Gastric hypomotility in Duchenne's muscular dystrophy. *N Engl J Med* 1988;319:15-18.

16. Oh JJ, Kim CH. Gastroparesis after presumed viral illness: clinical and laboratory features and

natural history. *Mayo Clin Proc* 1990;65:636-42.

17. Sonsino E, Movy R, Foucaud P, et al. Intestinal pseudo-obstruction related to cytomegalovirus infection of the myenteric plexus. *N Engl J Med* 1984;311:196-7.

18. Vassallo M, Camilleri M, Caron BL, Low PA. Intestinal pseudo-obstruction from selective cholinergic dysautonomia due to infectious mononucleosis. *Gastroenterology* 1990;98:A400.

19. Amarnath RP. Post infectious transient gastroparesis. *J Gastrointest Mot* 1991;4:A570.

20. Bardhan PK, Salam MA, Molla AM. Gastric emptying of liquid in children suffering from acute rotaviral gastroenteritis. *Gut* 1992;33:26-9.

21. Vanderwinden JM, Dassonvill E, VanderVeken E, et al. Post-necrotizing enterocolitis pseudo-obstruction treated with cisapride. *Z Kinderchir* 1990;45:282-5.

22. Kirshnamurthy S, Schuffler MD. Pathology of neuromuscular disorders of the small intestine and colon. *Gastroenterology* 1987;93:610-39.

23. Lake BD. Observations on the pathology of pseudo-obstruction. In: Milla P, ed. *Disorders of Gastrointestinal Motility in Childhood.* Chichester, England: J Wiley, 1988:81-90.

24. Schuffler MD. Chronic intestinal pseudo-obstruction: progress and problems. *J Pediatr Gastroenterol Nutr* 1990;10:157-63.

25. Smith B. *The Neuropathology of the Alimentary Tract.* London: Edward Arnold, 1972.

26. Garber A, Shohart M, Darti D. Megacystic-microcolon-intestinal hypoperistalsis syndrome in two male siblings. *Prenatal Diagnosis* 1990;10:377-87.

27. Devane SP, Coombes R, Smith VV, et al. Persistent gastrointestinal symptoms after correction of malrotation. *Arch Dis Child* 1991;218-21.

28. Berseth CL, McCoy HH. Birth asphyxia alters neonatal intestinal motility in term neonates. *Pediatrics* 1992;90:669-73.

29. Hyman PE. Absent postprandial duodenal motility in a child with cystic fibrosis: correction of the symptoms and manometric abnormality with cisapride. *Gastroenterology* 1986;90:1274-9.

30. McClung HJ, Murray R, Braden NJ, et al. Intentional ipecac poisoning in children. *Am J Dis Child* 1988;142:637-9.

31. Feldman KW, Christopher DM, Opheim KB. Munchausen syndrome/bulemia by proxy: ipecac as a toxin in child abuse. *Child Abuse & Neglect* 1989;13:257-61.

32. Liston TE, Levine PL, Anderson C. Polymicrobial bacteremia due to Polle Syndrome: the child abuse variant of Munchausen by proxy. *Pediatrics* 1983;72:211-3.

33. Malatack JJ, Wiener ES, Gartner JC, et al. Munchausen syndrome by proxy: a new complication of central venous catheterization. *Pediatrics* 1985;75:523-5.

34. Kleinhaus S, Boley SJ, Sheran M, Sieber WK. Hirschsprung's disease: a survey of the members of the surgical section of the American Academy of Pediatrics. *J Pediatr Surg* 1979;14:588-97.

35. Di Lorenzo C, Flores A, Reddy SN, Hyman PE. Colonic manometry differentiates causes of intractable constipation in children. *J Pediatr* 1992;120:690-5.

36. Vargas JH, Sachs P, Ament ME. Chronic intestinal pseudo-obstruction syndrome in pediatrics: results of a national survey by members of the North American Society of Pediatric Gastroenterology and Nutrition. *J Ped Gastro Nutr* 1988;7:323-32.

37. Glassman M, Spivak W, Mininberg D, Madara J. Chronic idiopathic intestinal pseudo-obstruction: a commonly misdiagnosed disease in infants and children. *Pediatrics* 1989;83:603-8.

38. Summers RW, Anuras S, Green J. Jejunal manometry patterns in health, partial intestinal obstruction, and pseudo-obstruction. *Gastroenterology* 1983;85:1301-6.

39. Camilleri M. Jejunal manometry in distal subacute mechanical obstruction: significance of prolonged simultaneous contractions. *Gut* 1989;30:468-75.

40. Di Lorenzo C, Flores AF, Reddy SN, et al. Colon manometry in children with chronic intestinal pseudo-obstruction. *Gut* 1993;34:807.

41. Bisset WM, Devane SP, Milla PJ. Gastric antral dysrhythmia in children with congenital idiopathic

intestinal pseudo-obstruction. *J Gastrointest Mot* 1989;1:A53.

42. Mayer EA, Raybould HE. Role of visceral afferent mechanisms in functional bowel disorders. *Gastroenterology* 1990;99:1688-1704.

43. Fone DR, Horowitz M, Maddox A, et al. Gastroduodenal motility during the delayed gastric emptying induced by cold stress. *Gastroenterology* 1990;98:1155-61.

44. Di Lorenzo C, Flores AF, Buie T, Hyman PE. Antroduodenal manometry predicts success of jejunal feeding in children with chronic intestinal pseudo-obstruction. *Gastroenterology* 1993;104:A497.

45. Hyman PE, Feldman EF, Ament ME, et al. Effect of enteral feeding on the maintenance of gastric acid secretory function. *Gastroenterology* 1983;84:341-5.

46. Dahms BB, Halpin TC Jr. Serial liver biopsies in parenteral nutrition-associated cholestasis of early infancy. *Gastroenterology* 1981;81:136-44

47. Roslyn JJ, Berquist WE, Pitt HA, et al. Increased risk of gallstones in children receiving total parenteral nutrition. *Pediatrics* 1983;71:784-9.

48. Di Lorenzo C, Reddy SN, Villanueva-Meyer J, et al. Cisapride in children with chronic intestinal pseudo-obstruction: an acute, double-blind cross-over placebo controlled trial. *Gastroenterology* 1991;101:1564-70.

49. Hyman PE, Di Lorenzo C, McAdams L, et al. Predicting the clinical response to cisapride in children with chronic intestinal pseudo-obstruc-tion. *Am J Gastroenterol* 1993:88;832-6.

50. Hyman PE, Garvey TQ, Abrams CE. Tolerance to intravenous ranitidine. *J Pediatr* 1987;110:794-6.

51. Hyman PE, Fiske ME, Di Lorenzo C, Diego A. North American Pediatric Pseudo-Obstruction Society (NAPPS) Survey. *Pediatr Res* 1993;31:108A.

52. Pitt HA, Mann LL, Berquist WE, et al. Chronic intestinal pseudo-obstruction: management with total parenteral nutrition and a venting enterostomy. *Arch Surg* 1985;120:614-18.

53. Di Lorenzo C, Flores A, Hyman PE. Intestinal motility in symptomatic children with fundoplication. *J Ped Gastro Nutr* 1991:12:169-73.

54. Ordein J, Di Lorenzo C, Flores A, Hyman PE. Diversion colitis in children with pseudo-obstruction. *Am J Gastroenterol* 1992;87:88-90.

55. Starzl TE, Rowe M, Todo S, et al. Transplantation of multiple abdominal viscera. *JAMA* 1989;26:1449-57.

56. Starzl TE, Todo S, Tzakis A, Fung J. The transplantation of gastrointestinal organs. *Gastroenterology* 1993;104:673-9.

57. Hyman PE, Di Lorenzo C. Chronic intestinal pseudo-obstruction. In: Wyllie R, Hymans JS, eds. *Pediatric Gastrointestinal Disease.* Philadelphia, PA: WB Saunders, 1993:641.

58. Reece RM. Unusual manifestations of child abuse. *Pediatr Clin North Am* 1990;37:905-21.

CHAPTER

8

Constipation

CARLO DI LORENZO

Constipation is variously defined on the basis of the frequency of defecation, the discomfort in passing stools, the delayed intestinal transit, and the weight of the stools. Patients complaining of constipation can describe stools that are too small, too big, too painful or difficult to expel, too infrequent, or which result in a feeling of incomplete evacuation after defecation. It is important to remember when discussing bowel habits that "normal" is not necessarily what most people do, and that the complaint of constipation should not be regarded in terms of epidemiology but as a state of well-being. Thus, every complaint of constipation—even within the "normal" range—should be addressed.[1]

The parameter most often used to define constipation in children is the frequency of defecation, which declines with age. In infants, the average number of bowel movements is approximately four per day at 1 week of age, with 97% of infants having between one and nine bowel movements per day during the first week of life.[2] Of 240 infants studied between 2 and 20 weeks of life, half of whom were fed breast milk and half of whom received cow's milk formula, 93% had between one and seven bowel movements per day.[3] Between the ages of 1 and 4 years, 85% of children defecate once or twice each day.

In Western countries, young adults have at least three bowel movements per week, with males defecating more often than females and whites more often than blacks.[1] Stool frequency correlates with gastrointestinal transit time. Mean intestinal transit time increases with age.[4] It is approximately 8.5 hours between 1 to 3 months of age, 16 hours from 4 to 24 months of age, and 26 hours between 3 and 13 years of age.[5,6] After puberty, transit times range from 30 to 48 hours. Determining total gastrointestinal transit time (ie, time needed for an ingested substance to appear in the stools) provides an objective measure of the severity of constipation in children. In one study, all the children with fewer than four defecations per week had a transit time of more than 33 hours, significantly slower than those with a normal frequency of defecation.[7] Weight and consistency of the stools are parameters which strongly correlate with the diet, are more difficult to quantify, and are rarely relied on in the evaluation of constipation in children.

Depending on the definition, 5% to 20% of the general population is constipated.[1] Constipation is the chief complaint in 3% of all pediatric outpatient visits,[8] and up to 25% of children referred to pediatric gastroenterologists have a disorder of defecation.[9] The ratio of females to males varies along the life span (Fig. 8.1). Young boys are more often constipated than young girls, but a reversal of the ratio occurs after puberty when women are much more often constipated than men.[1,10,11] In children, constipation is equally distributed among different social classes and there is no relation to family size, age of the parents, or ordinal position of the child in the family.[12] The incidence of constipation increases when a parent, sibling, or twin is constipated. It is four times more common in monozygotic than in dizygotic twins.[13]

Constipation is a symptom; it is not a disease, nor is it a sign. As a symptom, constipation can be caused by many different disorders. Organic disorders can cause constipation, although only a minority of children have organic or anatomic causes for constipation. The majority of children with constipation have functional or behavioral problems as the cause. In fact, in contrast to the high incidence of constipation in the pediatric population, the incidence of Hirschsprung's disease is only 1 in 6000 births and it is found in fewer than 1% of children presenting for the first time with constipation.[14] The incidence of anorectal malformations is 1 in 7000 births. Other organic causes of constipation in children are even more unusual. Table 8.1 summarizes most of the organic causes of constipation in children.

NONORGANIC CAUSES OF CONSTIPATION

Some breast-fed infants may produce stool as infrequently as every 5 to 20 days. In the absence of abdominal distention or other gastrointestinal symptoms, these children do not require any treatment. The frequency of bowel movements increases spontaneously, or when different milk formulas or solid foods are introduced into the diet. Some older children, apparently for constitutional reasons, pass large stools at intervals of 3 or 4 days. They do not develop stool retention, do not have soiling, and have no other symptoms. They also do not require treatment and will continue to have infrequent defecation throughout their lives without any distress.[15]

Three nonorganic clinical syndromes are

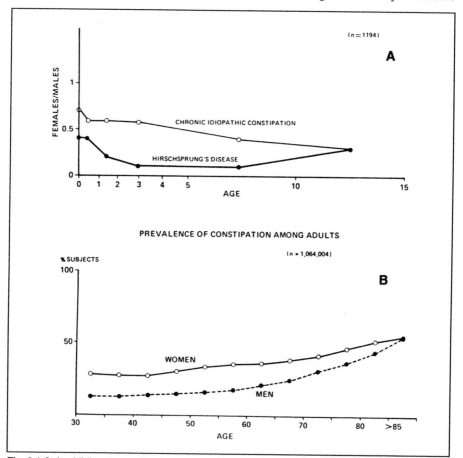

Fig. 8.1 **A**, In childhood, constipation is more common among boys than girls. **B**, In adulthood, it is more common among women. (Reprinted with permission from Devroede G, 1989[1])

TABLE 8.1 Organic Causes of Constipation in Children

Anatomic
  Anorectal malformations
    imperforate anus, anal stenosis,
    anterior displaced anus
  Acquired colonic strictures
    IBD, NEC

Metabolic
  Hypothyroidism
  Hypercalcemia
  Hypokalemia
  Multiple endocrine neoplasia
    type 2b
  Cystic fibrosis
  Diabetes mellitus

Neuropathic Conditions
  Spina bifida
  Myelomeningocele
  Spinal cord trauma
  von Recklinghausen's disease

Congenital Intestinal Nerve or Muscle Disorders
  Hirschsprung's disease
  Intestinal neuronal dysplasia
  Visceral myopathies
  Visceral neuropathies
    maturational arrest of
    myenteric plexus

Abnormal Abdominal Musculature
  Prune belly
  Gastroschisis
  Down syndrome

Connective Tissue Disorders
  Scleroderma
  Lupus erythematosus
  Amyloidosis

Drugs
  Opiates, sucralfate, antacids, anti-
    hypertensives
  Anticholinergics, tricyclic antide-
    pressants, sympathomimetics

Other
  Heavy-metal ingestion
  Vitamin D intoxication
  Botulism

associated with a presenting complaint of constipation in infants and children: 1) the grunting, purple-faced baby; 2) infant dyschesia; and 3) functional fecal retention.

Grunting Baby Syndrome

In the grunting baby syndrome, the parents of the affected child imagine that the act of defecation is associated with great effort for their infant. The infant is most commonly between 1 and 10 weeks old. Distressed parents describe a child with a red or purple face, straining for several minutes with agonizing cries. Crying may persist for 5 or 10 minutes before stool is produced. The stools, however, are soft and normal in appearance, and occur every day. After defecation, the baby appears comfortable again. The grunting baby is an infant who knows how to increase abdominal pressure by crying, but has not learned how to coordinate the increase in intra-abdominal pressure with relaxation of the pelvic floor to allow easy passage of stool. The grunting baby needs no treatment, but the parents of these infants require effective reassurance. Parents must be informed that infants will gradually learn to relax the pelvic floor to allow passage of stool. The learning process occurs faster in some newborns than in others, but always in the first few months of life. Parents are usually grateful that the physician recognizes a healthy child, and that there will be no need to perform tests on their newborn. It is important to emphasize that the use of enemas or suppositories is not indicated for this problem and should be discouraged for several reasons. First, manipulation of the anus may be painful or frightening to a child, and so further discourage defecation. Second, learning to defecate in a normal way takes practice, and interruptions in that practice may delay the learning process. After repetitive manipulations of the anal area, the infant may become fearful of defecation or learn that external intervention is required to pass stools.

Infant Dyschesia

Infants with dyschesia experience painful defecation as they pass firm pelletlike or highly segmented stools. This pattern often begins at weaning, when there is a change from breast milk to formula or cow's milk. Dyschesia is treated by softening the stools to ensure painless defecation. This may be accomplished by adding more fruit juices or prunes to the diet, or by using an osmotically active nonabsorbable sugar (eg, lactulose or Karo syrup), milk of magnesia, or mineral oil in emulsifier mixed with the milk or formula. Increasing the fiber content by adding whole grains, fruits, and vegetables to the diet or giving the children bulk-forming agents (eg, methylcellulose, malt soup extract, or psyllium) can also improve this condition.[16] Toddlers with dyschesia are at high risk for developing the third and most common cause of nonorganic disorder of defecation—functional fecal retention. Greater than half of school-age children with encopresis or fecal impaction had histories of painful defecation before 3 years of age.[17]

Functional Fecal Retention

Functional fecal retention is the most common chronic disorder of defecation in children, and may be responsible for nearly 25% of all visits to pediatric gastroenterologists. Functional fecal retention has been called psychogenic megacolon, or idiopathic or retentive constipation. The clinical features are listed in Table 8.2. Functional fecal retention is caused by fear of defecation and the voluntary withholding of stool. Children who suffer from functional fecal retention display retentive posturing. Instead of relaxing the pelvic floor during the Valsalva maneuver so that stool might pass, they contract the gluteal muscles in an attempt to avoid defecation. They consistently make a conscious decision to postpone defecation.

A child develops functional fecal retention when defecatory activities are associated with pain and fear. A history of magical thinking can often be found in toddlers with retentive soiling. The children imagine that painful stools are alive and dangerous. Also, an episode of painful defecation might elicit a response such as, "I'm never doing that again." Less commonly, the toddler fears the toilet. Functional fecal retention has been initiated by a television fantasy about a toilet bowl that swallowed people,[18] and after a child was frightened by seeing his mother's colostomy.[19] Fecal retention was found in a family with reflex seizures triggered by stimulation of the anoderm during defecation or wiping of the perineal area.[20]

There seem to be two peaks in the incidence of functional fecal retention. The first is during toilet training, and the second occurs when a child begins to attend a school

---

TABLE 8.2 Clinical Features of Functional Fecal Retention

- Symptoms begin after the first year of life
- Passage of enormous stools at intervals of 1 week or more
- Obstruction of the toilet by the stools
- Symptoms due to increasing fecal accumulation
  retentive posturing
  soiling
  irritability
  abdominal pain
  anorexia
- Dramatic disappearance of symptoms following passage of the enormous stool
- Behavior indicative of the child's irrational effort to cope with the soiling
  nonchalant attitude regarding soiling
  hiding of soiled underwear
  lack of awareness of soilage

(Reprinted with permission from Hyman PE, Fleisher D, 1992[14])

that does not permit trips to the lavatory as necessary, but only during specific times. During toilet training, the automatic, involuntary process of defecation becomes a voluntary act associated with morality and taboos at a time when patterns of behavior are labile and easily distorted. Attempts to accomplish toilet training at an inappropriately early age, coercive attitudes toward rectal continence, and placement of a high love premium on a perfect daily performance can cause the child to decide to "hold back."[21] In the older child, school, games, television, and social life can all detract from the need to defecate.[21] Children who defecate at home during the morning may decide on entering school to withhold defecation until they are back in the privacy of their own homes.

Functional fecal retention may be thought of as a maladaptive response of overcontrol. Educating both the child and parents about the act of defecation is the cornerstone to effective treatment. Figure 8.2 may be used to explain the normal act of defecation as well as the events during functional fecal retention. When a child decides not to have a bowel movement, a fecal mass accumulates in his rectum. Pain and fear prevent the effective relaxation of the pelvic floor muscles. The child may grunt and turn red in the face, but instead of relaxing the pelvic floor muscles during the Valsalva maneuver so that the stool may pass, the child contracts the pelvic floor muscles, buttocks, and thighs. The child may stand stiffly with a preoccupied facial expression, move around on tiptoes with stiff legs, or sit on his buttocks with his heels pressed against the perineum.[14]

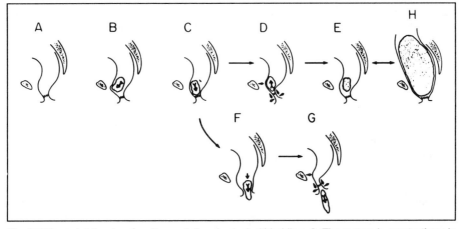

Fig. 8.2 Normal defecatory function and chronic stool withholding. **A,** The rectum is empty; there is no urge to defecate. The internal anal sphincter is closed. The resting tone of the pelvic floor muscles holds the sides of the anal canal in apposition, keeping it closed. **B,** Stool enters the rectum and presses on the rectal wall, causing a sensation of fullness. **C,** Distention of the rectal wall causes reflex relaxation of the internal anal sphincter, allowing the stool to descend into contact with the upper end of the anal canal. This causes conscious awareness that passage of stool is imminent. **D,** The pelvic floor muscles contract to maintain continence, moving the stool upwards. **E,** If the stool remains in this higher location after the pelvic floor returns to its resting tone, stool will no longer be in contact with the anoderm. Accommodation by the smooth muscle lessens rectal wall tension and the urge to defecate abates. **F,** Defecation occurs when the pelvic floor relaxes below the level of resting tone; this opens the anal canal to intrarectal pressure. The accompanying Valsalva maneuver propels the stool down the short, wide anal canal. **G,** An automatic contraction of the pelvic floor occurs when the stool is no longer in contact with the upper end of the anal canal, and this propulsive force expels the stool completely. **H,** If a child repeatedly responds to the defecatory urge by withholding (**C-D**), a fecal mass accumulates. It becomes more difficult to pass, especially if it is too firm to be extruded without painful stretching of the anal opening. It is too bulky to be shifted upwards, out of contact with the anoderm. As the pelvic floor muscles fatigue, anal closure becomes less competent and retentive fecal soiling with soft or liquid stool occurs. The child resorts to retentive posturing, attempting to preserve continence by vigorous contraction of gluteal muscles. (Reprinted with permission from Hyman PE, Fleisher D, 1992[14])

This experience may confuse parents, who insist that the child is "trying," when, in fact, the necessary pelvic floor relaxation is absent. As stools accumulate, mood and appetite deteriorate. The child complains of abdominal pain and experiences abdominal distention. Soiling may occur, especially during passage of flatus, due to the child's inability to control the overflow of stools. The parents often misinterpret the soiling as diarrhea and administer antidiarrheal agents, which worsen the constipation. This loss of control over defecation frightens the child and the parents. The parents often become angry and punish the child because they believe he is consciously responsible for soiling his underwear. The child may try to hide the soiling from his parents, assuming a nonchalant attitude about the resulting odor. The parents fail to realize that because the olfactory sensory apparatus accommodates to persistent smells and people have limited awareness of their own body odors, children with chronic incontinence are unaware of their offensive odor.[4] These children begin to believe they have a secret problem that no one else can understand. The longer this problem persists, the greater the risk that the child will develop a negative self-image, feeling "stinky" and "rotten inside."

The fear of pain may be caused by past experience with the passage of hard stools, an anal fissure, or from less common but even more important acute treatable sources, such as Group A beta hemolytic streptococcal perianal infection.[22,23] Sexual abuse with anal penetration is another important cause of painful defecation resulting in functional fecal retention. It should be suspected especially when there is a sudden onset of constipation. Occasionally, there will be large fissures, patulous anal sphincter, or venereal warts that suggest, but are not diagnostic for, sexual trauma.[24,25] The patulous anus may result from the large stool retained just above the anal verge, as well as from trauma. It is important to recognize that soiling exposes the perianal skin to liquid stools for prolonged periods, causing maceration and hyperkeratosis. The lesions caused by chronic soiling are called perianal pseudoverrucous papules and nodules, and must be differentiated from venereal warts and other dermatitis to avoid unnecessary diagnostic tests and therapy.[26]

A careful history that elicits characteristic behaviors, and a physical examination consistent with functional fecal retention may be the only evaluations that are required. Often the fecal accumulation filling the dilated rectum is appreciated by bimanual palpation as a mass on either side of the rectus sheath. The perianal area should be inspected after the child has been reassured that there will no "pokes" or pain. Painful procedures may be counterproductive to establishing a therapeutic doctor-patient relationship. Important findings on physical examination include the presence or absence of fecal soiling, dermatitis, perianal pseudoverrucous papules and nodules, a patulous anus, a rectoperineal fistula, an anteriorly placed anus, and vascular, pigmented, or hairy patches over the lumbosacral spine that suggest occult spinal dysraphism.[27] When the child is old enough to cooperate, light-touch sensibility in the sacral dermatomeres can be tested using a wisp of cotton at the end of an applicator. Reflex contraction of the external anal sphincter in response to stroking the perianal skin is evidence that the sensorimotor apparatus of fecal continence is functioning with integrity. Although rectal examination is an integral part of every physical examination, it is sometimes advisable to omit it from the first visit of a child with functional fecal retention. When the history is typical of this condition, the chances of diagnosing an anatomic or organic disease are very slim, and a rectal examination can compromise the attempt to establish communication and trust during the initial visit.

Once functional fecal retention is deemed likely, it is wise to treat it rather than embarking on a series of tests to rule out Hirschsprung's disease or other colonic neuromuscular diseases. Sufficient differences exist between these various entities (Table 8.3) so that in most cases endoscopic, manometric, and radiologic tests are unnecessary. These procedures serve only to reinforce the child's role as the "sick one in the family." If treatment for functional fecal retention fails, then the possibility that an

TABLE 8.3 Clinical Comparison of Functional Fecal Retention and Colonic Neuromuscular Disorders

Signs and Symptoms	Functional Fecal Retention	Colonic Neuromuscular Disorders
Soiling	Common	Rare
Obstructive symptoms	Rare	Common
Large-caliber stools	Common	Rare
Stool-withholding behavior	Common	Rare
Enterocolitis	Never	Possible
Associated upper - GI symptoms	Never	Common
Symptoms from birth	Rare	Common
Localization of stools	Rectum	Rectal and extra-rectal

unusual condition is causing the symptoms must be considered.

Although anorectal manometry has been studied extensively in children with fecal retention, results are conflicting. It is often unclear if the manometric abnormalities are the cause or result of the chronic fecal retention. Basal anal pressure has been reported to be increased,[9,28] decreased,[29] or similar to that of control children.[30] Thresholds of internal sphincter relaxation have also been higher than[28] or similar to[30] control children. An abnormal rectal sensation has been found by some authors[29] but not by others.[30] Anorectal manometry has also been used to predict outcome and response to treatment.[31]

The main indication for anorectal manometry in constipated children is still to rule out Hirschsprung's disease. The lack of rectoanal inhibitory reflex is diagnostic of Hirschsprung's disease. In a cooperative child with short-segment Hirschsprung's disease, anorectal manometry may be diagnostic when a suction rectal biopsy is not interpretable. In a dilated rectum, large volumes of balloon distention may be necessary to elicit a normal sphincter relaxation. More details on anorectal manometry may be found in Chapter 12. Barium enema studies provide little information in the child presenting with chronic constipation.[32,33]

Successful treatment of functional fecal retention depends on the ability of the clinician to draw the child and family into a therapeutic relationship. Virtually all management strategies for treating functional fecal retention are effective. Many are used together. Behavioral modification that emphasizes positive reinforcement schedules (eg, star charts),[34] stool softeners,[35] biofeedback training to improve conscious rectal sensitivity and anal sphincter relaxation skills,[36,37] cleansing enemas,[38] cisapride,[39] group therapy,[40] play with modeling clay,[41] and surgery,[10,42,43] are all effective in the majority of patients. Because no treatment appears to be superior to the others, surgery should be bypassed in favor of an approach that emphasizes the absence of organic disease.

Functional fecal retention is viewed as an acquired behavior in which the affected child has forgotten the mechanics of defecation. The child is asked to relearn effective toilet behavior by a sympathetic, knowledgeable pediatrician who promises to guide the child and the family through the training period. During the first outpatient visit, the examiner gains the patient's confidence by demonstrating an understanding of functional fecal retention and by explaining that the child is not alone with his problem. The patient should understand that many children are troubled by the same condition, and that physicians understand its cause and treatment. The pediatrician should draw pictures that demonstrate normal defecation and the abnormal choices that result in fecal accumulation (see Fig. 8.2). Next, the fears of the child and family should be addressed. A multitude of symptoms, such as fever, convulsions, nervousness, school failure, and bad breath have been attributed to constipation. It is extremely unlikely that failure to have a bowel movement results in any of these.[21] Toxins do not leak back into the body when stool is retained. Neither the colon nor the rest of the body is permanently damaged when stool is retained. Functional fecal retention does not cause cancer, and mineral oil does not cause clinically relevant vitamin deficiency.[44] These topics should be addressed directly by the physician because the family and the child are often too embarrassed to ask. Dispelling the myths surrounding constipation is fundamental for the treatment's success.

The physician, the family, and the child then enter into an informal contract. The physician agrees to provide guidance and prescribe stool softeners to ensure painless defecation. The parents are responsible for administering medication and securing private, unhurried lavatory time for the child twice daily—usually after breakfast and dinner—to take advantage of the gastrocolonic reflex.[45] The child assumes responsibility for taking the medication and responding to the defecatory urge rather than holding back.

In children over 5 years, it is a compliment to their maturity and self-reliance to offer a taste test of several stool softeners. It is important to use products that the child will drink without much confrontation. Forcing the child to drink an unpalatable solution may change the struggle from anal to oral, but keeps control issues in the forefront. The child is asked to choose a favorite, and the parents agree to purchase the chosen variety. The child is then reminded of his obligation to take the preparation. Mineral oil is all that is needed in most cases; enemas are required in only 2% of children during the initial clean-out.[46]

There are two phases to treatment: passage of the rectal mass and maintenance. Evacuation of the rectal fecal mass is the first step toward overcoming functional fecal retention. Almost every fecal mass, regardless of size, can be softened and liquefied with a sufficient quantity and duration of oral mineral oil and/or saline purgative. Enemas are best avoided. In one study, encopretic children undergoing psychotherapy indicated by the pictures they drew that they regarded enemas as a punitive measure.[47] Even if the element of discomfort that is associated with an enema is ignored, it must be expected that the child will react negatively to a procedure that is contrary to his original goal (ie, withholding stool).[4]

The administration of mineral oil preparations, osmotic agents, or magnesium salts can take two forms: the campaign and the routine. A campaign consists of administering large doses (50-60 ml) of mineral oil or lactulose a few times a day. Citrate of magnesia is also safe and effective. The preparation is continued until the mass liquefies or softens enough to be passed. The parents must be made aware that soiling will increase dramatically because the fecal mass softens from its surface inwards. Abdominal distention and cramping may also transiently increase, especially when lactulose is used. The campaign takes a few days and should not be initiated while the child is attending school. Weekends or school holidays are the best times. The child should be kept at home to have easy access to the toilet. Parents must be warned that the child's fearfulness and distress may increase as the ability to withhold stools lessens; the softer the stool becomes, the more difficult it is to withhold. The child's mounting distress constitutes a retentive crisis, a time of acute discomfort and apprehension. The retentive crisis culminates in the passage of an enormous amount of stool, followed by almost immediate relief and the disappearance of soiling within a day. Because large doses of mineral oil are used during this phase of the treatment, it may take a day or two for mineral oil leakage to cease. If parents become alarmed by the child's distress during the retentive crisis, they can be reassured that the distress is caused by fear rather than physical pain. The physician must remain accessible for reassessment and reassurance. After struggling with the passage of the rectal mass, the child will realize that the evacuation was easier than expected. Positive reinforcements are very important during this phase of treatment. After passage of each stool in the commode, the child should be complimented and tangible rewards should be provided.[34] When the attempts to eliminate the rectal mass with oral laxatives fail, it is probably wiser to disimpact the child manually under anesthesia rather than using enemas or nasogastric tubes with continuous infusion of electrolyte solutions. Both enemas and nasogastric tube placements can be interpreted by the child as unjustified punishment, hindering the therapeutic relationship with the physician. If sedatives with amnestic properties are used, the manual disimpaction is well tolerated by the child.

Once the mass is eliminated, the routine management phase can begin. Lower doses of the drugs used in the campaign are continued. The doses must be individualized and titrated to keep the stools soft and pudding-like. The child can be reassured that painless defecation will persist as long as he complies with the plan to take the stool softeners and respond to the urge to defecate. The child's fear of defecation often takes months to completely overcome. Every time the child has a painless, sometimes pleasurable defecation the fear lessens. Relapses are common. Changes in daily routines, such as vacation travel or weekend visits to a divorced parent, disrupt schedules and result in noncompliance. Parents can be coached to anticipate relapses in retentive behavior whenever control of defecation becomes an issue. Relapses tend to be handled more easily and quickly than the initial presentation.

Treatment should be continued for several months. After experiencing months of pain- and accident-free defecation, the child will indicate that there is no need for the medicine. Long-term use of mineral oil has been reported to be safe. A major concern about long-term mineral oil therapy had been its action as a lipid solvent, which could interfere with the absorption of fat-soluble vitamins. This concern has been dismissed by studies that show negligible reduction of the plasma levels of vitamins A and E after 6 months of mineral-oil treatment.[44] Leakage of mineral oil in the underwear can cause an orange stain. Parents should be reassured of its harmlessness.

Other authors have had success with cisapride in both open-labeled[48] and placebo-controlled trials[39] in the treatment of chronic constipation. It is unclear how cisapride increases frequency of defecation and improves stool consistency. It is possible that the decreased total intestinal transit time may raise the water content of the stool in the rectum, which facilitates defecation.

For children older than 6 years of age who can cooperate, biofeedback can be used with success. Some children have a paradoxical contraction of the external anal sphincter in response to rectal distention. This is probably a learned behavior, the manometric equivalent of holding back in response to the urge. It is possible to teach children to inhibit this contraction and normalize their manometric pattern, thereby resolving the symptoms.[4] When biofeedback was compared to mineral oil as a part of a program which included disimpaction and behavioral modification, biofeedback was found to be superior to mineral oil in children with paradoxical contraction, whereas mineral oil was superior in children with normal manometric readings.[49]

The role of dietary fiber in the treatment of functional fecal retention is controversial. Dietary fiber acts by increasing water retention and providing substrate for bacterial growth. Since some fibers—especially the insoluble fibers of wheat—are subject to little digestion by colonic bacterial enzymes and have hydrophilic properties, they increase water retention in the colon. Increased bacterial mass results in greater stool output and decreased transit time. Although some authors have shown that fiber can be beneficial,[50,51] its role in the treatment of childhood constipation has probably been overemphasized. Fiber might be effective in the maintenance phase of treatment to maintain fecal softness, but it does not help to diminish a fecal mass. Unfortunately, it is difficult to convince children to eat a high-fiber diet. Consistent stool softening is key to treatment of this condition.

Treatment failures occur in approximately 20% of children with functional fecal retention, regardless of the treatment. Children who are likely to fail are those who have suffered from functional fecal retention for several years and have developed a negative self-image, or those who find a secondary gain from the condition (eg, attention from a parent or avoidance of sexual abuse). Parents of these children may be offered two choices: 1) they can wait for the child to express interest in eliminating the problem, or 2) they may choose to enter psychotherapy with their child. Psychotherapy is not a substitute for treatment of functional fecal retention by the medical doctor; it is an additional therapy. Abandonment by the medical doctor might anger the child and family, making psychotherapy more difficult, and leaving the fecal mass untreated. The medical doctor and psychotherapist must work together.

Complications that require acute intervention sometimes arise. Rarely, the fecal accumulation is so rapid or massive that respiratory failure results from impaired diaphragmatic movement (Fig. 8.3), or repeated vomiting and dehydration are caused by bowel obstruction.[52] Many complications are related to fluid and electrolyte abnormalities precipitated by repeated enemas or other home remedies. Hypertonic enemas or excessive oral phosphates may cause dehydration, shock, hyper- and hyponatremia, and hyperphosphatemia.[53,54] Enema fluid has been documented to occasionally enter the circulatory system.[55]

Functional fecal retention is uncommon over the age of 12 years and is probably very rare in adults.[56] Those children who persist with functional fecal retention into early adolescence invariably rid themselves of the behavior when the urge to socialize overpowers the need to hold onto stool.

ORGANIC CAUSES OF CONSTIPATION
Colonic Neuromuscular Disorders

When mineral oil fails and retentive posturing is absent, when there is a history of

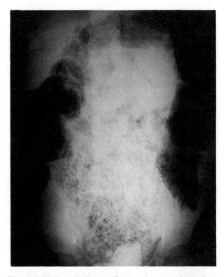

Fig. 8.3 Abdominal x-ray from a 9-year-old patient with functional fecal retention. The child suffered respiratory failure secondary to the accumulation of stools in the rectum.

constipation from birth and there are extrarectal fecal masses, when stools are soft but infrequent and soiling is absent, the child may have a colonic neuromuscular disorder. Rectoanal manometry is the most sensitive and specific test for Hirschsprung's disease, but only in a cooperative child. A barium enema in an unprepared colon may show a transition zone, with the narrowed Hirschsprung's segment located distally, and the segment proximal to the obstruction dilated. However, the characteristic radiographic features of Hirschsprung's disease are often absent in infants less than 3 months old, and in those with total colonic or short-segment Hirschsprung's disease. Biopsies demonstrating the absence of neuron cell bodies in the submucosal plexus are diagnostic for Hirschsprung's disease, but interpretation of biopsies in short-segment Hirschsprung's disease is difficult because there is normally a hypoganglionic area 2 to 3 cm proximal to the dentate line.

Radiopaque markers may be used to differentiate colonic inertia from outlet obstruction.[11] In healthy children, swallowed markers are excreted within 48 hours. In outlet obstruction, the markers remain in the rectum. Outlet obstruction can be found in functional fecal retention, short-segment Hirschsprung's disease, and anatomic obstruction. In colonic inertia, the markers are scattered throughout the colon for many days. If the radiopaque marker study suggests colonic inertia, full-thickness biopsies[57] or colonic manometry studies can differentiate between neuropathy and myopathy.

Colonic hypo- and hyperganglionosis have been associated with constipation.[58] The pathologic diagnosis of abnormalities of the myenteric plexus is difficult due to the paucity of pathologic specimens from age- and location-matched control subjects. The two characteristic features of colonic manometry in normal children and children with functional fecal retention are high-amplitude propagating contractions and an increase in motility following a meal.[59] Children with colonic myopathies have virtually no colonic contractions. Children with colonic neuropathies do not have the expected increase in motility following a meal, and often lack high-amplitude migrating contractions.[60] For more details on colonic manometry, see Chapter 13.

Children with Hirschsprung's disease are treated by resecting the segment of the bowel that lacks neuron cell bodies in the submucous plexus. In 10% to 20% of these children, constipation persists despite successful surgery. Recent manometric evidence suggests that a colonic neuropathy is sometimes present in the unresected proximal bowel.[61] Hirschsprung's disease is further discussed in Chapter 26.

Central Nervous System Disorders

Constipation in neurologically devastated children with developmental delay is common, and may result from several factors. In tube-fed children, the absence of dietary fiber may be constipating. The absence of normal skeletal muscle tone and coordination may result in a poor defecatory effort. There may be sensory or motor abnormalities due to affected enteric neurons, just as there are abnormalities in the central nervous system.

Treatment of constipation in children with chronic, static CNS disease may include attempts to introduce dietary fiber, behav-ioral modification techniques to teach toilet skills, daily administration of stool softeners such as mineral oil and lactulose, enemas, oral cathartics, rectal irrigations, and biofeedback.

In children with spinal cord injury or dysraphism, the external anal sphincter and levator ani muscles—which depend on sacral nerves 2, 3, and 4—are typically dysfunctional. Defects in innervation may affect both motor and sensory function in the rectum. Children with myelomeningocele have both constipation and fecal incontinence. Fecal continence is found only in 11% to 30% of children with myelomeningocele.[62-64] Biofeedback training has been helpful in patients who have preservation of some sensorimotor functions in the perianal region and who understand and cooperate during the process of biofeedback training.[62] The enema continence catheter has been used to empty the rectum every 48 hours in children with a variety of spinal cord impairments. It consists of a catheter with an inflatable balloon at the end, which prevents instant leakage of the enema solution from the incontinent anus, and an exterior baffle that locks the balloon in place within the rectum, preventing its displacement. When the total volume of the enema has been administered, the catheter is removed and the liquid contents of the abdomen are immediately evacuated.[63,65] Electric stimulation of the pudendal nerves with a neuroprosthetic device has also been used in some patients.[66] For the neuroprosthesis to be effective, the integrity of the pudendal and sacral nerves is essential. The pudendal nerve is stimulated continuously to achieve continence; stimulation is interrupted only for defecation and/or urination.

Anorectal Malformations

Anatomic disturbances of the anus and rectum are associated with constipation and fecal soiling. There is a wide range in the severity of these abnormalities,[67] as listed in Table 8.4. Anterior displacement of the anus is more common in females and is associated with a posterior rectal shelf as well as abnormalities in the angle of descent for the fecal mass, which causes constipation.[68]

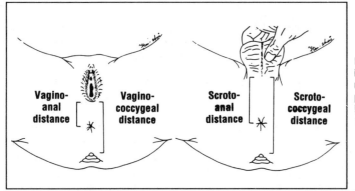

Fig. 8.4 The anogenital index in the female and male. (Reprinted with permission from Bar-Maor JA, Eitan A, 1987[69])

TABLE 8.4 Classification of Anorectal Malformations

MALE

A. Low (Translevator)
1. At Normal Anal Site
  a) Anal stenosis
  b) Covered anus—complete
2. At Perineal Site
  a) Anocutaneous fistula
     (Covered anus—incomplete)
  b) Anterior perineal anus

B. Intermediate
1. Anal Agenesis
  a) Without fistula
  b) With fistula
     rectobulbar
2. Anorectal Stenosis

C. High (Supralevator)
1. Anorectal Agenesis
  a) Without fistula
  b) With fistula
     1) rectourethral
     2) rectovesical
2. Rectal Atresia

FEMALE

A. Low (Translevator)
1. At Normal Anal Site
  a) Anal stenosis
  b) Covered anus—complete
2. At Perineal Site
  a) Anocutaneous fistula
     (Covered anus—incomplete)
  b) Anaterior perineal anus
3. At Vulvar Site
  a) Anovulvular fistula
  b) Anovestibular fistula
  c) Vestibular anus

B. Intermediate
1. Anal Agenesis
  a) Without fistula
  b) With fistula
     1) rectovestibular
     2) rectovaginal—low
2. Anorectal Stenosis

C. High (Supralevator)
1. Anorectal Agenesis
  a) Without fistula
  b) With fistula
     1) rectovaginal—high
     2) rectocloacal
     3) rectovesical
2. Rectal Atresia

D. Miscellaneous
Imperforate Anal Membrane
Cloacal Exstrophy
Others

(Reprinted with permission from Santulli T, et al, 1970 [67])

Anterior displacement of the anus can be determined with the anogenital index (Fig. 8.4),[69] which is the ratio of the distances between the vagina or scrotum, anus, and the coccyx. This index is constant and is not affected by age or ethnic differences. A ratio of less than 0.30 in females and less than 0.49 in males is diagnostic for this condition. Anal stenosis typically presents with thin ribbons of stool and fecal accumulations. Anal membranes and imperforate anus with or without fistulae are found during the newborn examination.

REFERENCES

1. Devroede G. Constipation. In: Sleisinger M, Fortrand JS, eds. *Gastrointestinal Disease: Pathophysiology, Diagnosis, Management*. Philadelphia, PA: WB Saunders 1989; 331-61.

2. Nyhan Wl. Stool frequency of normal infants in the first weeks of life. *Pediatrics* 1952;10:414-25.

3. Weaver LT, Ewing G, Taylor LC. The bowel habit of milk-fed infants. *J Pediatr Gastroenterol Nutr* 1983;7:568-71

4. Rosemberg AJ. Constipation and encopresis. In: Willie R, Hyams JS, eds. *Pediatric Gastrointestinal Disease: Pathophysiology, Diagnosis, Management*. Philadelphia, PA: WB Saunders, 1993:198-208.

5. Dimson SB. Carmine as an index of transit times in children with simple constipation. *Arch Dis Child* 1970;45:232-5.

6. Lesne E, Binet L, Paulin A. La traversee digestive chez ie nourisson: variation biologiques et pathologiques. *Arch Med Infant* 1920;23:449-56.

7. Corazziari E, Cucchiara S, Staiano A, et al. Gastrointestinal transit time, frequency of defecation, and anorectal manometry in healthy and constipated children. *J Pediatr* 1985;106:379-85.

8. Loening-Baucke VA, Younoszai MK. Abnormal anal sphincter response in chronically constipated children. *J Pediatr* 1982;100:213-8.

9. Molnar D, Taitz LS, Urwin OM, Wales JKH. Anorectal manometry results in defecation disorders. *Arch Dis Child* 1988;58:257-61.

10. Martelli H, Devroede G, Arhan P, Duguay C.

Mechanisms of idiopathic constipation: outlet obtruction. *Gastroenterology* 1978;75:623-31.

11. Wald A. Colonic transit and anorectal manometry in chronic idiopathic constipation. *Arch Intern Med* 1986;146:1713-6.

12. Anthony EJ. An experimental approach to the psychopathology of childhood: encopresis. *Br J Med Psychol* 1957;30:146.

13. Bakwin H, Davidson M. Constipation in twins. *Amer J Dis Child* 1971;121:179-81.

14. Hyman PE, Fleisher D. Functional fecal retention. *Practical Gastroenterology* 1992;16:29-37.

15. Fleisher D. Diagnosis and treatment of disorders of defecation in children. *Pediatr Ann* 1976;5:71-101.

16. Hamilton JW, Wagner J, Burdick BB, Bass P. Clinical evaluation of methylcellulose as a bulk laxative. *Dig Dis Sci* 1988;33:993-8.

17. Partin JC, Hamill SK, Fischel JE, Partin JS. Painful defecation and fecal soiling in children. *Pediatrics* 1992;89:1007-9.

18. Pilapil VR. A horrifying television commercial that lead to constipation. *Pediatrics* 1990;85:592-3.

19. De Vos I, Messer AP. Encopresis caused by mother's stoma. *Pediatrics* 1991;87:271-2.

20. Schubert R, Cracco JB. Familial rectal pain: a type of reflex epilepsy? *Ann Neurol* 1992;32:824-6.

21. Silverman A, Roy CC. Constipation, fecal incontinence, and other proctologic conditions. In: *Pediatric Clinical Gastroenterology* St. Louis, MI: CV Mosby, 1983:391-417.

22. Kokx NP, Comstock JA, Facklam RR. Streptococcal perianal disease in children. *Pediatrics* 1987;80:659-63.

23. Spear RM, Rothbaum R, Keating J, Biaufuss MC, Rosemblum JL. Perianal streptococcal cellulitis. *J Pediatr* 1985;107:557-9.

24. Agnarsson U, Warde C, McCarthy G, Evans N. Perianal appearances associated with constipation. *Arch Dis Child* 1990;65:1231-4.

25. Clayden GS. Reflex and dilation associated with chronic constipation in childhood. *Arch Dis Child* 1988;63:832-6.

26. Goldberg NS, Esterly NB, Rothman KF, et al. Perianal pseudoverrucous papules and nodules in children. *Arch Dermatol* 1992;128:240-2.

27. Anderson F. Occult spinal dysraphism: a series of 73 cases. *Pediatrics* 1975;55:826-35.

28. Meunier P, Marechal JM, deBeaugeu MJ. Recto-anal pressures and rectal sensitivity in chronic childhood constipation. *Gastroenterology* 1979;77:330-6.

29. Loening-Baucke VA, Younoszai MK. Effect of treatment on rectal and sigmoid motility in chronically constipated children. *Pediatrics* 1984;73:199-205.

30. Wald A, Chandra R, Chiponis D, Gabel S. Anorectal function and continence mechanisms in childhood encopresis. *J Pediatr Gastroenterol Nutr* 1986;5:346-51.

31. Loening-Baucke VA. Factors determining outcome in children with chronic constipation and soiling. *Gut* 1989;30:999-1006.

32. Meunier P, Louis D, Jaubert de Beaujeu M. Physiologic investigation of primary chronic constipation in children: comparison with the barium enema study. *Gastroenterology* 1984;87:1351-7.

33. Verduron A, Devroede G, Bouchoucha M, et al. Mega-rectum. *Dig Dis Sci* 1988;33:1164-74.

34. Steege MW, Harper DC. Enhancing the management of secondary encopresis by assessing acceptability of treatment: a case study. *J Behav Ther Exp Psychiatry* 1989;20:333-41.

35. Nolan T, Debelle G, Oberklaid F, Coffey C. Randomized trial of laxatives in treatment of childhood encopresis. *Lancet* 1991;338:523-7.

36. Benninga MA, Buller HA, Taminiau JA. Biofeedback training in constipation. *Arch Dis Child* 1993;68:126-9.

37. Keren S, Wagner D, Heldenberg D, Golan M. Studies of manometric abnormalities of the recto-anal region during defecation in constipated and soiling children: modification through biofeedback therapy. *Am J Gastroenterol* 1988;83:827-31.

38. Culp WC. Relief of severe fecal impactions with water-soluble contrast enemas. *Radiology* 1975;115:9-12.

39. Staiano A, Cucchiara S, Andreotti MR, Minella R, Manzi G. Effect of cisapride on chronic idiopathic constipation in children. *Dig Dis Sci* 1991;36:733-6.

40. Stark LJ, Owens-Stively J, Spirito A, Lewis A, Guevremont D. Group behavioral treatment of retentive encopresis. *J Pediatr Psychol* 1990;15:659-71.

41. Feldman PC, Villanueva S, Lanne V, Devroede G. Use of play with clay to treat children with intractable encopresis. *J Pediatr* 1993;122:483-8.

42. Kamm MA, Hawley PR, Lennard Jones JE. Lateral division of the puborectalis muscle in the management of severe constipation. *Br J Surg* 1988;75:661-3.

43. Vasilevsky CA, Nemer FD, Balcos EG, Christienson CE, Goldberg SM. Is subtotal colectomy a viable option in the management of chronic constipation? *Dis Col Rectum* 1988;31:679-81.

44. Clark J, Russell G, Fitzgerald J. Serum beta-carotene, retinol, and alpha tocopherol levels during mineral oil therapy for constipation. *Am J Dis Child* 1987;141:1210-2.

45. Lowery SP, Srour JW, Whitehead WE, Schuster MM. Habit training as treatment of encopresis secondary to chronic constipation. *J Pediatr Gastroenterol Nutr* 1985;4:397-401.

46. Gleghorn EE, Heyman MB, Rudolph CD. No-enema therapy for idiopathic constipation and encopresis. *Clin Pediatr* 1991;30:669-72.

47. Pinkerton P. Psychogenic megacolon in children: the implications of bowel negativism. *Arch Dis Child* 1958;33:371-80.

48. Murray RD, Li BUK, McClung HJ, Heitlinger L, Rehm D. Cisapride for intractable constipation in children: observation from an open trial. *J Pediatr Gastroenterol Nutr* 1990;11:503-8.

49. Wald A, Chandra R, Gabel S, Chiponis D. Evaluation of biofeedback in childhood encopresis. *J Pediatr Gastroenterol Nutr* 1987;6:554-8.

50. Marzio L, Lanfranchi GA, Bazzocchi G, Cuccurullo F. Anorectal motility and rectal sensitivity in chronic idiopathic constipation: effect of high-fiber diet. *J Clin Gastroenterol* 1985;7:391-9.

51. Cucchiara S, Devizia B, Staiano A, et al. Treatment of chronic functional constipation in children

by administration of vegetable fiber. *Minerva Pediatr* 1989;41:147-52.

52. McGuire T, Rothenberg MB, Tyler DC. Profound shock following intervention for chronic untreated stool retention. *Clin Pediatr* 1983;23:459-61.

53. Martin RR, Lisehora GR, Braxton M, Varcia PJ. Fatal poisoning from sodium phosphate enema. *JAMA* 1987;257:2190-2.

54. Ziskind A, Gellis SS. Water intoxication following tap water enemas. *AJDC* 1958;96:699.

55. Rabah R, Evans RW, Yunis EJ. Mineral oil embolization and lipoid pneumonia in an infant treated for Hirschsprung's disease. *Pediatr Path* 1987;7:447-55.

56. Abrahamian FP, Lloyd-Still JD. Chronic constipation in childhood: a longitudinal study of 186 patients. *J Pediatr Gastroenterol Nutr* 1984;3:460-7.

57. Achem SR, Owyang C, Shuffler MD, Dobbins WO. Neuronal dysplasia and chronic intestinal pseudo-obstruction: rectal biopsy as a possible aid to diagnosis. *Gastroenterology* 1987;92:805-9.

58. Wienberg AG. The anorectal myenteric plexus: its relation to hypoganglionosis of the colon. *Am J Clin Pathol* 1970;54:637-48.

59. Di Lorenzo C, Flores A, Reddy SN, Hyman PE. Colonic manometry differentiates causes of intractable constipation in children. *J Pediatr* 1992;120:690-5.

60. Di Lorenzo C, Flores AF, Reddy SN, Snape WJ Jr, Bazzocchi G, Hyman PE. Colonic manometry

in children with chronic intestinal pseudoobstruction. *Gut* 1993;34:803-7.

61. Di Lorenzo C, Flores AF, Reddy SN, Snape WJ Jr, Hyman PE. Colon motility in symptomatic children after surgery for Hirschsprung's disease: abnormalities in "healthy" colon. *Gastroenterology* 1991;100:A437.

62. Wald A. Use of biofeedback of fecal incontinence in patients with meningomyelocele. *Pediatrics* 1981;68:45-9.

63. Younoszai MK. Stooling problems in patients with myelomeningocele. *South Med J* 1992;85:718-23.

64. Cooper DGW. Detrussor action in children with myelomeningocele. *Arch Dis Child* 1968;43:427-32.

65. Liptak GS, Revell GM. Management of bowel dysfunction in children with spinal cord disease or injury by means of the enema continence catheter. *J Pediatr* 1992;120:190-4.

66. Schmidt RA, Kogan BA, Tanagho EA. Neuroprosthesis in the management of incontinence in myelomeningocele patients. *J Urol* 1990;143:779-82.

67. Santulli T, Kiesewetter WB, Bill AH. Anorectal anomalies: suggested international classification. *J Pediatr Surg* 1970;5:281-7.

68. Leape LL, Ramenofsky ML. Anterior ectopic anus: a common cause of constipation in children. *J Pediatr Surg* 1978;13:627-9.

69. Bar-Maor JA, Eitan A. Determination of the normal position of the anus. *J Pediatr Gastroenterol Nutr* 1987;6:559-61.

9

Irritable Bowel Syndrome

PETER J. MILLA

Irritable bowel syndrome (IBS) comprises a number of gastrointestinal symptoms—principally abdominal pain, constipation, and loose stools—for which no organic cause can be found. In some patients, all of these symptoms will eventually occur. In others, one symptom will predominate almost exclusively. In adults, the syndrome is a major cause of industrial absenteeism[1] and in children it is probably the single most common reason for referral to pediatric gastroenterology clinics. Nevertheless, information about the pathogenesis of IBS is fragmentary. Many of the symptoms may be associated with disturbances of intestinal motor activity,[2] but the cause of the dysmotility is almost certainly an interplay of psychogenic and organic disorders. Motility disorders are always found in IBS patients.

MECHANISMS OF DYSMOTILITY IN IBS

Disordered gastrointestinal motility is believed to result from a disturbance of the complex control mechanisms of gastrointestinal motor activity. Such disturbances may be produced by organic disease of the mechanisms themselves, producing conditions such as intestinal pseudo-obstruction, perturbation of the humoral environment of the nerves and muscle, and altered central nervous system (CNS) input. There is no evidence of organic disease directly affecting enteric nerve and muscle in IBS, but an accumulating body of evidence implicates an altered humoral environment and CNS input.

The Humoral Environment

A variety of disease processes, such as food allergies and other immune responses, may alter the humoral environment and produce disordered motor activity that might cause IBS-like symptoms. Studies of small intestinal motility during acute immediate hypersensitivity reactions in experimental animals have shown the presence of giant migrating complexes and clustered phasic activity,[3,4] both of which result in shortened transit. Such disordered motility could very well induce IBS-like symptoms, especially in those with toddler's diarrhea. No comparable studies have been performed in children with similar immune responses. Some preliminary studies of T-lymphocyte mediated responses in the small intestinal mucosa of both adults and children suggest that similar clustered phasic activity may be seen. Thus, a variety of immune responses in the gut may result in disordered motility, which could cause IBS-like symptoms.

The Central Nervous System and Stress

The CNS modulates intestinal motor activity. The effect of fear, anxiety, or other stressful emotions on gastrointestinal motility is supported by experimental and anecdotal evidence. Experimental studies show that a wide variety of stressors can induce disordered GI motor activity (Table 9.1). Stressful events such as family tensions, separation, changes of school or housing,[5] difficulty in peer relationships, or loss of important friends or relatives may induce

TABLE 9.1 **Effects of Laboratory Stressors on Gastrointestinal Motility**	
Region of GI Tract	**Stressor**
Esophagus	Noise increases peristalsis[44]
Stomach	Cold stress inhibits antral motility and gastric emptying[45]
Small intestine	Delayed auditory feedback, arcade games, and driving in traffic suppresses fasting activity[46]
Colon	Cold stress increases motility[47]

changes in motor activity that clinically present as IBS. Such stresses may be acute or chronic, overt or covert, minor or major. All too often, significant stresses are overlooked because they are not obviously traumatic, but are subtle, low-key, persistent, and sometimes far from clear to the observer. Some studies have also suggested that different emotions may have different effects. For example, fear and depression have been associated with inhibition of gastric acid secretion and delayed gastric emptying,[6] while resentment, anger, and aggression enhance motor activity and secretion.[7] The studies of the effects of neuropeptides in the CNS on intestinal motor activity show changes associated with particular peptides, lending credence to the notion that centrally determined events of different types may result in varied intestinal motor responses.[8]

Although many experimental studies have shown altered gastrointestinal motility in normal subjects under psychologic stress, IBS patients show a qualitatively different motility response. Richter et al[9] showed that patients with noncardiac chest pain had a lower threshold for reporting pain when a balloon was inflated in their esophagus. Similarly, Moriarty and Dawson[10] demonstrated that IBS subjects reported pain at lower levels of balloon distention in both the small and large intestines. Although the available data provides persuasive evidence that psychologic stress may exacerbate gastrointestinal motility disorders, the high frequency with which psychologic stress precipitates altered bowel habits in normal subjects must be taken into account. For example, Drossman et al[11] found that 68% of a large population without IBS symptoms reported that psychologic stressors caused constipation or diarrhea, and 47% reported that they caused abdominal pain. In contrast, those with IBS were significantly more likely to report stress-related changes in bowel patterns (85%) and abdominal pain (69%), but the base rate of such reports among the normals suggests that this is not a distinctive characteristic of IBS patients.

Studies of the effects of laboratory stressors and of naturally occurring stress generally agree in suggesting that these alter motility. Some indirect evidence implies that patients with IBS show a greater reactivity to stress than normal subjects, but the overlap is substantial. The physiologic mechanisms which mediate such effects are still unclear. Studies of gastrointestinal peptides, both centrally and peripherally, suggest that they are important in pathogenetic mechanisms.

SYMPTOMS OF IBS

In childhood, patients fall into three main groups: 1) those whose predominant symptom is abdominal pain; 2) those whose main complaint is of loose, frequent stools; and 3) those who present with constipation. These three groups will be discussed with regard to their etiology and pathophysiology.

Recurrent Abdominal Pain

Apley[12] found that approximately 10% of schoolchildren suffer from recurrent episodes of self-limiting recurrent abdominal pain (RAP) that last for longer than 3 months, interfere with their activities, and for which no cause can be found. The pain is usually colicky and periumbilical, but may also be dull, continuous, and found at other abdominal sites. Peak incidence is usually around 5 years of age in both sexes, with a further peak at puberty in girls. Complaints of pain are significantly more common in the families of affected children and seem to be most frequent in high-strung, anxious children. In Apley's study, psychogenic factors were more common than in control children. Those treated with informal psychotherapy showed a more rapid relief of symptoms. However, careful study of the data reveals that approximately 40% were unresponsive to psychotherapy.

The high proportion of patients who were unresponsive to psychotherapy suggests that obscure organic disease caused the symptoms. Claims have been made that reactions to food, such as allergies or lactose intolerance, play a role in this syndrome.[13,14] Some children respond to elimination diets, especially those that prohibit cow's milk, eggs, and wheat. A strong personal and/or family history of atopic-related disease and gastrointestinal disturbance, together with a prompt response to an elimination diet suggests a role for allergy in some patients. Food allergy may also account for many cases of migraine in which RAP is a feature.[15] Earlier suggestions by McMichael et al[14] that lactose intolerance would explain many cases has not been borne out in practice. Long-term studies suggest that over 50% of children who present with RAP have symptoms that persist into adulthood, and a diagnosis of IBS is made in approximately 33%.[16] In addition to abdominal pain, some children experience intermittent fluctuating episodes of diarrhea and constipation—which is reminiscent of adults with IBS[17]—in addition to nonspecific symptoms such as bloating, nausea, and abdominal tenderness.[12]

Pathophysiology. The pathophysiologic mechanisms operating in RAP are unknown, but some have been postulated. Attacks may represent the transient somatic correlates of anxiety, depression, or anger mediated by the autonomic nervous system, or may be simple physiologic responses. In some children, the pain may simply be the contractions of normal phase-3 activity of fasting small intestinal motility (ie, hunger pains). However, in other children with RAP, increased small intestinal pressure[18] and hyperactive colonic motor responses to cholinergic agonists have been found that resemble those in adults with IBS.[19] Studies of intestinal motor activity in experimental animals in whom immediate hypersensitivity responses are induced have shown the presence of giant migrating complexes which could also be responsible for abdominal pain in children with IBS.[3]

Toddler's Diarrhea

Although RAP is a common problem in general pediatric practice, it is the child with loose, frequent, foul-smelling stools that most often presents to the pediatric gastroenterologist. This symptom complex is known variously as toddler's diarrhea, chronic nonspecific diarrhea, and IBS of childhood. The condition usually occurs in children between the ages of 1 and 5 years and is more common in boys, who are typically described as overactive, destructive, and difficult to handle. The diarrhea is intermittent and characterized by the precipitous passage of loose, mucusy stools containing undigested food particles such as peas and carrots. Such stools are only passed during waking hours and are often exacerbated by stress. Despite the abnormal stools, failure to thrive is not a feature of this syndrome. The condition is self-limiting, but in one follow-up study[20] a high incidence of constipation was found later. The same study demonstrated a marked familial tendency, with recurrent functional bowel disorder in at least one parent of 67% of the patients. In those with unaffected parents, 55% had a sibling with a similar disorder. Thus, toddler's diarrhea is part of a spectrum of functional bowel disorders which present just as frequently in children as in adults.

Pathophysiology. A variety of mechanisms have been implicated in toddler's diarrhea, including changes in intestinal transport, brush-border enzymes, prostaglandin synthesis, food intolerance, and intestinal motor activity. Despite all of these investigations, the nature of this common, apparently self-limiting condition is still not entirely clear, although a hypothesis will be presented on the following page.

Intestinal Transport The diarrhea is not associated with malabsorption in either adults or children in the fasting state. There is no evidence of abnormal secretion of water and electrolytes in the small intestine[21] nor in glucose absorption in the proximal jejunum of children with toddler's diarrhea.[22]

Mucosal Enzymes Although the small intestinal mucosa is morphologically normal, Tripp et al[23] found a significant increase in the specific activities of Na K ATPase and basal adenylate cyclase in jejunal biopsies from children with toddler's diarrhea, as compared with those from children with postenteritis syndrome. In the active phase of postenteritis, adenylase cyclase activity was normal and Na K ATPase activity was reduced. During the recovery phase, the activity of both enzymes was increased in a proportion similar to that found in toddler's diarrhea. These findings add some credence to the clinical impression that toddler's diarrhea may follow an acute enteric infection. The increase in specific enzyme activity may be a response of normal villus cells to crypt cell secretion and might be mediated via prostaglandins.[23]

Prostaglandins Using a radioimmunoassay for prostaglandin E_2 (PGE_2) and prostaglandin F (PGF) in 30 patients with toddler's diarrhea and 26 healthy controls, Dodge et al[24] showed that PGF was raised in 17 and PGE_2 in four. Some patients showed good clinical response to aspirin (a prostaglandin synthetase inhibitor) or loperamide (an opiate analog). Although sequential data was not given, it was stated that aspirin therapy resulted in a decrease in plasma levels of prostaglandins but that loperamide had little effect. These observations may have some implications with respect to the pathogenesis of toddler's diarrhea and its treatment.

There is excellent evidence that prostaglandins induce secretion in the small intestine[25] and that loperamide can partially block this effect.[26] However, studies in children and adults suggest that the upper small intestine is not normally in a secretory state. If excessive secretion is involved, it might be taking place in either the lower small intestine or the colon.

Food Intolerance A study of adults with IBS suggests that some have unsuspected food allergies which may play a role in the pathogenesis of the condition.[13] Some children respond to elimination diets, especially those that prohibit allergens such as cow's milk, eggs, and wheat. However, these patients can nearly always be differentiated by their personal or close family history of atopy, peripheral blood eosinophilia, high IgE, positive radio-allergen absorbent tests (RAST) or skin prick tests, and ultimately by the response of their symptoms to the elimination of—followed by challenge with—the suspected allergens. Savilahti et al[27] surveyed children with chronic, nonspecific diarrhea and showed that one third had evidence of food allergy and all were atopic. Abnormal breath hydrogen tests have suggested that lactose maldigestion and malabsorption occurs commonly in IBS. However, few patients have clear-cut lactose intolerance, with the production of watery stools containing lactose in response to a lactose load.

Intestinal Motor Activity Abnormal breath hydrogen tests may provide evidence of lactose malabsorption and may also measure small intestinal transit. An abnormal breath test may result from the rapid delivery of a large quantity of lactose into the colon because of shortened small intestinal transit, which reduces contact time in the proximal jejunum. Corbett et al[28] showed decreased small intestinal transit times in adults with IBS, which was increased by treatment with loperamide. The previously reported beneficial effects of loperamide, therefore, may be related to an effect on small intestinal motility. It is well known that whole-bowel transit time is decreased in children with IBS. Davidson and Wasserman[20] showed that starch intolerance (ie, the presence of starch granules in the stool) was a manifestation of reduced whole-gut transit. The popular term "peas and carrots diarrhea" may be similarly explained. In studies of small intestinal absorption in toddler's diarrhea, it was repeatedly shown that transmural potential difference in over 40% of those with large-amplitude wave forms (ie, 8-13 mV) occurred during perfusion with glucose. In controls, these waves appear to be completely suppressed by glucose. Read et al[29] reported the presence of large-amplitude wave forms in recordings of small intestinal transmural potential difference and showed them to be associated with phase-3 activity of the migrating motor complex.[30] The recognition of the propulsive character of phase 3 in humans[31] and the change to continuous segmenting activity without phase-3 activity in the postprandial state prompted studies of small intestinal motility in children with IBS.[32] No differences in fasting activity could be found, but initiation of postprandial activity and disruption of the migrating motor complex with interduodenal dextrose was clearly defective in patients with IBS. Further studies show that patients in whom dextrose did not disrupt the motor complex were prone to abnormalities in postprandial activity induced by perfusion of the duodenum with soya milk.[33] Postprandial activity was weaker and shorter lived. In one third of patients, phase-3 activity occurred postprandially. Failure of the migrating motor complex to be disrupted by food has been documented in experimental animals subjected to vagotomy[34] and in adults who develop postvagotomy diarrhea.[35]

Previously isolated findings and the above studies of small intestinal motor activity in toddler's diarrhea can be coalesced to form a coherent hypothesis. When food fails to disrupt fasting interdigestive activity and the period of postprandial activity is weaker and shorter, propulsive phasic activity may result, leading to the rapid transit of small intestinal contents through the small intestine to the colon. The small intestinal efflu-ent dumped in the colon under these circumstances may contain partially digested food and excess bile salts. Further degradation by colonic bacteria might yield secretogogues such as unconjugated bile salts and hydroxy-fatty acids, which could adversely affect colonic absorption of water and electrolytes. Similarly, carbohydrates may be dumped in the colon, giving the illusion of lactose intolerance. The bacterial degradation of these substances may also be responsible for increased prostaglandin production, which might produce some of the patients' symptoms. Two studies provide evidence to support this hypothesis. Jonas and Diver Haber[36] studied stool output and composition in children with chronic nonspecific diarrhea and compared it to that from children with malabsorption due to cystic fibrosis or bacterial overgrowth of the small intestine, as well as controls. They found that sodium and bile acids in the extractable water phase were increased in the stool of children with chronic nonspecific diarrhea. These findings could reflect an effect of bile acids on the colonic handling of water and electrolytes. Alun Jones et al[13] showed that in adults with IBS, prostaglandin concentration in the rectal mucosa was increased when the patients were exposed to foods which precipitated their symptoms.

A body of evidence suggests that in children with the diarrheal variant of IBS, there is abnormal motor activity in the small intestine in which fasting activity is not suppressed by the motor response to food and this results in shortened small-bowel transit time. The cause of the inadequate postprandial response is unclear, although abnormal secretion of postprandial polypeptide hormones or disturbed populations or functioning of polypeptide hormone receptors are areas that require investigation.

Constipation

The term constipation refers to the infrequent passage of stools, which may be small, hard, and pelletlike or firm and very large. There may be associated leakage of liquid feces around compacted stools in a capacious rectum, associated with fecal incontinence. Constipation should be clearly distinguished from encopresis, which is the passage of stool in an inappropriate way or place. The frequency of stool passage varies with age. Weaver[37] has shown that the average baby passes 4 ± 1.8 stools per day during the first week of life. By 1 year, the rate falls to approximately 1.6 stools per day, then declines to one stool by the age of 5 years. Most children with idiopathic constipation present around the age of 3 to 4 years with a history of 6 to 24 months. Some are described by their parents as having always been constipated; others have never achieved bowel control. On closer questioning, however, it is rare for such infants to have had disturbed defecation since birth. It is of note that constipation is the only presenting symptom in 5% of patients subsequently proven to have Hirschsprung's disease.

Patients with chronic nonspecific diarrhea and abdominal pain may be intermittently troubled with constipation, but the majority who present with constipation do not experience diarrhea and do not have persistent abdominal pain. Their symptoms are solely those of constipation or soiling, secondary to overflow incontinence. Those who present from birth (ie, they fail to pass meconium in the first 24 h of life) or who experience persistent symptoms of episodic diarrhea and abdominal pain require further investigation to exclude neuromuscular disease of the rectum and colon. Rectal biopsy from clearly defined levels using both conventional histology and histochemistry is the definitive investigation for Hirschsprung's disease and its variants,[38] but anorectal manometry may also be useful. In patients who have a history suggestive of Hirschsprung's disease or who have a distended bladder, hydroureter, hydronephrosis, or a bladder that fails to empty completely, full-thickness biopsy to exclude less common disorders of smooth muscle or enteric nerves are required (see Chapter 22). Cystic fibrosis should be excluded in those who did not pass meconium in the first 24 hours of life or where there is developmental and growth delay, or hypothyroidism.

Pathophysiology. Children with constipation fall into two groups: 1) the majority, for whom no cause can be found and who may later develop megacolon but have no demonstrable physiologic or anatomic abnormality; and 2) the minority, who may have potentially serious pathology.

In those with functional constipation, the problem may stem from a number of factors, including a bout of constipation associated with loss of appetite due to an acute infection, moving to a new house, holidays, or pain from an anal fissure. Another cause may be difficult toilet training, which is either due to unpleasant facilities (eg, inadequate provision at school) or to a persistent, negative developmental phase experienced by some toddlers. Functional studies have focused mainly on the motility of the rectum and anal sphincters after recognition of the altered sphincteric reflexes in Hirschsprung's disease.[39] In the large majority of patients with functional constipation and an idiopathic megacolon—unlike those with Hirschprung's disease—the internal sphincter relaxes with rectal distention. In a study of anorectal physiology in 106 children with long-standing constipation, Clayden and Lawson[40] found 10 to have an ultra-short segment Hirschsprung's disease, which is failure of relaxation of the internal sphincter with distention of the rectum but no ganglia just above the anal verge. Ten others had similar physiologic abnormalities but normal ganglia and nerves were found on biopsy. In the remaining 86 cases, the physiologic findings differed from controls in that a high rectal distention pressure was required to induce relaxation of the internal sphincter, which showed high-amplitude, rhythmic fluctuations of pressure. They suggested that failure of the lower portion of the internal sphincter to relax caused functional obstruction and compensatory hypertrophy of the upper portion of the internal sphincter. About 40% of these patients had a dramatic response to a single anal dilation. A further 9% responded to repeat dilation and sphincterotomy.

Whether the physiologic abnormalities are primary or secondary remains to be determined. Davidson et al[41] showed a failure of some patients to increase colonic motility in response to acetylcholine. Subsequent failure to improve dramatically after an anal pull-through suggested that some form of neuromuscular disease was present. A dynamic test of colonic motor activity might be useful in children with chronic constipation to distinguish those more resistant cases who may have abnormal colonic function (see Chapter 13).

ETIOLOGIC FACTORS FOR IBS

An accumulating body of evidence suggests that feeding and the environment around birth may subsequently have a long-lasting effect on the function of infant gastrointestinal tracts. Evidence suggests that autonomic reactivity patterns are established early in infancy, but it is not clear what effects organic, mechanical, or emotional factors may have on the developing motor control systems of the infant gut. Several stages of development of intestinal motor activity in humans occur prenatally and in early infancy.[42,43] Both control and effector systems are involved in such developmental processes. Functional disorders of the gastrointestinal tract may start insidiously and be concurrent with the setting up of autonomic control patterns in the infant gut. Subsequently, some of these minor functional deviations may be more prone to exaggeration and will develop into lasting symptomatic disorders, such as IBS.

REFERENCES

1. Almy TP. Digestive disease as a national problem. *Gastroenterology* 1967;53:821-33.

2. Thompson DG, Laidlow JM, Wingate DL. Abnormal small bowel motility demonstrated by radiotelemetry in a patient with irritable colon. *Lancet* 1979;2:1321-3.

3. Scott RB, Diamant SG, Gall DG. The motility effects of IgE medicated intestinal anaphylaxis in the rat. *Dig Dis Sci* 1987;32:927.

4. Vermillon D, Scicchitano R, Ernst P. Immuno-modulation of gut motility: involvement of con-nective tissue mast cells. *Dig Dis Sci* 1987;32:931.

5. Berger MG. Somatic pain and school avoidance. *Clin Paediatr (Phila)* 1974;13:815-8.

6. Wolf S, Wolff HG. *Human Gastric Function*. London: Oxford University Press, 1943.

7. Cann P, Read N, Brown C. Psychological stress and the passage of a standard meal in man. *Gut* 1983;24:236-40.

8. Ewart WR, Wingate DL. Central representation and opioid modulation of gastric mechanoreception activity in the rat. *Am J Physiol* 1983;244:G27-32.

9. Richter JE, Barish CF, Castell DO. Abnormal sensory perception in patients with esophageal chest pain. *Gastroenterology* 1986;91:845-52.

10. Moriarty KJ, Dawson AM. Functional abdominal pain: Further evidence that whole gut is affected. *Br Med J* 1982;2:1670-2.

11. Drossman DA, Sandler RS, McKee D, Lovitz AJ. Bowel patterns among subjects not seeking health care. *Gastroenterology* 1982;83:529-34.

12. Apley J. *The Child With Abdominal Pains*. Oxford, England: Blackwell Scientific Publications, 1959.

13. Alun Jones V, McLaughlin P, Shorthouse M, Workman E, Hunter JO. Food intolerance: a major factor in the pathogenesis of irritable bowel syndrome. *Lancet* 1982;2:1115-7.

14. McMichael HB, Webb J, Dawson AM. Lactose deficiency in adults: cause of functional diarrhea. *Lancet* 1965;1:717-20.

15. Egger J, Carter CM, Wilson J, Turner MW, Soathill JF. Is migraine food allergy? A double blind controlled trial of oligoantigenic diet treatment. *Lancet* 1983;2:865-9.

16. Christensen MF, Mortenson O. The long term prognosis in children with recurrent abdominal pain. *Arch Dis Child* 1975;50:110-4.

17. Drossman DA, Powell DW, Sessions JT. The irritable bowel syndrome. *Gastroenterology* 1977;73:811-22.

18. Horowitz L, Farrar JT. Intraluminal mal-intes-

tinal pressures in normal patients and in patients with functional gastrointestinal disorders. *Gastroenterology* 1962;42:455-64.

19. Kopel FB, Kim JC, Barbero GJ. Comparison of recto-sigmoid motility in normal children, children with recurrent abdominal pain, and children with ulcerative colitis. *Paediatrics* 1967;39:539-45.

20. Davidson M, Wasserman R. The irritable colon of childhood (chronic non-specific diarrhea syndrome). *J Pediatr* 1966;69:1027-38.

21. Read NW. The migrating motor complex and spontaneous fluctuations of transmural potential difference in the human small intestine. In: Christensen J, ed. *Gastrointestinal Motility.* New York, NY: Raven Press, 1980;299-306.

22. Milla PJ, Atherton DA, Leonard JV, Wolff OH, Lake BD. Disordered intestinal functions in glycogen storage disease. *J Inherited Metab Dis* 1978;1:155-7.

23. Tripp JH, Muller DPR, Harries JT. Mucosal (Na + K +) ATPase and adenylate cyclase activities in children with toddler diarrhoea and postenteritis syndrome. *Paediatr Res* 1980;14:1382-6.

24. Dodge JA, Handi IA, Burns GM, Yamashiro Y. Toddler diarrhea and prostaglandins. *Arch Dis Child* 1981;56:705-57.

25. Matuchansky C, Bernier JJ. Effect of prostaglandin E_1 on glucose water and electrolyte absorption in the human jejunum. *Gastroenterology* 1973;64:1111-8.

26. Sandhu BK, Tripp JH, Candy DCA, Harries JT. Loperamide: studies on its mechanism of action. *Gut* 1981;22:658-62.

27. Savilahti E, Simell O. Chronic non-specific diarrhea. *Arch Dis Child* 1985;60:452-6.

28. Corbett CL, Thomas S, Read NW, Hobson N, Bergman I, Holdsworth CD. Electrochemical detector for breath hydrogen determination: measurement of small bowel transit time in normal subjects and patients with irritable bowel syndrome. *Gut* 1981;22:836-40.

29. Read NW, Small RH, Levin RJ, Holdsworth CD, Brown BH. Relationship between changes in intraluminal pressure and transmural potential dif-

ference in the human and canine jejunum in vivo. *Gut* 1977;18:141-5.

30. Read NW, Krejs GJ, Read MG, Santa Ana CA, Morowski SJ, Fordtran JS. Chronic diarrhea of unknown origin. *Gastroenterology* 1980;78:264-71.

31. Vantrappen G, Janssens J, Hellemans J, Shoos Y. The interdigestive motor complex of normal subjects and patients with bacterial overgrowth of the small intestine. *J Clin Invest* 1977;59:1158-66.

32. Fenton TR, Harries JT, Milla PJ. Disordered small intestinal motility: a rational basis for toddler's diarrhea. *Gut* 1983;24:897-903.

33. Fenton TR, Harries JT, Milla PJ. Abnormalities of postprandial small intestinal motor activity in childhood: their role in the pathogenesis of the irritable bowel syndrome. In: Labo G, Bortolotti M, eds. *Gastrointestinal Motility.* Verona, Italy: Cortina International 1983;207-13.

34. Diament NF, Hall K, Muir H, El Sharkaway TY. Vagal control of the feeding motor patterns in the lower esophageal sphincter, stomach, and upper small intestine of dogs. In: Christensen J, ed. *Gastrointestinal Motility.* New York, NY: Raven Press, 1980;365-70.

35. Thompson DG, Ritchie HD, Wingate DL. Patterns of small intestinal motility in duodenal ulcer patients before and after vagotomy. *Gut* 1982;23:517-23.

36. Jonas A, Diver Haber A. Stool output and composition in the chronic non-specific diarrhea syndrome. *Arch Dis Child* 1982;57:35-9.

37. Weaver LT. The bowel habit of young children. *Arch Dis Child* 1984;59:649-52.

38. Lake BD, Puri P, Nixon HH, Claireaux AE. Hirschsprung's disease: an appraisal of histochemically demonstrated acetylcholinesterase activity in section rectal biopsies as an aid to diagnosis. *Archives of Pathology and Laboratory Medicine* 1978;102:244-7.

39. Aaronson I, Nixon HH. A clinical evaluation of anorectal pressure, studies in the diagnosis of Hirschsprung's disease. *Gut* 1972;13:138-46.

40. Clayden GS, Lawson JO. Investigation and management of longstanding chronic constipation

tion in childhood. *Arch Dis Child* 1976;51:918-20.

41. Davidson M, Kugler MM, Bauer CH. Diagnosis and management in children with severe and protracted constipation and obstipation. *J Paediatr* 1963;67:261-75.

42. Bisset WM, Watt J, Rivers R, Milla PJ. The ontogeny of fasting small intestinal motor activity in the human infant. *Gut* 1988;483-8.

43. Bisset WM, Watt J, Rivers RPA, Milla PJ. Postprandial motor response of the small intestine to enteral feeds in preterm infants. *Arch Dis Child* 1989;64:1356-61.

44. Young LD, Richter JE, Anderson KO, Bradley LA, et al. The effects of psychological and environmental stressors on peristaltic esophageal contractions in healthy volunteers. *Psychophysiology* 1987;24:132-41.

45. Thompson DG, Richelson E, Malagelada J-R. Perturbation of upper gastrointestinal function by cold stress. *Gut* 1983;24:277-83.

46. Valori RM, Kuman D, Wingate DL. Effects of different types of stress and of "prokinetic" drugs on the control of the fasting motor complex in humans. *Gastroenterology* 1986;90:1890-1900.

47. Welgan P, Meshkinpour H, Hoechler F. The effect of stress on colon motor and electrical activity in irritable bowel syndrome. *Psychosom Med* 1985;47:139-49.

10

Visceral Pain in Children

LONNIE K. ZELTZER, SUSAN ARNOULT, ALISON HAMILTON, STEVEN DeLAURA

It has now been well documented that children's pain is rarely recognized and thus undertreated.[1] While great strides have been made in methods of treating postoperative and other acute pain in children, the assessment and therapies for visceral pain have lagged behind these advances. This undertreatment probably reflects the paucity of information about visceral pain, especially in children. Persistent and recurrent visceral pain has been implicated in the development of pathologic pain pathways and in the development of pathologic motor reflex arcs at the spinal cord level of action.[2] Thus, the clinical implication for children with intestinal dysmotility and pain is that pathologic, persistent pain may develop and be perpetuated unless the pain is adequately addressed and reduced. Since this pain is no longer simply based on the motor dysfunction, correction of the intestinal motor patterns may not provide relief. Further, the pain itself can alter motility. A vicious cycle of visceral pain and abnormal intestinal motor patterns becomes established, which is often refractory to common current approaches to management.

Because pain is a compelling symptom—especially in children—factors other than tissue injury contribute to the development of chronic pain. Parental reinforcement of pain behaviors, feelings of helplessness in both parents and the affected child, changes in the lifestyle of the child evolving from current and expected future pain, as well as sleep and eating disturbances are among the factors that exacerbate the pain. The health care team must sort out and attempt to effect change in a symptom that has complex origins and multifactorial perpetuators. Singular approaches aimed at correcting the motor abnormality or modifying family interactions are often met with failure or a high recidivism that takes its toll on the parents, child, and health care team alike. The child and family soon get the message that the child will have to "learn to live with the pain" or that the child's complaints are largely "attention-getting" manipulations that should be ignored or referred for psychiatric attention. These messages foster various reactions, including "doctor shopping" in which the child ultimately has increasing numbers of diagnostic and invasive procedures, typically without long-lasting benefits.

Physicians differ in their experiences with and approaches to evaluation and management of these children and their families, but the delimiting factor is time. To develop a sufficiently effective treatment plan takes significant amounts of time and a team that includes, but is not limited to, the pediatrician, pediatric gastroenterologist, nurse, and child psychologist or psychiatrist. Effective treatment also involves parental motivation and trust in the health care team. Various health care insurance plans may also play a role in dictating the type of treatment, often not for the betterment of the child. Some insurers limit psychologic services or hospitalizations, especially if the purpose of hospitalization is to remove the child from the home-reinforcers of pain behaviors and to establish new child and family patterns of behavior related to pain and eating. Some insurance companies view this type of hospitalization as "psychiatric" and will pay only for medical interventions, such as hospitalizations involving intravenous medications or invasive procedures.

To begin this chapter, a summary of the anatomy and mechanisms involved in pain transmission and inhibition is provided to help the reader understand the complexities of visceral pain, and also to delineate a framework for treatment approaches. Since new evidence for visceral pain mechanisms is evolving as this chapter is being written, and there are few studies of mechanisms or treatments in children, the proposed strategies are based on current data, the working theoretical model, and the experience of the authors.

PAIN TRANSMISSION AND INHIBITION

Pain is the subjective response of an individual to noxious stimuli. The noxious stimulus is sensed by a peripheral receptor and a pain message is then transmitted via afferent fibers to the spinal cord. After entering the central nervous system (CNS), the signal passes up ascending tracts in the spinal cord to synapse in specific areas of the midbrain, pons, and diencephalon. At any point along the path, reflex arcs may be stimulated to initiate aversion responses to the noxious event. From these lower brain centers, the nociceptive information may or may not be forwarded to the limbic and somatosensory areas of the telencephalon, where the subjective, conscious experience of pain originates.

Great variability in individual responses to nociceptive signaling is observed clinically. Identical nociceptive events, such as venipunctures, could produce severe pain in a patient who has had multiple invasive procedures and lives with chronic pain, while producing only mild discomfort in another child with no history of hospitalization or illness. Similarly, an event such as eating a meal would not initiate nociceptive signaling in a normal, healthy child, but might produce severe pain and nausea in a patient with chronic intestinal pseudo-obstruction. The great variability in pain perception can

be attributed to two mitigating categories of factors: physiologic and psychologic differences between individuals. Physiologic factors might include the baseline status of the autonomic nervous system and its range of available reactivity, threshold of sensory receptors (ie, level of stimulation required for nerve transmission or sensory perception), efficacy of synaptic connections, and health of the neuroendocrine axis. Psychologic factors can include cognitive maturation, language development, pain memories, coping ability, self-regulation capabilities, and cultural, familial, or individual beliefs about pain.

Receptors

The first component in the nociceptive pathway is the sensory receptor. There are two classifications of cutaneous nociceptors that respond only to noxious levels of stimulation: high-threshold mechanoreceptors and polymodal nociceptors. The concept of specific nociceptors, however, is relevant primarily to cutaneous somatic pain reception. Deep somatic and visceral pain are registered when a normal receptor (eg, mechano-, chemo-, thermo-, osmo-, or polymodal receptors) encounters supraphysiologic or noxious levels of stimulation.[3] At normal levels of stimulation, the receptors convey a message about the status of the viscera. At excessive levels of stimulation, the CNS translates the intensity to mean pain.

Afferent Fibers

Nociceptive signals are carried from the periphery to the spinal cord via A-d and C fibers. A-d fibers are the moderately myelinated, fast-conducting fibers that carry pain impulses from the high-threshold mechanoreceptors and polymodal receptors in visceral and somatic tissue. These fibers are involved in the transmission of "first pain," which is characteristically a sharp, well-localized pain that occurs immediately after the onset of injury. "Second pain" is carried in C fibers, which are unmyelinated and conduct impulses from cutaneous, deep, low-threshold sensory receptors. Their message is associated with the dull, poorly localized pain that ensues after the onset of injury. Many of the compounds released at the site of an injury are capable of stimulating nociceptors, although substance P appears to be the major neurotransmitter used by the primary afferent fibers.[4] Recently, cholecystokinin (CCK) has been shown to be hyperalgesic by antagonizing analgesia produced by opiates in the dorsal horn.[5] While both visceral and somatic afferents utilize A-d and C fibers in the transmission of pain messages, visceral afferent fibers travel within the sympathetic nerves to reach the spinal cord.

Spinal Cord and Ascending Tracts

Somatic pain transmission. When the afferent fibers reach the spinal cord, they synapse both ipsilaterally and contralaterally on second-order neurons within the gray matter of the spinal cord. The sensory information carried in the afferent fibers serves two basic functions. The first is protection. Many of the synaptic connections that the entering sensory neurons make are with motor neurons or interneurons in the ventral horn of the spinal cord. This gives rise to the protective reflex arcs that allow for immediate aversive action (such as withdrawal) against the noxious stimulus. In addition to the reflex connections, the sensory neurons may also connect with one or more of the ascending pain tracts that carry pain messages up to the brain for further processing. The major tracts involved are the spinothalamic, spinoreticular, and spinomesencephalic tracts.[6] These tracts terminate within the thalamus, the reticular formation, and the periaqueductal gray (PAG) regions of the brain. From these areas, the pain message can trigger arousal and initiate the motivational and affective aspects of pain, thereby bringing the noxious signal to conscious perception.

Visceral pain transmission. There are some differences between visceral and somatic pain transmission systems. Evidence for a subset of visceral receptors devoted solely to visceral nociception is lacking except in the bladder,[7,8] gallbladder, biliary ducts,[9] ureter,[10] and heart.[11] Most visceral afferent receptors subscribe to the intensity theory of pain transmission,[3] in which a more intense activation of a population of low-threshold receptors would result in pain.

Clinical observations indicate that patients have difficulty localizing abdominal pain and that visceral pain is often referred to a specific dermatome. The arrangement of the visceral pain transmission system provides some insight into these observations. First, spinal afferent receptive fields are much larger than those of cutaneous receptors, giving rise to greater visceral afferent information convergence within the spinal cord.[12] Second, the afferent fibers impinge on "somatovisceral" neurons within the spinal cord.[13] Thus, no second-order neuron within the spinal cord receives solely visceral input and no ascending tract devoted exclusively to visceral sensation has been found. These findings demonstrate that it is impossible to localize visceral pain and that somatic and visceral pain are intimately entwined.

Endogenous Pain Modulation and Descending Tracts

Since the introduction of the gate-control theory of pain by Melzack and Wall in 1965,[14] evidence has been amassed to demonstrate the existence of multiple pain modulation systems within the nervous system. Unlike its predecessors, this theory allows for pain modulation at multiple levels (Fig. 10.1). Ascending signal modulation occurs via an A-d excitatory collateral, the C-fiber inhibitory collateral, and descending fibers. In this model, integration of all inputs would determine the level of action taken by the organism. Three areas of the CNS have been identified as particularly important in the pain modulatory systems: 1) the midbrain PAG, 2) the rostral ventromedial medulla (RVM), and 3) the superficial layers of the dorsal horn.

A question has arisen as to how excitation (eg, with electrical stimulation) and inhibition (eg, with application of β-endorphins) of the PAG can both result in analgesia. A proposed explanation of this dichotomy is that the opioids repress an inhibitory

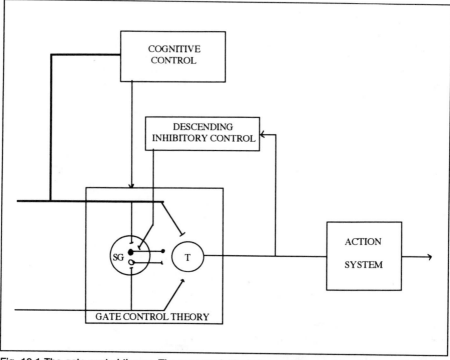

Fig. 10.1 The gate-control theory. The new model includes excitatory (white circle) and inhibitory (black circle) links from the substantia gelatinosa (SG) to the transmission (T) cells, as well as descending inhibitory control from brain stem systems. The round knob at the end of the inhibitory link implies that its action may be presynaptic, postsynaptic, or both. All connections are excitatory except the inhibitory link from SG to T cell. (Reprinted with permission from Zeltzer LK, et al, 1990[75])

interneuron within the PAG.[5] This shuts off the inhibition of the inhibitory projection neuron to the RVM. Thus, less inhibition equals more excitation. Increased release of serotonin or neurotensin from the RVM projections leads to excitation of inhibitory interneurons within the spinal cord. The enkephalin released from the inhibitory internuncial neurons then binds the nociceptive projection neuron,[15] thus producing postsynaptic inhibition of pain transmission. Although there are opioid binding sites on the primary afferent fibers, no endogenous opioid has been shown to exist at these sites.[5] The end result of the enkephalin-inhibition of the second-order neuron is a decrease in the nociceptive message transmitted from the C fiber to the second-order neuron of the ascending tract. Opiate analgesia ameliorates second pain more effectively than A-d first pain.

Endogenous opioids and their receptors, as they pertain to the descending pain modulatory mechanisms, have been studied in great detail. Opiate receptors are highly concentrated in laminae I to VII of the spinal cord, the limbic system, and respiratory centers of the brain. The binding of an opiate molecule to its receptor produces various pharmacologic effects including analgesia, euphoria or dysphoria, respiratory depression, inhibition of gastric motility, mydriasis, and bradycardia or tachycardia.[16] One reason for the variety of responses is that there are four distinct types of opiate receptors. The receptor that binds morphine with the greatest affinity is called the "mu" receptor (μ), of which the PAG contains significant quantities. The other receptor types are called "kappa," "delta," and "sigma." Each serves a specific function in pain analgesia. Endogenous peptides such as β-endorphin, leu- and met-enkephalin, and dynorphin are distributed between the PAG, RVM, and dorsal horn of the spinal cord. Some of the nonopiates are also involved in the pain modulation system, including serotonin (5-HT) and norepinephrine. Serotonin, the neurotransmitter released by descending long-tract fibers (DLF), is a necessary component of opiate-mediated analgesia. Norepinephrine, however, can antagonize or potentiate opiate analgesia, depending on where it is injected. Within the spinal cord it appears that norepinephrine potentiates morphine's ability to reduce nociception, but injection of norepinephrine into the RVM inhibits the analgesic system. There are separate norepinephrine and serotonin paths within the DLF, and blockade of opiate analgesia post-DLF lesion could be the result of damage from either of these two systems.

DEVELOPMENT OF PAIN SYSTEMS

Infant and childhood pain are often undertreated based on several faulty assumptions regarding the developmental age of a child's pain transmission system. Common clinical practice has been to perform major surgery on infants using only a paralytic agent and no analgesics or anesthetics. Additionally, postoperative pain was not acknowledged to exist in neonates. The rationale was based on two prevailing myths: 1) that the paucity of myelination at birth blunted neonatal pain transmission; and 2) due to the lack of cortical maturation, neonates did not yet have the cognitive abilities to remember pain and thus, the motivational/affective aspect of pain was not a factor.[17] If both of these assumptions were true, it would be reasonable to conclude that neonates, infants, and children would not experience pain in the same sense as adults. Unfortunately, overwhelming and chilling evidence in recent years has shown that not only are the pain transmission and associated cognitive systems in place and functional by birth, but that the lack of pain management in these patients has physiologic consequences that hamper clinical progress.

For pain perception to occur, several neural elements must be present: 1) functional afferent sensory receptors and fibers; 2) axons that can propagate action potentials; 3) neurotransmitters to carry the message between synapses; 4) proper connections between first-, second-, and third-order neurons that allow reflex aversive behavior and stimulation of conscious sensory centers of the brain; and 5) maturation of sensory and limbic cortices so that the noxious stimulus has meaning. New evidence shows that every one of these factors is present and working to some degree at birth, if not before. To begin with, cutaneous primary afferent endings have been shown to respond to stimulation from the earliest stages of skin innervation. Not only are these afferent endings capable of responding to stimulation, but they can do so in well-defined patterns with distinct receptive fields.[18] Second, the argument that fetuses and neonates cannot experience pain due to incomplete myelination of their afferent fibers is unsubstantiated.

Since unmyelinated C fibers play a major role in the transmission of both somatic and visceral pain in adults,[19] myelination of these afferent fibers is unnecessary for the successful reception and forwarding of a noxious stimulus to the CNS. Animal studies with rats have shown that C-fiber synaptic boutons begin to produce spikes in the second-order neurons of the dorsal horn around the first postnatal week.[20,21] Timetables comparing the rat and human nervous systems' development indicate that the first postnatal week of the rat corresponds to the 24th week of gestation in the human.[20] Neurotransmitters within the primary afferents appear at around 12 to 16 weeks in the human fetus.[22] The initial levels are fairly low, but increase throughout the rest of gestation and into the neonatal period. These findings suggest that fetal afferent fibers have the capacity to excite their second-order dorsal horn cells in predictable, mature-spiking patterns prior to birth. Even if human development did not correspond directly to the rat/human developmental timetable, it has been shown that, prior to the appearance of the synaptic boutons, C fibers are capable of producing long-lasting, subthreshold depolarizations in the spinal cord. Even with subthreshold stimulation, the dorsal horn targets become sensitized to subsequent stimulation.[20] Animal research, therefore, provides evidence that the neonate would have painful messages conveyed to the CNS.

In the adult, the pain message that reaches the CNS initiates protective reflexes and alerts the emotional/affective centers of the cortex to the noxious event. Exaggerated cutaneous reflexes, such as the flexor reflex, are observed in the newborn[23] and are probably due to two characteristics of the neonatal spinal cord. At first, the primary sensory neurons have a somewhat weak connection with their target spinal cells, but are capable of producing excitation that lasts several minutes.[24] Additionally, the receptive fields of the dorsal horn neurons are large in the newborn and diminish over the first 2 weeks postnatally.[24] Despite the differences in the neonatal spinal tracts when compared to the adult, signaling is still occurring. In fact, studies have shown that the whole complement of 10^9 cortical neurons is present by the 20th week and that thalamocortical connections are made by 29 weeks,[25] as evidenced by well-defined periods of wakefulness and sleep.[4] Myelination up to and including the thalamocortical connections is complete by the 37th week of gestation.[26] Taken together, these facts would indicate that the hard wiring for the detection, transmission, and reaction to noxious stimuli is present in the fetus. In fact, only the endogenous pain inhibition system is deficient at birth, probably because norepinephrine and serotonin appear at 6 weeks postnatally. Opiate receptors, however, are present at birth. Morphine is an effective analgesic in both full-term and premature newborns.[27]

In addition to the presence of the necessary wiring and neurochemicals at birth, neonates exhibit a stress response similar to that seen in adults.[28] The physiologic stress response observed in reaction to noxious stimuli includes release of catecholamines, growth hormone, glucogon, aldosterone, and other corticosteroids. As in adults, heart rate and blood pressure increase in newborns in pain, but these effects can be eliminated by administering anesthetics. The resultant, hormonally-driven breakdown of carbohydrate and fat stores, if prolonged, could lead to hyperglycemia and acidosis. These stress responses are dangerous in neonates, but administration of analgesia or anesthesia will decrease if not abolish the metabolic and hormonal responses to nociceptive stimuli.[29] Studies also demonstrate that infants given deep anesthesia during surgical procedures are more stable postoperatively than infants given minimal anesthetics.[30]

The idea that the neonate has no pain memory is also being refuted. Long-term memory requires the limbic system and the diencephalon,[31] both of which are well-developed and functional at birth.[32] The greatest period of learning and CNS plasticity (ie, capacity for change) occurs in the late prenatal and neonatal periods,[33,34] so it is somewhat ludicrous to think that repeated stimulation of an intact pain pathway would have no lasting effect on the developing CNS. Infants have many more synaptic connections and shorter distances for messages to travel than adults.[35] Additionally, individual sensory experiences dictate which paths are pruned out and which become permanent. In light of the plasticity and the effects of sensory experience on the development of the nervous system, it seems reasonable to conclude that unmanaged, severe, prolonged pain experiences in neonatal life could influence the development of the nervous system. If stimulation is the signal necessary for "fixing" a synaptic connection and repeated stimulation is required for increased synaptic efficacy and memory, untreated pain would serve to maintain connections within the pain transmission system that should have degenerated. Along with the immediate detrimental metabolic, hormonal, and cardiovascular effects of undertreated pain, the activation of pain pathways could also be initiated and their efficiency enhanced, leading to a much more dire, long-term clinical problem.

GASTROINTESTINAL INNERVATION AND VISCERAL PAIN

Pain is a common complaint with many gastroenterologic disorders in children. Bowel obstruction leads to distention of the gut wall, stretching of the mesentery, and pain. Infection within the gut lumen causes inflammation and can lead to peripheral receptor hyperalgesia (ie, lowered threshold for nociception and recruitment of mechanoreceptors as nociceptors) as well as stimulation of the afferent receptors by inflammatory products. Hormonal disorders (eg, hypothyroidism or cyclic changes associated with menstruation) can alter afferent transmission or affect gastrointestinal (GI) motility, both of which could lead to pain. Some treatments (eg, gastrotomy-tube placement or surgery) aimed at correcting the patient's nutritional deficits cause pain. Pain in the clinical setting is common and may be debilitating for the child.

The extrinsic and intrinsic sensory receptors are the two broad classes of sensory receptors in visceral structures. Extrinsic sensory reception comes via spinal afferent and vagal afferent receptors. It appears that only the spinal afferents are involved in the detection and transmission of pain signals from the viscera. The spinal afferent mechanoreceptors lie predominantly in the mesentery, although some are also located within the gut wall itself. These afferent endings are unimodal and detect a particular type of mechanical change, such as stretch or compression. The spinal cord transmissions are based on the intensity of the signal. Pain would be registered if the stimulus became excessive.

In contrast, vagal afferent terminals are polymodal and innervate both the gut mucosa and the smooth muscle of the gastrointestinal tract. Vagal afferent endings are designed for bowel proprioception because they continually relay information to the CNS about the degree of torsion, compression, or distention of the gut mucosa and muscle layers. Additionally, vagal afferents are chemo- and osmoreceptors, and are able to relay information about the chemical composition of the luminal contents as well as the GI blood supply. The CNS uses the vagal sensory information to initiate autonomic reflexes that control various GI functions, such as smooth-muscle contraction, secretion, absorption, and blood flow.

While autonomic afferent fibers do not directly regulate the GI tract, they influence the neurons of the enteric nervous system (ENS), which is the intrinsic neural system of the gut. Found within the ENS of the gut, intrinsic sensory receptors include fast-adapting and slow-adapting mechanoreceptors as well as the AH/type 2 neuron. The latter is a tonic type of unit that discharges despite intensity or duration of the stimulus. It also signals the occurrence of mechanical distortion.

Sensitization refers to a decrease in pain threshold which could be exhibited at the cellular level as well as by behavior. Sensory receptors can become sensitized to repeated mechanical, thermal, or chemical stimulation, thereby causing a decreased threshold for action potential firing and allodynia (ie, pain with any type of stimulation).[36,37] A child can become so sensitized to the emotional aspects of pain that fear, stress, and pain materialize at even the mention of a medical procedure. Both of these examples depend on the presence or expectation of the threatening stimulus—even at nonnoxious levels—for reaction to take place. Hyperalgesia (ie, pathologic pain), in contrast to sensitization, is manifested by an increased response to a noxious stimulus. This could occur at any level of message processing from the sensory receptor up to the sensory cortex.

Sensitization and hyperalgesia can be due to peripheral as well as central mechanisms. As mentioned above, sensory receptor thresholds may be reduced, thereby causing the afferent endings to be hypersensitive to noxious as well as nonnoxious stimulation.[38] While sensitization of a nociceptor is usually restricted to 5 to 10 mm from the site of injury,[39] cutaneous hyperalgesia spreads as far as 10 to 20 cm beyond the site of injury.[40] The increased sensitivity of these central neurons is seen by way of their increased spontaneous activity, increased response to afferent input, and decreased threshold for response,[41] as well by the expansion of receptive fields of dorsal horn second-order neurons.[42] Additional studies show that repeated C-fiber stimulation, which is found in chronic pain conditions, increases dorsal horn activity and leads to prolonged discharge of the cell,[43] known as "windup."[44] Studies have demonstrated that inflammatory lesions caused receptive-field expansion of projection cells within the ventrobasal thalamus.[45] Continual stimulation of the C-fiber afferents, therefore, has an effect in reshaping the peripheral receptors' responses as well as the central neurons' responses to pain. Central sensitization resulting in larger peripheral receptive fields, even after the damaged tissue heals, might explain the development of hyperalgesia.

Hyperalgesia, therefore, seems a likely candidate for some of the pathology observed in visceral pain associated with many GI disorders. Since visceral pain is registered within the CNS based on the intensity of signaling coming from the viscera to the spinal neurons, the development of a larger receptive field takes on significance for persistent visceral pain conditions. Dorsal horn neurons and even thalamic relay neurons would have considerably larger inputs following C-fiber sensitization. In this arena, doubling the normal afferent inputs to a single neuron would register as higher-intensity stimulation and, possibly, pain. This afferent signalling aberration could then translate into faulty control of GI function based on the fact that ENS neurons receive information from autonomic efferents.

Visceral pain signals travelling in the sympathetic afferent fibers activate or inhibit certain GI functions, such as gastric emptying.[46] Under normal conditions it would be important for the body to shut down its GI functions to attend to and control the noxious stimulation. With the pathologic condition, noxious stimulation does not come from the peripheral afferent endings but rather from the central, sensitized second-order neurons and, therefore, GI function does not

require alteration. For example, if gastric emptying were delayed due to a central pain message, nausea, vomiting, and distention could then follow. Distention of a viscus may lead to torsion or compression of the mesentery, and secondary pain messages could be transmitted, thus establishing an uninterrupted, escalating cycle of pain signaling.

There are other mechanisms by which pathologic visceral pain may develop. Disease of the mucosa or musculature of the GI tract could cause deafferentation. Some spinal and most vagal afferents terminate within the gut wall. Electrophysiologic studies in animals and humans indicate that 80% to 90%[47] of fibers in the abdominal vagi are afferent, predominantly unmyelinated fibers.[48,49] Damage to either of these afferent neural populations within the GI tract could potentially lead to a "phantom gut" syndrome, in which pain could persist or be triggered long after the primary intestinal condition has been cured, even after the offending part of the intestine has been surgically removed. Ronald Melzack, a leader in phantom limb pain research, has determined that once a central pain trace (ie, central memory of pain) is created, even amputation and complete deafferentation of the limb do not necessarily stop the pain.[50] Since vagal afferents are unmyelinated fibers similar to the C-fibers found in pain transmission, it stands to reason that they could also become sensitized by repeated stimulation. Since the receptors are polymodal, sensitization could result from chemical or mechanical overstimulation, both of which can accompany inflammatory, hormonal, or motility disorders of the GI tract. Even if the GI tissue has normalized, receptive fields of the vagal afferents might become enlarged, leading to hyperstimulation of the central neurons. This faulty signaling from the central neurons could result in inappropriate autonomic reflexes and efferent messages. Consequences might include cessation of bowel smooth-muscle contraction leading to distention and pain,[51] or augmentation of smooth-muscle contraction which could also be a potential cause of visceral pain.[52] Gastrointestinal disease states could also progress, causing further damage to the GI tract and the associated neurons, resulting in phantom gut syndrome.

With the emphasis on neural plasticity as a cause of visceral hyperalgesia and pathologic pain, it is important to focus on managing pain in patients whose nervous systems are at the height of their flexibility and development—infants and young children. Central hyperalgesia does not occur unless the injury information is allowed to reach the CNS. Administering analgesics prior to tissue damage could reduce the rate of rise of the excitatory postsynaptic potential (EPSP) that normally results from prolonged C-fiber input, thereby blocking the dorsal horn neuronal excitation in response to this input.[4] Development of hyperalgesia after cutaneous injury was prevented in one study by prior local anesthetic blocks of peripheral nerves proximal to the site of injury.[41] Wiesenfeld-Hallin et al[53] have demonstrated that once the flexor reflex has been conditioned by C-fiber afferent stimuli, it takes 10-fold higher doses of morphine to reverse. This potential for undertreated pain to cause central hyperalgesia, especially in early childhood, may have consequences for children with GI problems who require repeated, painful medical procedures for evaluation and treatment. Careful postoperative pain management and measures to reduce pain during medical procedures could potentially prevent the establishment of aberrant pain pathways and central pain memories, thereby eliminating some of the future avenues for pathologic pain in these children.

INDIVIDUAL DIFFERENCES IN PAIN VULNERABILITY

Given genetic differences in the development of the nervous system, potential intrauterine contributors, as well as postnatal environmental influences, it is not surprising that there are individual differences in pain perception and vulnerability to pathologic visceral pain.[54] This section will examine differences in pain perception and vulnerability from a clinical, rather than neuroanatomic or neurophysiologic, perspective.

Children differ in their visceral and somatic sensory awareness, with various thresholds for perception of pain. The same degree of stomach expansion for one child might not produce any sensations, for another it might produce "fullness," and for yet a third it might produce pain. Such differing sensory experiences may lead to different patterns of attention focus and arousal in relation to eating or drinking. The first child might eat without thinking about the process of eating. The second child might be cautious about the amounts consumed. The third child might become anxious in relation to any food—even small bites—so that eating anything immediately causes a focus of attention on visceral sensations and arousal as the child "waits for something bad to happen." These learned associations (ie, central cognitive processes) may lead to enhanced sympathetic nervous system signaling with reciprocal reduction in parasympathetic afferent input and subsequent GI contraction abnormalities. Thus, it is easy to understand how differing sensory thresholds may lead to a cascade of events that can reinforce a symptom such as visceral pain associated with eating.

Children also differ in their ability to tolerate a sensory experience. Some may experience a moderate amount of visceral pain and be able to distract themselves, ignore the pain, or use other coping strategies. Other children with the same or less discomfort may immediately find it intolerable and need rapid, dramatic measures to eliminate or reduce it. Level of pain tolerance has been shown to be a stable characteristic of children over a 2-year period.[55] While there may be some biologic substrate, the cognitive aspect of learning how to cope is likely learned, and thus influenced by a combination of early childhood and infancy pain experiences as well as parental responses to the child in pain.

Children also develop various coping styles for handling the anticipation of and their encounter with pain. Anticipatory extremes might include denying or not thinking about an upcoming event that is expected to be painful (eg, eating, defecating, or an anticipated medical procedure), or catastrophizing about it (eg, "It's going to be so bad that I will not be able to tolerate it!"). During the pain experience, children tend to either attend to it, focus on it, notice it, and dwell on it ("attenders") or distract themselves from it by using their imagination to think about or experience other things by watching television, playing, etc. ("distractors"). The status of anxiety/arousal may play an important role in attention regulation. A highly anxious child who normally can distract himself during pain may not be able to focus his attention on anything other than the pain during a medical procedure. Some children become so anxious during all pain experiences that they cannot change their focus of attention to other sensations.

As part of the evaluation process, therefore, it is important to learn about a child's typical visceral and somatic pain thresholds or perceptions, tolerance, and coping style. Assessment should also include the child's anxiety level during visceral pain episodes and associated pain behaviors.

ASSESSMENT OF PAIN

Assessment of the pain is critical for diagnosis and treatment. History should be obtained from both the child (for age 3 years or greater) and parents. Obviously, the extent of the child's self-report will depend on her age and developmental maturity. However, even a 3-year-old can at least indicate current pain through a variety of pain measurement tools. The simplest is a vertical 10-cm line anchored at the bottom with a "happy face" and at the top with a "sad face." The child is asked to point on the line to show how much she is "hurting now." The level of sophistication in self-report can increase with age to include the filling in of body diagrams with colors to indicate different types and intensities of pains in various locations. Location, intensity, type (pain descriptors), timing (duration, frequency, time of day), and factors that make the pain worse or better can all be assessed to some degree, depending on the child. It is also helpful to learn what the child believes is causing the pain and what the child believes will alleviate it.

Similar information should be obtained from the parents, in addition to the early childhood pain history and treatments. Although a history of parental pain problems may be helpful in individual cases, recent evidence suggests that children of adult chronic pain patients do not have more pain problems than other children.[56]

The history of the pain itself, combined with information about the contributory factors (which are described in the next section), should provide the basis for a working model of the etiology of the pain and the factors that probably contribute to its persistence, as well as those that help mitigate it. The differentiation can usually be made between the child's personal experience of pain and the child's pain-associated behaviors. It is usually the latter to which parents may be responding in ways that may enhance the pain.

The child's own description of the pain—especially if she can be taught to differentiate among types of pain — can be useful in understanding the etiology. While visceral pain is typically poorly localized compared with somatic pain, increasing evidence suggests that peripheral-referred pain (ie, referred hyperalgesia) is not an uncommon accompaniment.[57] In one study of adults with renal colic, ipsilateral back pain developed and persisted after the resolution of the colic (ie, after there was clinical and radiographic evidence that the stone had passed).[57] However, a lowered threshold for pain stimuli remained in the back muscles on the affected side. Electrical stimulation of these muscle groups and overlying subcutaneous tissue used to measure the pain threshold was enough to retrigger the renal colic pain that had been present earlier, even though the stone had been removed.

There are three aspects to pain assessment: 1) *ask*—self-report, parent report; 2) *look*—observation of the child for overall activity and focal limitation of movement or unusual body posturing; and 3) *examine*—physical findings, blood pressure, heart rate, respiratory rate, sweating, as well as skin temperature, texture, and color changes.

PLANNING A PAIN TREATMENT STRATEGY

There are a number of considerations in planning a pain treatment strategy. The multifactorial nature of pain requires that a variety of factors be assessed to develop a working model of a particular child's pain problem. Although it initially involves a somewhat lengthy history, this approach can be very helpful in guiding the pain treatment plan. Flexibility is a crucial element in effective pain control, including consideration of changes based on the child's and family's responses to the initial plan, new information that may not emerge until later during the treatment course, and unanticipated parental resistance to certain aspects of the treatment.

Parental resistance can be particularly frustrating and has the potential for damaging sequelae as a fallout from doctor/parent mutual anger. For example, parents may say—and believe—that they will "do anything" to relieve their child's suffering. However, requested changes in parental reinforcing behaviors around pain episodes, and/or temporary separations from the child in a hospital setting so that new coping responses can be established (eg, the father rather than the mother spend time with child), may be met with resistance. Mothers who have been primary caretakers of their children and have spent considerable time comforting their children during pain may have unconscious ambivalence about giving up that role. They may doubt their child's ability to cope without their help, and become anxious about changes in the family structure and their own value to the family if the pain resolves in their absence. It is also not uncommon for the child to develop nonpainful, asymptomatic eating, defecating, and sleeping patterns in the hospital without requiring "venting" of a gastrostomy tube, only to return home with the mother reporting numerous pain episodes, limited eating, and returned use of venting procedures. The goal of treatment in this case is to help the family adjust to new ways of thinking about the pain and to provide opportunities for the child to develop adaptive coping skills. A supportive system should be provided for the mother so that she does not feel blamed for, or dependent on, her child's pain.

It is also easy to recognize how irritated the physician may become with the child's mother when what she says and what she does conflict. The doctor needs to be aware of his or her own anger towards the mother so that punitive wishes do not creep into the child's treatment plan. Unnecessary invasive diagnostic procedures should not be performed to prove to the mother that factors other than intestinal disease may be contributing to the pain. Often, these children may be referred to another physician because the mother is seen as more of a "pain" than the child. However, a new physician often wishes to perform more diagnostic procedures to verify the diagnosis. Thus, many of these children are subjected to excessive procedures. Since evidence is emerging that repeated significant pain episodes in early childhood might be the triggers for the development of pathologic pain pathways, as noted previously, such unnecessary painful procedures may contribute to the development of chronic visceral pain.

Pain Contributors

For the above reasons, therefore, a complete initial history of pain contributors is important. The section below will summarize major factors to be evaluated.

Expectations of pain. Do the child and family anticipate pain in relation to certain events or situations (eg, eating a certain amount of food)? Does the child develop anxiety in certain situations because of expectations of pain? To what extent do the parents believe that certain factors will cause pain in their child, thereby initiating a self-fulfilling prophecy?

Ability to control pain. To what extent does the child feel that he or she can modify the pain experience via self-control? Does the child believe that others, such as parents or a doctor, can alleviate the pain? Does the child or parents believe that "no one or nothing can make it better" (ie, learned helplessness)?

Role of attention. Does the child tend to focus on visceral sensations? How readily can she change the focus of her attention on these sensory experiences (eg, ease of distraction from the pain)?

Role of arousal. How anxious does the child become during medical procedures, during acute, nonprocedural pain episodes, and during more intense episodes of persistent pain? Explore the relationship between arousal and attention regulation.

Memory. What is the history of the child's remembered past pain experiences? What does the parent report about early pain events (eg, procedures, pain episodes), especially during infancy? These inquiries are important because of the role that pain memories may play in the development of pathologic visceral pain.

Coping style. How does the child react in anticipation of pain? Does he seek information and talk about the event or does he avoid such talk and prefer not to think about it? How does the child react during pain? Does he tend to focus on the pain (attend) or away from the pain, trying to do or think about other things (distract)?

Duration of the pain problem. The longer the child's pain has endured, the more likely is the child to expect pain and develop habitual pain behaviors. With persistent pain, the child and family develop a host of beliefs about what makes the pain better or worse and begin to act on these beliefs. The child's environment changes as a result of the interaction between the pain behaviors and the family's responses to them. Over time, pain may become the major focus for the child and family, with a majority of child and family activities revolving around the child's pain. Thus, assessment should include the family's responses to the child's symptom. Is there enhancement of adaptive coping by the child or is there inadvertent reinforcement of maladaptive behaviors?

Family beliefs about medication. Do the parents (and thus the child) believe that the pain is not considered by the physican to be "real" unless it is treated with medication? Many families believe that only "real, physical" pain gets treated with medicine or surgery, and that psychologic, behavioral, or environmental treatments imply "psychologic" pain.

Family beliefs about psychologic therapies. To some extent, this factor is the corollary of the previous question. However, when families have experienced psychotherapy or counseling as the sole approach to pain management and the pain has not resolved, they may be more resistant to including psychologic intervention as part of a multimodal, integrated treatment plan. Also, as with medical treatments, children differ in their needs for specific psychotherapeutic approaches. Past experience with psychologic interventions and feelings or beliefs about these should be included in the initial history.

Meaning and practice of physical contact. Since some aspects of the treatment plan may include massage or other physical methods, it is important to know how physical contact is experienced within the family. Are the family members physically affectionate with one another? Do the parents ever perform massage on each other or on their children? Conversely, is there a history of sexual or nonsexual child abuse in the immediate family or in the parents' family of origin? This is often a difficult aspect of the history and can be initiated by a discussion of disciplining practices. Other aspects of the history might lead to suspicions about abuse. If abuse is suspected, further inquiry will necessitate separate interviews of each parent, the child, and probably the siblings as well.

The last topic also leads to the issue of *Munchausen's syndrome-by-proxy*, in which a parent (usually the mother or primary caretaker) either overreports symptoms in the child, reports factitious symptoms (eg, hematemesis), or causes the symptoms by what she does or gives to the child. Typically, the result is numerous unnecessary medical evaluations, diagnostic tests, clinic visits, hospitalizations, and treatments—often including surgery. In extreme cases, the child dies. The parents are usually intelligent, medically knowledgeable, and very convincing. Unless the parent is observed doing something to cause a symptom, the only way to confirm this diagnosis is to hospitalize the child, limit and supervise parental visitation, then see whether the symptoms resolve.

The diagnosis of this condition is complex in children with intestinal motility disorders, since symptoms typically appear early in infancy. At this time, it is necessary to sort out the differences between true intestinal motor pathology versus a mismatch between a mother and her infant. Examples include a mother who has a low tolerance for infant crying matched with an infant who cries excessively, or a mother who has high expectations for a certain timing of defecation for her infant matched with an infant who is normal but does not meet these specifications. The problem for the physician is to determine whether the reported infant behavior represents pathology in the infant or the concerns and tolerance of the mother. For physicians who do not see a patient until childhood, after a diagnosis of chronic intestinal dysmotility disorder has already been made, diagnosis may become more problematic. The child may have already undergone a host of diagnostic procedures and medical or surgical interventions. The diagnostic dilemma becomes one of sorting out parental factors (eg, overconcern, overcompliance, overreporting, overmanipulation), primary intestinal or neural pathology, and sequelae of the treatments themselves, each of which may contribute to the child's pain.

PAIN MANAGEMENT

The importance of obtaining a careful, detailed history, observing the child and family, and performing a complete physical examination cannot be overemphasized. These processes allow the development of an individualized treatment plan based on the child's pain with consideration of the interrelationships among the factors unique to that child and his or her family. This "biobehavioral approach" to treatment within a developmental context[56] differs from the more traditional medical approach, which is to treat the likely primary organic etiology of the pain first, and, if that fails, to refer the patient for psychotherapy. Effective pain treatment should reduce, alter, or eliminate the contributing pathophysiologic processes that may be causing, aggravating, or perpetuating the pain. These processes are often primarily neuroenteric in motility disorders, but sometimes secondary chemical and mucosal or transmucosal pathologies may contribute as well. The presence of referred somatic/peripheral pain also requires attention, since referred hyperalgesia may act as a trigger for the visceral pain. Finally, the child's emotional and cognitive contributors to the pain should be addressed. Those aspects of the child's environment that reinforce a focus on pain and contribute to maladaptive coping responses in the child must be altered.

A multipronged approach to pain management considers the multifactorial nature of pain transmission and inhibition, and holds more promise for initial success than a singular, targeted, trial-and-error strategy. This approach will likely require more intensive health care personnel time initially, either with the team at outset of therapy or through individual time spent by the primary treating physician who can assume these multiple roles. However, such initial expenditures should reduce the long-term costs to the child such as ongoing diagnostic evaluations, hospitalizations, school absences, and altered lifestyle. It should also ease the impact on siblings and other family members, as well as cut the costs of financing health care by minimizing expensive tests, hospitalizations, and procedures. The multipronged approach may include, in any combination, behavioral and psychologic components, physical methods, and pharmacologic interventions. The role of surgery in pain management will not be discussed here, since its indications are rare and selected (see Chapters 26 and 27). While not intended to indicate a stepwise approach, the different categories within the context of pain management will be discussed separately for clarity.

Behavioral and Psychologic Interventions

The cognitive/behavioral component of comprehensive pain management is extremely important to children with chronic pain problems[58,59] Behavioral interventions that improve children's coping skills can create positive expectations and give children a sense of control over their pain. Positive coping promotes self-efficacy, greater confidence, and altered beliefs about the pain experience, which can then alter the experience itself. Additionally, a simple, clear explanation by the physician of the likely causes and contributors to the pain can have the psychologic benefit of setting the stage for the multipronged treatment plan. Thus, families can understand more easily how psychologic interventions fit into this plan and the goals of this aspect of treatment.

The most common kinds of behavioral interventions for children with chronic pain involve teaching relaxation techniques, and helping them use distraction and imaginative involvement. Psychologic strategies are those aimed at enhancing children's coping abilities, thereby enhancing feelings of control and expectations of mastery over the pain. Family intervention is aimed at shaping the child's home environment to facilitate the child's attempts at adaptive coping. In general, intervention strategies are most effective when they are tailored to the child's needs and coping style; not all strategies are effective for all children.

Relaxation. Relaxation is an active cognitive/behavioral approach that promotes self-regulation by reducing the tension and anxiety that often accompany and increase pain.[60] With progressive muscle relaxation, the child is taught to alternately contract and relax the different muscle groups, often starting with the toes and progressing upward. This process allows the child to control her own body and to notice the difference between tightened and relaxed muscles. Another method of relaxation is to help the child to focus on

each body part, often beginning with the toes and methodically moving up the body. The child is told, "You notice your toes beginning to become warm and relaxed. With each breath, very slowly, feel how relaxed your toes can be." Controlled breathing can also help the child learn how to relax. The child can use counting to take "ten slow, deep breaths" or can be asked to picture himself slowly blowing up a big balloon. Sometimes young children need props, such as soap bubbles, to help them learn what deep breaths are. Older children and adolescents can be asked to "notice the warm air entering your nose, throat, and filling your lungs, while all the tension and any bad feelings leave your body as you breathe out."

Distraction and imaginative involvement. The goal of these techniques is to help the child learn how to shift attention away from pain and onto other, more enjoyable things. These attention-sustainers might be found in the child's environment such as video games, television, telephone, conversations, play activities with peers, or they may be internal to and created by the child. The latter might include helping the child to focus on nonpainful body parts and sensations (eg, concentrating on fingers or toes instead of the belly). Hypnosis (imaginative involvement) can be a potentially powerful tool to help capture attention, alter sensory experiences, and enhance feelings of mastery and self-control. As children notice their own abilities to alter sensory experiences, they begin to develop changing expectations of future pain.

There are a variety of ways to help children use their imagination to reduce pain. One method is called "hypnoanesthesia." The child is asked to imagine a specified body part (eg, a hand or arm in preparation for phlebotomy) beginning to "go to sleep" as if it were "heavy and numb." This could be accomplished by placing a "magic glove" or "magic lotion" on it or asking the child to remember the feeling of a hand "packed in snow, becoming more and more numb until it has no feeling at all." Another method is to help the child to dissociate from the pain by becoming increasingly involved in an imagined fantasy. Some scene or activity that is meaningful to the child, such as playing a favorite sport, swimming, riding a bike, or playing with friends can be used. To enhance involvement in the fantasy, the child could be asked to notice the sounds, colors, temperature of the air, clothes he is wearing, smells, texture of objects, or any other heightened sensory experience. The child should be an active manipulator of this fantasy so that it not only provides distraction, but also enhances feelings of mastery (eg, climbing a mountain, winning the soccer game for the team, etc). To help the child begin to alter expectations of future pain, another hypnotic technique involves the use of "central pain switches." The child is asked to find the part of her brain that "controls the feelings to all parts of the body...the control feeling station." It is suggested that the child might notice switches, lights, and knobs like the ones found in an airplane's cockpit. It is suggested that the child find the particular knob or switch that controls whatever body part hurts, such as the abdomen. The child is then asked to turn the knob or switch "just enough to stop some of the feelings from getting to the brain, but not all the feelings...just as much as you want." Through a variety of hypnotic strategies, the child begins to learn that she can have some control over pain. How these hypnotic techniques work from a neurophysiologic standpoint is unclear. However, some children are able to turn off pain even when pathologic organic processes causing the pain are evident. For more information on hypnotic control of pain in children, readers are referred to Zeltzer and LeBaron.[61]

Psychotherapy is indicated if it appears that there are significant psychologic contributors to the pain and to pain behaviors, such as problems in separating from parents or a need for attention when only pain behaviors bring about the desired result. Through the development of a trusting relationship with a therapist, the child can learn to trust herself and can develop confidence over time in her abilities to cope with and reduce pain. Psychotherapy may also incorporate some of the cognitive-behavioral interventions noted above. Family therapy may be brief and oriented towards helping parents understand how they can reinforce and facilitate their child's coping abilities. Family therapy can also be more extensive when the dynamics of the family are such that parental behaviors may be reinforcing maladaptive child behaviors and there is resistance to change. For some families, a focus on the child's pain may permit an avoidance of parental attention to marital difficulties, resulting in a reluctance for pain resolution.

Psychologists, social workers, and other health care professionals can help a family alleviate stress. Often it is helpful for a family to have positive coping behavioral models so that they have examples of how to react to the variety of situations encountered over the duration of the pain condition. Psychotherapeutic support can help the family to cope with all the stresses that contribute to a maladaptive environment. Positive family coping methods emphasize open communication, an optimistic outlook, social contact, and return to normal, day-to-day living, thus minimizing the disruption caused by the chronic pain condition.[62,63] Support groups can also help families to adopt positive strategies by advocating healthy behavior for all family members.

Mechanical intervention. Many nonpharmacologic interventions can result in behavioral, cognitive, and physical modulation. Although hypnosis, for instance, is primarily a cognitive tool, it can also result in physical relaxation and behavioral modification. Similarly, massage, which is primarily a mechanical or physical intervention, can result in psychologic relaxation and behavioral modification. Mechanical interventions for the relief of chronic pain include massage, electrical nerve stimulation, trigger-point injections, applications of heat or cold, and biofeedback.

Although massage has not been extensively studied in children, those with chronic pain benefit from physiotherapeutic massage techniques.[64] Massage can relax the muscles that contribute to visceral pain or that act as triggers for pain. Massaging stimulates the mechanoreceptors, thus overloading spinal cord nociceptive transmission.

The physiologic mechanism for massage is closely linked to the gate-control theory. In summary, the gate-control theory suggests that a neurophysiologic mechanism located in the cells of the substantia gelatinosa of the spinal cord's dorsal horn acts as a gate that can regulate the flow of pain impulses from peripheral nerve fibers to spinal cord transmission cells that project to the brain. Accordingly, activity in the large, nonnociceptive primary afferents can inhibit the spinal effects of primary nociceptive afferents. Psychologic variables play an integral role in the transmission of pain. Perceived pain consists of both physiologic and psychologic inputs. Initial nociception rarely bears a unilateral relationship to the ultimate perception of pain.[65]

The gate-control theory led to a great deal of research on the analgesic effects of electrical nerve stimulation therapy. While several nerve stimulation techniques have been explored, the most popular is transcutaneous electrical nerve stimulation (TENS). Electrodes are placed on the surface of the skin and mild electric currents, measured in milliamps, are administered through small, 9-volt, battery-operated units. The patient can vary the intensity, frequency, width, and shape of the pulses, depending on her needs and desired sensations. TENS has three possible physiologic mechanisms: 1) it may activate large, low-threshold peripheral (nonnociceptive) afferents that can suppress excitatory effects of the small, high-threshold primary nociceptive afferents on the second-order neurons in the dorsal horn; 2) it may activate the endogenous endorphin-mediated analgesia system; and 3) it may decrease abnormal excitability of damaged parts of peripheral nerves, because the stimulation causes nerve impulses to travel centrally and peripherally towards the damaged area on the nerve.[66] TENS has many advantages because it is noninvasive and is continuous without causing respiratory depression or sedation. Unfortunately, it has not been used extensively for pain control in children. Its application to visceral pain control, in particular, remains unexplored. For a pediatric protocol for TENS administration, and several pediatric case studies, see Eland J, 1993.[66]

If musculocutaneous referred pain is evident in the child with visceral pain, and the above strategies are ineffective, other mechanical therapies, such as heat, ice, or vibratory methods, may be useful. With heat and ice, the physiologic mechanism is much the same as with other mechanical interventions. The application of extreme temperatures activates both types of thermal afferents, possibly inhibiting the second-order nociceptive neurons and suppressing pain through the spinal gating mechanism discussed above.

If specific focal points of muscle pain are evident on physical examination, trigger-point injections might be helpful. Because visceral pain, like myofascial pain, transmits in predictable patterns, the constant, concurrent, referred pain patterns can be used to locate the trigger points responsible for the primary pain.[67] Trigger points can be injected with local anesthetic (eg, lidocaine) to eliminate the pain signals. Trigger-point injections can ultimately restore the normal resting muscle length and full range of motion. Dry needling, wherein no anesthetic is injected, has also been explored. The needle serves as a substitute pain stimulus that can override the existing nerve pathway transmission of pain by breaking up the nerve bundle.[68] In myotherapy, trigger points are pressed deeply, depriving them of oxygen and resulting in the relief of pain. In one of the few studies with children, trigger points were easily located and erased using myotherapy. The results of this research, however, are anecdotal.[65]

Biofeedback may also aid some children with visceral pain. Biofeedback combines the hypnotic techniques described above with a mechanical device that provides visual or auditory feedback to the child when the desired cognitive action is approximated. Examples of such cognitive action include skeletal muscle relaxation, and vasodilation or vasoconstriction that results in peripheral skin temperature changes, as well as rectal muscle contraction and relaxation. Biofeedback has also been found to have the positive side effect of altering children's internal locus of control. The process and knowledge of self-regulation techniques help the child to unlearn chronic pain symptoms and to develop more positive coping skills.[69,70]

Pharmacologic interventions. The pharmacologic plan described in this section should be adjusted to the child's responses. The recommendations are based on the current theories of visceral pain that have arisen from animal and human adult studies, general knowledge of pain in children, and the senior author's clinical experience. Unfortunately, visceral pain mechanisms in children have received little attention. Future studies may prove current recommendations to be erroneous. For details on drug types within a drug category and drug dosages, readers are referred to the appropriate chapters in the comprehensive pediatric pain textbook by Schechter, Berde, and Yaster.[71]

If a specific, likely contributor to chronic pain can be identified (eg, postprandial hypomotility, intestinal bacterial overgrowth), it should be addressed directly with appropriate specific pharmacologic agents such as cisapride or antibiotics. When pain persists despite an attempt at specific treatment for the presumed overwhelming contributor to the pain, however, then the pharmacologic approach must be based on more general mechanisms of visceral pain transmission and inhibition. Although opiates may have a role for specific children at specific times (eg, to reduce postoperative pain), they should be avoided for long-term use because they may contribute to abnormal motility and transit, and thus paradoxically contribute to pain processes.

The pharmacologic treatment strategy tends to be based on a neuropathic pain model, especially for children in whom neuroenteric pathologic processes are believed to be major contributors to abnormal motility and pathologic visceral sensory processing. Drugs in this category include those aimed at serotonergic systems (eg, tricyclic antidepressants, including amitriptyline and disipramine), α-adrenergic systems (eg, clonidine), and neural membrane stabilization (eg, calcium channel blockers such as verapamil and sodium channel blockers such as mexiletine). Because evidence suggests that prostaglandins may play a role in sensitizing both nociceptive and nonnociceptive neural fibers to become active pain transmitters with low thresholds for nociception, nonsteroidal anti-inflammatory agents (NSAIDs) may also play a role in the treatment of persistent visceral pain. These and other anti-inflammatory agents (eg, steroids) may play special roles when ongoing mucosal inflammation is believed to contribute to the child's pain. Inflammation itself may cause increased production of nerve growth factors which, in turn, may cause sensitization in primary visceral nociceptive afferents, as well as dorsal horn sensitization.[72,73] Such dorsal horn sensitization can then lead to increased peptide production in the neuronal cell bodies. This in turn may alter central processing of pain (ie, enhancing nociceptive transmission to the brain, reducing efficacy of inhibitory systems) as well as enhancing transmission in spinal motor reflex arcs that may themselves contribute to the abnormal motility. It should be emphasized that there are no clinical studies of the efficacy of NSAIDs in children with pain and motility disorders. NSAIDs have their own local GI side effects, but a clinical trial may be warranted for selected children.

The treatment of visceral pain by treating peripheral pain in children with referred hyperalgesia rests on even thinner ice. For example, if persistent back-muscle pain exists—even if visceral pain is the primary complaint—after initial treatment with heat and massage, muscle relaxants may be worthwhile to determine whether reduction of back pain minimizes visceral pain. Similarly, if there is an area of cutaneous hyperalgesia, local application of capsaicin cream (Zostrix, GenDerm Corp., Lincolnshire, IL), which causes a reduction in local substance P, may be warranted to determine the role of peripheral pain in maintaining the visceral pain.

Finally, ongoing visceral pain may cause

the development of pathologic pain pathways in the spinal cord and brain. Epidural anesthetics (0.125% bupivacaine) is one approach to turning off sensory processing while leaving motor systems intact for a limited period of time. The temporary turning off of pain in this manner can be used as a window of opportunity for intensive child and parent psychologic and behavioral therapy that reframes the child's and family's understanding of pain, proving that it can go away and helping the child to develop effective coping skills. In addition to its use as a pain respite for the child, the epidural anesthetic can be viewed as a way to cause major shifts in thinking and behavior that lead to more rapid progress in pain reduction and enhanced functioning. It should not be viewed as a singular treatment; rather, it is best used in conjunction with psychologic treatment.

A treatment strategy was used for two children, ages 6 and 14 years, who were admitted to UCLA Medical Center with intense visceral pain associated with stomach wall expansion. Barostat evaluation demonstrated that even a small volume of food or drink produced pain. The 6-year-old boy presented with a 2-year history of such pain following fundoplication for gastroesophageal reflux associated with documented esophagitis. After surgery, he required gastrostomy nighttime drip feedings to maintain an appropriate nutritional status. His oral intake consisted of miniscule amounts of food or drink in a grazing pattern throughout the day. The 14-year-old girl presented with a 3-year, similar history related to pain with oral intake of even small volumes. She maintained her nutrition by the nightly self-insertion of a nasogastric tube, through which she had 8 hours of drip feeding.

Hospitalization consisted of the self-administration of local anesthetic—via gastrostomy in the boy and nasogastric tube in the adolescent girl—immediately prior to each of three meals a day under monitoring conditions and with considerable verbal reinforcement for expected sensory changes. Initial meals were observed and patient awareness of new feelings was positively reinforced. The goal, as explained to the patients and

their families, was to turn off pain and allow other sensory experiences. Patients could then experience eating without pain, while still feeling full when they had enough to eat. This approach was combined with behavioral strategies aimed at altering cues that previously may have reinforced expectations of pain with eating. In this regard, we asked the fathers to play a more active role in their child's care, asked the mothers to spend less time in the hospital, and encouraged nonfamily time so that the child could be without parents and could interact with peers. Parents were asked to not be present during mealtimes over the first few days of hospitalization. In each case, the children were rapidly able to increase their oral intake without pain. Midway through their week of hospitalization, each patient was eating three meals per day with adequate volumes of food. Nightly drip feedings were reduced substantially by the end of the week. The anesthetic prefeed installations were reduced to half dose by the fourth hospital day and discontinued on the fifth day without any return of symptoms with eating.

Although the boy did not require any venting of his gastrostomy tube in the hospital, his mother reported that during the month at home after discharge he "of course" required venting on occasion "to prevent pain," although he continued to eat. He also had some pain episodes not associated with eating, but used the imagination techniques learned in the hospital to resolve these symptoms. Continued family therapy was recommended after discharge. A longer hospital stay would have been preferable—especially since the child was home for a month before the insurance-approved psychiatrist could see him—but the insurance company denied a longer stay.

The adolescent had a similar course relative to her eating and pain resolution. However, it was more difficult to separate her mother from her. It took active efforts by the adolescent, with team support, to convince her mother to go home at night. Despite minimal changes in the mother, this patient made excellent use of the hospitalization for exploring adolescent individuation needs, developing new coping skills for relaxation and pain control, and changing her beliefs and expectations related to eating. As stated initially, however, the effects may have been placebo-related or secondary to the local installation of the anesthetic. Further studies of this treatment modality for this special population of children will be conducted.

Before ending this section, we wish to emphasize the importance of reducing pain and anxiety during any and all medical procedures. These acute pain episodes trigger and aggravate persisting visceral pain and enhance the development of pathologic pain pathways. The memories of these procedure-related pain episodes also may play a role in enhancing visceral pain. For major painful procedures, we typically use midazolam and propofol, although we have also used midazolam and ketamine. Results with midazolam and an opiate, typically fentanyl, have been more variable, and thus this combination is not the best choice. For all procedures, we use psychologic intervention, with or without pharmacologic treatment depending on the child and procedure.[74-77] For needle insertions, we use EMLA cream (Astra Pharmaceutical Products, Westborough, MA).

CONCLUSION

Pain in children with intestinal motility disorders is multifactorial and necessitates a multipronged treatment strategy. Because of the condition's complexity and the lack of studies of visceral pain in children, pain in these children is often underevaluated and undertreated. Its undertreatment is indicated by the fact that 60% of children with chronic intestinal pseudo-obstruction report pain.[78] It is hoped that evolving research in visceral pain mechanisms and clinical treatment studies, especially in children, will supply the information necessary for adequate prevention and pain management for children with intestinal neuroenteric disorders.

The authors would like to thank the Pediatric Research Summer Student Research Program 1993 and the UCLA Student Research Program for their support and assistance.

REFERENCES

1. Schechter NI. The undertreatment of pain in children: an overview. *Pediatr Clin North Am* 1989;36:781-94.

2. Schmidt RF. Silent and active nociceptors: structures, functions, and clinical implications. *International Association for the Study of Pain,* 1993.

3. Janig W, Morrison JFB. Functional properties of spinal visceral afferents supplying abdominal and pelvic organs, with special emphasis on visceral nociception. In: Cervero F, Morrison JFB, eds. *Progress in Brain Research: Visceral Sensation.* New York, NY: Elsevier Press, 1986;67:87-111.

4. Anand KJS, Carr DB. The neuroanatomy, neurophysiology, and neurochemistry of pain, stress, and analgesia in newborns and children. *Pediatr Clin North Am* 1989;36:795-822.

5. Fields HL, Basbaum AI: Endogenous pain control mechanisms. In: Wall PD, Melzack R, eds. *Textbook of Pain,* 1989;206-14.

6. Willis WD. The origin and destination of pathways involved in pain transmission. In: Wall PD, Melzack R, eds. *Textbook of Pain.* New York, NY: Churchill Livingstone, 1989;112-123.

7. McMahon SB. Neuronal and behavioural consequences of chemical inflammation of rat urinary bladder. *Agents Actions* 1988;25:231-3.

8. Habler HJ, Jaenig W, Koltzenburg M. A novel type of unmyelinated chemosensitive nociceptor in the acutely inflamed urinary bladder. *Agents Actions* 1988;25:219-25.

9. Cervero F. Afferent activity evoked by natural stimulation of the biliary system in the ferret. *Pain* 1982;13:137-51.

10. Cervero F, Sann H. Mechanically evoked responses of afferent fibers innervating the guinea pig's ureter: an in vitro study. *J Physiol* 1982;412:245-66.

11. Baker DG, Coleridge HM, Nergrum T. Search for a cardiac nociceptor: stimulation by bradykinin of sympathetic afferent nerve endings. *J Physiol* 1980;306:519-36.

12. Cervero F. Mechanisms of acute visceral pain. *Br Med Bull* 1991;47:549-60.

13. Cervero F, Tattersall JEH. Somatic and visceral sensory integration in the thoracic spinal cord. In: Cervero F, Morrison JFB, eds. *Progress in Brain Research.* New York, NY: Elsevier Press, 1986;67:189-205.

14. Melzack R, Wall PD. Pain mechanism: a new theory. *Science* 1965;150:971.

15. Glazer EJ, Basbaum AI. Opioid neurons and pain modulation: an ultrastructional analysis of enkephalin in the cat. *Neuroscience* 1983;10:357-76.

16. Zeltzer LK, Anderson CTM, Schechter NL. Pediatric pain: current status and new directions. In: Lockhart JD, ed. *Current Problems in Pediatrics.* St Louis, MI: Mosby Yearbook, 1990;20(8):411-86.

17. Berde CB, Sethna NF, Anand KS. Pediatric pain management. In: Gregory GA, ed. Pediatric Anesthesia. New York, NY: *Churchill Livingstone,* 1989;2:679-727.

18. Fitzgerald M Spontaneous and evoked activity of fetal primary efferents in vivo. *Nature* 1987;326:603-5.

19. Schulte FJ. *Neurophysiological aspects of brain development.* Mead Johnson Symposium on Perinatal Development 1975;6:38-47.

20. Fitzgerald M. The developmental neurobiology of pain. In: Bond M, Woolf CJ, Charlton M, eds. *Proceedings of the VIth World Congress on Pain* 1990.

21. Fitzgerald M. The development of activity evoked by fine- diameter cutaneous fibers in the spinal cord of the newborn rat. *Neurosci Lett* 1988;86:161-6.

22. Marti E, Gibson SJ, Polak JM, et al. Ontogeny of peptide- and amino-containing neurons in motor, sensory, and autonomic regions. *J Comp Neurol* 1987;266:332-59.

23. Fitzgerald M, Shaw A, MacIntosh N. Postnatal development of the cutaneous flexor reflex: comparative study of preterm infants and newborn rat pups. *Med Child Neurol* 1988;30:520-6.

24. Fitzgerald M. The postnatal development of cutaneous afferent fibre input and receptive field organization in the rat dorsal horn. *J Physiol* 1985;364:1-18.

25. Klimach VJ, Cook RWI. Maturation of the neonatal somatosensory evoked response in preterm infants. *Dev Med Child Neurol* 1988;30:208-14.

26. Gilles FH, Shakle W, Dooling EC. Myelinated tracts: growth patterns. In: Gilles FH, Leviton A, eds. *The Developing Human Brain.* Boston, MA: Wright & Co. 1983:117.

27. Fitzgerald M, McIntosh N. Pain and analgesia in the newborn. *Arch Dis Child* 1989;64:441-3.

28. Anand KJS, Brown MJ, Causon RC, Christofides ND. Can the human neonate mount an endocrine and metabolic response to surgery? *J Pediatr Surg* 1985;20:41-8.

29. Bregman BS. Development of serotonin immunoreactivity in the rat spinal cord and its plasticity after neonatal spinal lesions. *Dev Brain Res* 1987;34:245-64.

30. Anand KJS, Hickey PR. Pain and its effects in the human neonate and fetus. *N Engl J Med* 1987;317:1321-6.

31. Squire LR. Mechanisms of memory. *Science* 1986;232:1612-9.

32. Prechtl HFR. *Continuity of Neural Functions from Prenatal to Postnatal Life.* Oxford, England: Blackwell, 1984.

33. Will B, Schmitt P, Dalrymple-Alford J. Brain plasticity, learning, and memory: historical background and conceptual perspectives. *Adv Behav Biol* 1985;28:1-11.

34. Bischof JH. Influence of developmental factors on imprinting. *Adv Behav Biol* 1985;28:51-9.

35. Shepherd GM, ed. *The Synaptic Organization of the Brain.* New York, NY: Oxford University Press, 1990.

36. Campbell JN, Meyer RA. Sensitization of unmyelinated nociceptive afferents in monkey varies with skin type. *J Neurophysiol* 1983;49:98-110.

37. Koltzenburg M, Kress M, Reeh PW. The nociceptor sensitization by bradykinin does not depend on sympathetic neurons. *Neuroscience* 1992;46:465-73.

38. Fitzgerald M, Millard C, MacIntosh N. Hyperalgesia in premature infants. *Lancet* 1988:292.

39. Fitzgerald M. The spread of sensitization of polymodal nocicepetors in the rabbit from nearby injury and by antidromic nerve stimulation. *J Physiol* 1979;297:207-16.

40. Hardy JD, Wolff HG, Goodell H. Experimental evidence on the nature of cutaneous hyperalgesia. *J Clin Invest* 1950;29:115-40.

41. Coderre TJ, Katz J, Vaccarino AL, Melzack R. Contribution of central neuroplasticity to pathological pain: review of clinical and experimental evidence. *Pain* 1993;52:259-85.

42. Cook AJ, Woolf CJ, Wall PD, McMahon SB. Dynamic receptive field plasticity in rat spinal cord dorsal horn following C-primary afferent input. *Nature* 1987;325:151.

43. Schouenbourg J, Dickenson AH. The effects of a distant noxious stimulation on A and C fiber evoked flexion reflexes and neuronal activity in the dorsal horn of the rat. *Brain Res* 1985;328:23-32.

44. Mendell LM. Physiological properties of unmyelinated fiber projections to the spinal cord. *Exp Neurol* 1966;16:316-22.

45. Lumb BM. Brainstem control of visceral afferent pathways in the spinal cord. In: Cervero F, Morrison JFB, eds. *Progress in Brain Research: Visceral Sensation.* New York, NY: Elsevier, 1986;67.

46. Bojo L, Cassuto J, Nellgard P. Pain-induced inhibition of gastric motility is mediated by adrenergic and vagal non-adrenergic reflexes in the rat. *Acta Physiol Scand* 1992;146:377-83.

47. Andres PRL. Vagal afferent innervation of the gastrointestinal tract. In: Cervero F, Morrison JFB, eds. *Progress in Brain Research: Visceral Sensation.* New York, NY: Elsevier, 1986;67:65-86.

48. Andrews PRL, Wood KL. An electrophysiological study of the posterior abdominal vagus nerve in man. *Clin Sci* 1982;63:169-173.

49. MacKay TW, Andres PRI. A comparative study of the vagal innervation of the stomach in man and the ferret. *J Anat* 1983;136:449-81.

50. Katz J, Vaccarrino AL, Coderre TJ, Melzack R. Injury prior to neurectomy alters the pattern of autotomy in rats: behavioral evidence of central

neural plasticity. *Anesthesiology* 1991;75:876-83.

51. Mayer EA, Raybould H. Role of neural control in gastrointestinal motility and visceral pain. In: Snape WJ, ed. *Pathogenesis of Functional Bowel Disease.* New York, NY Plenum Medical Book Co, 1989:13-35.

52. Pineiro-Carrero VM, Andres JM, Davis RH, Mathias JR. Abnormal gastroduodenal motility in children and adolescents with recurrent functional abdominal pain. *J Pediatr* 1988;113:820-5.

53. Wiesenfeld-Hallin Z, Durant R. Effects of intrathecal cholecystokinin, substance P, and morphine on the nociceptive flexion reflex in the rat. *Pain* 1987;supp:455.

54. Boyce T, Barr RG, Zeltzer LK. Temperament and the psychobiology of childhood stress. *Pediatrics* 1992;90:483-6.

55. Mizell T, Fanurik D, Zeltzer L. Stability of children's responses to cold pressor pain: a two-year follow-up. *Clin Research* 1993.

56. Roy R, Mogilevsky I, Chenhall P, Cook A, Thomas M. *Impact of parental chronic pain on children.* VIIth World Congress on Pain (Paris, France) 1993.

57. Marchettini P. *Mechanisms of referred muscle pain.* VIIth World Congress on Pain (Paris, France) 1993.

58. Anderson CTM, Zeltzer LK, Fanurik D. Procedural pain. In: Schechter NL, Berde C, Yaster M, eds. *Pain Management in Infants, Children, and Adolescents.* Baltimore, MD: Williams & Wilkins, 1993;435-58.

59. Bush JP, Harkins SW, eds. *Pain in Children: Clinical and Research Issues from a Developmental Perspective.* New York, NY: Springer Verlag, 1991.

60. Zeltzer LK. Pain and symptom management. In: Bearison D, Mulhern R, eds. *Pediatric Psychooncology: Psychological Research in Children with Cancer.* New York, NY: Oxford University Press, 1994 (In press).

61. Zeltzer LK, LeBaron S. The hypnotic treatment of children in pain. In: Routh D, Wolraich M, eds. *Advances in Development and Behavioral Pediatrics.* JAI Press, 1986;7:197-234.

62. Patterson SM, McCubbin HI. Chronic illness: family stress and coping. In: Figley CR, McCubbin HI, eds. *Stress and the Family, Vol II: Coping with Catastrophe*. New York, NY: Brunner/Mazel, 1983:21-36.

63. Kupst MJ. Long-term family coping with acute lymphoblastic leukemia in childhood. In: La Greca AM, Siegel JL, Wallender JL, Walker CE, eds. *Stress and Coping in Child Health*. New York, NY: Guilford Press, 1993:242-61.

64. McGrath PA. *Pain in Children: Nature, Assessment and Treatment*. New York, NY: Guilford Press, 1990:136-8.

65. Ross DM. *Childhood Pain*. Baltimore, MD: Urban & Schwarzenberg, 1988:14.

66. Eland J. The use of TENS with children. In: Schechter NL, Berde CB, Yaster M, eds. *Pain in Infants, Children, and Adolescents*. Baltimore, MD: Williams & Wilkins, 1993:331-9.

67. Travell J. Myofascial trigger points: clinical view. In: Bonica JJ, Albe-Fessard, eds. *Advances in Pain Research and Therapy* 1976;1:919-26.

68. Raj PP. Myofascial trigger point injection. In: Raj PP, ed. *Practical Management of Pain*. Chicago, IL: Yearbook Medical Publishers, 1986;569-77.

69. Attanasio V, Andrasik F, Burke EJ, Blake DD, Kabela E, McCarran MS. Clinical issues in utilizing biofeedback with children. *Clin Biofeedback Health* 1985;8:134-41.

70. Conners CK. Application of biofeedback to treatment of children. *Am Acad Child Psychiat* 1979;143-53.

71. Schechter NL, Berde CB, Yaster M, eds. *Pain in Infants, Children, and Adolescents*. Balitmore, MD: Williams & Wilkins, 1993.

72. Steen AE, Reeh PW, Kreysel HW, Steen KH. *Experimental tissue acidosis potentiates pain induced by inflammatory mediators*. VIIth World Congress on Pain (Paris, France), 1993.

73. Stein C. *Interaction of immune-competent cells and nociceptors*. VIIth World Congress on Pain (Paris, France), 1993.

74. Zeltzer LK, Jay SM, Fisher DM. The management of pain associated with pediatric procedures. *Ped Clin North Am 1989;36:1-24*.

75. Zeltzer LK, Anderson CTM, Schechter NI. Pediatric pain: current status and new directions. In: Lockhart JD, ed. *Current Problems in Pediatrics* Mosby Year Book 1990;20:415-86.

76. Steward DJ, ed. Management of childhood pain: new approaches to procedure-related pain. *Journal of Pediatrics* 1993;122:supp.

77. Hyman PE, Fiske ME, DiLorenzo C, Diego A. North American Pediatric Pseudo-obstruction Society (NAPPS) survey. *Pediatr Res* 1992;31:108A.

Motility
Testing

11

Esophageal Manometry in Children

ANNAMARIA STAIANO

Manometric studies were first performed more than a century ago by Kronecker and Meltzer.[1] Since that time, esophageal manometry has evolved to the point where it is widely used in the clinical pediatric evaluation of esophageal function.[2-4] Esophageal manometry has been a valid and reliable technique to test the efficacy of medical and surgical interventions, and it has also been used to establish the effect of gastrointestinal hormones or pharmacologic agents on esophageal function.

FUNCTIONAL ANATOMY AND PHYSIOLOGY OF THE ESOPHAGUS

There are three functional regions of the esophagus: the upper esophageal sphincter (UES), the esophageal body, and the lower esophageal sphincter (LES).

The Upper Esophageal Sphincter

The muscles of the UES are striated, with the cricopharyngeus, adjacent portions of the esophagus, and inferior constrictor contributing to sphincteric function. The cricopharyngeus inserts bilaterally at the inferolateral margins of the cricoid lamina, giving the lumen a slitlike configuration. This accounts for the pressure asymmetry that produces greater values anteriorly and posteriorly than laterally.[5] Since the only insertion of the cricopharyngeus is anterior to the cartilages of the larynx, the sphincter and larynx move together during axial laryngeal movement.[6] Intraluminal UES pressure is comprised of an active component—related

to cricopharyngeal contraction—and a passive component on the order of 10 mm Hg, which is attributable to collapse of the lumen.[7,8]

Substances in the pharynx stimulate sensory receptors, which send impulses to the swallowing center in the brain stem.[9] The central nervous system then initiates a series of involuntary responses that determine the passage of the bolus from the pharynx, across the UES, and into the proximal esophagus. This complex act is controlled by the afferent excitation of the glossopharyngeal nerve, the trigeminus, and the superior laryngeal nerve. Efferent impulses are transmitted by the trigeminus, the vagus, glossopharyngeal, and hypoglossal nerves.

Swallowing is associated with manometric relaxation of the sphincter.[10] Deglutitive relaxation of the UES is difficult to record accurately because the brisk movement of the larynx and sphincter is discordant with the movement of the intraluminal recording device.[11] However, videofluoroscopic studies performed concurrently with intraluminal manometry have shown that UES relaxation occurs during the swallow-associated laryngeal elevation, and that relaxation precedes the opening of the sphincter by about 0.1 second.[12]

Contraction of the superior constrictor muscle of the pharynx represents the beginning of the peristaltic wave that propels food into the esophagus.

The Esophageal Body

The body of the esophagus is a tube composed of skeletal and smooth muscle.

The proximal third of the esophagus is striated muscle, the middle third is mixed, and the distal third is exclusively smooth muscle. The striated portion of the esophageal body begins at the inferior border of the cricopharyngeus muscle. Generally, there is a longitudinal outer muscle layer and a circular inner layer. There is a myenteric nerve plexus in both the striated and smooth-muscle segments of the esophagus; this is less well developed in the striated portion. The extrinsic innervation of the esophagus is via the vagus nerve. Fibers innervating the striated muscle are axons of lower motor neurons of the ambiguous nucleus, whereas the innervation of the smooth muscle is provided by the dorsal motor nucleus of the vagus.[13] The vagus nerves also provide sensory innervation via the superior laryngeal nerve and the recurrent laryngeal nerve, or via the esophageal branches of the vagus. The intrinsic enteric neurons function as the relay neurons between the nerve and the smooth muscle.

Peristalsis in the esophagus differs from peristalsis in the intestine in that it is not governed by an intrinsic myogenic slow wave and can be initiated voluntarily. Smooth-muscle contraction and its control are characterized by an "off-response." Electrical stimulation results in muscle contraction after the cessation of the stimulus, a phenomenon that is abolished by tetrodotoxin. Thus, swallowing provides an inhibitory vagal input to the esophageal body, with peristaltic contraction occurring when the input ceases.[14]

The coordinated motor pattern of the esophagus is initiated by the act of swallowing, and is called primary peristalsis (Fig. 11.1). A rapidly progressing pharyngeal contraction transfers the bolus through a relaxed UES into the esophagus. As the UES closes, a progressive circular contraction begins in the upper esophagus and proceeds distally along the esophageal body to propel the bolus through a relaxed LES.

Secondary peristalsis is a progressive contraction in the esophageal body that is not induced by a swallow, but rather by stimulation of sensory receptors in the esophageal body. Secondary peristalsis is usually induced in two ways: by luminal distention with refluxed gastric contents, or following incomplete clearing of the esophageal contents by a primary swallow.

The Lower Esophageal Sphincter

The human LES is a ring of thickened, circular muscle angling obliquely upward from the lesser to the greater curvature of the stomach.[15] The LES is normally situated within the diaphragmatic hiatus, typically formed by the right diaphragmatic crus. Recently, it has been suggested that a component of LES pressure results from extrinsic compression by the crural diaphragm, and that contraction of the crural diaphragm may determine the increase of the LES pressure that accompanies inspiration.[16] This increase correlates with crural EMG activity.

Physiologically, the LES in children is a 2- to 3-cm long segment of tonically contracted smooth muscle at the distal end of the esophagus. Intra-abdominal pressure, gastric distention, peptides, hormones, various foods, and many drugs modify the LES pressure. When swallowing, LES relaxation is mediated via preganglionic, cholinergic vagal fibers in addition to postganglionic, noncholinergic, nonadrenergic nerves.[17] However, the LES transiently relaxes independent of swallowing, and an increased proportion of this type of inappropriate relaxation has been reported in children with gastroesophageal reflux.[18,19]

INDICATIONS FOR THE TEST

Esophageal manometry, measuring peristalsis at all levels of the esophagus, is the only method capable of detecting focal motor abnormalities and analyzing motor activity along the entire esophageal length. However, in clinical practice the major value of esophageal manometry is in the diagnosis and management of esophageal motility disorders.

Esophageal manometry should be performed and interpreted by a well-trained physician or technician and interpreted by a supervising physician. The limitations of esophageal manometry are primarily technical.

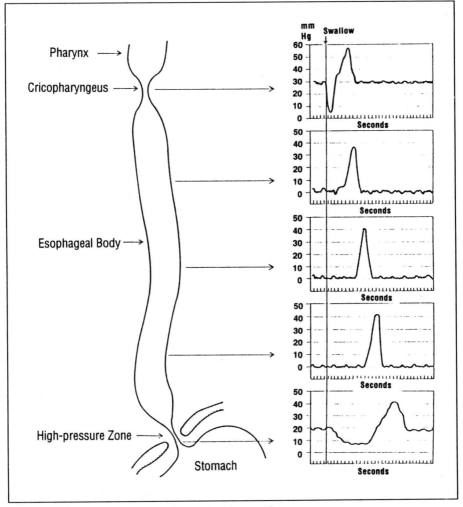

Fig. 11.1 Esophageal motor events in response to a swallow.

Because premedications are not employed, the study may be poorly tolerated by some children. In addition, the manometry catheter does not measure alterations in longitudinal muscle contraction following the swallow.[11] Resultant axial displacement is not detected by the rigid catheters, and thus inadvertent changes in catheter position may produce artefactual results.[20] Completely distinct disorders, such as one affecting intramural nerves and one affecting muscle cells, could both result in loss of esophageal peristalsis; both disorders could nevertheless have identical manometric diagnoses. Finally, UES disorders are diagnosed more satisfactorily with cineradiography or nasopharyngeal endoscopy.

TECHNIQUES

A manometric examination provides an accurate description of esophageal contractions, but only if physical principles and equipment characteristics are respected. In the evaluation of each esophageal region, the recording accuracy of the equipment, the appropriateness of sensor design and configuration, and the technique of data acquisition must be considered.

The frequency content and waveform of esophageal contractile waves define the re- •

quired characteristics of manometric recording equipment. In order to produce a high-fidelity recording, the apparatus must be capable of faithfully reproducing these waveforms. According to Orlowski et al,[21] to reproduce esophageal pressure waves with 98% accuracy the manometric systems should have a frequency response of 0 to 4 Hz. To reproduce pharyngeal pressure waves accurately, the frequency response should be 0 to 56 Hz. Because the characteristics of the manometric system as a whole are only as good as those of the weakest element within that system, each element (pressure sensor, transducer, recorder) must possess these response characteristics if high-fidelity recordings are to be obtained.

The basic equipment for esophageal manometry includes the esophageal manometry catheter, the infusion system, the transducers, and the physiograph. The esophageal manometry catheters are available in two general designs: either water-perfused catheters with volume displacement transducers or strain-gage transducers with solid-state circuitry. In children, the most commonly utilized technique involves a catheter composed of 3 to 6 capillary tubes (0.6-0.8 mm or less internal diameter) joined together. The catheter diameter is 3 mm or less. Small side holes are spaced 2.5 cm apart and oriented radially at 90° angles. Radial orientation helps to accurately measure LES pressure, which often has an asymmetric pressure profile. Each catheter is perfused with water from a low-compliance perfusion device connected to the external transducers. The transducers are usually set at the same height as the child's esophagus in the supine position and are connected to both the infusion pump and the physiograph. The resistance imposed by a fine capillary wire reduces water pressure to nearly zero at the diaphragm of the pressure transducer. Obstruction of the catheter port by an esophageal contraction wave produces a rapid pressure increment in the dome of the transducer. Pressure in the water reservoir sufficiently exceeds pressures created by typical esophageal waves, enabling the flow of water into the transducer dome to continue. Low compliance in this system produces a rapid increase in recorded pressure until perfusion pressure exceeds the contraction squeeze pressure at the orifice. Pressures are subsequently converted to electrical signals by the transducer and printed out on the chart recorder.

A solid-state esophageal manometry catheter contains small transducers. This non-perfused system has excellent recording fidelity and patient tolerance, yet the perfused catheters are used more often because they are much less expensive.

Squeeze pressure and relaxation characteristics of the upper and lower sphincters should also be monitored. Standard perfused catheters or imbedded microtransducers are suboptimal because of the radial and axial asymmetry of contraction pressures within the sphincters. Both the UES and LES exhibit profound orad excursion (2-3 cm) during swallowing, owing to laryngeal elevation and contraction of the longitudinal muscle of the esophageal body.[10,20] A manometric assembly passed transnasally, on the other hand, will move to a lesser degree (1-2 cm) and in a discordant fashion, coincident with soft-palate elevation early in the swallow. If a sensing element is initially positioned at the peak of the sphincter high pressure zone, its position may change during the swallow. As a result, the sensing element will register a diminished pressure suggesting complete relaxation, whether or not relaxation has actually occurred. This problem decreases the accuracy of a point sensor for detecting dynamic sphincter activity, including the completeness of sphincter relaxation. A single point sensor can, however, be used for a static determination of sphincter pressure using a pull-through technique in which the sensing element is pulled across the sphincter in steps, yielding an axial pressure profile.

A sleeve sensor[22] is an experimentally validated method for the dynamic recording of intraluminal sphincter pressure. Typically, a sleeve sensor contains a 4 to 6 cm long silicone membrane through which water is perfused. When pressure is applied anywhere along the length of the membrane, the resistance to water flow beneath it increases and pressure registers on that manometric channel. The physical properties of a sleeve sensor are based on the fact that it measures the highest pressure acting anywhere along its length—ideal for tracking the contractile activity of a mobile sphincter. However, a sleeve sensor has a limited frequency response, making it unsuitable for the recording of brisk contractile activity.

PATIENT PREPARATION AND MANOMETRIC STUDY

The patient should fast for at least 3 to 5 hours before the study, depending on age. If the child is able to communicate, it is important to talk with him/her at the beginning of the study and explain to him what will happen. The patient should understand that the passage of the tube through the throat can be uncomfortable, but after the first few swallows it will feel better. Children less than 5 years old should be awakened early in the morning, at least 5 to 6 hours before the study, so that they nap spontaneously during the test. Sedation should not be employed for routine studies, because the sedative may interfere with swallowing and influence pressures.[23]

For recording respiratory movements, a belt pneumograph is placed around the chest. Swallowing may be recorded by a sensor belt around the neck or a pressure sensor in the mouth.

The intubation through the nose should be gentle and careful: lubricate the tube immediately prior to insertion with a lubricating jelly and let the child bend his neck down (chin to chest) to help the tube drop into the back of the throat. Through a small syringe, give the child a sip of water and as the child swallows, advance the tube into the esophagus. Tape the tube to the nose and wait until the child quiets.

To begin the study, first verify that all perfused ports are in the stomach. Viewed at a paper speed of 2.5 mm per second, all channels will show a relatively flat, smooth tracing with a small pressure increase moving upward on inspiration. To measure the lower esophageal sphincter, slowly pull the tube out (0.5-1 cm/s) while watching the tracing. The catheter may be left in one position throughout the study, or it may be withdrawn in a stepwise manner so that additional areas of the esophagus are sampled by the recording orifices.

Measurement of resting lower sphincter pressure is obtained first, before proceeding with evaluations of peristalsis and UES.

The Lower Esophageal Sphincter

Lower esophageal sphincter pressure (LESP) is assessed by a rapid pull-through technique (RPT), a station pull-through technique (SPT), or a sleeve recording. A rapid pull-through is performed by withdrawing adjacent recording sites across the high pressure zone at a rate of about 1 cm per second, with respiration suspended at mid-expiration. A station pull-through differs from a rapid pull-through in that the recording assembly is withdrawn 0.5 cm at a time and held at each station for 30 to 60 seconds. Respiration is not suspended during a station pull-through, and one or more swallows is obtained at each station, which allows deglutitive LES relaxation to be assessed. Sleeve recordings of LES pressure are obtained by first localizing the LES high pressure zone via a rapid pull-through, then centering the high pressure zone on the sleeve sensor. A continuous recording of basal LES pressure is obtained for 5 to 10 minutes, during which swallowing is kept to a minimum.

During both the RPT and the SPT, each pull-through is terminated about 5 cm above the proximal margin of the LES. The catheter is then advanced again into the stomach. Usually, three pull-throughs are performed; the mean of these values is the resting LES pressure. With the sleeve method, LES pressure is recorded continuously. In children, SPT is used much more than the RPT, because the latter is uncomfortable and requires that the patient not breathe or swallow.

With the SPT technique, the catheter is moved through the LES 0.5 cm at a time, with a pause at each point or station to closely observe LES pressure and relaxation.

Pull the tube out of the stomach 0.5 cm at a time. Attempt to remain at each station for at least 5 respiration cycles. As you move further into the LES, the bottom of the pressure complex will usually rise above the gastric baseline and sphincter relaxation can be assessed. With a wet swallow, the normal lower sphincter should always relax completely to gastric pressure. As the catheter is pushed through the LES, stopping at 0.5-cm intervals, a point is reached where the pressure decreases, rather than increases, with inspiration. This is the pressure inversion point (PIP), which occurs as the recording orifice moves from the abdominal cavity into the thoracic cavity. If you are measuring a very weak or low pressure sphincter, this reversal point may be the only way to locate the LES. In a hiatal hernia, the fundus and the gastric cardia lie in an intrathoracic position. When a hiatal hernia is present, the PIP may be several centimeters below the LES. It is generally agreed that manometry is not a useful technique for diagnosing a hiatal hernia.

The study of the esophageal body evaluates the esophageal response to a series of swallows. Swallows are monitored and controlled carefully to ensure reproducibility of the study. Water swallows (1-2 ml) are used because more vigorous peristaltic response results with water swallows than with saliva swallows.[24] The catheter may be left in one position throughout the study, or it may be withdrawn in a stepwise (mapping) manner so that additional areas of the esophagus are sampled by the recording sites. The stationary technique is only slightly less sensitive than the mapping technique but is considerably abbreviated. Focal motor disturbances are more likely to be detected by the mapping process, but such abnormalities are uncommon.

Using a small syringe, place 1 to 2 ml of water in the child's mouth and, if he is older than 3 years, ask him to swallow once. In younger or uncooperative children, place the water in the child's mouth while he is using a pacifier, then move the pacifer to let the child swallow. If the child has not swallowed spontaneously after 20 seconds, give another sip of water with the same method. Do not forget to label all wet swallows, dry (saliva only) swallows, and anything else that affects the tracing. Give at least two swallows for each station and pull forward.

In an attempt to induce esophageal symptoms in adult patients, many provocative tests have been devised that are commonly done in conjunction with esophageal manometry. Provocative tests in adults include edrophonium (Tensilon) injection, intraesophageal balloon distention, and hydrochloric acid perfusion (Bernstein test). In children, only the Bernstein test is employed in clinical practice.[25] This test was initially described as a patient-blinded perfusion of the esophageal lumen with acid or gastric aspirate, aimed at reproducing symptoms associated with gastroesophageal reflux. The most common technique for the Bernstein test is to perfuse 0.1 N HCl for 5 to 15 minutes at the end of a manometric evaluation.

Upper Esophageal Sphincter

The assessment of the UES is the final part of the esophageal manometric study and is done during withdrawal of the catheter. At present, there are many limitations associated with UES measurements. Indeed, the small length of the various segments (pharynx, upper esophageal sphincter, and striated muscle portion of the esophagus), the very rapid pressure changes, and the upward and downward anatomic movements of the region during swallowing all suggest that special devices and specific techniques of recording are required.[26] This does not mean that a manometric investigation of the esophagus may ignore the striated muscle region of the esophagus. A minimal requirement for esophageal manometry is a quantitative study of the LES and esophageal body, and a qualitative study of the upper part of the esophagus.

To accurately monitor the upper esophageal sphincter pressure, a miniaturized UES sleeve can be used.[27] A less satisfactory option is a slow pull-through of an infused catheter or transducer sensor, stopping 1 minute or more at each station.

Although the UES relaxes with swallowing, the recording of this phenomenon with conventional manometric instrumentation is largely artefactual. Because swallow-induced UES relaxation usually occurs during the orad UES excursion, accurate manometric recording of UES relaxation remains elusive. Recent testing of a sleeve device positioned across the UES segment suggests that this device accurately records the onset of the nadir of UES relaxation, but its offset is obscured by the oncoming pharyngeal peristaltic wave, which squeezes the proximal part of the sleeve and obscures the post-relaxation UES contraction.[28]

ANALYSIS OF RECORDINGS
Adults

Despite the seeming complexity of the examination, the interpretation of clinical manometric examinations is relatively simple. In adults, it has been reported that four types of measurements in two esophageal regions (the distal esophageal body and the LES) generally are sufficient for manometric interpretation. These required measurements are: 1) peristaltic performance, 2) contraction wave parameters, 3) LES basal pressure, and 4) LES relaxation. Peristaltic performance refers to the percentage of swallows that are followed by normally propagating (peristaltic) waves. Failed motor responses also can be recorded. Contraction wave parameters refer to the amplitude, duration, and shape of the wave at any one esophageal level. On the basis of these four measurements, the use of a categorical scheme for making manometric diagnoses has been proposed for adult patients.[29] Advantages to this approach include: 1) easy use in clinical practice, 2) improved communication between gastroenterologists who interpret tracings, and 3) potential research utility for those studying and categorizing both minor and major manometric abnormalities. This classification is mainly due to the wide variety of manometric diagnoses that can be made in adults.

In children, a categorical scheme for manometric classification has not been proposed because most of the esophageal motor disorders deviate markedly from normal and represent motor disorders with defined pathology (eg, achalasia, esophageal atresia).

Children

In children, the esophageal motility parameters that should be analyzed include:

Basal LES pressure. Measurements of LES pressure are made in millimeters of mercury (mm Hg), using the gastric baseline as the reference point (0 mm Hg). Peak LES pressure is the sum of the tonic sphincter muscle contraction plus a phasic respiratory component related to diaphragmatic contraction. Basal LES pressure may be defined as the mean LES pressure at the midpoint of amplitude of the phasic respiratory component (mid-expiratory pressure), or as the tonic component alone (end-expiratory pressure). The manometry report should describe whether mid-expiratory or end-expiratory pressures were used to measure LES pressure. If the respiratory component is greater than the tonic component (often the case in chronic respiratory diseases such as bronchopulmonary dysplasia), then the report should include a description of the tonic and respiratory components.

LES relaxation with swallow. The percentage of relaxation (mean percentage reduction in basal LES pressure) and residual sphincter pressure can be used as parameters of completeness. To determine the nadir of relaxation, an approximated smooth line is drawn through the fine respiratory and cardiac oscillations. The pressure difference between the nadir value and fundic pressure represents the residual pressure barrier.

Swallow: To assess esophageal body motility, only waves induced by wet swallows preceded by at least 20 seconds of motor silence should be considered. The following measurements are recoded:

Amplitude—determined in mm Hg from the mean resting esophageal pressure to the peak of the pressure wave;

Duration—measured in seconds from the onset of the major upstroke of the wave to its return to the baseline.

Velocity. Velocity is measured in cm per second by dividing the distance between the proximal and distal recording orifices (5 cm) by the time required for the beginning of a wave's upstroke to traverse this distance.

Furthermore, qualitative analysis of the manometric tracings should be made to detect the number of abnormal motor responses as percentage of assessable swallows. Abnormal motor responses consist of:

1) Simultaneous contraction sequences with a velocity over 6.25 cm per second;

2) Double-peaked or multi-peaked waves. If the descending limb of the deglutitive pressure waves descends over a length greater than the respiratory swing at that level, but does not reach the baseline before giving rise to another up-stroke, it is double peaked;

3) Failed peristalsis, noted as a wet swallow followed by no activity in the distal esophagus.

The usefulness of information obtained for the UES with intraluminal manometry depends on appropriate manometric instrumentation and technique. However, the following parameters should be measured:

1. *Basal UES pressure:* UES pressure is best measured with a sleeve sensor; measurements are made in mm Hg, using the esophageal baseline pressure as the reference point (0 mm Hg);

2. *UES relaxation with swallows:* Relaxation of the UES to the esophageal baseline (taken as zero) with swallows can be assessed using a continuous recording lasting at least 2 minutes at a paper speed of 5 mm per second. The first side hole is stationed in the pharynx and the second—or the sleeve sensor—is in the UES. The percent of UES relaxation is determined by multiplying the fractional decrease in UES pressure to the esophageal baseline by 100;

3. *Pharyngoesophageal coordination:* This value is arrived at by comparing the timing sequence between the spike of the pharyngeal contraction and the UES relaxation. Peak pharyngeal pressures normally occur during the trough of UES relaxation.

Normal Values for Esophageal Manometry

Large population-based studies are unavailable because of the difficulty in recruiting normal children for manometric study. Consequently, some variability related to small sample size can be expected in the reported values. Variability also relates to differences in technique and methods. Table 11.1 compares normal values of the esophageal

	TABLE 11.1 **Normal Values for Esophageal Manometry**		
Parameter	Hillemeier et al (1983) n = 15 mean age: 7.9 mo	Cucchiara et al (1985) n = 16 mean age: 11 mo	Mahony et al (1988) n = 9 age range: 3 mo-2 y
Abnormal motor response* (% of swallows)	17.4	4.3 ± 6.3	—
Amplitude (mm Hg)	50.2 ± 3.2	59 ± 20	72 ± 17.2
Duration (s)	—	2.4 ± 0.2	3.9 ± 1.0
Velocity cm/s	—	3 ± 0.9	2.9 ± 2.1
LES basal pressure (mm Hg)	22.4 ± 4.7	15 ± 2	21.9

Values represent M ± SD
* Simultaneous contraction sequences and double-peaked waves

body and LES parameters in the three series.

The practitioner should either establish normal values for the laboratory or adhere to a set of values obtained using similar techniques.

DISORDERS OF THE UPPER ESOPHAGEAL SPHINCTER

Dysphagia in children may be secondary to neurogenic or structural abnormalities, and may be congenital or acquired. These disorders can also produce nasal regurgitation, failure to thrive and aspiration secondary to oral, pharyngeal, and esophageal involvement (see Chapter 3).

Cricopharyngeal dysfunction should be suspected when saliva pools at the back of the pharynx and passage of barium at the UES is delayed. Motility studies suggest two main defects: abnormalities in cricopharyngeal resting pressure and relaxation. Incomplete relaxation and incoordination of UES has been demonstrated in response to swallowing in children with disorders of deglutition complicated by pulmonary aspiration.[30]

Sondheimer[31] examined UES and pharyngeal motor function in infants with gastroesophageal reflux. She found no difference in resting UES pressures and pharyngeal motor function in patients compared with normal controls. Recently, Willing et al[32] used a sleeve recording device and reported that the esophageal distention caused by gastroesophageal reflux is a stimulus of transient UES relaxation in children. These relaxations are more likely due to an esophagopharyngeal reflux than defective UES pressure. Unfortunately, recording the response of the pharyngoesophageal region during deglutition is complicated by a large number of factors.[33] UES dysfunction is best evaluated with videofluoroscopy and nasopharyngeal endoscopy.

DISORDERS OF THE ESOPHAGEAL BODY AND LOWER ESOPHAGEAL SPHINCTER

A variety of diseases that affect esophageal muscle result in disordered motor function. Primary esophageal motility disorders, in which the esophagus is the major site of involvement, encompass a spectrum of conditions including achalasia, diffuse esophageal spasm, and intermediate types (Table 11.2). Achalasia is the most common primary esophageal motor disorder in children. The others include diffuse esophageal spasm and nutcracker esophagus, although diffuse esophageal spasm and achalasia were the most common esophageal motility disorders identified in children with chief complaints of chest pain.[34] Diffuse esophageal spasm was defined according to the criteria of Rich-

---

TABLE 11.2 **Esophageal Motor Disorders of the Smooth Muscle**

Primary Esophageal Motor Disorders
Achalasia
Diffuse esophageal spasm
Nutcracker

Secondary Esophageal Motility Disorders
Congenital malformation
Collagen vascular diseases
Metabolic disorders
Neuromuscular disorders
Iatrogenic
Chronic intestinal pseudo-obstruction
Gastroesophageal reflux disease
Surgery

ter et al;[35] nutcracker esophagus was defined by peristaltic pressures of increased amplitude (>180 mm Hg) and prolonged duration (>6) with normal propagation (mean of 10 wet swallows).

In secondary disorders, the esophageal abnormalities are due to more generalized neural, muscular, or systemic diseases, to metabolic disturbances, or to inflammatory lesions of the esophageal wall.

In children with gastroesophageal reflux-associated esophagitis, manometric abnormalities include impaired peristalsis[36] and LES hypotension,[37] or excessive transient relaxations.[19] However, the detection of any of these manometric aberrations has not been demonstrated to predict either the occurrence of gastroesophageal reflux-associated disease or the appropriateness of a particular therapeutic agent. Abnormal peristalsis and gastroesophageal reflux have been found in children after successful surgical repair of esophageal atresia. It is likely that esophageal motor incoordination is an intrinsic part of the congenital abnormality.[38]

A mass that is extrinsic to the esophagus may be associated with unusual manometric findings. Figure 11.2 shows a manometry of an aberrant right subclavian artery in an 18-month-old girl with dysphagia. The diagnosis was made by aortic arch angiography, after a barium swallow demonstrated a persistent filling defect from a structure posterior to the esophagus (Fig. 11.3).

Abnormal esophageal motor responses to swallows are highly prevalent in children with Hirschsprung's disease who have not yet undergone operations (Fig. 11.4). These abnormalities do not resolve following resection of the aganglionic segment of colon. These data suggest that diffuse gastrointestinal motor dysfunction may be a feature of Hirschsprung's disease.[39]

The three motility disorders of the esophagus that affect children are achalasia, as well as neuromuscular and connective tissue diseases.

ACHALASIA

Achalasia is a disease of esophageal innervation with features that include discoordination of peristalsis, incomplete lower sphincter relaxation, and eventual motor failure in the esophageal body (Fig. 11.5). Although this condition is uncommon at any age, fewer than 5% of those affected develop symptoms before the age of 15 years.[40] The disease involves both the submucosa and myenteric plexus. Degeneration of neurons occurs, often in association with a chronic inflammatory perineural infiltrate. Progression of symptoms is accompanied by steady loss of neurons.

Ultrastructural studies can confirm the intrinsic nerve damage and also show abnormality of the vagal innervation of the lower esophageal sphincter.[41]

The most prominent symptom is pro-

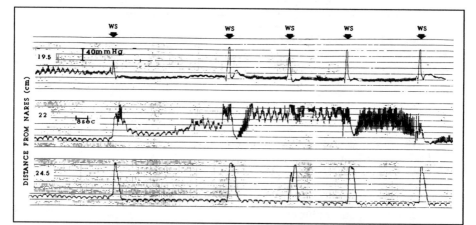

Fig. 11.2 Esophageal manometry in an 18-month-old with an aberrant right subclavian artery. In the proximal two leads, a pulsatile area with an elevation of the baseline can be seen. (WS, wet swallow)

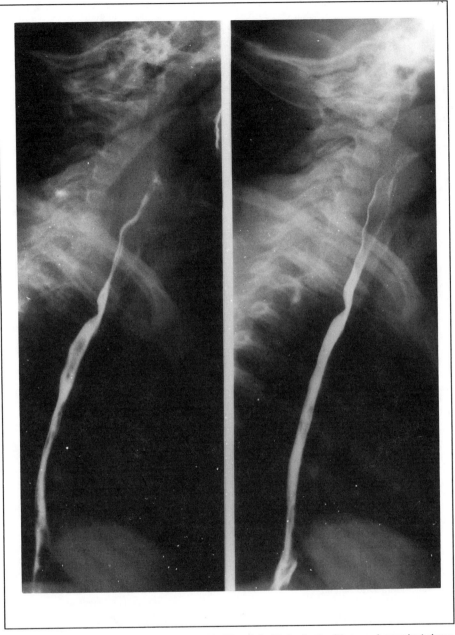

Fig. 11.3 Barium swallows revealing a persistent filling defect in the body of the esophagus just above the aortic arch from extrinsic compression due to an aberrant right subclavian artery.

gressive dysphagia, but children may present with recurrent emesis, failure to thrive, or respiratory symptoms.

Radiology and esophageal manometry remain the diagnostic methods of choice. The barium swallow shows a dilated esoph-agus that ends in a pointed "beak," which represents the nonrelaxing LES. Fluorosco-py during the swallow reveals no meaning-ful peristalsis in the esophageal body.

Manometric findings in achalasia in-clude: 1) absence of distal esophageal body

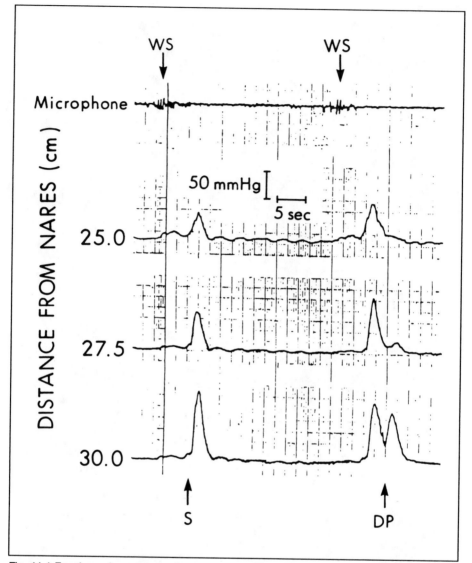

Fig. 11.4 Esophageal manometry in a 5-year-old boy with Hirschsprung's disease. Note a simultaneous contraction sequence following one wet swallow and a double-peaked response (DP) on subsequent swallow(s).

peristalsis, 2) incomplete LES relaxation, 3) hypertensive basal LES pressure, and 4) elevated intraesophageal pressure. The latter two features are less consistently observed, but incomplete relaxation of the LES and failure of at least distal esophageal body peristalsis are required for confident diagnosis.

Apart from Chagas' disease in endemic areas, the differential diagnosis of dyspha-

gia in childhood includes strictures, benign neoplasms, vascular rings, webs, foreign bodies, and severe esophagitis (peptic, infectious, chemical, or drug-induced).

The aim of treatment is to relieve the esophageal obstruction. The two accepted methods of treatment have been pneumatic dilation, and myotomy of the LES.[42] Complications for both include perforation, hemorrhage, and gastroesophageal reflux. Be-

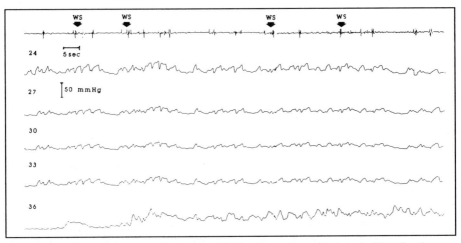

Fig. 11.5 Esophageal manometry in a 5-year-old girl with esophageal achalasia. Note the absence of peristalsis after swallowing. The most distal site records LES pressure measured by pediatric Dent sleeve.

cause of the high incidence of the latter complication after myotomy, it has been suggested that an antireflux procedure should be done at the same time as the myotomy.[43]

Recently, sublingual nifedipine has been effective in some children with achalasia.[43] Nifedipine is a calcium channel blocker that relaxes esophageal spasm and the LES. Treatment with sublingual nifedipine 10 mg 15 minutes before each meal may induce a remission of symptoms, although drug tolerance develops after weeks to months of use.[44]

COLLAGEN-VASCULAR DISEASES

The esophagus may be affected by almost any of the collagen diseases, although involvement is most commonly seen with progressive systemic sclerosis, mixed connective-tissue disease, polymyositis, and dermatomyositis. Scleroderma and mixed connective-tissue disease are rare in childhood, but esophageal motor disorders have been documented in most adult patients with

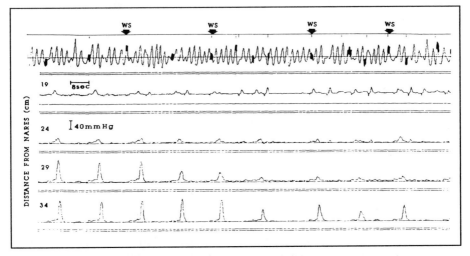

Fig. 11.6 Esophageal motility tracing from a 10-year-old girl with dermatomyositis. After wet swallows, the amplitude of contractions was less than expected in the proximal two recording sites but normal in the most distal recording site.

these diseases. Esophageal motor abnormalities were found in 73% of pediatric patients with progressive systemic sclerosis or mixed connective-tissue disease.[45] The esophageal motility abnormalities included low to absent LES pressure, weak to absent distal esophageal peristalsis, and normal upper esophageal peristalsis and sphincter pressure. Manometry is more sensitive than radiography for detecting early esophageal involvement. The most common esophageal symptoms are heartburn and regurgitation, which result from gastroesophageal reflux.

The pathogenesis of esophageal motor abnormalities in patients with scleroderma remains unknown. Atrophy and sclerosis of esophageal smooth muscle as well as local ischemia have been hypothesized.

In patients with mixed connective-tissue disease, manometric findings are similar to scleroderma, with a decrease in both LES pressure and distal esophageal peristalsis.

The esophagus is involved in approximately 60% to 70% of adults with dermatomyositis or polymyositis. Since the upper third of the esophagus is mainly involved in both diseases, esophageal symptoms are related to upper esophageal dysfunction, with aspiration, nasopharyngeal regurgitation, and oropharyngeal dysphagia.

Recently, two children underwent esophageal manometry due to feeding problems and failure to thrive. Both children had normal LES pressure and relaxation, and normal peristalsis in the distal esophageal body. However, in the proximal esophagus a marked decrease in the amplitude of the contraction waves and an increase in the number of swallows followed by simultaneous waves was observed (Fig. 11.6). In both patients the final diagnosis was dermatomyositis. Subsequently, esophageal manometry allowed assessment of the disease's progression and response to medical treatment.

NEUROLOGIC DISEASE

Gastroesophageal reflux-related diseases such as recurrent vomiting, pulmonary aspiration, and failure to thrive occur frequently in children with central nervous system diseases. Children with psychomotor retardation may show no esophageal motility abnormalities aside from those associated with gastroesophageal reflux.[46] In particular, children with mild to moderate psychomotor retardation often exhibit normal esophageal motility or mild degrees of esophageal motility abnormalities. The esophageal motility abnormalities and associated symptoms do not persist after effective treatment for GER or after 6 months of follow-up. In children with severe psychomotor retardation, UES and esophageal body abnormalities (decreased amplitude of the esophageal waves and abnormal motor responses) do not improve after treatment of gastroesophageal reflux. From these observations, it can be supposed that GER disease in severely handicapped children is exacerbated by impaired esophageal motor function that persists even after healing of esophagitis and may predispose to frequent relapses.

In 1989, two children evaluated for hypotonia and a presumptive disorder of esophageal motility and/or GER due to recurrent respiratory tract infections and feeding problems were reported. In both, further evaluation led to a diagnosis of a primary myopathy.[47]

Recently, low amplitude of the contraction waves in the proximal esophagus was reported in children with muscular dystrophy early in the course of the disease, even when gastrointestinal symptoms were absent and skeletal muscle symptoms were minimal.[48] The delayed gastric emptying and the low amplitude of the contraction waves in the proximal portion of the esophagus are probably caused by weak, diseased muscle. Gastrointestinal motor abnormalities in the patients were not age-related or related to the type of muscular dystrophy. In adults, smooth-muscle involvement of the gastrointestinal tract may be prominent in the muscular dystrophies, and may be asymptomatic or give rise to symptoms.

CONCLUSION

Esophageal manometry is best suited to study the distal esophagus. Manometric recordings from the pharyngoesophageal junction do not provide reliable information; motor activity in this area is therefore better evaluated by videofluoroscopy.

The primary indication for esophageal pressure studies in adults is to investigate dysphagia or chest pain of unknown origin. The most frequent indication for esophageal manometry in children is to evaluate the pathophysiologic mechanism underlying gastroesophageal reflux-associated disease. Esophageal manometric studies in the evaluation of patients before antireflux surgery offer important information regarding the decision for surgery or the outcome of the operation. For example, demonstration of abnormal motor patterns is often followed by poor results. Antireflux surgery does not appear to alleviate symptoms secondary to motor disorders not caused by reflux itself.[49]

Esophageal manometry can also be used to evaluate the results of medical and surgical treatments. This technique has been used to establish the efficacy of drugs, pneumatic dilations, extramucosal myotomies, and antireflux operations.

REFERENCES

1. Kronecker H, Meltzer SJ. Der schluckmechanismus, seine erregung und seine hemmung. Arch Ges Anat Physiol 1883;(Suppl 7):328-32.

2. Euler AP, Ament ME. Value of esophageal manometric studies in the gastroesophageal reflux in infancy. Pediatrics 1977;59:58-61.

3. Moroz SP, Espinoza J, Cumming WA, Diamant NE. Lower esophageal sphincter function in children with and without gastroesophageal reflux. Gastroenterology 1976;71:236-41.

4. Whitington PF, Shermeta DW, Seto SY, Jones L, Hendrix TR. Role of lower esophageal sphincter incompetence in recurrent pneumonia after repair of esophageal atresia. Pediatrics 1977;91:550-4.

5. Winans CS. The pharyngoesophageal closure mechanism: A manometric study. Gastroenterology 1972;63:768-77.

6. Nilsson ME, Isaccsson G, Isberg A, Schiratzki H. The mobility of the upper esophageal sphincter in relation to the cervical spine - a morphological study. Doctoral Thesis, Karolinska Institute, Huddinge, Sweden, 1988.

7. Jacob P, Kahrilas PJ, Herzon G, McLaughlin B.

Determinant of upper esophageal sphincter pressure in dogs. Am J Physiol 1990;259:G245-51.

8. Asoh R, Goyal RK. Manometry and electromyography of the upper esophageal sphincter in the opossum. Gastroenterology 1978;74:514-20.

9. Weisbrodt NW. Neuromuscular organization of esophageal and pharyngeal motility. Arch Intern Med 1967;136:524-31.

10. Kahrilas PJ, Dodds WJ, Dent J, Logemann JA, Shaker R. Upper esophageal sphincter function during deglutition. Gastroenterology 1988;95:52-62.

11. Dodds WJ, Stewert ET, Hogan WJ, Stef JJ, Arndorfer RC. Effect of esophageal movement on intraluminal esophageal pressure recording. Gastroenterology 1974;67:592-7.

12. Jacob P, Kahrilas PJ, Logemann JA, Shah V, Ha T. Upper esophageal sphincter opening and modulation during swallowing. Gastroenterology 1989;97:1469-78.

13. Higgs B, Kerr FWL, Ellis FH. The experimental production of esophageal achalasia by electrolytic lesion in the medulla. J Thorac Cardiovasc Surg 1965;50:613-25.

14. Crist J, Gidda JS, Goyal RK. Intramural mechanism of esophageal peristalsis: role of cholinergic and noncholinergic nerves. Proc Natl Acad Sci USA 1984;81:3593-9.

15. Liebermann-Meffert D, Allgower M, Schmidt P, Blum AL. Muscular equivalent of the lower esophageal sphincter. Gastroenterology 1979;76:31-8.

16. Boyle JT, Altsculer SM, Nixon TE, Tuchman DN, Pack AI, Cohen S. Role of the diaphragm in the genesis of lower esophageal sphincter pressure in the cat. Gastroenterology 1985;88:723-30.

17. Conklin JL, Du C, Murray JA, Baker JN. Characterization and mediation of inhibitory junction potentials from opossum lower esophageal sphincter. Gastroenterology 1993;104:1439-44.

18. Werlin SL, Dodds WJ, Hogan DJ, et al. Mechanisms of gastro-esophageal reflux in children. J Pediatr 1980;97:244-9.

19. Cucchiara S, Bortolotti M, Minella R, Auricchio S. Fasting and postprandial mechanisms of gas-

troesophageal reflux in children with gastroesophageal reflux disease. *Dig Dis Sci* 1993;38:86-92.

20. Edmundowicz SA, Clouse RE. Shortening of the human esophagus in response to swallowing. *Am J Physiol* 1991;260:g512-16.

21. Orlowski J, Dodds WJ, Linehan JH, Dent J, Hogan WJ, Arndorfer RC. Requirements for accurate manometric recording of pharyngeal and esophageal peristaltic pressure waves. *Invest Radiol* 1982;17:567-72.

22. Dent J. A new technique for continuous sphincter pressure measurement. *Gastroenterology* 1976;71:263-7.

23. Reveille RM, Goff JS, Hollstrom-Tarwater K. The effect of intravenous diazepam on esophageal motility in normal subjects. *Dig Dis Sci* 1991;36:1046-51.

24. Dodds WJ, Hogan WJ, Reid DP, Stewart ET, Arndorfer RC. A comparison between primary esophageal peristalsis following wet and dry swallows. *J Appl Physiol* 1973;35:851-6.

25. Berezin S, Medow M, Glassman M, Newman LJ. Use of the intra-esophageal acid perfusion test in provoking nonspecific chest pain in children. *J Pediatr* 1989;115:709-12.

26. Dodds WJ, Kahrilas PJ, Dent J, Hogan WJ. Considerations about pharyngeal manometry. *Dysphagia* 1987;1:209-17.

27. Davidson GP, Dent J, Willing J. Monitoring of upper esophageal sphincter pressure in children. *Gut* 1991;32:607-11.

28. Kahrilas PJ, Dent WJ, Dodds WJ, Hogan WJ, Arndorfer RC. A method for continuous monitoring of upper esophageal sphincter pressure. *Dig Dis Sci* 1987;32:121-8.

29. Clouse RE, Staiano A. Manometric patterns using esophageal body and lower sphincter characteristics. Findings in 1013 patients. *Dig Dis Sci* 1992;37:289-96.

30. Staiano A, Cucchiara S, De Vizia B, Andreotti MR, Auricchio S. Disorders of upper esophageal sphincter motility in children. *J Pediatr Gastroenterol Nutr* 1987;6:892-8.

31. Sondheimer JM. Upper esophageal sphincter and pharyngoesophageal motor function in infants with and without gastroesophageal reflux. *Gastroenterology* 1983;85:301-5.

32. Willing J, Davidson GP, Dent J, Cook I. Effect of gastroesophageal reflux on upper esophageal sphincter motility in children. *Gut* 1993;34:904-10.

33. Dodds WJ, Kahrilas PJ, Dent J, Hogan WJ. Considerations about pharyngeal manometry. *Dysphagia* 1987;1:209-14.

34. Glassman MS, Medow MS, Berezin S, Newman LJ. Spectrum of esophageal disorders in children with chest pain. *Dig Dis Sci* 1992;37:663-6.

35. Richter JE, Wu WC, Johns DN, Blackwell JN, Newson JL, Castell JA, Castell DO. Esophageal manometry in 95 healthy adult volunteers: Variability of pressure with age and frequency of abnormal contractions. *Dig Dis Sci* 1987;32:583-92.

36. Cucchiara S, Staiano A, Di Lorenzo C, D'Ambrosio R, Andreotti MR, Prato M, De Filippo P, Auricchio S. Esophageal motor abnormalities in children with gastroesophageal reflux and peptic esophagitis. *J Pediatr* 1986;198:907-10.

37. Hillemeier AC, Grill BB, McCallum R, Gryboski J. Esophageal and gastric motor abnormalities in gastroesophageal reflux during infancy. *Gastroenterology* 1983;84:741-6.

38. Whitington PF, Shermeta DW, Seto DSY, Jones L, Hendrix TR. Role of lower esophageal sphincter incompetence in recurrent pneumonia after repair of esophageal atresia. *J Pediatr* 1977;91:550-4.

39. Staiano A, Corazziari E, Andreotti MR, Clouse RE. Esophageal motility in children with Hirschsprung's disease. *AJDC* 1991;145:310-3.

40. Boyle JT, Cohen S, Watkins JB. Successful treatment of achalasia in childhood by pneumatic dilation. *J Pediatr* 1981;99:35-40.

41. Casella RR, Ellis FH, Brown AH. Fine structural changes in achalasia of the esophagus. I. Vagus nerves. *Am J Pathol* 1965;46:279-88.

42. Milla PJ. Achalasia and disorders of swallowing. In: Buts JP, Sokal EM, eds. *Management of Digestive and Liver Disorders in Infants and Children.* New York, NY: Elsevier 1993;8:95-102.

43. Buick RS, Spitz L. Achalasia of the cardia in children. *Br J Surg* 1985;72:341-3.

44. Maksimak M, Perlmutter DH, Winter HS. The use of nifedipine for the treatment of achalasia in children. *J Pediatr Gastroenterol Nutr* 1986;5:883-6.

45. Flick JA, Boyle JT, Tuchman DN, Athreya BH, Doughty RA. Esophageal motor abnormalities in children and adolescents with scleroderma and mixed connective tissue disease. *Pediatrics* 1988;82:107-11.

46. Staiano A, Cucchiara S, Del Giudice E, Andreotti MR, Minella R. Disorders of oesophageal motility in children with psychomotor retardation and gastroesophageal reflux. *Eur J Pediatr* 1991;150:638-41.

47. Staiano A, Cucchiara S, Del Guidice E, Andreotti MR, Francica D, Auricchio S. Oesophageal motor involvement in minimal change myopathy. *Ital J Gastroenterol* 1989;21:159-63.

48. Staiano A, Del Giudice E, Romano A, et al. Upper gastrointestinal tract motility in children with progressive muscular dystrophy. *J Pediatr* 1992;121:720-4.

49. Spitz L, Kirtane J. Results and complications of surgery for gastro-oesophageal reflux. *Arch Dis Child* 1985;60:743-7.

12
Antroduodenal Manometry

TAKESHI TOMOMASA

MEASURING MOTILITY

The physiologic role of gastrointestinal motility comprises more than sweeping the intraluminal contents down to the anus. To obtain the maximal nutrition from ingested food and avoid bacterial overgrowth inside the canal, complex coordination by each part of the system is required. The stomach holds food until it is adequately mixed with acid and pepsin and is broken down into small particles. The proximal jejunum, which has many propagating contractions, spreads food particles quickly as they exit the pylorus so that a large area of intestinal mucosa is contacted for a long time, making digestion more efficient. In contrast, the ileum does not have many propagating contractions and retains food longer to ensure maximal absorption of nutrients. Occasionally, toxic substances or bacteria must be eliminated by specially coordinated actions of the entire upper gastrointestinal tract, or by vomiting.

To carry out these complicated objectives, the coordination of muscle contractions is controlled by a hierarchy of mechanisms, including myocytes as well as neural and hormonal controls. These mechanisms respond to external stimuli, such as food, toxins, and stress. Muscle contractions force the intestinal wall to produce forward, backward, or rolling movements of the intraluminal contents.

Full understanding of gastrointestinal motility therefore requires evaluation of regulatory mechanisms, sensory nerves, enteric reflexes, muscle contractions or wall motion, and transit of intraluminal contents. The evaluation of muscle contractions, or

motility in its narrow sense, should provide key physiologic or pathophysiologic information. Several methods of examining gastrointestinal contractile movements are available, each with advantages and disadvantages.

Fluoroscopy

Fluoroscopy has been providing visual access to intestinal wall motion since Cannon first used a contrast medium mixed with a meal to observe feline gut motility more than 90 years ago.[1] Fluoroscopy records the wall motion and the movement of the intraluminal materials that were mixed with the contrast medium. This method sometimes provides useful information concerning the causes of abnormal motility. For example, it may reveal an esophageal hernia in a patient with gastroesophageal reflux, or a mechanical obstruction in a patient with intractable vomiting. Fluoroscopy, however, has a few critical shortcomings. Several hours of observation are necessary to complete a study of gastric and intestinal motility, requiring an exposure to radiation that is unacceptable for human subjects. Also, it shows wall motion only, not the muscle contractions themselves. Finally, due to the overlying loops of the small bowel, the observation of the entire intestine is difficult, if not impossible.

Ultrasonography

Recent efforts to observe gastric motility with ultrasonography have had some success. As with fluoroscopy, this method shows both the contractions and movements of intraluminal materials, such as gastroesophageal reflux, gastric emptying, and duodeno-antral reflux. This technique, however, is time-consuming, subjective, and cannot be performed when the stomach is empty (see Chapter 20).

Myoelectrography

Myoelectric recordings have been applied in humans[2] with serosal and mucosal electrodes. Surgery is necessary to implant serosal electrodes, thus limiting the usefulness of this method. For mucosal recordings, surgical invasion is unnecessary. Peroral mucosal recording devices are fitted with a pair of needle electrodes and a suction cup that keeps electrodes attached to the mucosal surface.[2] It is technically difficult, although possible, to use many mucosal (suction) electrodes to record the propagation of contractions. The validity of these techniques is based on the proven assumption that spike potentials indicate the presence of mechanical contractile movements. The validity of the electrogastrography (EGG), the percutaneous recording of electrical events in the stomach, is currently under study (see Chapter 19).

Manometry

Manometry measures changes in intraluminal pressure. Unlike fluoroscopy or ultrasonography, it does not necessarily reflect wall motion. Fone et al[3] used a special catheter which had side holes for manometry and an elliptical wire transducer for detecting wall motion, so that antral pressure changes and wall motion could be recorded simultaneously. Only 51% of antral transducer deflections were associated with antral side-hole pressure, presumably because manometry did not detect nonlumen-occluding contractions. Nevertheless, manometry directly reflects the physical consequence of contractile movements or pressure changes, and is therefore useful for investigating the physiology of gastrointestinal motility as well as the pathophysiology of motility disorders. In some diseases, such as hollow visceral myopathy, manometry is one of the best diagnostic tests. It can also help clinicians

predict the effect of drugs, or the best form of nutritional support.

Manometry is not yet a routine clinical tool because it is difficult to use and requires special training. The most critical problem arises when interpreting the recorded data, due to a lack of validation in normal children and patients. For example, the frequency or specificity of a finding in a disease is often unclear. Most reports of abnormal motility patterns that describe findings in children with symptoms are not compared with studies of healthy children. Also, the physiologic or clinical implications of most abnormal findings have not been explored. Only a few cases[4,5] have demonstrated the temporal correlation between the motility finding and the clinical symptom, thus suggesting that the abnormal pattern was related to the patient's symptom.

HISTORY OF MANOMETRY

Around the turn of the century, Vasili Nikolaivich Boldyreff[6] measured the periodicity of canine gastric contractions with balloon manometry. He noted a series of contractions lasting 20 to 30 minutes, alternating with periods of quiescence lasting 1.5 to 2 hours. Although small intestinal contractions were not recorded, rumblings in the dog's abdomen coincident with gastric contractions suggested that the small intestine was also contracting. After feeding, these periodic contractions stopped. Boldyreff also noted secretions from both the pancreas and the small intestine when the stomach contracted. This periodicity, which was later observed by others,[7] stimulated little interest at the time. His discovery of the periodicity of motility, however, made it clear that brief recordings were insufficient to evaluate fasting gastrointestinal motility patterns.

In 1968, when Szurszewski[8] was studying the frequency gradient of the slow wave by implanting 20 electrodes at equidistant intervals along the small intestine, he happened to find that periodic contractions—later called phase 3 or the activity front—moved down the entire length of the small intestine. As one episode ended in the ileum, another arose in the duodenum. He called the entire sequence of electrical events the "interdigestive migrating myoelectric complex" (IMMC). Later, Code and Marlett[9] made detailed descriptions of the IMMC. Code called the activity front the "interdigestive housekeeper" of the small bowel, because he believed it swept the bowel clean in preparation for the next meal. It later became clear, however, that herbivores experienced similar movement in postprandial periods. The phenomenon, therefore, is usually referred to as the migrating motor complex (MMC).

Vantrappen[10] first demonstrated the MMC in humans in 1976, recording gastrointestinal motility for a long period of time with manometry. Although the physiologic significance of MMCs remains uncertain, it is clear that it represents intact motility-controlling mechanisms. The discovery of the MMC demonstrated that gastrointestinal motility investigations should encompass distance, in addition to time.

In 1977, Arndorfer[11] developed a pneumohydraulic pump with a low compliance for manometry, which transformed manometry to a very sensitive technique that required minimal water infusion. The pump enabled pressure changes to be recorded much longer than the previous system, which used syringe-type pumps. Arndorfer's system became a popular tool for investigating gastrointestinal motility. Prolonged ambulatory recordings are now possible using a catheter with multiple strain-gauge transducers implanted in its lateral surface.[12-14]

Manometry has also been used to study the pathophysiology of motility disorders. More than a decade has passed since antroduodenal manometry was used as a diagnostic test in selected adults[15] and children.[16]

Gastrointestinal motility in children is a relatively new topic. In 1958, Barbero[17] observed duodenal motility in 31 children and infants using a primitive manometric method. Although phase 3 was clearly demonstrated in one of his figures, he did not focus on the analysis of the MMC, because it had not yet been described. In 1981, Milla and Fenton[18] recorded phase-3 activity in the duodenum of infants using a single lumen tube, which did not allow them to confirm the migration of phase 3s. Later, others[19-22] used manometric assemblies with much lower perfusion rates to study human infants and found that real phase 3s that migrate can be seen after 32 to 35 weeks of postconceptual age. It is now accepted that gastrointestinal motility in infants differs from that in adults (see Chapter 1). Only a few reports are available on gastrointestinal motility in healthy older children.[23,24] Much more work is necessary to establish the normal values for gastrointestinal motility patterns in children at various stages of development.

INDICATIONS FOR MANOMETRY

In addition to its value as a research tool, antroduodenal manometry is useful in certain clinical situations. Almost all patients with chronic symptoms that suggest motility disturbance can benefit from an antroduodenal manometry test. Manometry can be helpful for making the diagnosis, understanding the pathophysiology, and determining the physiologic response to drugs or other interventions (eg, hypnosis or guided imagery). However, one must be aware of the limitations of information gained through manometry. As will be discussed below, many qualitative abnormalities are found in more than one condition, even in healthy subjects. Information about the specificity of these abnormalities is currently limited. Therefore, the manometric results often only determine whether or not the motility patterns of the patients are abnormal.

In children, the disease for which manometry is the most reliable diagnostic test is chronic intestinal pseudo-obstruction (CIP). One or more abnormal findings, listed in Table 12.1, are found in most CIP patients, especially in severe cases.[16,25,26] However, the absence of abnormality does not necessarily exclude this disease; most findings in CIP are not specific to the disease.

Manometry can predict the prognosis or course of a disease in certain situations. For example, antroduodenal motility predicts feeding intolerance in preterm infants. Infants in whom the motility index — Log e

TABLE 12.1 Abnormal Findings in Antroduodenal Manometry

Fasted State
 Absence of phase 3 or long interval of phase 3s
 Short interval of phase 3
 Absence of phase 1
 Short phase 2
 Abnormal phase-3 migration
  Stationary phase 3
  Retrograde phase 3
 Tonic contraction
 Prolonged phasic contraction
 Nonmigrating cluster of contractions
 Low amplitude of contraction (myopathy pattern)

Postprandial State
 Failure to change to postprandial motility
 Postprandial hypomotility
  Low frequency of contraction
  Low amplitude of contraction (myopathy)
 Nonmigrating cluster of contractions

(sum of amplitudes of all contractions + 1) — increased after a test feeding are likely to tolerate enteral feedings.[21] Unfortunately, both the sensitivity and the specificity of that criterion are unsatisfactory.

The effect of drugs can also be predicted by manometry. The acute effect of prokinetic drugs, such as cisapride, metoclopramide, domperidone, erythromycin, and somatostatin can be ascertained during motility tests. Some manometric findings might predict the effect of a drug without provocation. The presence of the MMC, for instance, predicts a good response to cisapride in patients with functional upper-gut symptoms.[27]

Manometry can demonstrate which organs are involved in patients who have diseases that may affect gastrointestinal motility, such as progressive systemic sclerosis and diabetes mellitus.[28] Such information helps clinicians select appropriate therapies. Patients with CIP who have small-intestinal MMCs are more likely to tolerate jejunal feeding than those without MMCs.[29] Fundoplication is contraindicated in patients who vomit frequently and in whom manometry reveals abnormal gastrointestinal motility.[30]

Parents ask pediatricians, "What is wrong with my child?" Often their question goes unanswered because radiology and transit studies are descriptive rather than diagnostic. Antroduodenal manometry testing may be able to provide a pathophysiologic explanation for the child's symptoms. If the manometry is inconsistent with the degree of disability shown by the child (ie, a child with normal manometry who requires TPN) there may be a psychiatric problem.

RECORDING TECHNIQUE
Assembly

Perfused catheters or strain-gauge catheters are available for manometry. In the first method, a catheter with various lumina — each connected to a pressure transducer — is perfused with distilled water. Outside the body, the pressure in the system is transformed into an electrical signal by the transducers. The system includes a catheter, transducers, infusion pumps, amplifiers, and a polygraph. Various types of catheters are commercially available. The size and number of lumens or number of recording sites must be decided depending on the patient's age and the test's purpose.

For adequate sensitivity, the catheter must be perfused with water.[31,32] Recording fidelity is determined primarily by the total compliance or deformability of the system and by the catheter infusion rate.[32,33] The stainless steel capillary perfusion tubes inside Arndorfer's pump creates a huge pressure gradient, and makes the system very sensitive, with a slow water infusion rate. This pump has been the most popular infuser in esophageal and gastrointestinal motility testing.

One of the advantages of the infused catheter method is that the required equipment is relatively inexpensive and sturdy. Another is that catheter modifications are not difficult. A long, polyvinyl catheter can record ileal motility.[34,35] A perfused sleeve attached to the catheter can record lower esophageal sphincter pressure and pyloric pressure.[36,37]

The strain-gauge catheter has one or more strain gauge transducers on the lateral surface of the catheter, which transform pressure changes into electrical signals inside the body. Data can be stored in a portable memory unit, which makes ambulatory monitoring possible.[13,14] Since no water infusion is required, recording over a long period of time is also possible. Comparing simultaneous recordings made by a strain-gauge catheter and a perfused catheter, Valori et al[12] found no difference in accuracy when recording tonic or phasic contractions. Strain gauges, however, recorded bifid, negative, or biphasic contractions more often than perfused tubes.[13,14] In addition to the catheter, amplifiers and a polygraph are necessary in this method. The need for a polygraph is overridden if data can be put into a computer for later analysis (see Chapter 23).

Assemblies for Children

Catheter. Assemblies for adults are appropriate in children older than 1 year. When studying infants, several modifications must be considered. First, catheters must be thin and soft. The effect of catheters on motility has not been well investigated, especially in small children. Even if the catheter is soft enough, it might partially obstruct the pylorus, causing slow gastric emptying. Moreover, rare cases have been reported in which duodenal perforation occurred during duodenal tube alimentation.[38,39] No data is available on how thin the catheter must be. Although the catheter should be as thin and soft

as possible, thinner catheters limit the number of possible recording sites.

Three lumen tubes can be used in infants, with one or two recording sites in the antrum and the remainder in the duodenum.[19] Three recording sites are often sufficient to determine phase-3 migration. When only one recording site is placed in the antrum, it is sometimes difficult to record the antral motility continuously because the recording site might move forward into the duodenum or back into the fundus during recording. On the other hand, when two sites are placed in the antrum, it is impossible to determine if a duodenal cluster migrated.

Three or four lumen soft catheters with a diameter of less than 2mm are recommended in infants younger than 6 months. Four to six lumen tubes are best for toddlers and older children; either of these tubes can be used in children between 6 months to toddlers, depending on the purpose of manometry. The volume of water infused must be calculated, with care taken not to cause overhydration or electrolyte imbalance during tests of infants with a water-perfused system. The strain-gauge transducer-catheter is relatively hard and is not appropriate for infants.

Distance Between Recording Sites

The stomach and small intestine in children are several times shorter than in adults. The catheter must be thinner in children, thus limiting the number of recording sites. Special consideration is therefore necessary to determine the distances between recording sites.

Due to bending of the catheter in the stomach and the change in the stomach's size with meals, the catheter slides up or down through the pylorus during the test, making it difficult to record antral motility constantly. When there are no pressure changes it is unclear whether the recording site moved into the fundus (which is manometrically silent) if there are no antral contractions. Since the catheter cannot be held in the same place in the stomach, the only way to record antral motility is to place many recording sites close together (eg, 1 cm apart).

In recording duodenal motility, the greater

the distance between recording sites, the longer the total length of the catheter beyond the pylorus and, therefore, the less likely it is to miss phase-3 activities which start from the distal duodenum. It is also less likely that the catheter will become dislodged from the pylorus during recording. It is more difficult, however, to put the tube into the most desirable position. The farther apart the recording sites, the more difficult it will be to evaluate the propagation of contractions that propagate over short distances.

For the reasons described above, distances between recording sites must be decided based on the purpose of the manometry. Six lumen catheters with side holes 6 cm apart, or four lumen catheters, with side holes 10 cm apart, can be used in routine evaluations of motility, where the main interest is the presence and migration of phase 3. Two side holes should be placed in the antrum. With toddlers, a six-lumen catheter with side holes 3 cm apart can be used. If the most distal recording site is at the ligament of Treitz, there are usually four duodenal sites, one antral, and one fundic site. With infants, a 3-lumen catheter with 3 side holes, 3 cm apart can be used, placing one or two side holes in the stomach.

Infusion Rate

The infusion rate for adults, usually about 0.4 ml/min or 24 ml/h per recording site, is too rapid for small children and must be reduced. It is impossible to get a very low infusion rate for several recording sites with Arndorfer's system, because when the infusion rate is reduced, the rates of each route become uneven. For instance, when the infusion rate is 0.1 ml/min for one recording site, it may be significantly higher or lower at other recording sites.

Several methods can be used to reduce the infusion rate. The best method is to replace the pneumohydraulic pump in Arndorfer's system with syringe-type infusion pumps, or to add the stainless capillaries of Arndorfer's pump to the conventional manometry system. In this way, a very low rate for each recording site can be obtained constantly. One study showed that when the

infusion rate was higher than 1.5 ml per hour or 0.025 ml per minute, the peak amplitude of contraction recorded on the polygraph was more than 90% of that recorded simultaneously with an Arndorfer's system that had an infusion rate of 24 ml per hour.[19]

The fidelity of a system is directly related to the infusion rate.[11,31,32] When recorded at a very high paper speed, it is noticeable that the system outlined above cannot respond to sudden pressure changes, so that the configurations of pressure waves recorded are smoother and the peaks are recorded slightly late, as shown in Fig. 12.1. This difference is not detectable at normal paper speed (eg, 1.0 or 0.5 mm/s). Fidelity is inversely related to wave amplitude and directly related to wave duration. Therefore, when evaluating gastrointestinal motility, the relatively slow response of the system might be acceptable, as long as the number and peak amplitude of the contractions are being assessed.

Another way to reduce the infusion rate is to replace the stainless capillaries of Arndorfer's system with capillaries that are twice the length of the original (2 x 610 mm). At a very low infusion rate, however, the compliance of the catheter and transducer should be dominant, and it seems illogical to prefer high-pressure pneumohydraulic pumps to the syringe-pumps because of their extremely low compliance. This method is less than ideal because it is still difficult to obtain exact infusion rates for all recording sites with this system.

PATIENT PREPARATION

Preparation depends on the patient's condition and the purpose of the study. In general, diet and drugs must be altered prior to testing.

The presence or absence of MMCs and their abnormalities is easily determined. It is reasonable to assume that a normal phase 3 guarantees intact intrinsic motility control mechanisms, at least to some extent. It follows that most current knowledge about motility focuses on the motility pattern in the fasting period. The adequate duration of fasting depends on the subject. In a healthy subject, an overnight fast is enough. If the subject has delayed gastric emptying or in-

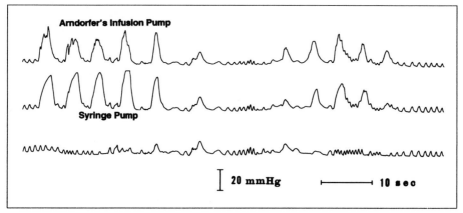

Fig. 12.1 A comparison of the record with an Arndorfer's infusion pump and a recording system in which the pneumohydraulic pump was replaced with conventional syringe-type pumps. The catheter had three side holes, two of which were placed 1 mm apart. One of the two holes was perfused with the Arndorfer's pump at an infusion rate of 0.4 ml/min (top) and the other was perfused with an infusion rate of 0.025 ml/min (middle). The third hole was 5 cm apart from the other two. Note that although response to pressure changes is slower in the revised system, resulting in slightly late peaks, all contractions were recorded with almost the same amplitudes.

testinal transit, longer fasting might be necessary. In newborn infants, MMCs often appear more than 3 hours after ingestion of breast milk. Longer fasting is necessary in infants fed with cow's-milk formula.[40]

Administration of drugs that might affect motility must be discontinued prior to the study. Prokinetic drugs, adrenergic and cholinergic drugs, narcotics, and hormones might affect motility. Even drugs which do not have any direct action on the myocyte or its control mechanisms might have some effect. For instance, omeprazole influences motility by reducing gastric juice secretion, even though its receptor is absent in muscles and nerves. With most drugs, it has not been established how long administration must be stopped. Generally, 2 to 3 days' withdrawal is adequate. Drugs with short half-lives might need shorter washout times.

The effects of intravenous infusions must be observed. Blood glucose levels higher than 140 mg/dl reduce the occurrence of gastric phase 3.[41] Hyperglycemia inhibits gastric emptying.

TUBE PLACEMENT

It is often difficult to position the motility tube at an appropriate place. The tip of the tube must be inserted deep enough in the duodenum to preclude its falling back into the stomach from duodenal contractions or gastric distention during meals. Even when only gastric contractions are recorded, the tip must be placed in the duodenum to stabilize tube direction during the recording.

It is common to use fluoroscopy when inserting the tube. The part of this procedure requiring the most skill is the transpyloric passage. In general, it is easier to insert a hard tube through the pylorus than a soft tube. It is often difficult, however, to advance a hard tube through the duodenal bulb, especially in infants, because of the acute angles in gastroduodenal anatomy. In addition, hard tubes cause greater discomfort for patients and might affect motility. Heavy metal attached to the tip of the tube can help guide the tube with its gravity. A small balloon at the tip of the catheter will lead the catheter, if inflated in the duodenum.[14] Prokinetic drugs such as metoclopramide and erythromycin increase gastric motility and help to advance the tube. Intravenous erythromycin 1 mg/kg infused over 30 minutes induces repetitive propagating contractions in the gastric body and antrum, usually within 20 minutes after infusion.[42] It is, however, unclear how long the effects of these drugs last. Some investigators, therefore, record

TABLE 12.2 **Normal Values for Fasted Motility**			
	Infants	**Children[24]**	**Adolescents[23]**	**Adults**
Duration of phase 1 (min)				
antrum				46[88]
small intestine		12		25 (12-20)[45, 65, 75, 78]
Duration of phase 2 (min)				
antrum				107[88]
small intestine		40		70 (30-130)[45, 65, 68, 75, 78, 79]
Duration of phase 3 (min)				
antrum	3.5 (3-4)[19]			3 (1.5-5)[45, 48, 86]
small intestine	3.5 (3-7)[19, 20, 64]	4.4	5.0	6 (3-9)[14, 45, 48, 57, 65, 75, 78]
Amplitude of phase 3 contractions (mm Hg)				
antrum			131.8	
small intestine	20 (15-30)[19, 63, 64]		55.3	35 (30-40)
Frequency of phase 3 contractions (cont/min)				
antrum	3.3 (3-3.5)[19]			3 (2.5-3.5)[48, 57, 86]
duodenum	12 (11-12.5)[19, 20]			11.3 (10.8-11.6)[10, 14, 48, 57, 75]
Migration velocity of phase 3 (cm/min)				
stomach to the duodenum	2 (1-4)[19, 22]			12 (7-30)[48, 64]
in the duodenum or jejunum	2.5 (1-5)[19, 64]			9 (3-15)[10, 14, 45, 74-76]
Interval of phase 3 (min)	30 (20-50)[19, 20, 63]	55	103.9	100 (40-240)[5, 14, 45, 48, 75, 76, 78, 79,86, 87]
Values are the mean and range (parentheses).			

the motility on the day after tube insertion when they administer these drugs.[43]

An endoscope is another tool used to position the tube. As little air as possible must be delivered to prevent distention of the intestinal wall, which might affect motility. Sedatives affect motility, so it is best to study motility the day after sedation.[43a]

In infants, it may be possible to position a tube without fluoroscopic guidance.[19] When the baby is fasted, a tube is inserted from the nose to stomach and advanced less than 0.1 cm per minute. The tube is judged to be in the duodenum when the typical duodenal clusters of contractions are recorded or when bile exits from the tube. This procedure should be repeated if proper placement is not first obtained. The procedure is successful in more than 90% of cases.

RECORDING

In the perfused catheter method, subjects should maintain the same posture (eg, supine) during recording, to stabilize the baseline. When a strain-gauge catheter is used, the subject is free to choose any position. Restriction of body posture may or may not influence gastrointestinal motility.

It is unclear how long motility must be recorded. Some investigators record motility for 3 hours in outpatient routines and find that phase 3s are lacking in many healthy subjects.[44] Normal values for intervals of phase 3 vary considerably.[45] Mean interval length is about 100 minutes and its deviation is considerable (Table 12.2). Therefore, it is likely that 3-hour recording is insufficient to determine the presence of phase 3s. Other investigators record for 4 hours.[23] The provocation tests mentioned below will help to determine if phase 3s are absent in a shorter period of time.

It is also important to evaluate postprandial motility because several abnormal patterns in the postprandial period are known (see below). A meal inhibits the MMC and induces postprandial motility patterns. In routine examinations at the Mayo clinic, motility is recorded for 2 hours after a 535-kcal solid meal.[46] In a study with healthy preterm infants, the conversion of motility from fasted to fed patterns depended on caloric strength. Threshold concentration was about 22 cal/dl, when 5 ml/kg milk was given.[47] However, it is often impossible to give predetermined volumes to patients who have severe gastrointestinal motility disorders and do not tolerate much food.[25]

PROVOCATION

In addition to regular recordings of fasted and fed motility, it is possible to test the effects of some treatments, including drugs. Intravenous erythromycin, which induces phase 3 of the MMC in the stomach of healthy subjects,[48] can be used to provoke phase 3s in the stomach and assess migration into the small intestine.[43] Recently, erythromycin derivates with no antibacterial activity have been developed and can be used for the same purpose.[49] Somatostatin, which induces phase 3s in the small intestine, can also be used. Erythromycin-induced antral contractions are not propagated in children without spontaneous phase 3s, but somatostatin analog induces phase 3s in the duodenum regardless of spontaneous phase-3 status. Testing the effectiveness of prokinetic drugs such as cisapride[50] and metoclopramide in a particular patient might help determine the treatment.

DATA ANALYSIS

Currently, most investigators evaluate data visually. Most abnormal features, including the absence of phase 3s or tonic elevation of baseline, are easily recognizable to the experienced eye. For quantitative analyses, however, computers can save time and ensure objective evaluations. Methods for computerized data evaluation are discussed in Chapter 23.

NORMAL ANTRODUODENAL MOTILITY

As described in Chapter 1, the normal range of gastrointestinal motility varies with age. In this section, normal adult motility patterns are described first, followed by children's patterns.

Migrating Motor Complex in Adults (Interdigestive Pattern)

Gastrointestinal motility patterns in fasted, healthy humans are characterized by the cyclic occurrence of repetitive, strong phasic contractions and quiescence known as the migrating motor complex. The MMC consists of three distinctive contraction patterns or phases (Fig. 12.2, see also Fig. 1.1). Phase 1 is a motor quiescence which follows phase 3 and precedes phase 2. Phase 2 is a period of irregular contractions, varying in amplitude and periodicity. Phase 3 is a distinctive pattern of regular, high-amplitude contractions repeating at a maximal rate for several minutes. Each phase migrates proximal to distal. The term MMC best describes the entire cycle, although it has been occa-

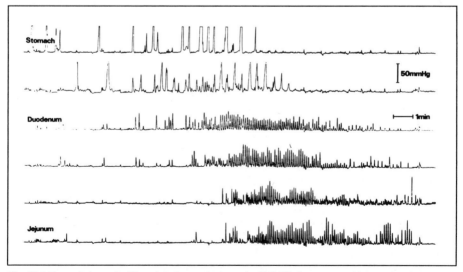

Fig. 12.2 Normal phase 3 of the migrating motor complex (MMC). Strong repetitive contractions occur in the stomach and migrate down the duodenum aborally.

sionally used interchangeably with phase 3.

During Phase 1, contractions are not recorded and intraluminal contents move very little. Contractions in phase 2 either propagate or do not. Nonpropagating contractions probably mix intestinal contents and bring chyme into contact with the mucosa. Propagating phasic contractions move forward at a rate that is similar to the ECA or slow wave, with durations of a few seconds to half a minute. Propagating contractions progress through several loops of bowel, moving the intestinal contents forward rapidly. The length of the bowel traversed by propagating contractions determines the speed of transit of intraluminal materials.[51] Quantitative information about the number, amplitude, and propagation rate of normal phase-2 contractions is insufficient at present. Computer programs should help to evaluate these values in the near future (see Chapter 23).

Phase 3, the most distinctive contraction pattern in the fasting subject, may start from anywhere proximal to the ileum.[34] Approximately 50% to 70% of all phase 3s begin in the esophagus or the stomach; the remainder begin in the small intestine. Phase 3 propagates at a rate of 3 to 10 cm per minute to the ileum (see Table 12.2). Phase 3s often stop migrating before reaching the terminal ileum.[34] Phase 3 contractions repeat at a rate of approximately 11 per minute in the duodenum, slowing gradually to 7 to 9 per minute in the terminal ileum. Intestinal transit is fastest when the luminal marker is just distal to the segment that is in phase 3.[42,52]

Phase 3s that start in the stomach are presumably under different control mechanisms than those that begin in the small intestine. Peptides and chemicals, such as somatostatin,[53,54] pancreatic peptide,[55] morphine,[56] and metoclopramide, which induce phase 3s in the small intestine, never induce phase 3s beginning in the stomach. Much evidence indicates that motilin is involved in the initiation of phase 3s that start in the stomach. The level of motilin fluctuates, and the initiation of phase 3 coincides with the peak concentration of motilin.[57,58] Intravenous infusion of motilin[57] or the motilin receptor agonist erythromycin[48] induces premature phase 3s that start in the stomach and propagate into the small intestine. Intravenous infusion of motilin antiserum inhibits phase 3 arising from the stomach in dogs.[59]

Motilin plays little role in initiating phase 3 in the small intestine.[60] Somatostatin and other peptides might be responsible for the initation, and also for the migration, of phase 3.[53,54,61] Extrinsic nerves, such as the vagus and sympathetic system, can modulate the initiation of intestinal phase 3s. However, the persistence of MMC after vagotomy or complete removal of extrinsic nerves suggests that extrinsic nerve systems play a limited role.[62] Intrinsic nerves are probably involved in its migration.

Some have speculated that phase 3 sweeps undigested food and mucosal debris down to the ileum, like an interdigestive housekeeper.[7] In fact, an absence of phase 3 is associated with bacterial overgrowth in the small intestine.[10] During gastric phase 3, the pylorus relaxes, facilitating the passage of undigested solids greater than 2 mm in diameter, including swallowed coins and other ingested objects.

Migrating Motor Complex in Infants

Premature infants with postconceptional age less than 32 weeks do not have MMC patterns. In premature infants in whom phase 3s are absent, there are no cyclical changes in the motility patterns. Both sporadic contractions and clusters of contractions occur randomly in the antrum and duodenum.

As they develop, phase 3s in premature infants differ from those in adults (see Table 12.2). The migration velocity in infants is slower than in adults, the mean interval between phase 3 episodes is shorter, and the peak amplitude of contractions is smaller.

Clustered contractions, which occur 0 to 2 times an hour and last 3 to 7 minutes in the antrum and occur 10 to 15 times an hour and last 1 to 2 minutes in the duodenum, are the dominant motility pattern in fasted and fed infants.[40] These clustered contractions have the same frequency as phase 3s, but do not migrate caudally. They comprise 70% of total duodenal contractions in newborns during phase 2 and after meals.[19,63,64] The duration of these clusters varies widely, as the mean duration is shorter than that of phase 3s.[19] The amplitude of the clusters are slightly less than those of mature phase 3s.[19,63,64]

The frequency of clusters in the duodenum decreases with postconceptional age (13.5 ± 0.8/h in preterm infants versus 10.5 ± 1.4/h in term infants), whereas its duration increases (1.4 ± -0.1 min in preterm versus 2.1 ± 0.1 min in term).[64] The mean amplitude of contractions in clusters in preterm infants (15.8 ± 1.0 mm Hg) is less than that in term infants (22.2 ± 2.0 mm Hg).

Clusters are either absent or less than 10% of total phase-2 recording time in the adult proximal intestine. They sometimes dominate phase 2 in adults with motility disorders, such as mechanical obstruction,[65] diabetic gastroparesis,[66] and chronic intestinal pseudo-obstruction.[26] It is unknown at what age these clusters disappear.

Normal values for phase 3s in each age group are summarized in Table 12.2. As will be discussed, values outside of these normal ranges do not necessarily indicate abnormal motility.

Digestive Pattern

The normal digestive pattern in gastrointestinal motility is an irregular occurrence of contractions with various amplitudes. After solid meals, strong repetitive contractions are often induced in the antrum. In the small intestine, postprandial motility appears similar to phase 2 to the naked eye. With careful analysis, however, both qualitative and quantitative differences become apparent.[67] Both the amplitude and the frequency of contractions are greater in the fed state than during phase 2. Most contractions after meals propagate over short distances, and the percentage of propagating contractions is less in the fed pattern than during phase 2. Hormones, such as cholecystokinin, are involved in changing the fasting motility pattern to the fed pattern after a meal. Otherwise, little is known about the controlling mechanisms in the digestive state.

In infants, phase 3s do not appear for a while after feeding. In a study with healthy neonates, phase 3 appeared within 3 hours after feeding in 10 out of 12 breast-fed infants, whereas it appeared in 2 out of 12 infants fed with cow's-milk formula. As during phase 2, many clusters of contractions as well as sporadic contractions, are present postprandially.[40]

ABNORMAL MOTILITY

Abnormal findings as demonstrated by antroduodenal manometry are outlined in Table 12.1.

Interdigestive Period

The absence of phase 3 or long intervals between phase 3s has been reported in various motility disorders. No antral phase 3s were recorded during 3-to 5-hour recording periods in patients with idiopathic delay in gastric emptying (20 of 22 patients),[68] orthostatic hypotension (9 of 9),[69] and systemic sclerosis (7 of 8).[70] Antral phase 3s were less frequent in postsurgery patients (0.1/h) and those with diabetic gastroparesis (0.2/3 h) than in healthy subjects (2.0/3 h).[71] Fewer phase 3s started from the stomach in patients with gastric ulcers (9%) than in healthy subjects (42%).[72]

Both antral and intestinal phase 3s were absent for the recording period of 4 to 8 hours in 6 to 13 children with pseudo-obstruction,[25] for 7 hours in patients with bacterial overgrowth (4 of 12),[10] for 24 hours in an adult patient with the same disease,[73] and for 8 hours in adults with functional upper-gut symptoms.[74] Intestinal phase 3s are less frequent in patients with systemic sclerosis (0.1/3 h),[70] duodenal ulcers (mean interval, 174 ± 23 min),[75] and bile reflux with and without gastritis (mean interval, 163-185 min).[76] In CIP, the absence of phase 3 during a 4-hour recording period is more frequent in children who required total parenteral nutrition (65%) than in those who did not (8%) (Tomomasa, unpublished data).

Absent or less frequent phase 3s have been seen in various types of disorders. It is therefore clear that these findings do not specifically indicate any particular disease. The cause and effect relationship between the absence of phase 3 and motility disorders is unclear. In a rare case, such as bacterial overgrowth, the absence of phase 3 is assumed to be a cause, not the consequence, of bacterial overgrowth, because even after overgrowth is treated, the phase 3 remains absent or reduced.[10,73]

The presence of phase 3s guarantees—at least to some extent— healthy motility-controlling mechanisms. In a preliminary report correlating manometry and biopsy in children with a clinical diagnosis of pseudo-obstruction, MMCs were absent in patients with histologically abnormal myenteric plexuses.[77] At present, therefore, the absence or reduced occurrence of phase 3s should be regarded as an indicator of disturbed intestinal function.

The presence or absence of MMCs can predict the effect of certain treatments. In one study, children with MMCs more often responded to cisapride clinically than those without MMCs.[27] Children with CIP who had required parenteral nutrition underwent manometric studies and later received jejunostomies. All patients who had MMCs in 4-hour manometry tolerated jejunal feeding, eliminating the need for parenteral nutrition, whereas less than half of patients who had lacked MMCs did so.[29]

Some investigators who record fasting motility for 3 hours routinely claim that the absence of phase 3s can be seen in normal subjects and therefore does not have high diagnostic value.[46] As mentioned above, however, phase-3 intervals vary considerably.[45] Therefore, the absence of phase 3s is an important manometric finding in children that provides much prognostic information when the recording period is long enough.

Very short intervals between intestinal phase 3s are noted in CIP patients (Fig. 12.3). Disrupted phase 3, characterized by the interruption of contractions, was noted in 4 of 10 myotonic dystrophy patients.[78] Disrupted phase 3 (which cannot be differentiated clearly) combined with phase 3 with intervals shorter than 30 minutes apart is seen in about 30% of pseudo-obstruction patients (unpublished data). Phase-3 intervals are reported to be shorter in patients with irritable

bowel syndrome with diarrhea (77 ± 10 min),[5] short bowel (71 ± 16 min),[79] diabetic motility disorders (69 ± 6 min), and postvagotomy diarrhea (86 ± 6 min).[80] The difference between these values and controls, however, is not great. It is unlikely that disease can be diagnosed based solely on short phase-3 intervals.

Phase 1 is absent in about 50% of CIP patients (unpublished data), including those with familial visceral myopathy.[81] Short phase 1 (10 ± 4 min) has been reported in myotonic dystrophy.[78]

Short phase 2 has been reported in patients with short bowel (19 ± 7 min).[79] Phase 2 is inhibited by somatostatin. Phase 2s are abnormally long in myotonic dystrophy (136 ± 20 min)[78] and duodenal ulcer (160 ± 21 min).[75] Since the length of phase 2 varies widely in normal subjects,[65] the diagnostic value of this finding is questionable.

Abnormal propagation of phase 3 includes nonpropagating (stationary) (Fig. 12.4), retrograde, and slow-propagating phase 3s. Nonpropagating and retrograde phase 3s were reported in patients with functional upper-gut symptoms,[74] myotonic dystrophy,[78] and chronic intestinal pseudo-obstruction.[16,26] Propagation of phase 3 was slow in a patient with brainstem encephalitis (0.9 cm/min)[76] and in a patient with bacterial overgrowth (0.9 cm/min).[82] In patients with Chagas' disease, the mean propagation velocity of phase 3 (4.7 cm/min) was less than in controls (9.4 cm/min), although there was overlap.[83]

Tonic contractions (>30 s duration, >10 mm Hg amplitude) are usually seen during clusters of phasic contractions, with some rare exceptions. In some pseudo-obstruction patients, the phasic contractions during phase 3 are superimposed on a marked tonic rise (>30 mm Hg, >3 min) of baseline.[26] Nonmigrating burstlike activity with tonic elevation of baseline is seen in some patients with functional upper-gut symptoms,[74] systemic sclerosis,[70] and orthostatic hypotension.[69] Although slight elevation of the baseline for short periods of time during clusters of phasic contractions is not uncommon in healthy subjects, marked and sustained elevations

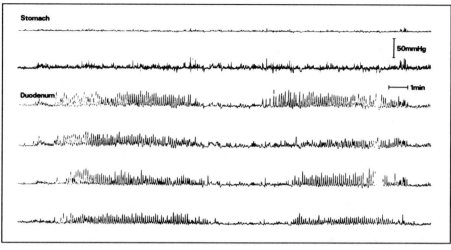

Fig. 12.3 Two-minute interval between phase 3s in the duodenum of a child with chronic pseudo-obstruction (CIP).

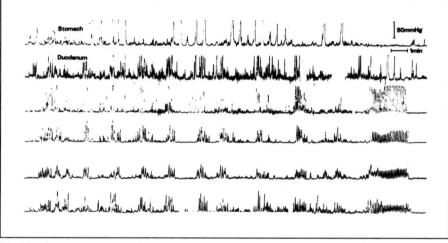

Fig. 12.4 Stationary phase 3 (right end), and phase 2 with many nonpropagating clusters of phasic contractions.

should be regarded as abnormal.

Prolonged phasic contractions (>20 s) have been reported in several motility disorders (Fig. 12.5). Prolonged contractions occur simultaneously in recording sites at least 20 cm apart in patients with subacute mechanical obstruction.[46] In irritable bowel syndrome[5] and a novel type of chronic diarrhea,[82] rapidly propagating and high-pressure prolonged (>15 s and 12-48 s, respectively) contractions might be present in the small intestine. Single or double pressure waves lasting approximately 10 sec-

onds and migrating 60 cm or more at a rapid rate of 2 cm per second can occur in healthy subjects (0.3 times/h), but occur significantly more frequently in patients who have proctocolectomy with ileal pouch anastomosis (2.1 times/h).[84]

Nonmigrating clusters of contractions that last longer than 2 minutes are rare in the adult upper small intestine, although they account for more than half of total contractions in newborns (see Fig. 1.4). Frequent clusters of contractions with or without tonic elevations of baseline have been reported in

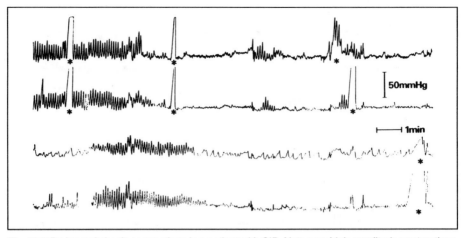

Fig. 12.5 Prolonged phasic contractions in a patient with CIP. Note very high-amplitude contractions lasting 10 to 20 s during phases 3 and 2 (asterisks).

patients with motility disorders, including: 1) more than half of pseudo-obstruction cases,[26] 2) orthostatic hypotension,[69] 3) diabetic gastroparesis[66] 4) mechanical obstruction patients;[65,84] 5) some cases of systemic sclerosis,[70] 6) functional upper-gut symptoms;[74] and 7) some cases of chronic diarrhea.[82]

Discrete clustered contractions, or groups of phasic waves, occurring at a rate of 10 to 12 per minute and lasting 5 minutes or longer, were observed in 15 of 16 irritable bowel syndrome patients, and 9 of 16 healthy controls.[5] Prolonged clustered contractions at some manometric sites coexisting with almost complete quiescence at other sites have been observed in patients with functional upper-gut syndromes[74] and pseudo-obstruction (Fig. 12.6). The Q-complex, or bursts of high-frequency (15.4 ± 2.6/min), short-duration pressure activity, is seen with irritable bowel syndrome, diabetes, and postvagotomy diarrhea.[80]

In addition to these qualitative abnormalities, quantitative abnormalities, or hyper- and hypomotility, can be seen. Relative hypomotility of the gastric antrum has been reported in patients with orthostatic hypotension,[69] systemic sclerosis,[70] and gastric ulcer.[72] Long-lasting, constant antral phasic activity was seen in 3 of 104 patients with functional upper-gut symptoms.[74] Low-amplitude intestinal contractions have been seen in myotonic dystrophy[78] and the myo-

pathic varieties of chronic intestinal pseudo-obstruction.[25,85] An increased frequency of contractions is present in myotonic dystrophy.[76] Since these findings are only quantitative, and considerable variation exists in both sick and healthy subjects, their diagnostic value is limited, except for low-amplitude contractions in visceral myopathy, which can be seen with the eye[17] (Fig. 12.7).[19,25]

Abnormal Digestive Patterns

Failure to change to a postprandial pattern or a premature appearance of phase-3 activities after meals has been reported in patients with pseudo-obstruction[25,26] and diabetic gastroparesis.[66] A certain amount of food is necessary to induce postprandial patterns in healthy subjects. The volume and caloric value required to induce postprandial motility in healthy subjects remains to be determined.

Postprandial duodenal hypomotility is the only finding in some children who present with clinical findings consistent with pseudo-obstruction.[26] Antral hypomotility has been reported in some patients with functional upper-gut symptoms,[74] systemic sclerosis,[70] and orthostatic hypotension.[69] Similar findings have been reported in diabetic gastroparesis in adults[66] and children,[28] as well as adults with myotonic dystrophy.[78]

Clustered contractions lasting longer than 2 minutes, which are similar to those in the interdigestive period, are rare in healthy subjects,[65] but frequent in patients with mechanical obstruction,[46,65] orthostatic hypotension[69] diabetic gastroparesis,[66] and irritable bowel syndrome.[65] As with clusters in the interdigestive state, they might be a normal finding in infancy. Moreover, the presence of clusters does not correlate with the severity of the symptoms in CIP patients (unpublished data). The implication of these findings, therefore, is not clear.

Although many findings have been reported as abnormal, none were found in all patients of a given disease, nor were they specific to any disease. These findings may clarify the pathophysiology of the disease, but their diagnostic value is limited and the overinterpretation of data must be avoided.

Age-related differences present another difficulty. The findings that are abnormal in adults but might be normal in children are the absence of phase 3 in preterm infants, and abundant clusters of contractions in early infancy.

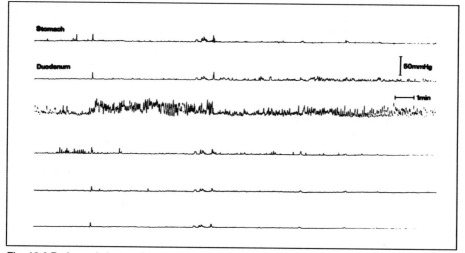

Fig. 12.6 Prolonged cluster of small intestinal contractions in the duodenum of CIP patients. Note continuous occurrence of phasic contractions at only one recording site with quiescence at other sites.

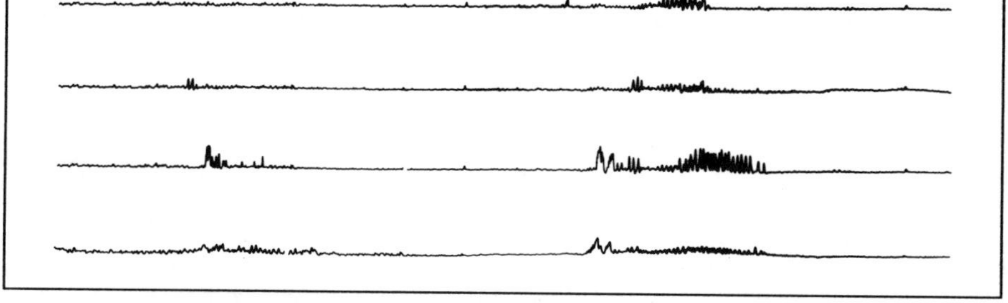

Fig. 12.7 Low-amplitude contractions in a patient with myopathic variant of CIP. Amplitude of contractions in phases 2 and 3 was remarkably low.

PITFALLS

Technical Problems

When using the perfused catheter method, one of the most common technical problems is the presence of air bubbles in either the transducer or the catheter. A single, very small air bubble reduces the sensitivity dramatically, especially when the infusion rate is low. Air-free, distilled water must be used, and the insides of the transducer and the catheter must be checked carefully for bubbles. Sensitivity can also be compromised by an obstructed stainless steel capillary. The flow of water through every hole must be checked before each study. A simple, primitive method to check sensitivity during recording is to watch the baseline change with respiration. When respiration is not apparent at a recording site, the path to the hole is probably obstructed.

There is no good way to hold the catheter in the same place during the entire recording period. The hole for the duodenum slides back into the antrum after meals due to dilation of the stomach. The catheter can be pushed back into the stomach by the duodenal contractions that accompany retching or vomiting. The catheter might advance by peristaltic waves, and antral recording sites might move into the duodenum. Therefore, recording sites must be checked carefully; when there is doubt, an x-ray is indicated to ascertain the location of the catheter.

Difficulties in Data Interpretation

Whether extended fasting affects phase 3s is unclear. In dogs, Boldyreff[6] found that phase 3s stopped after 2 or more days of fasting. Abnormal motility findings in patients with severe motility disturbances might be either the cause or result of long starvation.

Some artificial waves can be recorded and confused with real pressure changes. In children, motion artefacts are the most common. If pressure waves with almost the same amplitudes and configurations are recorded simultaneously at all recording sites, it is likely that the pressure changes recorded are motion artefacts. Simultaneous recording of electrogastrogram or pneumographs in the same polygraph often helps differentiate motion artefacts from real gastrointestinal contractions.

In rare cases, respirations are recorded as great pressure changes by unknown mechanisms. Wave amplitude can be as high as 30 mm Hg (Fig. 12.8).

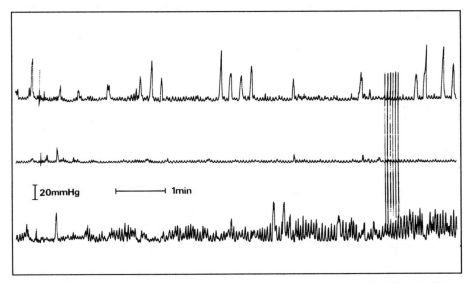

Fig. 12.8 Respiration artefacts. Note that the high-pressure waves recorded in the bottom tracing — with peak amplitude up to 30 mm Hg—coincided exactly with respirations recorded in the top and middle tracings.

REFERENCES

1. Cannon WB. The movements of the intestines studied by means of the roentgen rays. *Am J Physiol* 1902;6:251-77.

2. Hamilton JW, Bellahsene B, Reichelderfer M, Webster JG, Bass P. Human electrogastrograms: comparison of surface and mucosal recordings. *Dig Dis Sci* 1986;31:33-9.

3. Fone DR, Akkermans MA, Dent J, Horowitz M, Schee EJVD. Evaluation of patterns in human antral and pyloric motility with an antral wall motion detector. *Am J Physiol* 1990;258:G616-23.

4. Sarna SK. Motor correlates of functional gastrointestinal symptoms. *Viewpoints on Dis Des* 1988;20:1-4.

5. Kellow JE, Phillips SF. Altered small bowel motility in irritable bowel syndrome is correlated with symptoms. *Gastroenterology* 1987;92:1885-93.

6. Boldyreff VN. La travail periodique de l'appareil digestif en dehors de la digestion. *Arch Des Sci Biol* 1905;11:1-157.

7. Code CF, Schlegel JF. The gastrointestinal interdigestive housekeeper: motor correlates of the interdigestive myoelectric complex of the dog. In: Daniel EE, ed. *Proceedings of the 4th International Symposium on Gastrointestinal Motility.* Vancouver: Mitchell Press, 1974;631-4.

8. Szurszewski JH. A migrating electric complex of the canine small intestine. *Am J Physiol* 1969;217:1757-63.

9. Code CF, Marlett JA. The interdigestive myoelectric complex of the stomach and small bowel of dogs. *J Physiol (Lond)* 1975;246:289-309.

10. Vantrappen G, Janssens J, Hellemans J, Ghoos Y. The interdigestive motor complex of normal subjects and patients. *J Clin Invest* 1977;59:1158-66.

11. Arndorfer RC, Steff JJ, Dodds WJ, Linehan JH, Hogan WJ. Improved infusion system for intraluminal esophageal manometry. *Gastroenterology* 1977;73:23-7.

12. Valori RM, Collins SM, Daniel EE, Reddy SN, Shannon S, Jury J. Comparison of methodologies for the measurement of antroduodenal motor activity in the dog. *Gastroenterology* 1986;91:546-53.

13. Gill RC, Kellow JE, Browning C, Wingate DL. The use of intraluminal strain gauges for recording ambulant small bowel motility. *Am J Physiol* 1990;258:G610-5.

14. Lindberg G, Iwarzon P, Stal P, Seensalu R. Digital ambulatory monitoring of small-bowel motility. *Scand J Gastroenterol* 1990;35:216-24.

15. Camilleri M. Disorders of gastrointestinal motility in neurologic diseases. *Mayo Clin Proc* 1990;65:825-46.

16. Hyman PE, Napolitano JA, Diego A, et al. Antroduodenal manometry in the evaluation of chronic functional gastrointestinal symptoms. *Pediatrics* 1990;86:39-44.

17. Barbero GJ, Kim IC, Davis J. Duodenual motility patterns in infants and children. *Pediatrics* 1958;12:1054-63.

18. Milla PJ, Fenton TR. Small intestinal motility patterns in the perinatal period. *J Pediatr Gastroenterol Nutr* 1983;2(suppl 1):S141-4.

19. Tomomasa T, Itoh Z, Koizumi T, Kuroume T. Nonmigrating rhythmic activity in the stomach and duodenum of neonates. *Biol Neonate* 1985;48:1-9.

20. Bisset WM, Watt JB, Rivers RPA, Milla PJ. Ontogeny of fasting small intestinal motor activity in the human infant. *Gut* 1988;29:483-8.

21. Berseth CL, Ittmann PI. Antral and duodenal motor responses to duodenal feeding in preterm and term infants. *J Pediatr Gastroenterol Nutr* 1992;14:182-6.

22. Ittmann PI, Amarnath R, Berseth CL. Maturation of antroduodenal motor activity in preterm and term infants. *Dig Dis Sci* 1992;37:14-9.

23. Pineiro-Carrero VM, Andres JM, Davis RH, Mathias JR. Abnormal gastroduodenal motility in children and adolescents with recurrent functional abdominal pain. *J Pediatr* 1988;113:820-5.

24. Cucchiara S, Bortolotti M, Colombo C, et al. Abnormalities of gastrointestinal motility in children with nonulcer dyspepsia and in children with gastroesophageal reflux disease. *Dig Dis Sci* 1991;36:1066-73.

25. Hyman PE, McDiamid SV, Napolitano J, Abrams CE, Tomomasa T.Antroduodenal motility in children with chronic intestinal pseudo-obstruction. *J Pediatr* 1988;112:899-905.

26. Stanghellini V, Camilleri M, Malagelada J-R. Chronic idiopathic intestinal pseudo-obstruction: clinical and intestinal manometric findings. *Gut* 1987;28:5-12.

27. Hyman PE, DiLorenzo C, MacAdams L, Flores AF, Tomomasa T, Garvey TQ. Predicting the clinical response to cisapride in children with chronic intestinal pseudo-obstruction. *Am J Gastroenterol* 1993;88:832-6.

28. Reid B, DiLorenzo C, Travis L, Flores AF, Grill BB, Hyman PE. Diabetic gastroparesis due to postprandial antral hypomotility in childhood. *Pediatrics* 1992;90:43-6.

29. Di Lorenzo C, Flores AF, Buie T, Hyman PE. Antroduodenal manometry predicts success of jejunal feeding in children with chronic intestinal pseudoobstruction (CIP). *Gastroenterol* 1993;104:A497.

30. Di Lorenzo C, Flores A, Hyman PE. Intestinal motility in symptomatic children with fundoplication. *J Pediatr Gastroenterol Nutr* 1991;12:169-73.

31. Pope CE. Effect of infusion on force of closure measurements in the human esophagus. *Gastroenterology* 1970;58:616-24.

32. Dodds WJ, Steff JJ, Hogan WJ. Factor determining pressure measurement accuracy by intraluminal esophageal manometry. *Gastroenterology* 1976;70:117-23.

33. Steff JJ, Dodds WJ, Hogan WJ, Linehan JH, Stewart ET. Intraluminal esophageal manometry: an analysis of variables affecting recording fidelity of peristaltic pressures. *Gastroenterology* 1974;67:221-30.

34. Kellow JE, Borody TJ, Phillips SF, Tucker RL, Haddad AC. Human interdigestive motility: variations in patterns from esophagus to colon. *Gastroenterology* 1986;91:386-95.

35. Quigley EMM, Boroday TJ, Phillips SF, Wienbeck M, Tucker RL, Haddad A. Motility of the terminal ileum and ileocecal sphincter in healthy humans. *Gastroenterology* 1984;87:857-66.

36. Dent J. A new technique for continuous sphincter pressure measurement. *Gastroenterology* 1976;71:263-7.

37. Houghton LA, Read NW, Heddle R, et al. Motor activity of the gastric antrum, pylorus, and duodenum under fasted conditions and after a liquid meal. *Gastroenterology* 1988;94:1276-84.

38. Perez-Rodrigues L, Quero J, Frias EG, Omenaca F, Martinez A. Duodenorenal perforation in a neonate by a tube of silicone rubber during transpyloric feeding. *J Pediatr* 1978;92:113-6.

39. Chen JW, Wong PWK. Intestinal complications of nasojejunal feeding in low-birth weight infants. *J Pediatr* 1974;85:109-10.

40. Tomomasa T, Hyman PE, Itoh K, et al. Gastroduodenal motility in neonates: response to human milk compared to milk formula. *Pediatrics* 1987;80:434-8.

41. Barnett JL, Owyang C. Serum glucose concentration as a modulator of interdigestive gastric motility. *Gastroenterology* 1988; 94:739-44.

42. Di Lorenzo C, Lachman R, Hyman PE. Intravenous erythromycin for postpyloric intubation. *J Pediatr Gastroenterol Nutr* 1990;11:45-7.

43. Di Lorenzo C, Reddy SN, Villanueva-Meyer J, Mena I, Martin S, Hyman PE. Cisapride in children with chronic intestinal pseudo-obstruction. An acute, double-blind, crossover, placebo-controlled trial. *Gastroenterology* 1991;101:1564-70.

43a. Di Lorenzo C, Mohan O, Hoon A, Hyman PE. Effect of conscious sedation on antroduodenal manometry in children. *Gastroenterology* 1994 (In press).

44. Malagelada J-R, Camilleri M, Stanghellini V. *Manometric Diagnosis of Gastrointestinal Motility Disorders.* New York, NY: Theime Medical Publishers, 1986.

45. Dooley CP, DiLorenzo MC, Valenzuela JE. Variability of migrating motor complex in humans. *Dig Dis Sci* 1992;73:723-8.

46. Camilleri M. Jejunal manometry in distal subacute mechanical obstruction: significance of prolonged simultaneous contractions. *Gut* 1989;30:468-75.

47. Amarnath RP, Berseth CL, Abell TL, Perault J, Malagelada J-R. The effect of nutrient concentration on small intestinal motility in pre-term infants. *Gastroenterology* 1986;91:1043.

48. Tomomasa T, Kuroume T, Arai H, Wakabayashi K, Itoh Z. Erythromycin induces migrating motor complexes in the human gastrointestinal tract. *Dig Dis Sci* 1986;31:157-61.

49. Kawamura O, Sekiguchi T, Itoh Z, Onura S. Effect of erthromycin derivative EM 523L on human interdigestive gastrointestinal tract. *Dig Dis Sci* 1993; 38:1026-3.

50. Di Lorenzo C, Dooley CP, Valenzuela JE. Role of fasting gastrointestinal motility in the variability of gastrointestinal transit time assessed by hydrogen breath test. *Gut* 1991;32:1127-30.

51. Schemann M, Ehrlein HJ. Effects of neurohormonal agents on jejunal contraction spread and transit in the fed dog. *Gastroenterology* 1986;90:1950-5.

52. Kerlin P, Zinsmeister A, Phillips S. Relationship of motility to flow of contents in the human small intestine. *Gastroenterology* 1982;82:701-6.

53. Peeters TL, Janssens J, Vantrappen GR. Somatostatin and the interdigestive migrating complex in man. *Regul Pept* 1983;5:209-17.

54. Soudah HC, Hasler WL, Owyang C. Effect of octreotide on intestinal motility and bacterial growth in scleroderma. *N Engl J Med* 1991;325:1461-7.

55. Bueno L, Fioramonti J, Rayner V, Ruckebusch Y. Effect of motilin, somatostatin, and pancreatic polypeptide on the migrating myoelectric complex in pig and dog. *Gastroenterology* 1982;82:1395-1402.

56. Sarna S, Condon RE, Cowles V. Morphine versus motilin in the initiation of migrating myoelectric complexes. *Am J Physiol* 1983;245:G217-20.

57. Vantrappen G, Janssens J, Peeters TL, Bloom SR, Christofides ND, Hellemans J. Motilin and the interdigestive migrating complex in man. *Dig Dis Sci* 1979;24:497-500.

58. Rees WDW, Malagelada J-R, Miller LJ, Go VLW. Human interdigestive and postprandial gastrointestinal motor and gastrointestinal hormone patterns. *Dig Dis Sci* 1982;27:321-9.

59. Lee KY, Chang TM, Chey WY. Effect of rabbit antimotilin serum on myoelectric activity and plasma motilin concentration in fasting dog. *Am J Physiol* 1983;245:G547-53.

60. Jannsens J, Vantrappen G, Peeters TL. The activity front of the migrating complex of the human stomach but not of small intestine is motilin-dependent. *Regul Pept* 1983;6:209-27.

61. Hostein J, Janssens J, Vantrappen G, Peeters TL, Vandewood M, Leman G. Somatostatin induces ectopic activity fronts of the migrating motor complex via a local intestinal mechanism. *Gastroenterology* 1984;87:1004-8.

62. Weisbrodt NW. Motility of the small intestine. In: Johnson LR, ed. *Physiology of the Gastrointestinal Tract,* 2nd ed. New York: Raven Press, 1987;631-63.

63. Amarnath RP, Berseth CL, Malagelada J-R, Perrault J, Abell TL, Hoffman AD. Postnatal maturation of the small intestinal motility in preterm and term infants. *J Gastrointest Motil* 1989;1:138-43.

64. Berseth CL. Gestational evolution of small intestine motility in preterm and term infants. *J Pediatr* 1989;115:646-51.

65. Summers RW, Anuras S, Green J. Jejunal manometry patterns in health, partial intestinal obstruction and pseudo-obstruction. *Gastroenterology* 1983;85:1290-1300.

66. Camilleri M, Malagelada J-R. Abnormal intestinal motility in diabetics with the gastroparesis syndrome. *Eur J Clin Invest* 1984;14:420-7.

67. Sarna SK, Soergel KH, Harig JM, et al. Spatial and temporal patterns of human jejunal contractions. *Am J Physiol* 1989;257:G423-32.

68. Labo G, Bortolotti M, Vezzadini P, Bonora G, Bersani G. Interdigestive gastroduodenal motility and serum motilin levels in patients with idiopathic delay in gastric emptying. *Gastroenterology* 1986;90:20-6.

69. Camilleri M, Malagelada J-R, Stanghellini V., Fealey RD, Sheps SG. Gastrointestinal motility disturbances in patients with orthostatic hypotension. *Gastroenterology* 1985;88:1852-9.

70. Greydanus MP, Camilleri M. Abnormal postcibal antral and small bowel motility due to

neuropathy or myopathy in systemic sclerosis. *Gastroenterology* 1989;96:110-5.

71. Malagelada J-R, Rees WDW, Mazzotta LJ, Go VLW. Gastric motor abnormalities in diabetic and postvagotomy gastroparesis: effect of metoclopramide and bethanechol. *Gastroenterol* 1980;78:286-93.

72. Miranda M, Defilippi C, Valenzuela JE. Abnormalities of interdigestive motility complex and increased duodenogastric reflux in gastric ulcer patients. *Dig Dis Sci* 1985;30:16-21.

73. Kellow JE, Gill RC, Wingate DL, Calam JE. Small bowel motor activity and bacterial overgrowth. *J Gastrointest Motil* 1990;2:180-3.

74. Malagelada J-R, Stanghellini V. Manometric evaluation of functional upper gut symptoms. *Gastroenterology* 1985;88:1223-31.

75. Itoh Z, Sekiguchi T. Interdigestive motor activity in health and disease. *Scand J Gastroenterol* 1983;18:121-34.

76. Bortolotti M, Mattioloi S, Alampi G, Giangaspero G, Barbara L. Brainstem viral-like encephalitis as a possible cause of a gastroduodenal motility disorder: a case report. *J Gastrointest Motil* 1989;1:99-104.

77. Hyman PE, DiLorenzo C, Hoon A, Krishnamurthy S, Dean P, Schuffler MD. Antroduodenal manometry and intestinal pathology correlate in congenital chronic intestinal pseudo-obstruction (CIP). *Gastroenterology* 1993;104:A525.

78. Nowak TV, Anuras S, Brown BP, Ionasescu V, Green JB. Small intestinal motility in myotonic dystrophy patients. *Gastroenterology* 1984;86:808-13.

79. Remington M, Malagelada J-R, Zinsmeister A, Fleming CR. Abnormalities in patients with short bowels: effect of a synthetic opiate. *Gastroenterology* 1983;85:629-36.

80. Foster GE, Arden-Jones J, Beattie A, Evans DF, Hardcastle JD. Disordered small bowel motility in gastrointestinal disease. *Gastroenterology* 1982;84:1059.

81. Anuras S, Mitros FA, Nowak TV, et al. A familiar visceral myopathy with external ophthalmoplegia and autosomal recessive transmission. *Gastroenterology* 1983;84:346-53.

82. Kellow J, Phillips S, Miller M, Osterholm M, MacDonald K. Abnormalities of motility and absorption in an outbreak of chronic diarrhea. *Gastroenterology* 1985;88:1442.

83. Oliveira RB, Meneghelli UG, De Godoy RA, Dantas RO, Padovan W. Abnormalities of interdigestive motility of the small intestine in patients with Chagas' disease. *Dig Dis Sci* 1983;28:294-9.

84. Chaussade S, Merite F, Hautefeuille M, Valleur P, Hautefeuille P, Couturier D. Motility of the jejunum after proctocolectomy and ileal pouch anastomosis. *Gut* 1989;30:371-5.

85. Anuras S, Anuras J, Bozeman T. Small intestinal manometric studies in patients with familial visceral myopathies. *J Gastrointest Motil* 1990;2(3):190-3.

86. Achem-Karam SR, Funakoshi A, Vinik AI, Owyang C. Plasma motilin concentration and interdigestive migrating motor complex in diabetic gastroparesis: effect of metoclopramide. *Gastroenterology* 1985;88:492-9.

87. Testoni PA, Fanti L, Bagnolo F, Passaretti S, Guslandi M, Masci E, Tittobello A. Manometric evaluation of the interdigestive antroduodenal motility in subjects with fasting bile reflux, with and without antral gastritis. *Gut* 1989;30:443-8.

88. Oberle RL, Chen TS, Lloyd C, et al. The influence of the interdigestive migrating myoelectric complex on the gastric emptying of liquids. *Gastroenterology* 1990; 99:1275-82.

13

Colonic Manometry

CARLO DI LORENZO

The lack of an appropriate animal model and the relative inaccessibility of the colon to studies in vivo are among the reasons why the motor activity of the colon has been poorly understood. The human colon is unusual because it exhibits characteristics associated with both herbivores and carnivores. It is haustrated like the colons of most herbivores, and relatively simple and short compared to the rest of the bowel, as in carnivores.[1]

The best animal model for the study of colon physiology is the pig because its dietary habits and large-bowel structure are similar to those of humans. Both porcine and human colons contain a cecum, taenia coli, and an arrangement of circular muscle in bundles, with similar microscopic anatomy.[2,3] Unfortunately, the pig's size and bellicose temperament limited its use in research. Instead, the canine colon has become the most studied, although its motility patterns are different from those of humans.[4] For example, the dog has colonic migrating motor complexes (MMCs) that are independent of gastrointestinal MMCs, but the human colon does not. This absence of a cyclical, easily recognizable motor pattern in the adult human colon accounts for some of the difficulty in the interpretation of colonic motor activity. Also, data on colonic motility were gathered under dissimilar experimental conditions (eg, unprepared v. cleaned colon), or using different recording devices (eg, perfused and solid-state catheters or intraluminal balloons) so that comparing studies is difficult.

Until recently, colonic pressure studies in children were limited to the rectosigmoid area,[5] and most of the data concerning colonic motility were obtained by indirect measurement, such as the movement of radiopaque markers[6] or barium.[7] The availability of small-diameter, flexible pediatric colonoscopes has facilitated the placement of motility catheters in the proximal colon, making it feasible to study motility of the entire colon in children of any age.[8,9] There are age-related differences in colonic motility and some of the criteria used to analyze colonic manometry in adults do not apply to children.

In adults, the colon is divided into two functionally diverse segments. The ascending and transverse colon serves as a site for storage, as well as for fluid and electrolyte absorption. The descending and sigmoid colon functions as a conduit.[10] Feces empty rapidly from the cecum and proximal ascending colon and are retained for several hours in the transverse colon.[11] The distal colon is responsible for propelling the fecal material into the rectum, where it can be stored prior to defecation. This functional difference between the proximal and distal colon is less marked in children. Colonic motility in infants and young children is characterized mostly by the presence of propagated contractions which sweep luminal contents to the distal colon.[12] In the child who is not toilet trained, the arrival of stools in the rectum is usually accompanied by defecation.

NORMAL MOTILITY

The interdigestive cycling motor activity, observed in adults and children from the lower esophagus to the terminal ileum, does not propagate into the human colon.[13] Noncyclic features of colonic motility in adults include irregular alternation of quiescence with nonpropagating and propagating contractions, producing a flow of luminal contents through the colon which is not steadily progressive. Some contractions last more than 30 seconds and are considered *tonic*; others are shorter and are considered *phasic*. Most of the tonic contractions have phasic contractions superimposed. Nonpropagating, segmental contractions move fecal material in a retrograde and antegrade direction.[7] This motility pattern probably mixes and shifts intraluminal contents over short distances, permitting adequate absorption of water and electrolytes.[2] Segmental, nonpropagating contractions are rare in infants but are more common in toddlers.[12] An area of high pressure with a high frequency of phasic contractions is found at the level of the rectosigmoid junction.[14] Specialized motility at this site could prevent the uncontrolled caudad progression of stools from the sigmoid colon to the rectum. It is doubtful, however, that a true sphincter exists at the rectosigmoid junction.[15]

High-amplitude propagated contractions (HAPCs) are another feature of normal colonic motility. During colonic manometry, the visual identification of HAPCs is based on an amplitude of more than 80 mm Hg that does not overlap other contractions, a duration greater than 10 seconds, and unequivocal propagation over at least 30 cm. HAPCs can reach amplitudes of more than 200 mm Hg and represent the strongest contractions recorded distal to the gastric antrum. Because the fecal material in the colon becomes progressively harder and thicker as water is absorbed, colonic contractions, which are stronger and last longer than contractions in the small intestine, are probably required to move contents in a caudad direction.[16] In adults, HAPCs occur 4 to 6 times a day in a colon cleansed with cathartics[17] and more infrequently (no more than 2/d) in a normal, unprepared colon.[18] They originate most often in the proximal colon and propagate to the distal sigmoid colon. Retrograde HAPCs rarely occur in the sigmoid colon of healthy individuals.[19]

Most HAPCs are associated with mass movements — a term used by radiologists to describe the movement of barium over long colonic distances — and passage of stools or gas.[20,21] Children have more frequent HAPCs than adults, and HAPCs are associated with defecation or tenesmus more often in children than in adults. The increased number of HAPCs probably correlates with the larger number of bowel movements commonly observed in infants and children.[22] Not all HAPCs are associated with defecation in adults and in toilet-trained children, and not all defecations are immediately preceded by HAPCs; subjects sometimes delay the act of defecation until it is convenient. In healthy adults[23] and children, the frequency of HAPCs increases after meals and upon awakening. In children, one HAPC is often followed by other HAPCs at 3 to 4 minute intervals in the postprandial period (Fig. 13.1). It is not clear what initiates HAPCs. There is some evidence that HAPCs can be induced by distention of the lumen[24] or by luminal irritants such as olive oil,[25] bisacodyl,[26] and glycerol.[27] Cholinergic stimulation does not evoke HAPCs, although it does increase the number and strength of segmental contractions.[28,29]

The only colonic cyclic activity occurs distal to the rectosigmoid junction as a rectal motor complex (RMC), which is not synchronous with or related to the intestinal MMC.[30,31] The RMC occurs in normal adults every 90 to 300 minutes during the day and every 50 to 90 minutes at night and lasts an average of 10 minutes. Within each complex, contractions have a mean frequency of 3 to 4 per minute. Unlike the intestinal MMCs, the RMCs are not abolished by feeding, although it should be noted that the colon is in a continuous digestive state and is seldom empty. The physiologic role of the RMCs remains unknown. The RMCs may keep the rectum empty, especially at night, thereby avoiding the sensation of rectal fullness and promoting undisturbed sleep.[30] Because it is more frequent during sleep, the RMC might be a function of intrinsic rather

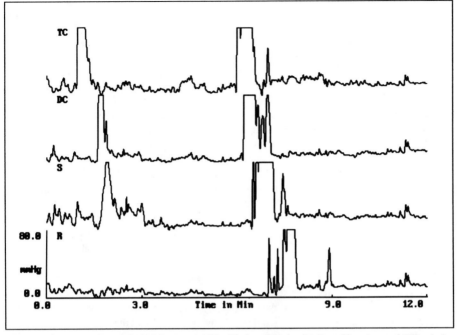

Fig. 13.1 Two postprandial HAPCs in a child with functional retention. (Courtesy of Narasimha Reddy, PhD) (TC, transverse colon; DC, descending colon; S, sigmoid colon; R, rectum)

than extrinsic innervation, as is the MMC. It is not known if the absence of RMCs is diagnostic of abnormal colonic motility.[31]

Because no recognizable motility patterns other than HAPCs and RMCs are present, most investigators calculate the area under the pressure tracing,[32,33] to obtain a crude, quantitative measure of colonic motor activity known as the motility index. The motility index is relatively low before meals and during nighttime sleep or afternoon naps but increases after meals and upon awakening.[17,34] In children, it is unusual to observe colonic contractions during sleep. Eating stimulates colonic motility in healthy subjects.[17] Normal adults experience the gastrocolonic response or gastrocolonic reflex,[35] which are increases in colonic motility that occur within 20 to 40 minutes after beginning a meal. There seem to be early and late postprandial responses, occurring 20 and 60 minutes after the meal, respectively.

Though clearly demonstrable in the distal colon, the gastrocolonic reflex is less prominent in the cecum and ascending colon.[36] The term gastrocolonic reflex is a misnomer because it is not a reflex and does not require the stomach (it sometimes occurs in gastrectomized patients).[37] A more appropriate but less popular term is "colonic response to food."[38] There is no cephalic phase of the colonic response to food. Sham feeding does not stimulate colonic motor activity.[39] Gastric or intestinal contact of the meal with the mucosa is necessary for the colonic response to food. Intravenous administration of lipids does not stimulate colonic motor activity[40] and pretreatment of the gastric mucosa with a local anesthetic delays the response. Administration of food into the duodenum[41,42] and infusion of a complex liquid meal through a jejunostomy (personal observation) also increase colonic motor activity. The magnitude of the colonic response to eating increases as the fat content and the total number of calories of the meal increase. In adults, a 350 kcal meal did not stimulate colonic motility, but a 1000 kcal meal did.[43] Fat was a potent stimulant of colonic motility, carbohydrates had a minimal effect, and amino acids inhibited colonic motility.[43] The minimum amount of calories needed to stimulate colonic motility in children is unknown. Based on data from adults, a meal with at least 40% fat should be used to test colonic response to food.[33] Physical exercise,[44] physical[45] or mental[21] stress, emotional arousal,[46] and caffeinated or decaffeinated coffee[47] increase colonic motility in adults. In children, an increase in motility is observed 5 to 10 minutes after eating. In the younger child, it is characterized mainly by an increase in the frequency of HAPCs. In older children, both the number of HAPCs and segmental contractions are increased. The duration of the response is proportional to the caloric content of the meal and is shorter than in adults. There seems to be no late postprandial response in children.[12]

Ontogeny of Colonic Motility

It is abnormal for defecation to occur before birth. Meconium is usually passed within the first 24 hours of life in healthy newborns. Severely distressed babies can pass meconium prior to delivery. Children with Hirschsprung's disease or other anatomic or functional disorders may have a delayed passage of meconium. Infants and young children have an increased frequency of HAPCs and a more rapid but shorter duration of the colonic response to food than adults. There is a negative correlation between the child's age and the number of HAPCs during fasting and after feeding. There is a positive correlation between postprandial motility index and age when HAPCs are excluded from the motility index analysis (Fig. 13.2), indicating that non-HAPC contractions increase with age. The duration of the gastrocolonic response also increases with age, lasting 30 minutes after a meal in infants[12] and up to 2 hours in adults.[45]

INDICATIONS FOR COLONIC MANOMETRY

Colonic manometry is a useful diagnostic test for evaluating children with intractable, undiagnosed constipation or a generalized motility disorder. Most children with constipation have functional fecal retention (FFR), a condition due to a maladaptive response to painful defecation (see Chapter 8). Children with FFR have normal colon physiology and colonic manometry is normal, provided that the areas under study are not dilated. In generalized colonic motility disorders, the colonic manometry differentiates between neuropathy or myopathy. In children with neuropathies, contractions are present, but uncoordinated. No colonic contractions are found in myopathies.[9] Children with Hirschsprung's disease who continue to be constipated following resection of the aganglionic segment have neuropathic changes in the motor activity of the remaining

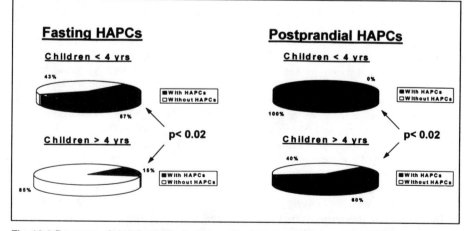

Fig. 13.2 Presence of HAPCs during fasting and in the postprandial period in children less than 4 years old and more than 4 years old. A significantly higher percentage of children in the younger group had HAPCs.

colon.[48] Uncoordinated colonic manometry correlates with neuropathies found with silver-stain examinations of the myenteric plexus.[49] A full-thickness biopsy is necessary for a pathologic diagnosis of enteric neuromuscular disease (see Chapter 22). Colonic manometry, which is less invasive than a surgical biopsy, should be considered part of the evaluation for children with undiagnosed intractable constipation.

In children with pseudo-obstruction, anorectal manometry is usually normal and constipation may be due to abnormal motility in the small bowel or the colon, or both (see Chapter 7). Colonic manometry provides information that can help determine whether or not to perform a colectomy. A child with pseudo-obstruction and normal colonic motility does not benefit from a total colectomy. Prolonged studies of colonic motility coupled with small-bowel recordings have also been used to select surgical options in adults with severe constipation.[50]

Colonic manometry can also provide insights in the decision of whether to reconnect a diverted colon. Surgeons commonly divert the colon and place an ileostomy in infants whose symptoms are consistent with colonic pseudo-obstruction. Once the child has grown and the symptoms have improved, the decision to reconnect the colon can be based on the results of colonic manometry.

METHOD OF STUDY
Type of Recording System

Most manometric catheters used to record colonic pressures have water-perfused, radially oriented side openings.[8,9,29,51,52] The distance between openings varies from 5 cm[26] to 15 cm.[8,53] Having several recording sites close to one another allows assessment of contraction propagation over short distances. Greater distances between recording sites are used to monitor longer colon segments, but often miss contractions occurring between recording sites. Motility catheters with side openings spaced 15 cm apart can be used whenever the tip of the catheter can be positioned at least 60 cm from the anus. A catheter with recording sites 5 cm apart is used when the catheter cannot be advanced

more than 60 cm from the anus. This method allows recording from at least five sites.

Water-perfused catheters with side openings or open-tipped tubes only record contractions that occlude the lumen or squeeze a confined region with sufficient force to increase the intraluminal pressure, and might underestimate the true contractile activity within the bowel wall.[54] A direct comparison between serosal strain gauges and water-perfused catheters showed that water-perfused tubes detected 87% of all tonic contractions and 80% of all phasic contractions detected by serosal strain gauges.[55] The catheters can be perfused with distilled water by means of a pneumohydraulic pump at a rate of 10 ml/h per recording site. When used in more than 100 colonic manometries in children, this method avoided occlusion of catheter orifices by stools. An infusion rate of 10 ml/h was chosen because there is no difference in colonic motility recorded with infusion rates of 10, 20, or 30 ml/h.[56]

Thin-walled balloons record wall movement more accurately than perfused catheters[32] but cause artefacts by distending the colon and obstructing the movements of colonic contents.[57,58] Small intraluminal strain-gauge transducers are ideal for studying subjects for prolonged periods of time, without water perfusion or bed restraint. The transducers are connected to a battery-operated data logger. The patient is free to leave the motility suite, returning only at the end of the study. With this technique it is possible to study the patients under more physiologic conditions. The disadvantages to ambulatory monitoring are that solid-state transducers are more expensive and more fragile than water-perfused catheters, and the investigator is unable to constantly monitor the pressure changes. Printing the study only at the end of the test makes it impossible to perform provocative studies in response to specific contractile patterns. Solid-state transducers have not been used for colonic manometry in children. In adults, studies with solid-state transducers reported the same motility patterns that were found with water-perfused catheters.[19]

Radiotelemetry is an alternative method that utilizes a swallowed capsule which emits radio signals in response to pressure changes. The signal is detected by a receiver worn around the waist, and is converted into a voltage proportional to the intraluminal pressure as the capsule moves caudad.[59,60] The problems with this technique are that 1) pressure is recorded at only one site, 2) there is no control over capsule position, and 3) its inevitable

caudad progress cannot be arrested.[33]

Placement of the Recording Device

Endoscopy aides in the placement of the tip of the catheter into the transverse colon. Since the splenic flexure is an anatomic region easily reached and identified by an experienced endoscopist, this region is accessed so that a guidewire can be advanced into the transverse colon. A Teflon®-coated

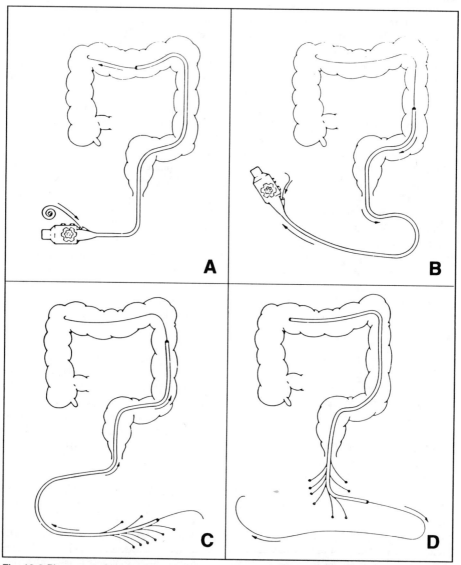

Fig. 13.3 Placement of the motility catheter. **A,**The colonoscope is advanced beyond the splenic flexure and a guidewire is passed through the endoscope. **B,**The endoscope is withdrawn. **C,**The motility catheter is placed over the guidewire. **D,** The guidewire is then removed.

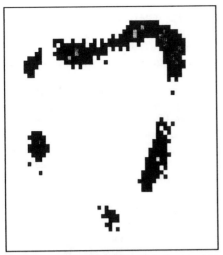

Fig. 13.4 Nuclear medicine can be used to delineate the placement of a colonic manometry catheter. The radioactive marker is sequentially infused at the level of each recording site. The tip of the catheter is at the level of the ascending colon. (Courtesy of Narasimha Reddy, PhD)

guidewire designed for biliary endoscopy can guide the manometry catheter. The guidewire has a diameter of 0.052 cm and a very soft tip, which minimizes the risk of trauma to the colon. Thinner guidewires coil easily, usually at the rectosigmoid or the splenic flexure. After withdrawing the endoscope, the manometry catheter is advanced over the guidewire (Fig. 13.3). During colonoscope withdrawal, air is aspirated as completely as possible. Finally, the guidewire is removed and the catheter is securely taped to the child's buttocks. Properly taping the catheter maintains its position while transferring the patient from place to place if the child is combative or uncooperative. One side of the buttocks should be cleaned and dried before applying a 7 x 10 cm piece of DuoDerm® (ConvaTec, Squibb) to the skin. The motility catheter is then placed across the DuoDerm and secured with a 10 x 13 cm piece of transparent dressing (Bioclusive®, Johnson & Johnson).

Custom-made manometry catheters with a 1-mm central lumen allow the catheter to slide easily over the guidewire. Using this system, most catheter placements take 15 to 30 minutes and can be performed with minimal sedation. A different endoscopic tech-

nique is sometimes used in adult subjects. A silk thread in the catheter is held by a biopsy forceps inside the operational channel of the endoscope. Once the catheter reaches the planned location, the biopsy forceps is opened and the endoscope is withdrawn, leaving the catheter in situ.

After the catheter has been placed, its position must be confirmed. It is impossible to predict the position of the recording sites from the manometric pattern. Unlike antroduodenal manometry, in which antral contractions clearly differ from duodenal contractions, the amplitude, shape, and frequency of the contractions are similar throughout the entire colon. Either radionuclide imaging or brief fluoroscopy can be used to assess the position of the catheter and the recording sites. If the motility suite is equipped with a gamma camera, it is easy to infuse a radionuclide marker mixed with a small amount of water, either through the central lumen or through each recording site (Fig. 13.4). The marker may be recovered by gentle aspira-

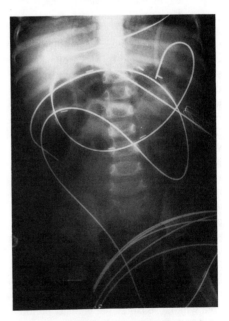

Fig. 13.5 Radiology can delineate the placement of antroduodenal and colonic manometry catheters. The tip of the antroduodenal manometry catheter is at the ligament of Treitz. The tip of the colonic manometry catheter is at the level of the hepatic flexure.

tion or can be used to perform a simultaneous colonic manometry and colonic transit study.[52,53] Fluoroscopy or an x-ray of the abdomen can confirm the catheter position (Fig 13.5). Leaving the guidewire in place before taking the x-ray facilitates the visualization of the catheter. The guidewire can then be removed under fluoroscopic vision to verify that the catheter remains in position. The same steps can be performed at the end of the test to assess the possibility of catheter migration.

The endoscopic placement of the catheter requires a relatively clean colon. In adults, a flexible sigmoidoscopy without bowel preparation can be used to place a motility catheter in the descending colon.[33] Such an approach would probably increase the duration, sedation requirements, and risks of the procedure if used in children. The colon is prepared with a liquid diet for 48 hours prior to the procedure and a standard, balanced oral electrolyte solution on the day before the study. Enemas should be avoided because they increase contractile activity.[56]

Colon preparation has been criticized as altering the normal state, which may affect the accuracy of the recorded motility. Those claims are balanced by the argument that studying an unprepared colon may introduce more variables, since different patients would have variable stool volumes of unknown composition in their colons. Bowel preparation removes one cause of interindividual variation, clarifying the differences in colonic motility that are responsible for the variable character of stools.[33] Differences in motility that explain the symptoms of patients with diarrhea or constipation can be consistently recorded after bowel preparation, indirectly supporting the validity of the studies performed after colon cleansing.[2,20,51]

Another variable to consider is the effect of sedation on motility. It is sometimes possible to endoscope older, cooperative children without sedation, but younger children require sedation during placement of the manometry catheter. Narcotics should be avoided because they decrease motor activity throughout the entire gastrointestinal tract.[61] Short-acting benzodiazepines are preferred. The child should be completely awake and fully recovered from the procedure before the study is begun. Diazepam increases gastric contractions and accelerates gastric emptying[62] but it is unclear what effect, if any, benzodiazepines have on colonic motility. Anger and discomfort associated with the procedure may alter colonic motility.[63] When the catheter placement has been particularly laborious and the child has required deeper sedation and is asleep when the study is scheduled, the manometry catheter should be left in place and the motility study performed on the following day.

Peroral placement of both water-perfused and solid-state manometry catheters in an unprepared colon has been achieved in adults.[18] A radiopaque polyvinylchloride (PVC) catheter with a balloon at the end is introduced transnasally. When the tip of the tube has passed the pylorus, the balloon is inflated. The catheter is then allowed to advance to the colon. Once the balloon has been delivered through the anus, the manometry catheter is tied to the proximal end of the PVC tube protruding from the nose. Gentle traction of the distal end of the PVC tube protruding from the anus moves the tip of the manometry catheter throughout the length of the gastrointestinal tract to the anus. The advantages of this system are that the colon can be studied under more physiologic conditions, the bowel is unprepared, and defecation does not terminate the test. In a child with severe constipation, this total body intubation will require several days to position the catheter. The technique will undoubtedly also fail in children with intestinal pseudo-obstruction, who have very delayed gastric emptying and very slow intestinal transit.

Performing the Study

The choice of performing colonic manometry in an inpatient or outpatient setting must be based on the child's age, clinical condition, and ease of achieving satisfactory colon cleansing. Children who receive nasogastric infusion of the colon lavage solution and central venous catheter antibiotic prophylaxis should be hospitalized on the day prior to the procedure. Older children who are able to drink the colon lavage solution can be studied as outpatients.

After catheter placement, the colonic manometry can be initiated as soon as the child recovers from sedation. Entering a room full of medical equipment can be frightening for the child. Being immobilized on a bed among strangers and in intimidating surroundings increases the child's anxiety. Trained pediatric nurses in a child-friendly setting are an important factor to ensure success of the study. Anxiety related to the testing can be diminished by an assistant who has previously met the child and parents, explained the procedure, showed them to the motility suite before the study, and greeted them in the endoscopy suite. The same person should be present as the child recovers from sedation and during the motility study. We encourage the parents to be present during the motility study.

Children adapt well to having a tube taped to their buttocks and often become unaware that they are undergoing a test. Although colonic manometry is a painless procedure, it may be boring for the child. The child may talk, laugh, and eat during the study, but movements should be kept to a minimum. Movements and crying create artefacts in the recording. We ask the parents to bring the child's favorite "quiet time" toys to the motility suite for play during the study. A VCR with age- and gender-related videotapes and videogames keep children (and parents) engaged.

A colonic manometry study usually lasts about 4 hours. The children are allowed to leave the hospital after the test is completed and the results are discussed with the parents. The study duration varies depending on the motility pattern the child exhibits. Fasting, unstimulated motility is studied for 1 hour. The patient is then fed, and motility is recorded for another hour. Few investigators have found fasting recordings useful in distinguishing between different groups of patients. Recording fasting motility, however, helps determine if motility is increased after feeding. When the child falls asleep during the study, it is useful to observe if motility is increased upon awakening. Characteristics of the ideal meal have already been discussed (see pages 3-4). The child can eat his or her favorite meal, providing it is complete and balanced. Eating constitutes the first of several provocation tests that can be performed during the study.

Provocation tests are useful because there is a great interindividual variability in basal recording of colonic motility. By using provocation tests which elicit clear differences between patient groups, the duration of the study can be shortened and diagnostic confidence is improved.

A bisacodyl stimulation test, for instance, is routinely performed. Bisacodyl appears to stimulate submucosal nerves, and its effect is blocked by local anesthetic agents.[21] Infusion though the manometry catheter into the transverse colon of 0.2 mg/kg bisacodyl diluted in 5 ml of 0.9% NaCl induces HAPCs in all children with normal colonic motility.[30] The HAPCs induced by bisacodyl occur within 5 minutes after infusion and are identical to the spontaneous HAPCs exhibited by the same subject. Often, cramping and the urge to defecate accompany the presence of the HAPCs. Absence of response to bisacodyl has been correlated with abnormalities of the myenteric plexus in adults with severe constipation and slow colonic transit.[64,65] Cholinergic agents, such as edrophonium, can be used to increase the motility index without inducing HAPCs.[28,29] Other pharmacologic agents have been rarely used to stimulate colonic motility. Prokinetics such as metoclopramide, domperidone, and erythromycin have little or no effect on colonic motility. Cisapride has been reported to accelerate colonic transit,[66] but the lack of an available parenteral preparation hinders its uses as a provocative drug.

Balloon distention has been used to stimulate colonic motility in adults. Balloon stretching of the transverse colon induces HAPCs more than the stretching of the sigmoid colon,[58] and distention of the sigmoid colon induces more propagating contractions in adults with diarrhea than in subjects with constipation.[57] Unfortunately, the use of balloon distention requires the introduction of another catheter in the colon, and the response to balloon distention is less reproducible than the response to bisacodyl.

Different softwares are available for data acquisition and analysis, but most programs were designed for esophageal and anorectal motility. Often a careful visual inspection of the recording is all that is needed for diagnosis. Software can be used to calculate the motility index and is especially useful for research trials when the effect of drugs on colonic motility is being evaluated. Software analysis of manometry in pediatric

patients poses a special problem, because children tend to move frequently during the study, causing discontinuous changes in the baseline. Unless the record is meticulously edited, the motility index provided by the personal computer may be inaccurate.

Colonic transit studies are often performed simultaneously with colonic manometries.[52,53,67] The most commonly used radioisotopes are ^{99m}Tc and [111]In. The former is inexpensive, readily available, and has a half-life of approximately 6 hours. Indium is expensive and has a half-life of 3 days, and

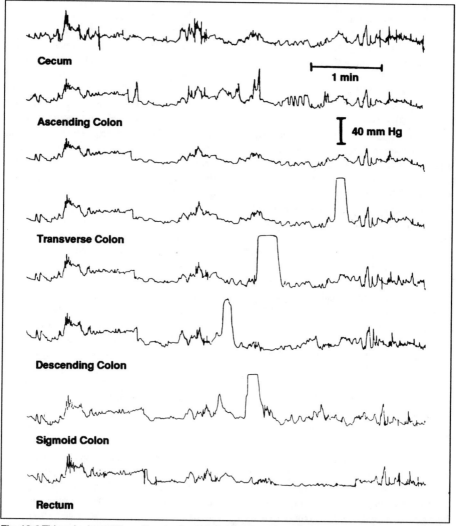

Fig. 13.6 This colonic motility pattern is characterized by HAPCs starting in the descending colon and migrating both proximally and distally. (Reprinted with permission from Di Lorenzo, et al,1993 [71])

so is appropriate for studies of longer duration. The estimated whole-body radiation when using 9 MBq of ^{99m}Tc is 0.1 mSv, less than the dose received from a plain abdominal x-ray.[68] It has been noted that in the postprandial period adults have a backward flow of a radioactive marker injected at the splenic flexure in the absence of retrograde contractions.[52] The movement of the marker is thought to be due to the difference in intraluminal pressures between the descending and transverse colon. In children, markers rarely move during fasting, but the marker quickly migrates to the rectum after feeding. Often the radioactive marker is found in the diaper, following an HAPC, immediately after feeding.[67] A simultaneous transit study, which causes children additional discomfort because they must lie motionless for hours under a gamma camera, provides little clinically relevant information over that gained from colonic manometry.

INTERPRETATION

When examining a colonic motility tracing, the features of normal colonic motility and the absence of abnormal motility patterns should be distinguished. The presence of HAPCs and a gastrocolonic response with normal amplitude contractions, in the absence of abnormal features, is diagnostic of normal colonic motility. In most children with severe constipation and a neuropathy involving the colon, HAPCs are absent and there is no gastrocolonic response.[8,49] No precise quantization defines increased motility after a meal. A twofold increase in the motility index is found in all children with functional fecal retention, but not in most children[9] and adults[69] with chronic intestinal pseudo-obstruction involving the colon. A postprandial gastrocolonic response is also absent in patients with diabetes mellitus and severe constipation.[70] The lack of a gastrocolonic response and HAPCs may suggest disease and also may contribute to the pathogenesis of constipation.[51] Reduced colonic propulsive activity may be responsible for a slower shifting of colonic contents and be directly responsible for constipation. The complete absence of colonic contractions is associated with a visceral myopathy.[9]

Due to the variety in shape, duration, and frequency of normal colonic contractions, abnormal motility patterns are difficult to identify. The presence of retrograde HAPCs is considered abnormal, although they can occur rarely in healthy adults.[19] Retrograde HAPCs in children without symptoms have not been observed. One child with a recur-

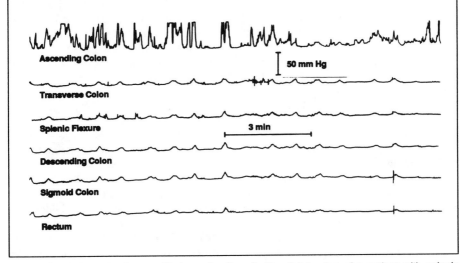

Fig. 13.7 Simultaneous low-amplitude contractions in the distal colon of a patient with colonic neuropathy. (Reprinted with permission from Di Lorenzo, et al, 1992 [8])

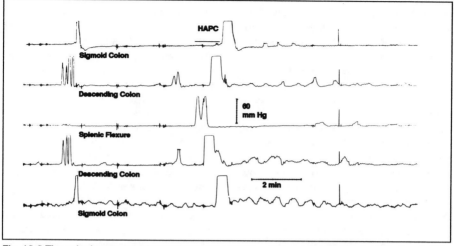

Fig. 13.8 The colonic manometric tracing shows HAPCs, which seem to originate at the level of the splenic flexure and migrate both proximally and distally. An x-ray of the abdomen showed the catheter coiled in the descending colon.

rent fecal bezoar had retrograde HAPCs, a probable cause for his condition (Fig. 13.6).[71] A monotonous pattern characterized by simultaneous low-amplitude contractions was identified in a nondilated colon in some children with colonic neuropathy (Fig. 13.7)

There are several sources of error in interpreting colonic manometry. A catheter which is partially coiled will record contractions that seem to have both oral and aboral migration (Fig.13.8). A catheter completely coiled in a dilated rectum will show only simultaneous low-amplitude contractions.

In children with a dilated colon it is still possible to record contractions but their amplitude is lower than normal. It is important to aspirate all the air used during colonoscopy as the endoscope is withdrawn to avoid distention, which interferes with the fidelity of the recording.

Since little motor activity occurs during fasting and sleeping, it is essential to perform the study while the child is fully awake. It is not uncommon for children to fall asleep immediately after being fed. When this happens, the gastrocolonic response does not occur and the test is not interpretable. It is sometimes difficult to evaluate the gastrocolonic response in patients with intestinal pseudo-obstruction. The amount of food the child is able to eat can be insufficient to

trigger the response and the very delayed gastric emptying can produce a delayed gastrocolonic response.

The presence or absence of diversion colitis should be determined before performing a study in a diverted colon. Colitis develops when a colonic segment is excluded from the fecal stream.[72] Colonic inflammation is associated with abnormal motility[73] and may prevent an interpretation of the manometry; if colonic manometry is abnormal, it may reflect a primary motility abnormality or the effect of inflammation. In the presence of diversion colitis, therefore, an abnormal colonic manometry may not be sufficient cause to reject reanastomosis of the diverted segment.

CONCLUSIONS

Several years ago, N. W. Read asked, "Does the study of colonic pressure help to make clinical decisions?"[54] His answer at the time was an emphatic "No," but the knowledge of normal and abnormal colonic motor activity in adults and children has since expanded. Improved recording techniques, reliable provocation tests, and correlations between clinical presentations and pathology have added to our knowledge of colonic motility in health and disease. Differences between the colonic motility of children and adults are recognized, and the interpretation of colonic manometry is probably easier in children. Thus, at least in children, the answer to the question is now "Yes."

Colonic manometry in children should be performed by investigators who have a special interest in motility and are willing to invest personnel, time, and energy to ensure accuracy and reliability. In the future, prolonged ambulatory and computerized motility studies in children should help correlate symptoms with specific motility patterns. Future studies should also identify colonic motility patterns that predict prognosis and response to drugs.

REFERENCES

1. Christiansen J. Motility of the colon. In: Johnson LR, ed. *Physiology of the Gastrointestinal Tract.* New York, NY: Raven Press; 1987:665-93.

2. Bassotti G, Crowell MD, Whitehead WE. Contractile activity of the human colon: lessons from 24 hours study. *Gut* 1993;34:129-33.

3. Huizinga JD, Daniel EE. Control of human colonic function. *Dig Dis Sci* 1986;31:865-77.

4. Shuurkes JAJ, Tukker JJ. The interdigestive colonic motor complex of the dog. *Arch Int Pharmacodyn Ther* 1980;247:329-34.

5. Davidson M, Bauer CH. Studies of colonic motility in children. *Pediatrics* 1958;21:746-51.

6. Hinton J, Lennard-Jones J, Young A. A new method of studying gut transit times using radioopaque markers. *Gut* 1969;10:842-7.

7. Ritchie JA. Mass peristalsis in the human colon after contact with oxyphenisatin. *Gut* 1972;13:211-9.

8. Di Lorenzo C, Flores AF, Reddy SN, Hyman PE. Colonic manometry differentiates causes of intractable constipation in children. *J Pediatr* 1992;120:690-5.

9. Di Lorenzo C, Flores AF, Reddy SN, Snape WJ Jr, Bazzocchi G, Hyman PE. Colonic manometry in children with chronic intestinal pseudo-obstruction. *Gut* 1993;34:803-7.

10. Proano M, Camilleri M, Phillips SF, Brown ML, Thomforde GM. Transit of solids through the human colon: regional quantification in the unprepared colon. *Am J Physiol* 1990;258:G856-62.

11. Krevsky B, Malmud LS, D'Ercole F, Maurer AN, Siegel AJ, Fisher RS. Colonic transit scintigraphy: a physiologic approach to the quantitative measurement of colonic transit in humans. *Gastroenterology* 1986;91:1102-12.

12. Di Lorenzo C, Watanabe F, Flores AF, Hyman PE. Inhibition of high-amplitude propagated contractions (HAPCs) characterized maturation of colonic motility. *Gastroenterology* 1993;104:A617.

13. Kellow JE, Borody TJ, Phillips SF, Tucker RL, Haddad AC. Human interdigestive motility: variation in patterns from the esophagus to colon. *Gastroenterology* 1986;91:386-95.

14. Connell AM. The motility of the pelvic colon. *Gut* 1961;2:175-86.

15. Phillips SF. Physiology of colonic motility. In: McCallum RW, Champion MC, eds. *Gastrointestinal Motility Disorders—Diagnosis and Treatment.* Baltimore, MD: Williams and Wilkins; 1990:37-47.

16. Sarna SK. Physiology and pathophysiology of colonic motor activity (Part one). *Dig Dis Sci* 1991;36:827-62.

17. Narducci F, Bassotti G, Gaburri M, Morellia A. Twenty-four hour manometric recording of colonic motor activity in humans. *Gut* 1987;28:17-25.

18. Soffer EE, Scalabrini P, Wingate DL. Prolonged ambulant monitoring of human colonic motility. *Am J Physiol* 1989;257:G601-6.

19. Crowell MD, Bassotti G, Cheskin LJ, Shuster MM, Whitehead WE. Method for prolonged ambulatory monitoring of high-amplitude propagated contractions from colon. *Am J Physiol* 1991;261:G263-8.

20. Torsoli A, Ramorino ML, Ammaturo MV, Capurso L, Paoluzzi P, Anzini F. Mass movement and intracolonic pressure. *Am J Dig Dis* 1971;16:693-6.

21. Hardcastle JD, Mann CV. Study of large-bowel peristalsis. *Gut* 1968;9:512-20.

22. Weaver LT. Bowel habit from birth to old age.

J Ped Gastroenterol Nutr 1988;7:637-40.

23. Bassotti G, Gaburri M. Manometric investigation of high-amplitude propagated contractile activity of the human colon. *Am J Physiol* 1988;255:G660-4.

24. Narducci F, Bassotti G, Gaburri M, Solinas A, Fiorucci S, Morelli A. Distension simulated motor activity of the human transverse, descending, and sigmoid colon. *Gastroenterology* 1985;88:1515.

25. Spiller RC, Brown ML, Phillips SF. Decreased fluid tolerance, accelerated transit and abnormal motility of the human colon induced by oleic acid. *Gastroenterology* 1986;91:100-7.

26. Preston DM, Lennard Jones JE. Pelvic motility and response to intraluminal bisacodyl in slow-transit constipation. *Dig Dis Sci* 1985;30:289-94.

27. Delvaux M, Camman F, Staumont G, et al. Glycerol induces a recto-colonic reflex associating a stimulation of colonic myoelectrical activity and a decrease in colonic tone in man. *J Gastrointest Motil* 1993;5:186.

28. Di Lorenzo C, Flores AF, Buie T, Hyman PE. Bisacodyl but not edrophonium stimulates high-amplitude propagated colon contractions (HAPCs) in children. *Gastroenterology* 1993;104:A498.

29. Bassotti G, Imbimbo BP, Betti C, et al. Edrophonium chloride for testing colonic contractile activity in man. *Acta Physiol Scand* 1991;141:289-93.

30. Orkin BA, Hanson RB, Kelly KA. The rectal motor complex. *J Gastrointest Motil* 1989;1:5-8.

31. Kumar D, Williams NS, Waldron D, Wingate DL. Prolonged manometric recording of anorectal motor activity in ambulant human subjects: evidence of periodic activity. *Gut* 1989;30:1007-11.

32. Ritchie JA, Ardran GM, Truelove SC. Motor activity of the sigmoid colon in humans: a combined study by intraluminal pressure recording and cineradiography. *Gastroenterology* 1962;43:642-68.

33. Spiller RC. Colonic manometry. In: Read NW, ed. *Gastrointestinal Motility: Which Test?* Sheffield, England: Wrightson Biomedical Publishing Ltd; 1989:191-203.

34. Bassotti G, Bucaneve G, Betti C, Morelli A. Sudden awakening from sleep: effect on proximal and distal colonic contractile activity in man. *Eur J*

Gastroenterol Hepatol 1990;2:475-8.

35. Wright SH, Snape WJ Jr, Battle W, Cohen S, London RL. Effect of dietary components on gastrocolonic response. *Am J Physiol* 1980;238: G228-32.

36. Kerlin P, Zinsmeister A, Phillips SF. Motor responses to food of the ileum, proximal colon, and distal colon of healthy humans. *Gastroenterology* 1986;91:1102-12.

37. Holdstock DJ, Misiewicz JJ. Factors controlling colonic motility and colonic pressures and transit after meals in patients with total gastrectomy, pernicious anemia, or duodenal ulcer. *Gut* 1970;11:100-10.

38. Phillips SF. Physiology of colon motility. In: *Physiology, Diagnosis, and Therapy in GI Motility Disorders.* Toronto: MES Medical Education Services 1988;37-47. MEDICINE Publishing Foundation Symposium Series, 22.

39. Sun EA, Snape WJ Jr, Cohen S, Renny A. The role of opiate receptors and cholinergic neurons in the gastrocolonic response. *Gastroenterology* 1982;83:689-93.

40. Levinson S, Bhasker MK, Gibson TR, Morin R, Snape WJ Jr. Comparison of intraluminal and intravenous mediators of colonic response to food. *Dig Dis Sci* 1985;30:33-9.

41. Wiley J, Tatum D, Keinath R, Owyang C. Participation of gastric mechanoreceptors and intestinal chemoreceptors in the gastrocolonic reponse. *Gastroenterology* 1988;94:1144-9.

42. Meshkinpour H, Dinoso VP Jr, Lorber SH. Effect of intraduodenal administration of essential amino acids and sodium oleate on motor activity of the sigmoid colon. *Gastroenterology* 1974;66:373-7.

43. Wright SH, Snape WS, Battle W, Cohen J, London RL. Effect of dietary components on gastrocolonic response. *Am J Physiol* 1980;238:G228-32.

44. Bingham SA, Cummings JH. Effect of exercise and physical fitness on large intestine function. *Gastroenterology* 1989;97:1389-99.

45. Sarna SK. Physiology and pathophysiology of colonic motor activity (Part two). *Dig Dis Sci* 1991;35:998-1018.

46. Narducci F, Snape WJ Jr, Battle WM, London RL, Cohen S. Increased colonic motility during exposure to a stressful situation. *Dig Dis Sci* 1985;30:40-4.

47. Brown SR, Cann PA, Read NW. Effect of coffee on distal colon function. *Gut* 1990;31:450-3.

48. Di Lorenzo C, Flores AF, Reddy SN, Snape WJ Jr, Hyman PE. Colon motility in symptomatic children after surgery for Hirschsprung's disease: abnormalities in "healthy" colon. *Gastroenterology* 1991;100:A437.

49. Hyman PE, Di Lorenzo C, Krishnamurthy S, Dean P, Schuffler MD. Pathology validates colonic manometry in neuropathic constipation. *Ped Res* 1993;33:102A.

50. Bassotti G, Betti C, Pelli MA, Morelli A. Extensive investigation of colonic motility with pharmacological testing is useful for selecting surgical options in patients with inertia colica. *Am J Gastroenterol* 1992;87:143-7.

51. Bassotti G, Gaburri M, Imbibo BP, et al. Colonic mass movements in idiopathic chronic constipation. *Gut* 1988;29:1173-9.

52. Moreno-Osset E, Bazzocchi G, Lo S, et al. Association between postprandial changes in colonic intraluminal pressure and transit. *Gastroenterology* 1989;96:1265-73.

53. Bazzocchi G, Ellis J, Villanueva-Meyer J, et al. Postprandial colonic transit and motor activity in chronic constipation. *Gastroenterology* 1990;98:686-93.

54. Read NW. Tests of colonic motility: summary and conclusions. In: Read NW, ed. *Gastrointestinal Motility: Which Test?* Sheffield, England: Wrightson Biomedical Publishing Ltd; 1989;213-23.

55. Cook IJ, Reddy SN, Collins SM, Daniel EE. The influence of recording techniques on measurement of canine colon motility. *Dig Dis Sci* 1988;33:999-1006.

56. Dinoso VP, Murthy SNS, Goldstein J, Rosner B. Basal motor activity of the distal colon: a reappraisal. *Gastroenterology* 1983;85:637-42.

57. Whitehead WE, Engel BT, Shuster MM. Irritable bowel syndrome: physiological differences between diarrhea-predominant and constipation-predominant patients. *Dig Dis Sci* 1980;25:404-13.

58. Lo SK, Yanni GS, Di Lorenzo C, Reddy SN, Snape WJ Jr. Motility and symptomatic responses to balloon distension of the colon. *Am J Gastroenterol* 1991;86:1362.

59. Browning C, Valori R, Wingate DL, MacLachlan D. A new pressure-sensitive ingestible radio-telemetric capsule. *Lancet* 1981;2:504-5.

60. Reynolds JR, Clark AG, Evans DF, Hardcastle JD. Investigation of colonic motility patterns in the irritable bowel syndrome using radiotelemetry. *Gut* 1985;26:A1131.

61. Kaufman PN, Krevsky B, Malmud LS, et al. Role of opiate receptors in the regulation of colonic transit. *Gastroenterology* 1988;94:1351-6.

62. Schurizek BA, Kraglund K, Andreasen F, Jensen LV, Juhl B. Gastrointestinal motility and gastric pH and emptying following ingestion of diazepam. *Br J Anaesth* 1988;61:712-9.

63. Welgen P, Meshkinpour H, Beeler M. Effect of anger on colon motor and myoelectric activity in irritable bowel syndrome. *Gastroenterology* 1988;94:1150-6.

64. Preston DM, Butler MG, Smith B, Lennard-Jones JE. Neuropathology of slow transit constipation. *Gut* 1983;24:A997.

65. Kamm MA, Lennard Jones JE, Thompson DG, Sobnack R, Granowska M. Dynamic scanning defines a colonic defect in severe idiopathic constipation. *Gut* 1988;29:1085-92.

66. Krevsky B, Maurer AH, Malmud LS, Fisher RS. Cisapride accelerates colonic transit in constipated patients with colonic inertia. *Am J Gastroenterol* 1989;894:882-7.

67. Di Lorenzo C, Reddy SN, Villanueva-Meyer J, et al. Simultaneous colonic manometry and transit in children. *Gastroenterology* 1990;98:345.

68. Kamm MA. Colonic scintigraphy. In: Read NW, ed. *Gastrointestinal Motility: Which Test?* Sheffield, England: Wrightson Biomedical Publishing Ltd; 1989:181-9.

69. Snape WJ, Sullivan MA, Cohen S. Abnormal gastrocolic response in patients with intestinal pseudo-obstruction. *Arch Intern Med* 1980;140:386-7

70. Battle WM, Snape WJ Jr, Alavi A, Cohen S, Braunstein S. Colonic dysfunction in diabetes mellitus. *Gastroenterology* 1980;79:1217-21.

71. Di Lorenzo C, Ordein JJ, Hyman PE. Cecal fecal bezoar. *J Pediatr Gastroenterol Nutr* 1993;16:212-5.

72. Ordein JJ, Di Lorenzo C, Flores A, Hyman PE. Diversion colitis in children with severe gastrointestinal motility disorders. *Am J Gastroenterol* 1992;87:88-90.

73. Reddy SN, Bazzocchi G, Chan SS, et al. Colonic motility and transit in health and ulcerative colitis. *Gastroenterology* 1991;101:1289-97.

14

Anorectal Manometry And Biofeedback Training

VERA LOENING-BAUCKE

The major structures responsible for continence and defecation are the external anal sphincter, the puborectalis muscle, the internal anal sphincter, and the rectum. The function of these structures can be evaluated with anorectal manometry. This chapter will cover techniques for anorectal manometry, their application in the investigation of disorders of anorectal continence in children, and the methods and outcome of biofeedback treatment for constipation and fecal incontinence in children. The appendix at the end of this chapter lists suppliers and manufacturers of the equipment and other products discussed throughout the text.

ANORECTAL MANOMETRY
Equipment

Many techniques are available for anorectal manometry. There is no uniformity of technique, and results in part reflect the use of different recording devices and study procedures. All instruments and techniques for anorectal manometry, when properly used, are able to provide reproducible and useful measurements.

Anorectal devices. Many investigators[1-7] use a water-perfusion technique for anorectal manometric testing. Either several open-ended tubes or assemblies containing tubes with side holes can be bought or made. Perfused catheters are inexpensive and simple to use. The thin, flexible, multilumen catheters induce fewer artefacts than balloon devices. Sidehole catheters allow multiple simultaneous recordings from different sites in the longitudinal and radial axes. This is

advantageous when studying the anal canal. Numerous technical constraints, however, affect accuracy. The compliance of the recording device is critical, the deformity of the catheters must be minimal, and a hydraulic capillary infusion system for perfusion and pressure transducers for pressure measurement are necessary. The flow rate of the infusion system should be between 0.1 and 0.5 ml per minute for each sidehole. The water that is instilled into the anal canal during the investigation may induce abnormal reflexes and voluntary contraction of anal muscles in children who are afraid to soil the examination table.

A double-balloon device[8] is used by some investigators in the USA.[9-16] A latex balloon is tied at the ends and in the middle of a hollow metal cylinder, creating a two-balloon system. Both balloons are inflated with 7 to 10 ml air after placement in the anal canal. The more proximal balloon is surrounded mostly by the internal anal sphincter and the distal balloon mostly by the external sphincter. One balloon is inserted through the hollow core of the cylinder for rectal distention, but it can also be used for recording rectal activity. This relatively large device is available in two smaller sizes, but is still too big for the investigation of small infants.

A smaller balloon system is used by other investigators, especially in Canada and France.[17-21] The balloons are filled with water instead of compressible air. The advantage of this device is that results can be duplicated in other laboratories. It can also measure a nonradial pressure representing the sum of all pressures from each direction.

No fluid is instilled into the anal canal with this method. It is necessary, however, to eliminate all air bubbles from the balloon to avoid dampening the recorded pressure. Large balloons may induce reflex relaxation of the anal muscles. The recording location is also restricted to two locations, one in the upper, and one in the lower anal canal.

Balloons for rectal distention are usually cut from unlubricated condoms. Anorectal manometry and biofeedback training can be performed with a probe containing three microtransducers.[22,23] The Dent sleeve device[24] can be used for the saline continence test. A self-made perfused catheter assembly is appropriate for premature infants, and Schuster's balloon system[8] can be used for biofeedback training in fecally incontinent patients.

Commercially available probes can be used for the anorectal manometric evaluation.[22,23] Standardization of the investigation is easy, and investigators using this technique can compare results. Microtransducers are convenient. No water leakage occurs, the set-up and calibration are easy, and the pressures are recorded directly from the area rather than transmitted through a water column. Stimulation artefacts are minimal with this probe due to its small diameter (5 mm). This flexible, silicone-rubber tube contains three intraluminal transducers, which are staggered at 120-degree intervals around the probe and are spaced 5 cm apart at the distal end. One disadvantage is the

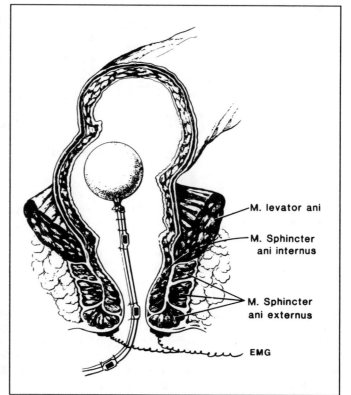

Fig. 14.1 Recording technique for anal and rectal pressure. One transducer of the motility probe is placed into the lower part of the anal canal and one is placed in the rectum. The rectal distention balloon is shown expanded. Two surface electrodes are placed over the external anal sphincter. Another is placed on the buttock to evaluate anal response to straining for defecation and voluntary squeeze. (EMG, electromyogram)

fixed location of the pressure transducers, which restricts recording locations to two or three. Fragility is often cited as a disadvantage, but with careful handling these motility probes can last for more than 10 years.

The probe can be marked in 1-cm increments to provide external reference for the intraluminal transducer position in the anal canal and rectum. A latex balloon (2.5 cm x 3 cm), cut from the finger of a latex glove, is attached to the end of a thin polyethylene tube and tied to the tip of the motility probe, 5 cm above the distal transducer (Fig. 14.1). Pressure from the latex balloon is transmitted via the polyethylene tube to a pressure transducer. The outputs for all four transducers are fed into a recorder and graphed on running paper.

In older children, the electromyogram (EMG) can be recorded from the external anal sphincter. Two surface electrodes are attached over the external anal sphincter as close as possible to the anal orifice. A third serves as a ground and is attached to the buttock (see Fig. 14.1).

Polygraphs. All 21 participants of an International Consensus Meeting in Lyon in 1989[7] used conventional polygraphs. Pressure recordings require DC amplifiers, which do not modify the shape of the signal. Alternate-current amplifiers are used for EMG recording.

Computerized polygraphs are also available, as is a combination of recorder and computerized motility system. They offer the advantage of precise calculations, easy computer storage of the recordings, as well as minimal maintenance and set-up time. Computerized polygraphs are best for those who use anorectal manometry exclusively for routine investigations. Disadvantages are that the software is restrictive, predetermined for a routine investigation, and can only be modified by the company.

Indications for Anorectal Physiologic Testing

The two common disorders of anorectal function, constipation and fecal incontinence, occupy extremes of a continuum. Pediatric patients with functional fecal retention, neuromuscular disorders, and even those operated on for anal atresia often present with both disorders. Anal resting pressure, anal squeeze pressure, rectosphincteric reflex, constant relaxation of anal pressure produced by inhibition of both anal sphincters with rectal distention, degree of rectal sensation abnormality and rectal contractility, defecation dynamics, as well as continence and incontinence can all be assessed. These measurements allow us to explain what went wrong to children and their parents. The anorectal physiologic tests help the physician to plan effective management by either medical intervention, biofeedback treatment, or surgery. Anorectal physiologic testing is useful in disorders of constipation due to

functional fecal retention with or without soiling, Hirschsprung's disease, and fecal incontinence due to myelomeningocele, anorectal anomalies, anorectal trauma, and neuromuscular diseases.

Preparation for Testing

Anorectal manometry and the other studies are only performed after complete clearance of the lower bowel. Bowel preparation is not performed for very sick newborns. Unfortunately, this may be the reason for false-negative and false-positive results in patients with symptoms that suggest Hirschsprung's disease.[3,25] Sedating a child should not be necessary. Restless newborns or infants usually relax while sucking on a pacifier or drinking from a bottle. Preschool-age children can be distracted by having their parents read a story to them. It is rarely necessary to wait until an infant falls asleep to perform manometry. Manometric studies are performed with the child lying on its left side, with the hips and knees flexed. The motility probe and balloon are well lubricated.

Measurements

Performance of a series of tests to provide a profile takes approximately 1 to 1½ hours, and analysis requires experience.

Anal resting pressure, squeeze pressure, and anal canal length. The external and internal anal sphincters envelop the anal canal in a sleevelike fashion, and are responsible for maintaining resting pressure and generating squeeze pressure. The internal anal sphincter contributes up to 85% of the anal resting pressure.[26] Anal resting pressure and maximal squeeze pressure are determined during stepwise retraction (0.5 cm/min) of one intraluminal pressure transducer of the motility probe from the rectum through the anal canal. Anal resting pressure is defined as the pressure in mm Hg at the troughs of the waves. It is highest 1 to 2 cm above the anal verge. The mean ± SD of highest anal resting pressure is given in Table 14.1. The maximal squeeze pressure in mm Hg is generated by contraction of the

TABLE 14.1 Anal Measurements in Children, Ages 5 to 16 Years*			
	Healthy Controls	Chronic Constipation	Functional Fecal Retention With Encopresis
	n = 20	n = 12	n = 97
Anal resting pressure (mm Hg)	67 ± 12	62 ± 12	54 ± 16**
Maximal squeeze pressure (mm Hg)	140 ± 52	Not done	127 ± 63
Anal pull-through pressure (mm Hg)	143 ± 36	143 ± 37	134 ± 33
Anal canal length (cm)	3.3 ± 0.8	3.6 ± 0.7	3.6 ± 0.7

*Mean ± SD
** p< 0.05 from healthy children (Wilcoxon nonpaired rank sum test)

external anal sphincter and puborectalis muscle and is measured as the highest pressure increase above anal resting pressure. The mean ± SD of maximal squeeze pressure is also given in Table 14.1. Sustained squeezes can be examined, but fatigue is rapid and exponential and, therefore, sustained squeeze pressure is currently of limited clinical usefulness. The station pull-through method can determine anal resting pressure, as can a continuous withdrawal technique. Normal values depend on the speed of withdrawal. Table 14.1 gives the pull-through pressures for a withdrawal speed of 1 cm per second.

The anal canal is the region with resting pressure at least 5 mm Hg higher than the pressure in the rectum. Its motor activity pattern is different than that in the rectum, and it has a reflex relaxation of anal pressure during rectal distention. Anal canal length is determined by recording the anal resting pressure, motor activity pattern, and reflex relaxation at each position during stepwise retraction of 0.5 cm per minute of the pressure transducer assembly from the rectum through the anal canal. The mean length of the anal canal in healthy children over 4 years old is 3 cm.

Effects of rectal distention. The response of the anal canal to rectal distention and rectal sensation can be evaluated with the base of the distending balloon 11 cm above the anal verge, one pressure transduc-

er in the rectum 6 cm above the anal verge, and another in the anal canal 1 cm above the anal verge (see Fig. 14.1). With sudden rectal distention, the external sphincter contracts and the internal anal sphincter relaxes. This relaxation of the internal sphincter results in reduced anal pressure (Fig. 14.2A). This phenomenon is referred to as the rectosphincteric reflex or anorectal inhibitory reflex. It is hypothesized that the transient relaxation of the internal sphincter allows rectal contents to contact the mucosa of the upper anal canal. Its contents can then be recognized as gas, liquid, or solid, and a decision can be made to allow the gas to escape, evacuate the rectal contents, or delay evacuation. Transient rectal distention produces a rectosphincteric reflex in healthy children and in patients with chronic constipation due to a variety of causes, including functional fecal retention, but the rectosphincteric reflex is absent in patients with Hirschsprung's disease (Fig. 14.2B).

The minimal amount of air required to elicit the threshold of the rectosphincteric reflex (>5 mm Hg relaxation of anal pressure) is determined by rapidly inflating the balloon two to three times with volumes between 5 and 60 ml of air in random order, starting each time at 0 ml. In infants, distention volumes up to 30 ml are used. In newborns, the balloon lies in the rectum, 5.5 cm to 6 cm above the anal verge. Only one of the three intraluminal transducers is placed in the anal canal, 0.5 cm to 1 cm above the anal

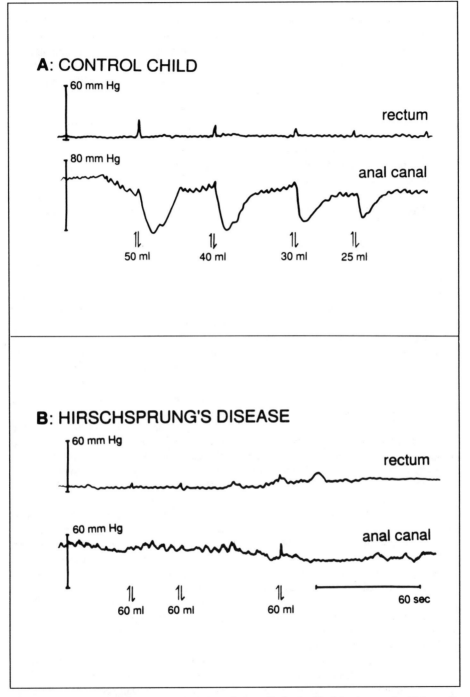

Fig. 14.2 The double arrows indicate distention of a rectal balloon with air for 1 second, which results in decreased anal pressure (the rectosphincteric reflex). **A,** this recording is from a healthy 10-year-old boy. **B,** Distention of a rectal balloon with air for 1 second produces no decrease in anal pressure. The absent rectosphincteric reflex in this 14-year-old boy with severe constipation and intermittent encopresis is due to Hirschsprung's disease.

TABLE 14.2 **Anal Responses and Rectal Sensation with Rectal Distention***

	Controls	Functional Fecal Retention with Encopresis
	n = 16	n = 97**
Rectal balloon volume (ml air):		
Threshold of rectosphincteric reflex	11 ± 5	19 ± 8
Volume of constant relaxation	104 ± 49	179 ± 88
Threshold of rectal sensation	14 ± 7	26 ± 14
Critical volume	101 ± 39	172 ± 91
Threshold of rectal contractility	54 ± 28	106 ± 88

* Mean ± SD
**p < 0.005 as compared to controls (Wilcoxon nonpaired ranked sum test)

verge. The distention volumes used in the newborn to elicit the rectosphincteric reflex range from 5 to 15 ml. Mean rectal distention volumes for the threshold of the rectosphincteric reflex in children over 5 years of age are given in Table 14.2.

The motility probe is too long for the premature newborn. A three-lumen perfused catheter assembly can be constructed with the first side hole 10 mm below the tip; each of the 3 side holes are spaced 2 mm apart. This water-perfused catheter assembly is placed into the anal canal so that 2 or 3 of its side holes lie in the anal canal. A small 1 cm by 1 cm balloon is inserted as far up into the rectum as possible—usually 4 to 5 cm. Volumes to elicit the rectosphincteric reflex are 2 to 10 ml of air.

The minimal amount of air required to produce a sustained complete relaxation of the internal and external anal sphincters (constant relaxation) is determined by adding 10 ml air stepwise up to 60 ml, then 30 ml each 10 to 15 seconds into the rectal balloon (Fig. 14.3A). When the critical volume has been reached, but constant relaxation has not occurred, the next higher volume is used as the volume of constant relaxation. The mean ± SD for constant relaxation is given in Table 14.2.

Rectal sensitivity is evaluated with the base of the distending balloon 11 cm above the anal verge and one pressure transducer in the rectum and the other in the anal canal, 6 cm and 1 cm above the anal verge, respectively (see Fig. 14.1). The threshold amount of air required to elicit a transient rectal sensation is determined by inflating the rectal balloon two to three times transiently with volumes between 5 and 60 ml in random order, starting each time at 0 ml. Results in control children are given in Table 14.2.

The minimal amount of air required to produce a sensation of a lasting urge to defecate (critical volume) is determined by stepwise adding 10 ml air up to 60 ml, then 30 ml every 10 to 15 seconds into the rectal balloon (see Fig. 14.3A).

Rectal contractility induced by rectal distention is recorded from the simultaneous rectal intraluminal pressure reading during the test, which determines the critical volume and the volume of constant relaxation (see Fig. 14.3A). Rectal contractility is expressed as the threshold volume that produces rectal contractility of greater than or equal to 10 mm Hg (see Table 14.2).

Evaluation of defecation dynamics.
Continence depends on the ability to defer defecation to a socially convenient time and place. Fecal material can be retained in the rectum by contraction of the external sphincter and puborectalis muscle. Fecal material can be expelled by the combination of in-

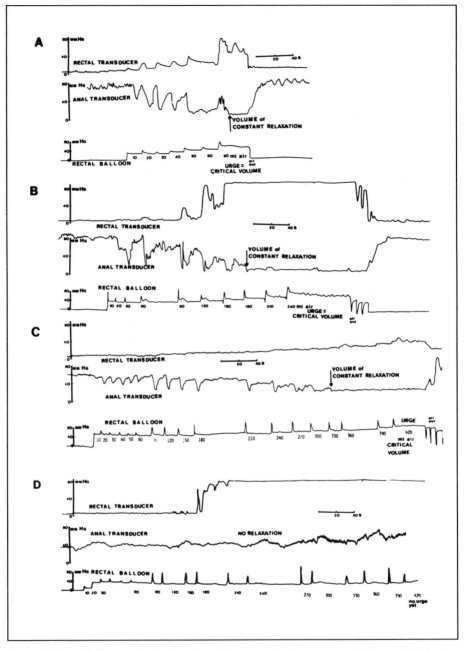

Fig. 14.3 The tracings show the changes in rectal, anal, and balloon pressure during rectal distention by stepwise adding initially 10 ml air up to 60 ml, then 30 ml every 10 to 15 seconds in 10-year-old children. **A,** Healthy control child. **B,** Functional fecal retention with encopresis and mild impairment of rectal sensation and rectal contractility. **C,** Functional fecal retention with encopresis, and severe impairment in rectal sensation and rectal contractility, indicating rectal atony. A sustained, complete relaxation of the internal and external anal sphincters occurs in healthy children and patients with functional fecal retention. **D,** This patient had previous surgery for Hirschsprung's disease but continued with stool retention and fecal incontinence. The internal anal sphincter does not relax in patients with Hirschsprung's disease, hindering defecation.

creased intra-abdominal pressure (produced by closure of the glottis, fixation of the diaphragm, and contractions of the abdominal, perineal, and hamstring muscles), relaxation of the internal and external sphincters, and rectal contractions. Defecation dynamics can be tested with two methods: 1) by evaluating the combined external and internal anal sphincter pressures, the external sphincter EMG, and the abdominal pressure exerted onto the rectum during defecation attempts; and 2) by evaluating the ability to defecate an object from the rectum.

External Anal Sphincter and Pelvic Floor During Straining Myoelectrical activity from the external anal sphincter is recorded at a speed of 10 mm per second with three surface electrodes. Two electrodes are placed over the external anal sphincter and a third on the buttock (see Fig. 14.1). The raw EMG data is recorded and the primary signal is integrated with an EMG averaging coupler. The area under the wave form of the action potentials—an index of total activity—is obtained by this integration. External sphincter EMG activity, the combined function of the external and internal anal sphincters measured with the transducer in the anal canal, and intra-abdominal pressures transmitted onto the transducer in the rectum are evaluated during straining for defecation (Fig. 14.4A) and voluntary squeeze. While lying in the left lateral position, the child is asked to strain down as if defecating and to squeeze in random order. During a normal defecation attempt, the integrated EMG activity from the external anal sphincter decreases. During an abnormal defecation attempt, it increases (Fig. 14.4B). Abnormal defecation dynamics have been termed paradoxical pelvic floor contraction during straining, rectoanal dyssynergia, rectosphincteric dyssynergia, abnormal defecation dynamics, abnormal defecation patterns, anismus, and spastic pelvic floor syndrome. All healthy control children are able to

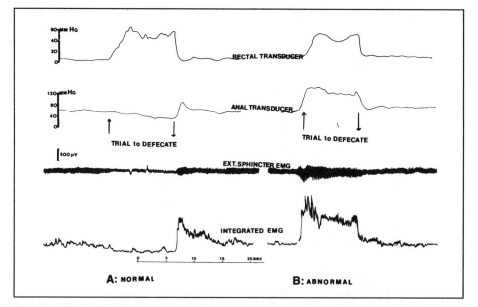

Fig. 14.4 These tracings depict the pressure changes in the rectum and anal canal, and the electromyographic changes from the external anal sphincter during a trial to defecate. The duration of the defecation trial is indicated by arrows. **A,** Normal defecation consists of increased rectal (intra-abdominal) pressure, decreased anal pressure, and decreased direct and integrated EMG activity. **B,** Abnormal defecation is characterized by increased rectal (intra-abdominal) pressure, anal pressure, as well as direct and integrated EMG activity. (Reproduced with permission from Loening-Baucke V, 1990[29])

relax the external sphincter during straining for defecation.

Ability to defecate. The ability to defecate can be determined by the use of materials such as spheres, barium paste, slurs, and saline. Water-filled balloons can simulate defecation of a stool from the rectum. Children 5 years of age or older are asked to defecate a rectal balloon filled with 100 ml water while sitting on a toilet chair, allowing five minutes for defecation. Balloon defecation is evaluated during the first minute and during five minutes. The 100 ml balloon is defecated by 100% of healthy children during the first minute. Intra-abdominal pressure exerted on the rectal balloon during attempts to defecate is transmitted via a polyethylene catheter to a pressure transducer and recorded. The child's defecation effort is evaluated by measuring the highest intra-abdominal pressure generated and the duration of the straining effort.

Saline Continence The saline continence test[5] is used to objectively measure continence in patients with expected weak sphincter pressure or poor voluntary squeeze (eg, those with spina bifida, post-repair of anal atresia, anal trauma, neuromuscular disease). A small, 8 Fr feeding tube or the Dent sleeve device[24] is inserted into the rectum and anal canal, with its open tip positioned 10 cm above the anal verge. Saline maintained at 37° C is infused into the rectum at a rate of 60 ml per minute up to 240 ml, while the child sits upright in a specially designed chair with a central, round aperture.[20] If no leakage occurs, the child is instructed to retain the saline for 5 minutes. The volume of leakage is determined by a funnel and collecting cylinder which sits on top of a weight transducer. A measurement is taken of the volume infused into the rectum when 10 ml or more saline first leaks. When this test was performed in 12 healthy controls, 7 to 13 years of age, eight children did not leak, while four leaked saline at 120, 125, 175, and 210 ml, respectively. Children with weak or no external anal sphincter

function leak as soon as saline infusion is started.[20]

Functional Fecal Retention With or Without Soiling

Functional fecal retention is a common problem, affecting up to 10% of children. Most often, fecal soiling occurs in long-standing fecal retention. Several anorectal physiologic abnormalities can be found during anorectal function testing in these children, including impaired rectal and sigmoid sensations to balloon distention,[2,17,22,23,27-32] decreased spontaneous rectal and sigmoid motility,[33] and decreased or no rectal contractility induced by rectal distention.[30] The external anal sphincter and pelvic floor muscles are abnormally contracted during straining for defecation instead of being relaxed in up to 53% of these patients.[12,13,27-31,34]

The highest anal resting pressure is decreased in a group of children with fecal retention and soiling, but normal in those with fecal retention only (see Table 14.1).[23,35] Maximal anal squeeze, anal pull-through pressures, and anal canal length were similar to control data. Anal resting pressure has been reported as increased in some of these children, particularly in those without soiling.[1,36,37]

Distention of the rectum reveals that the rectosphincteric reflex is present in all patients, but the threshold volume for the rectosphincteric reflex is significantly increased in children with fecal retention and soiling as compared with controls (see Table 14.2).

The air volumes required in the rectal balloon to inhibit both the external and internal anal sphincters (constant relaxation) are significantly larger in these patients than in control children. In many children with functional fecal retention and stool incontinence, complete inhibition of the internal and external anal sphincters occurs before feces is perceived in the rectum (Fig. 14.3 B,C).[22] Therefore, no contraction of the external anal sphincter is initiated.[4,37] The threshold for rectal sensation is significantly increased in patients with or without encopresis.[1,2,4,22,27,28,37] The critical volume, the volume to produce rectal contractility, and rectal compliance were significantly increased in children with fecal retention and soiling as compared with control children (see Table 14.2).[1,2,4,22,27] These abnormalities are shown in the anal and rectal tracings of Figure 14.3B,C. Apparently, the cerebral cortex does not perceive sensations when a normal-sized fecal bolus enters the rectum in many patients. In some with impaired rectal sensation, vigorous contractions of the rectal smooth musculature are absent. In others, they were observed only after the rectal balloon was inflated to volumes which produced pain or a strong urge to defecate. Vigorous contractions are necessary to empty the rectum. These contractions may play a part in bringing receptors into action so that the degree of distention can be sensed, possibly by comparing afferent activity with the efferent command signal.

Studies of defecation dynamics show that 31% to 53% of the patients contracted the pelvic floor and external anal sphincter abnormally, making defecation or balloon expulsion more difficult or impossible.[13,19,27-32,34,38-40] Patients generate similar intra-abdominal pressures and strain longer than healthy control children, but are significantly less likely to defecate the 100 ml water-filled balloon from the rectum (patients: 59% in 5 min; controls: 100% in 1 min).[31] These abnormal defecation dynamics persisted after 12 months of laxative treatment. Patients with abnormal defecation dynamics were significantly less likely to recover after 1 year of conventional laxative treatment (26%) than patients with normal defecation dynamics (61%; p<0.01).[27]

Hirschsprung's Disease

When a child presents with severe constipation, it is important to exclude Hirschsprung's disease. Several extremely rare conditions resemble Hirschsprung's disease but have ganglion cells in the rectal biopsy. These poorly understood conditions include the small left colon syndrome in infants,[41] pseudo-Hirschsprung's disease in older children,[42] and neuronal intestinal dysplasia.[43] In the vast majority of cases of childhood constipation, no rec-

ognizable organic cause can be determined.

Patients may present with constipation or signs of intestinal obstruction in the immediate newborn period or with enterocolitis. Older patients often complain of intractable constipation. Children noted to have constipation starting in the first year of life, constipated children who fail to respond adequately to conventional laxative treatment, and children with a huge abdominal fecal mass should undergo anorectal manometry to exclude Hirschsprung's disease.

Anorectal manometry reveals certain characteristics in patients with Hirschsprung's disease. The rectosphincteric reflex is absent (Figs. 14.2B, 14.5C) and no decrease of anal pressure occurs because the ganglion cells that would normally transmit this distention reflex are absent.[3,9,25,44] In addition, rectal elasticity is decreased.[45] Anorectal manometry is safe and noninvasive in the diagnosis of Hirschsprung's disease in the neonate,[25] but the utmost care is necessary. The recording device should be placed precisely. The smallest distention volumes possible will prevent short-duration displacement of the transducer from the high anal pressure zone during rectal distention. Recordings from two newborns with delayed stooling, vomiting, and abdominal distention not due to Hirschsprung's disease are shown in Figures 14.5A and B. Recordings from a newborn with Hirschsprung's disease is shown in Figure 14.5C.

Balloon volumes used for rapid rectal distention range from 2 to 10 ml for the premature newborn and 5 to 15 ml for the full-term newborn. It is difficult to use anorectal manometry for diagnostic studies in the neonatal period when rhythmic activity is absent or anal pressure is low (see Fig. 14.5A). These findings have been encountered frequently in the stressed infant[46] and have led to the wrong diagnosis in neonates suspected of having Hirschsprung's disease.[3,25,47,48] The maturity of the patient does not seem to be a factor that influences the success or failure of manometry as a diagnostic method.[25] The diagnosis of Hirschsprung's disease is made by anorectal manometry and an unprepped barium enema,

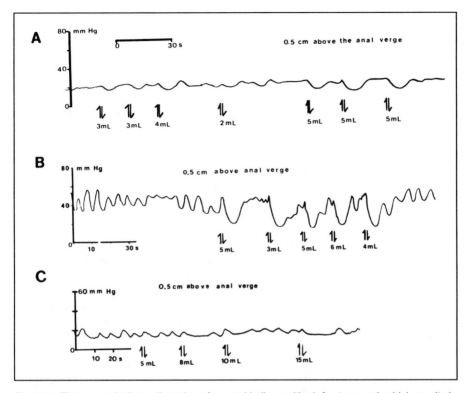

Fig. 14.5 The arrows indicate distention of a rectal balloon with air for 1 second, which results in decreased anal pressure. **A, B:** These recordings are from two newborns with delayed meconium passage, abdominal distention, and vomiting. The presence of the rectosphincteric reflex rules out Hirschsprung's disease as a cause of these newborns' symptoms. Anal resting pressure for the first infant is low and the rectosphincteric reflex is not as easily seen as that in the second, where higher anal resting pressure was present. **C,** Distention of a rectal balloon produces no decrease in anal pressure. The absent rectosphincteric reflex in this newborn indicates that the vomiting, abdominal distention, and diarrhea is due to Hirschsprung's disease.

and confirmed by the rectal suction biopsy.

Surgery is the only effective therapy for Hirschsprung's disease. Unfortunately, many children will have postoperative problems, including constipation (21-42%), fecal soiling (19-47%), and enterocolitis (15-35%),[45,49] all of which can be assessed with anorectal manometry. In one study, constipation was still present in 10% and fecal soiling in 14% of patients 5 years after surgery.[45,50] Anorectal testing reveals that most continue with no rectosphincteric reflex and some will have an incomplete rectosphincteric reflex. The nonrelaxing internal anal sphincter can be demonstrated with anorectal manometry. With larger rectal distention volumes of air or stool, a sustained complete relaxation of the internal and external anal sphinc-

ters occurs in healthy children, as well as in those with functional fecal retention with and without encopresis (see Fig. 14.3). The internal anal sphincter does not relax, hindering defecation in patients who have had surgery for Hirschsprung's disease and have continuous problems with stool retention and fecal incontinence. The rectum accommodates the stool retention, and the development of a megarectum is secondary to the distal obstruction. In others, the megarectum develops due to neuronal intestinal dysplasia, a ganglionosis with hyperganglionosis, which is found in 25% of patients with Hirschsprung's disease.[51] Sometimes an anastomotic stricture is responsible for obstructive symptoms and further surgery is required.

Fecal Incontinence

In humans, very specialized control mechanisms prevent the unintentional loss of wind, stool or urine. Fecal incontinence may be defined as a loss of control of solid, liquid, or gaseous matter. Incontinence can be separated into major and minor categories, each secondary to neurologic or anatomic causes.

Visual study of the anus and perineum and simple neurologic examination of the anus with determination of perianal sensation should be part of a good physical examination. Loss of perianal skin sensation can be associated with various neurologic diseases of the spinal cord and lumbosacral roots. Increased stool volume and decreased stool consistency contribute to fecal incontinence in those with anorectal functional abnormalities.

A healthy person is able to voluntarily contract the external anal sphincter, has a short reflex contraction of the external anal sphincter before reflex relaxation of the internal anal sphincter with balloon distention, and can override the reflex relaxation of the internal anal sphincter when balloon distention is perceived (Fig. 14.6 A-C). Patients with fecal incontinence due to weak anal sphincters have low anal resting pressure and squeeze pressure. Their voluntary contractions of the external sphincter are weak and short; they cannot contract the external sphincter by reflex with balloon distention, and are unable to override the reflex relaxation of the internal anal sphincter when told to squeeze as soon as rectal distention is perceived (Fig. 14.6 D-F).

Myelomeningocele. As a result of aggressive medical and surgical treatment, 80% to 90% of children with myelomeningocele survive. Rehabilitation is therefore increasingly important in their management. Neurologic impairment causes fecal incontinence in 90% of children with myelomeningocele. Many suffer from severe constipation with overflow fecal incontinence; others have incontinence due to diarrhea.

Varying degrees of nerve impairment exist in patients with myelomeningocele, the most common being loss of anal and/or rectal sensation.[10,11,14,15,20,21,52] Such patients usually are unable to differentiate sensations produced by gas from those produced by liquid or solid feces. Using rectal balloon distention, the threshold of rectal sensation in children with myelomeningocele is significantly greater than that of control children.[20] The level of the sensory motor deficit does not correlate with rectal sensation thresholds.[10,20] Abnormal rectal sensation is not explained by a megarectum, because an increased critical volume or increased rectal wall elasticity in patients with myelomeningocele is not present.

The second most common impairment in children with myelomeningocele is loss of function of the external anal sphincter.[11,15,20] The external sphincter cannot be squeezed voluntarily. External anal sphincter contraction is absent during reflex relaxation of the internal anal sphincter because rectal distention allows a rectal contraction to propel a fecal bolus through the anal canal.[10,11,15,20,21] Loss of external anal sphincter function results in a significant decrease in anal resting pressure, squeeze pressure, and leak volume during saline infusion.[20] The rectosphincteric reflex is present.

The results of anorectal function evaluation influence the design of an appropriate treatment plan, incorporating medical therapy (eg, stool softeners, laxatives, suppositories, phosphate enemas, or large-volume saline enemas), frequent manual removal of feces, a constipating diet or medication, behavior modification, biofeedback training, or a combination of these.

Anorectal anomalies. Anorectal atresias can be classified as low, intermediate, or high. Many patients treated for anorectal anomalies have postoperative difficulties in defecation, constipation and/or fecal incontinence. Most previous reports have stressed the treatment of fecal incontinence after surgery, while constipation after surgery was dismissed or not fully addressed. Despite an adequately sized neoanus, patients with low- and intermediate-type anomalies often suffer from severe constipation and overflow fecal incontinence, which should be man-

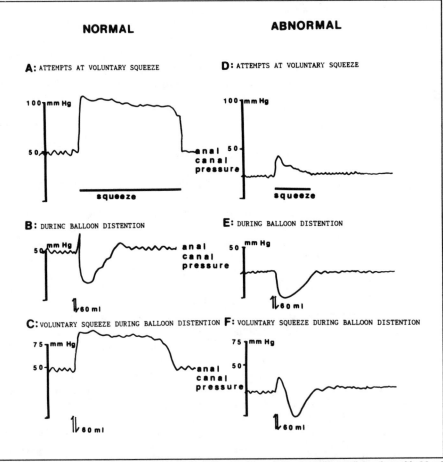

NORMAL

A: ATTEMPTS AT VOLUNTARY SQUEEZE

B: DURING BALLOON DISTENTION

C: VOLUNTARY SQUEEZE DURING BALLOON DISTENTION

ABNORMAL

D: ATTEMPTS AT VOLUNTARY SQUEEZE

E: DURING BALLOON DISTENTION

F: VOLUNTARY SQUEEZE DURING BALLOON DISTENTION

Fig. 14.6 Intraluminal pressure recordings from the anal canal. Rectal balloon distention with 60 ml air for 1-2 seconds (semiarrows). A healthy child is able to voluntarily contract the external anal sphincter (**A**); has a reflex contraction of the external anal sphincter prior to the reflex relaxation of the internal anal sphincter after balloon distention (**B**); and can override the reflex relaxation when balloon distention is perceived (**C**). A child with weak anal sphincter can accomplish only a weak and short voluntary contraction of the external anal sphincter (**D**); has no reflex contraction of the external anal sphincter after balloon distention (**E**); and is unable to override the reflex relaxation when told to squeeze as soon as rectal distention is perceived (**F**). (Reproduced with permission from Loening-Baucke V, 1990[64])

aged with laxatives or stimulants and a toilet-sitting routine. Long-term functional results, 5 to 25 years after surgery, have been reported by Iwai et al.[53] Good results and adequate continence was accomplished in 87% of patients with low anomalies, but in only 28% of those with high anomalies. Children with low anomalies are more likely to be continent, while children with high anomalies have frequent problems with incontinence. Continence after repair of anorectal malformations depends on many ano-

rectal function parameters. Incontinence is associated with abnormal function of the anal sphincters or the rectum: 1) abnormal, low anal resting pressure; 2) abnormal, low squeeze pressure; 3) abnormal neoanal sensation; and 4) abnormal rectal sensation and rectal reservoir function in those with high abnormalities.[18,53-56]

Anorectal trauma. Anorectal trauma may be related to an impalement injury or child abuse. Presentations are rectovaginal tears that often extend through the anal sphincters, rectovaginal fistula, or even destruction of the rectum. Anorectal manometry helps assess the functioning of the external and internal anal sphincters and puborectalis muscle. In addition, electromyographic mapping of the external anal sphincter with a needle electrode may be necessary.[57,58]

Neuromuscular disease. Occasionally, a child may have fecal incontinence due to neuromuscular disease, such as myotonic dystrophy, Duchenne muscular dystrophy, and congenital myopathy. Some of these children may have a fecal impaction. Most have low anal-resting and squeeze pressures.

Myotonic dystrophy is a myopathy of the smooth muscle and also involves the striated muscles of the anal canal. Colonic involvement manifests as megacolon in childhood, but sometimes is severe enough to cause symptoms of chronic intestinal pseudo-obstruction.[59] Some children with myotonic dystrophy have fecal impaction with fecal incontinence. Patients with myotonic dystrophy have low anal-resting and squeeze pressures. They can accomplish only a weak, short, voluntary contraction of the external sphincter and have a prolonged reflex contraction of the external sphincter after balloon distention. Some have a myotonic contraction of the upper anal canal after reflex relaxation.[60]

Treatment with laxatives is often not very successful. The constipation is relieved, but fecal incontinence is exacerbated. Increasing dietary fiber and establishing a regular toilet routine improve incontinence in most of these children. The regular use of stimulants such as senna preparation or emptying the rectum regularly with enemas or suppositories is sometimes necessary.

BIOFEEDBACK

Biofeedback has been successful in treating a variety of illnesses. Biofeedback training teaches patients self-control over bodily functions. During biofeedback training of the anal sphincter, the patient is instantly provided with information on the current function of the physiologic activity of the external anal sphincter. The physiologic response is probably not an unconscious reflex function but is under voluntary control, such as the external sphincter's response to rectal distention or to straining for defecation. The patient is provided with visual and/or auditory information about the function of the external anal sphincter using an electronic device. The patient learns to recognize the physiologic response of the external anal sphincter, and may be able to learn to respond appropriately and gain control. Depending on the particular type of sphincter dysfunction, training goals may be focused on helping the patient to contract the external sphincter and pelvic floor muscles, relax the external sphincter and pelvic floor muscles, or inhibit the spastic action of these muscles.

Four conditions must exist for biofeedback to be successful: 1) there must be a well-defined, readily measurable response (eg, a contraction or relaxation of the external anal sphincter); 2) the end organ must be capable of responding (a completely paralyzed, denervated external anal muscle would not respond during biofeedback); 3) there must be a perceptible cue that signals the patient to initiate control (distention of the rectum); and 4) there must be adequate patient motivation to carry out the biofeedback training.

Anorectal Devices

Biofeedback training can be performed with any device that records anal pressure or external anal sphincter EMG activity and incorporates a balloon for rectal distention. Biofeedback training can be provided with a multitude of instruments that either give pressure feedback, EMG feedback, or a combination of both. Anorectal instruments that are used for anorectal manometry include water-perfused tubes, Schuster's balloon instrument, the small balloon probe by Arhan, or the Dent sleeve. A simple biofeedback training apparatus with anal plug can be bought. Simpler, less expensive biofeedback devices were constructed by Loening-Baucke[20] and Constantinides and Cywes.[61]

Commercially available anorectal probes

come with visual display instruments. Visual biofeedback can be provided by having the patient watch the recording obtained with conventional polygraphs. Biofeedback treatment can also be provided with computers requiring special software.

Biofeedback for Functional Fecal Retention

A healthy child can voluntarily initiate the actions connected with defecation. In this process, an increase in intra-abdominal pressure is produced by 1) closure of the glottis; 2) fixation of the diaphragm; 3) contractions of the abdominal, perineal, and hamstring muscles; and 4) relaxation of the external and internal anal sphincters (see Fig. 14.4A). During defecation attempts, approximately 50% of children 5 years of age or older with fecal retention and encopresis abnormally close the anal canal by contracting the external anal sphincter as well as the puborectalis and pelvic floor muscles (see Fig. 14.4B).[29,38] Other studies indicate an incidence rate of 25% to 33% for abnormal defecation dynamics in children with fecal retention.[13,32] The abnormal defecation dynamics persisted after 12 months of laxative treatment.[27,28] Patients with abnormal defecation dynamics were significantly less likely to recover after 1 year of conventional laxative treatment (26%) than patients with normal defecation dynamics (61%; p<0.01).[27]

For biofeedback training of patients with abnormal defecation dynamics, the equipment used for anorectal manometry can be employed (see Fig. 14.1). The motility probe can evaluate the combined function of the external and internal anal sphincters and rectal pressure changes. One of the transducers is placed into the rectum, a second into the anal canal, and the balloon for rectal distention is inserted 11 cm into the rectum. Simultaneously, the myoelectrical activity from the external sphincter is recorded at a speed of 10 mm per second with three surface electrodes. Two electrodes are placed over the external sphincter, as close as possible to the anal opening, and a third is placed on the buttock. The area under the wave form of the action potentials—an index of total activity—is obtained by integrating the primary signal with an EMG averaging coupler. The outputs of the transducers and surface electrodes are fed into amplifiers of an eight-channel dynograph recorder and are graphed on paper.

A manometric and EMG tracing from an individual with normal defecation dynamics is shown to the patient (see Fig. 14.4A). The difference in the healthy child's external sphincter relaxation and the patient's external sphincter contraction during defecation trials is explained. The patient lies on his or her side and observes the record as it is registered. Initially, the rectal balloon is inflated with 50 ml air and the patient is instructed to increase intra-abdominal pressure (to push as if defecating) and to inhibit contraction of the external sphincter, in attempts to produce relaxations or tracings approximate to the normal external sphincter relaxations. Constant verbal, visual (recording), and sound reinforcements (the EMG recording stylus produces less noise) are given when correct responses are made. The patient tries to modify the external sphincter responses to make them appear more normal until relaxations of the external sphincter are finally accomplished. After the patient is able to relax the external sphincter, he or she is encouraged to increase the duration of the relaxation without rectal balloon distention. Sometimes children will perform a few partial relaxations before finally doing it right. Most patients can develop completely normal defecation dynamics. After relaxation of the external sphincter is accomplished, the visual, and later the verbal feedback is withdrawn.

A biofeedback training session includes approximately 30 to 35 defecation trials and lasts approximately 45 minutes. At least two and up to six weekly training sessions are given. The number of training sessions depends on how soon the child learns to relax the external sphincter. Biofeedback training is stopped after 10 relaxations of the external anal sphincter without visual feedback can be accomplished in each of two successive sessions.

Results of training. In two studies, the benefits of biofeedback training on defecation dynamics and outcome in children with functional fecal retention, encopresis, and abnormal defecation dynamics were evaluated.[29,30] Patients 5 to 16 years of age with functional fecal retention, encopresis, and abnormal defecation dynamics were randomly assigned to receive conventional treatment alone or conventional plus biofeedback treatment.[29] Conventional treatment consisted of clearing the fecal impaction, preventing future impaction with the aid of laxatives, and promoting regular bowel habits with frequent toilet sitting. Approximately 80% of patients learned normal defecation dynamics. On follow-up, 13% of patients in the conventional group and 77% in the biofeedback group had normal defecation dynamics.[29] At the 12th month, 16% of conventionally treated and 50% of additional biofeedback-treated patients had recovered (p<0.05).[29] Seventy-one percent of those who learned normal defecation dynamics with biofeedback treatment recovered. This is similar to the 61% 1-year recovery rate after conventional treatment alone in the patients with normal defecation dynamics.[27] This study demonstrates that biofeedback treatment complements good conventional therapeutic regimen in patients with abnormal defecation dynamics. A second study was composed of 38 children with fecal retention, encopresis, and abnormal defecation dynamics who had failed a previous treatment program.[30] Biofeedback was given in addition to conventional laxative treatment. The overall recovery rate was 37%. Seventy-four percent learned to relax the external anal sphincter and pelvic floor in up to six biofeedback training sessions, and 26% did not learn to relax these muscles in six sessions. Of the 28 children who learned to relax the external anal sphincter and the pelvic floor muscles, 14 recovered and 14 did not. Anorectal function testing showed that, compared to control children, recovered and nonrecovered successful biofeedback-treated patients initially required significantly larger balloon volumes to produce a rectal sensation, an urge to defecate (criti-

cal volume), a rectosphincteric reflex, constant relaxation, and a rectal contraction of 10 mm Hg or more.[30] These balloon volumes were notably increased in patients who later did not recover as compared to those of patients who recovered (p<0.05).[30] Follow-up manometric evaluations at 7 months showed no improvement in the parameters of rectal function testing in recovered and nonrecovered patients. Nonrecovered patients continued with significantly more impairment of rectal and anal function than recovered patients.[30]

Many studies[13,32,34,38-40,62] show that relaxation of the pelvic floor during straining can be taught, even to those who have failed a previous conventional treatment program. Learning to relax the pelvic floor during straining is significantly correlated with recovery (p<0.02). Others report that 67% of children markedly improve or recover 12 months after biofeedback training,[13] 58% clinically recover 2 to 18 months after biofeedback training,[34] and 55% recover 12 months later.[38] Even better outcome has been reported by others.[32,39] Nine of 12 children who had failed prior treatment recovered after biofeedback treatment, three experienced a self-limited relapse,[39] and all seven (7-14 years of age) achieved a bowel movement daily or every other day after learning to relax the pelvic floor with biofeedback.[32]

Biofeedback for Fecal Incontinence

Causes of fecal incontinence in children include complications of anorectal surgery (eg, that for Hirschsprung's disease or imperforate anus syndrome), spinal cord injuries or birth defects (eg, spinal trauma, spinal surgery, meningomyelocele, or imperforate anus syndromes), traumatic disruption of the puborectalis, external, or internal sphincter during impalement injuries or child abuse.

Auditory and/or visual biofeedback has been used for the training of children ages 5 years and older with fecal incontinence.[10,11,14-16,20,40,52,63,64] The most commonly employed biofeedback procedure incorporates three separate and potentially effective components: 1) exercise of the external sphincter muscle, 2) training in discrimination of rectal sensations, and 3) training synchrony of the internal and external sphincter responses to rectal distention.

During biofeedback, children are made aware of the abnormal, weak, or absent anal pressure increases during voluntary external anal sphincter or pelvic floor contraction (see Fig. 14.6D), rectal sensations during distention, absent or weak external sphincter contraction prior to the internal sphincter relaxation (see Fig. 14.6E), and the inability to override reflex relaxation of the internal sphincter with external sphincter squeeze (see Fig. 14.6F) in their anorectal manometric recordings. The patients are also shown tracings from a healthy control child (see Fig. 14.6A-C). The children are instructed to contract the external anal sphincter, including muscles in the anal area that surround the anal canal, such as the muscles of the pelvic floor and nearby gluteal muscles. Constant visual, auditory, and verbal reinforcements are given when correct responses are made. In approximately 50 training trials per session, the children are encouraged to try harder or to modify their efforts to produce tracings similar to normal tracings. In addition, rectal balloon distention volumes large enough to be felt by the children are used to train the patients to recognize smaller and smaller distention volumes and to synchronize voluntary anal sphincter contraction with the distention. The children are encouraged to increase the amplitude and duration of the voluntary anal sphincter squeeze. In some children, an abnormal increase in intra-abdominal pressure during attempted anal squeeze is recorded. These children are also instructed to inhibit the intra-abdominal pressure increase. Biofeedback is withdrawn when the child can increase the squeeze amplitude and duration.

Many investigators encourage their patients to practice external sphincter contraction between sessions. In some patients, a portable biofeedback device is used.[20,61] Such practice is probably essential if the procedure is to be transferred from the laboratory to the home. Patients with fecal incontinence secondary to meningomyelocele can practice at home using a self-made biofeedback device,[20] which consists of a 2.5 by 3-cm balloon placed into the anal canal and connected via small and large water-filled tubing to an upright, standing, water-filled, graded measuring device. By varying the height of placement of the device, individual differences in anal sphincter pressure and strength can be taken into account. The patient should practice anal sphincter and pelvic floor contraction for 20 to 30 minutes at least every other day. Instruments for home biofeedback training are also commercially available.

Results of training. In a number of uncontrolled studies, biofeedback training has been reported to result in continence or markedly reduced frequency of fecal incontinence.[16,63] Therapeutic gains appear to be maintained at 1 to 2 years' follow-up. Biofeedback's apparent safety, physiologic appeal, and minimal training sessions suggest that it is contributing to the treatment of fecal incontinence, although its effects on anorectal function may not be measurable.

Myelomeningocele Several authors have reported on the efficacy of biofeedback in training patients with fecal incontinence secondary to myelomeningocele.[10,11,14-16,52,63] However, control groups were not used to separate the effects of biofeedback from those of behavioral treatment and changes in bowel habits, which might occur either spontaneously or through medication and/or diets. In contrast, when patients were randomized to a comparison treatment group who received the same behavior modification and follow-up attention, biofeedback patients had no better clinical outcome than those treated with conventional therapy alone.[20] These findings agree with a study by Whitehead et al[14] in incontinent patients with myelomeningocele, which reported that patients who received only behavioral modification therapy for 3 months showed as much clinical improvement as those who received behavioral modification plus biofeedback. Patients with myelomeningocele did not improve their anal squeeze pressure and were not able to retain a significantly larger volume of rectal infused saline without leakage after three biofeedback training sessions and perineal exercises using a home biofeedback device. None of these patients learned a normal anal sphincter squeeze. These findings conflict with previous studies,[15,16,52] probably because of recent improvements in recording techniques using intraluminal pressure transducers.

Anal atresia. The anatomic development of the anal sphincters and rectum determines the degree of fecal incontinence in patients who have undergone surgery for anal atresia. Cerulli et al[63] did not improve fecal incontinence of their patient with biofeedback training. The best results after biofeedback training were reported by Olness et al[65] in 10 patients, ages 4 to 18 years, who had little or no fecal control following repair of supralevator-type anal atresia. Patients were taught to increase anal pressure in a 20-minute period. Additional biofeedback was given until bowel control was complete or until it was judged that the patient was not responding. Patients practiced anal muscle contraction at home. Six patients achieved normal bowel habits within a few weeks. Four patients continued with incontinence; two had not cooperated with the biofeedback treatment. Biofeedback treatment seems to improve the fecal incontinence in children with repair of high- or intermediate-type anorectal malformations,[54,66-68] but children do not become symptom-free. It appears that most children with fecal incontinence from high anal atresia or meningomyelocele do not achieve continence with biofeedback training. Most investigators have suggested medical treatment with laxatives, fiber, or constipating medications in addition to biofeedback. These additional treatments may have been responsible for the decrease in the frequency of soiling.

Only a few studies reported anorectal manometric measurements pre- and post-biofeedback treatment. Some studies showed a significant improvement in squeeze pressure after biofeedback treatment.[15,16,52,54,56] Others showed mild or no improvement in anal squeeze pressure.[18,20,66] Adequate anal resting pressure before biofeedback therapy is correlated with good response to biofeedback.[60]

The mechanisms of action of biofeedback for fecal incontinence are complex. There are several components to the treatment: 1) squeeze training of the external sphincter muscle for those with fecal incontinence due to a weak anal sphincter; 2) training in discrimination of rectal sensations; and 3) synchronizing of the internal and external sphincter responses during rectal distention. Each of these components may be effective for some patients. It is conceivable, for example, that patients who have an impaired external sphincter muscle and normal rectal sensation will respond to exercise so that reflexive response to rectal distention will be adequate. In contrast, children with an elevated sensory threshold to rectal distention may respond by learning to sense smaller volumes of rectal distention. There are other cases in which there is adequate sensation and muscular strength, but the appropriate synchrony of the sphincteric response does not occur, as in the contraction of the external anal sphincter and pelvic floor muscles when defecation needs to be delayed.

CONCLUSION

Anorectal physiologic testing is useful in disorders of constipation due to functional fecal retention with or without soiling and Hirschsprung's disease, as well as in fecal incontinence due to myelomeningocele, anorectal anomalies, anorectal trauma, and neuromuscular disease. Many techniques are available for anorectal manometry and results partially reflect the use of different recording devices and study procedures. All instruments and techniques for anorectal manometry, when properly used, are able to provide reproducible and useful measurements.[7]

Four conditions must exist for biofeedback to be successful: 1) a well-defined, readily measurable response—either a contraction or relaxation of the external anal sphincter; 2) the end organ must be capable of responding; 3) the patient must be able to perceive a rectal distention that signals the patient to initiate control; and 4) the patient must be motivated. Depending on the particular type of sphincter dysfunction, training goals may focus on helping the patient to activate the external sphincter and pelvic floor muscles, induce relaxation of the external sphincter and pelvic floor muscles, or inhibit the spastic action of these muscles.

REFERENCES

1. Meunier P, Louis D, Jaubert de Beaujeu M. Physiologic investigation of primary chronic constipation in children: comparison with the barium enema study. *Gastroenterology* 1984;87:1351-7.

2. Meunier P, Marechal JM, Jaubert de Beaujeu M. Rectoanal pressures and rectal sensitivity studies in chronic childhood constipation. *Gastroenterology* 1979;77:330-6.

3. Meunier P, Marechal JM, Mollard P. Accuracy of the manometric diagnosis of Hirschsprung's disease. *J Pediatr Surg* 1978;13:411-5.

4. Meunier P, Mollard P, Jaubert de Beaujeu M. Manometric studies of anorectal disorders in infancy and childhood: an investigation of pathophysiology of incontinence and defaecation. *Br J Surg* 1976;63:402-7.

5. Haynes WG, Read NW. Anorectal activity in man during rectal infusion of saline: a dynamic assessment of the anal continence mechanism. *J Physiol* 1982;47:57-65.

6. Read NW, Harford WV, Schmulen AC, Read MG, Santa Ana C, Fortram JS. A clinical study of patients with fecal incontinence and diarrhea. *Gastroenterology* 1979;76:745-56.

7. Meunier PD. Anorectal manometry: a collective international experience. *Gastroenterol Clin Biol* 1991;15:697-702.

8. Schuster MM, Hookman P, Hendrix TR, Mendeloff A. Simultaneous manometric recording of internal and external anal sphincteric reflexes. *Bull Johns Hopkins Hosp* 1965;116:79-88.

9. Tobon F, Nigel C, Talbert J, Schuster MM. Non-surgical test for the diagnosis of Hirschsprung's disease. *N Engl J Med* 1986;278:188-194.

10. Wald A. Biofeedback for neurogenic fecal incontinence: rectal sensation is a determinant of outcome. *J Pediatr Gastroenterol Nutr* 1983;2:302-6.

11. Wald A. Use of biofeedback in treatment of fecal incontinence in patients with meningomyelocele. *Pediatrics* 1981;68:45-9.

12. Wald A, Chandra R, Chiponis D, Gabel S. Anorectal function and continence mechanisms in childhood encopresis. *J Pediatr Gastroenterol Nutr* 1986;5:346-51.

13. Wald A, Chandra R, Gabel S, Chiponis D. Evaluation of biofeedback in childhood encopresis. *J Pediatr Gastroenterol Nutr* 1987;6:554-8.

14. Whitehead WE, Parker LH, Bosmajian L, et al. Treatment of fecal incontinence in children with spina bifida: comparison of biofeedback and behavior modification. *Arch Phys Med Rehabil* 1986;67:218-24.

15. Whitehead WE, Parker LH, Masek BJ, Cataldo MF, Freeman JM. Biofeedback treatment of fecal incontinence in patients with myelomeningocele. *Dev Med Child Neurol* 1981;23:313-22.

16. Engel BT, Nikoomanesh P, Schuster MM. Operant conditioning of rectosphincteric responses in the treatment of fecal incontinence. *N Engl J Med* 1974;290:646-9.

17. Arhan P, Faverdin CL, Thouvenot J. Anorectal motility in sick children. *Scand J Gastroenterol* 1972;7:309-14.

18. Arhan P, Faverdin C, Devroede G, Dubois F, Coupris L, Pellerin D. Manometric assessment of continence after surgery for imperforate anus. *J Pediatr Surg* 1976;11:157-66.

19. Devroede G. Mechanisms of constipation. In: Read NW, ed. *Irritable Bowel Syndrome*. New York, NY: Grune and Stratton, 1985;127-39.

20. Loening-Baucke V, Desch L, Wolraich M. Biofeedback training in patients with meningomyelocele and fecal incontinence. *Dev Med Child Neurol* 1988;30:781-90.

21. Arhan P, Faverdin C, Devroede G, Pierre-Kahn A, Scott H, Pellerin D. Anorectal motility after surgery for spina bifida. *Dis Colon Rectum* 1984;27:159-63.

22. Loening-Baucke V. Sensitivity of the sigmoid colon and rectum in children treated for chronic constipation. *J Pediatr Gastroenterol Nutr* 1984;3:454-9.

23. Loening-Baucke V. Abnormal rectoanal function in children recovered from chronic constipation and encopresis. *Gastroenterology* 1984;87:1299-1304.

24. Dent JA. A new technique for continuous sphincter pressure measurement. *Gastroenterology* 1976;71:263-7.

25. Loening-Baucke V, Pringle KC, Ekwo EE. Anorectal manometry for the exclusion of Hirschsprung's disease in neonates. *J Pediatr Gastroenterol Nutr* 1985;4:596-603.

26. Freckner B, Euler CV. Influence of pudendal block on the function of the anal sphincters. *Gut* 1975;16:482-9.

27. Loening-Baucke V. Factors determining outcome in children with chronic constipation and fecal soiling. *Gut* 1989;30:999-1006.

28. Loening-Baucke V. Factors responsible for persistence of childhood constipation. *J Pediatr Gastroenterol Nutr* 1987;6:915-22.

29. Loening-Baucke V. Modulation of abnormal defecation dynamics by biofeedback treatment in chronically constipated children with encopresis. *J Pediatr* 1990;116:214-22.

30. Loening-Baucke V. Persistence of chronic constipation in children after biofeedback treatment. *Dig Dis Sci* 1991;36:153-60.

31. Loening-Baucke V, Cruikshank B. Abnormal defecation dynamics in chronically constipated children with encopresis. *J Pediatr* 1986;108:562-6.

32. Louis D, Valancogne G, Loras O, Meunier P. Techniques et indications du biofeedback dans les constipations chez l'enfant. *Psychol Méd* 1985;17:1625-7.

33. Loening-Baucke V, Younoszai MK. Effect of treatment on rectal and sigmoid motility in chronically constipated children. *Pediatrics* 1984;73:199-205.

34. Veyrac M, Granel D, Parelon G, Michel H. Constipation idiopathique de l'enfant. Intérêt du traitement par biofeedback. *Pédiatrie* 1987;42:719-21.

35. Loening-Baucke V, Younoszai MK. Abnormal anal sphincter response in chronically constipated children. *J Pediatr* 1982;100:213-8.

36. Mischalany HG, Wooley MG. Chronic constipation: manometric patterns and surgical considerations. *Arch Surg* 1984;119:1257-9.

37. Molnar D, Taitz LS, Urwin OM, Wales JKH. Anorectal manometry results in defecation disorders. *Arch Dis Child* 1983;58:257-61.

38. Benninga MA, Büller HA, Taminiau JAJM. Biofeedback training in chronic constipation. *Arch Dis Child* 1993:68:126-9.

39. Keren S, Wagner Y, Heldenberg D, Golan M. Studies of manometric abnormalities of the rectoanal region during defecation in constipated and soiling children: modification through biofeedback therapy. *Am J Gastroenterol* 1988;83:827-31.

40. Shephard K, Hickstein R, Rose V, Nasser C, Cleghorn GJ, Shephard RW. Faecal incontinence in childhood: a multidisciplinary approach including biofeedback. *Aust Paediatr J* 1989;25:351-5.

41. Berdon WE, Baker DH, Blanc WA, Gay B, Santulli TV, Donovan C. Megacystis-microcolon intestinal hypoperistalsis syndrome: a new cause of intestinal obstruction in the newborn: report of radiologic findings in five newborn girls. *Am J Roentgenol* 1976;126:957-64.

42. Nixon HH. What is pseudo-Hirschsprung's disease? *Arch Dis Child* 1966;41:147-9.

43. Bussmann H, Roth H, v Deimling O, Nuetzenadel W. Clinical variability in neuronal intestinal dysplasia. *Monatsschr Kinderheilkd* 1990;138:184-7.

44. Callaghan RP, Nixon HH. Megarectum: physiological observations. *Arch Dis Child* 1964;39:153-7.

45. Holschneider AM. Elektromanometrie des Enddarms. *Diagnostik und Therapie der Inkontinenz und der chronischen Obstipation.* Munich: Urban and Schwarzenberg, 1983.

46. Howard ER, Nixon HH. Internal anal sphincter: observations on the development and mechanism of inhibitory responses in premature infants and children with Hirschsprung's disease. *Arch Dis Child* 1968;43:569-78.

47. McParland FA, Olness K. Diagnostic uses of anorectal manometry in pediatrics. *Minn Med* 1979;62:447-0.

48. Morikawa Y, Donahoe PK, Hendren WH. Manometry and histochemistry in the diagnosis of Hirschsprung's disease. *Pediatrics* 1979;63:865-71.

49. Mishalany HG, Woolley MM. Postoperative functional and manometric evaluation of patients with Hirschsprung's disease. *J Pediatr Surg* 1987;22:443-6.

50. Holschneider AM, Börner W, Buurman O, et al. Clinical and electromanometrical investigations of postoperative continence in Hirschsprung's disease: an international workshop. *Z Kinderchir* 1980;29:39-48.

51. Fadda B, Pistor G, Meier-Ruge W, Hofmann-von Kap-herr S, Müntefering H, Espinoza R. Symptoms, diagnosis, and therapy of neuronal intestinal dysplasia masked by Hirschsprung's disease. *Pediatr Surg Int* 1987;2:76-80.

52. Shepherd K, Hickstein R, Shepherd R. Neurogenic faecal incontinence in children with spina bifida: rectosphincteric responses and evaluation of a physiological rationale for management, including biofeedback conditioning. *Aust Paediatr J* 1983;19:97-9.

53. Iwai N, Hashimoto K, Goto Y, Majima S. Long-term results after surgical correction of anorectal malformations. *Z Kinderchir* 1984;39:35-9.

54. Iwai N, Nagashima M, Shimotake T, Iwata G. Biofeedback therapy for fecal incontinence after surgery for anorectal malformations: preliminary results. *J Pediatr Surg* 1993;28:863-6.

55. Nagashima M, Iwai N, Yanagihara J, Shimotake T. Motility and sensation of the rectosigmoid and the rectum in patients with anorectal malformations. *J Pediatr Surg* 1992;27:1273-7.

56. Rintala R, Lindahl H, Louhimo I. Biofeedback conditioning for fecal incontinence in anorectal malformations. *Pediatr Surg Int* 1988;3:418-21.

57. Chantraine A. EMG examination of the anal and urethral sphincters. In: Desmedt JE, ed. *New Developments in Electromyography and Clinical Neurophysiology.* Basle, Switzerland: Karger, 1973;2:421-32.

58. Swash M, Snooks SJ. Electromyography in pelvic floor disorders. In: Henry MM, Swash M, eds. *Coloproctology and the Pelvic Floor.* London, England: Butterworths, 1985:88-103.

59. Nowak TV, Ionasescu V, Anuras S. Gastrointestinal manifestations of the muscular dystrophies. *Gastroenterology* 1982;82:800-10.

60. Hamel-Roy J, Devroede G, Arhan P, Tétreault J-P, Lemieux B, Scott H. Functional abnormalities of the anal sphincters in patients with myotonic dystrophy. *Gastroenterology* 1984;86:1469-74.

61. Constantinides CG, Cywes S, Fecal incontinence: a simple pneumatic device for home biofeedback training. *J Pediatr Surg* 1983;18:276-7.

62. Emery Y, Descos L, Meunier P, Louis D, Valancogne G, Weil G. Constipation terminale par asynchronisme abdomino-pelvien; analyse des données étiologiques aprés rééducation par biofeedback. *Gastroenterol Clin Biol* 1988;12:6-11.

63. Cerulli MA, Nikoomanesh P, Schuster MM. Progress in biofeedback conditioning for fecal incontinence. *Gastroenterology* 1979;76:742-6.

64. Loening-Baucke V. Biofeedback therapy for fecal incontinence. *Dig Dis* 1990;7:112-24.

65. Olness K, McParland F, Piper J, Biofeedback: a new modality in the management of children with fecal soiling. *J Pediatr* 1980;96:505-9.

66. Allen ML. Biofeedback for fecally incontinent children with repaired imperforate anus. *Practical Gastroenterology* 1990;14:53-62.

67. Herold A, Bruch H-P, Hocht B, Müller G. Biofeedback-training and funktionelle elektrostimulation zur verbesserung der inkontinenz bei kindern mit analatresie. *Langenbecks Arch Chir* 1989;(2):991-5.

68. Koltai JL. Kontinenzverbesserung durch biofeedback-konditionierung. *Langenbecks Arch Chir* 1989;(2):987-9.

APPENDIX 14.1: Commercially Available Equipment

Open-Ended Tubes or Assemblies With Side Holes
Arnsdorfer, Inc., Greendale Wisconsin, USA
Mui Scientific, Mississauga, Canada

Hydraulic Capillary Infusion System
Arnsdorfer, Inc., Greendale, Wisconsin, USA
Mui Scientific, Mississauga, Canada

Pressure Transducers
P23 ID, Gould Statham, Gould Inc., Cleveland, Ohio

Motility Probes
Model P31-D3, Sandhill Scientific, Littleton, Colorado, USA
Konigsberg Instruments Inc., Pasadena, California
Medical Measurements, Inc., Hackensack, New Jersey, or Gaeltec, Scotland

Electrodes
Disposable, ECG
  Abco Dealers, Inc., Milwaukee, Wisconsin, USA
  Andover Medical Supply, Bloomington, Minnesota

Polygraphs
Conventional
  Beckman Recorder, SensorMedics, Anaheim, California
  ES 1000B Electrostatic Chart Recorder, Gould, Inc., Cleveland, Ohio
  TDS-4000, Sandhill, Littleton, Colorado
Computerized
  PC Polygraph, Synectics Medical, Irving, Texas

Combined Recorder and Motility System
Sandhill, Littleton, Colorado

EMG Averaging Coupler
SensorMedics, Type 9852A, Anaheim, California

Anorectal Probes With Visual Display
PerryMeter Systems, Biotechnologies, Inc., Stratford, Pennsylvania
The Biofeedback Meter, Sandhill, Littleton, Colorado
The Dobbhoff Anorectal Biofeedback System 5, Biosearch Medical Products,Inc.,
  Somerville, New Jersey
Orion Pelvic Floor Muscle Rehabilitation System,
Self-Regulation Systems, Inc., Redmond, Washington

Biofeedback Computers (suitable for home use)
I-330 System, J & J Enterprises, Pousbo, Washington

Biofeedback Trainer with Anal Plug
Farrell Instruments, Inc., Grand Island, Nebraska

15

Esophageal pH Monitoring

YVAN VANDENPLAS

Gastroesophageal reflux (GER) is a physiologic phenomenon that occurs occasionally in every human being, especially in the postprandial period. Reflux occurs so frequently in infants that physicians and other health care practitioners are often reluctant to accept it as a possible cause of clinical problems. Nevertheless, any parent of a "regurgitating baby" can appreciate the social discomfort induced by the phenomenon. It is difficult to believe that the normal function of the stomach and esophagus is to reflux ingested material back into and out of the esophagus. Moreover, recent literature has implicated "occult" GER (ie, without regurgitation or emesis) as a relatively frequent cause of severe morbidity (see Chapter 4) and even mortality; GER is a possible cause of fatal apnea. Although esophageal pH monitoring doesn't actually measure GER, it is the only investigative technique able to detect reflux episodes beyond the postprandial period.

INDICATIONS FOR pH MONITORING

Two major but totally different indications for esophageal pH monitoring exist: 1) in clinical and laboratory research, and 2) as a routine clinical procedure in the diagnosis and treatment of GER. Its popularity in clinical research contributed substantially to an overconsumption in daily practice.

Esophageal pH monitoring should not be performed as a first diagnostic approach in patients with so-called physiologic or uncomplicated regurgitations or emesis.[1] Whatever the result of the recording, it will have little effect on therapeutic management. As a diagnostic investigation, pH monitoring is indicated for patients with unusual presentations (Table 15.1) in whom the classic causes of the symptoms are not apparent. Even in these patients, results should be interpreted with great care. A patient with chronic wheezing might be allergic and not improve with classic antiallergic treatment because he also suffers from primary or secondary GER that

---

TABLE 15.1 Symptoms of Gastroesophageal Reflux (GER) Disease

Esophageal Manifestations
Specific symptoms
  regurgitation
  nausea
  vomiting
Symptoms possibly related to reflux esophagitis
  symptoms related to anemia (iron-deficiency anemia)
  hematemesis, melena
  dysphagia (as a symptom of esophagitis and/or due to stricture formation)
  weight loss and/or failure to thrive
  epigastric or retrosternal pain
  "noncardiac, anginalike" chest pain
  pyrosis or heartburn, pharyngeal burning
  belching, postprandial fullness
  irritable esophagus
  general irritability in infants ("colic")

Unusual Presentations
GER related to chronic respiratory disease
  (bronchitis, asthma, laryngitis, pharyngitis, etc.)
Cystic fibrosis
Sandifer Sutcliffe syndrome
Rumination
Apnea, apparent life-threatening event, sudden infant death syndrome (SIDS)

Associated With Congenital and/or Central Nervous System Abnormalities
Intracranial tumors, cerebral palsy, psychomotor retardation, etc.

TABLE 15.2 Advantages and Disadvantages of pH Monitoring in Diagnosing GER Disease

Technique	Advantages	Disadvantages
	physiologic conditions normal ranges good reproducibility long duration (24 hours)	physiologic conditions social discomfort (electrode)
Diagnosis	quantification number of pH changes quantification duration pH changes time-relation symptom-pH change	measures pH change, not GER alkaline GER (?) no neutral GER
Complications	area under pH 4: related to esophagitis	no direct information, tissue damage
Treatment	contributes to choice of treatment evaluation of treatment	no acid secretion if H_2-blocker

was induced by treatment with xanthine-derivatives.[2]

In research, the situation is different. Esophageal pH monitoring is the investigation of choice to study GER beyond the immediate postprandial period (Table 15.2). However, since feeding neutralizes intragastric acidity, postprandial reflux might not be detected with pH monitoring.

HARDWARE AND SOFTWARE

The greatest advantage of pH monitoring as compared with other techniques for GER is probably the development of ambulatory recording systems that enable the evaluation of GER in physiologic conditions, even in young children. Recorders smaller than a credit card (although a little thicker) are commercially available. Before a facility acquires this equipment, its intended applications should be considered. For routine diagnostic clinical use, the simplest device with automated analysis will probably be sufficient. As to the commercial aspects, the relation between quality and price is difficult to assess. Purchase costs, system abilities, costs in use, number of measurements, and durability of the material are all factors to consider before purchasing equipment. The device should have a 1) power back-up; 2) time-indication on the display (eg, number of data recorded, real time, duration of investigation); 3) light but solid construction, 4) at least one, but not too many, event

markers (a simple but precise diary minimizes confusion and errors) and 5) capacity to refuse to collect data if not calibrated adequately.[3] This last point is very important. All too often the operator forgets to calibrate the system. The time-indication on the display ensures that the diary will be as precise as possible. The latter allows a comparison between the manual diary and the recorded data.

Currently antimony or glass electrodes are most popular, although other types do exist (eg, capsules, ion-sensitive field-effect transistors, and plastic electrodes with polymeric membranes). Glass electrodes appear to be slightly more precise than antimony electrodes.[4] Glass electrodes with an internal reference electrode are preferable, but have an inconveniently large diameter (3.0-4.5 mm), making them less suitable for infants and small children. The problem is not so much the passage through the nostrils, but that an electrode of 4.0 mm diameter might influence esophageal function in a 6-month-old baby. In a recent unpublished study with combined pressure-pH recordings, it became clear that the larger the diameter of the electrodes, the more frequently the patient had to swallow. Frequent swallowing might have a normalizing effect on pH monitoring data, since the more the patient swallows, the more primary peristalsis will be induced and the better the esophageal clearance will be. The small diameter of glass micro-electrodes (approximately 1.2 mm) or antimony electrodes (approximately 2.1 mm) make them preferable for infants. Antimony electrodes with a diameter of approximately 1.5 mm exist for premature babies, but are too flexible for older infants.

Glass and antimony electrodes also inconveniently require an external cutaneous reference electrode, which is one more possible cause of erroneous measurement, resulting from transmucosal potential differences. It is important that the cutaneous electrode and the contact gel used for the calibration are identical to those used for the recording, since all these factors will influence the pH measured.[5] If the environmental temperature is high or the patient sweats profusely, the contact gel might dry, resulting in a less accurate conduction of the electric potential.

The cost of the electrodes depends both on the local situation and the frequency with which they are used. Antimony is cheaper, but more measurements can be performed with a glass electrode, resulting in a comparable cost in most situations.

Recently, antimony electrodes with a diameter of approximately 2.0 mm and an internal reference electrode have been developed (Synectics, Stockholm, Sweden; M.I.C., Solothurn, Switzerland). A comparative study between the latter type and glass microelectrodes provided comparable results (Table 15.3), suggesting this new type of electrode might become the electrode of choice in the future. It is accurate, thin, flexible, easy to place in the esophagus, and does not require a cutaneous reference electrode. The cost is also comparable to that of other electrodes (in Belgium, it is approximately \$35 per investigation for Synectics and \$20 for M.I.C.).

Whichever electrode is chosen, a medical center should use only one type, since each electrode has its own characteristics. One can tell by looking at the tracing if glass or antimony has been used.

The placement of the electrode has an important influence on the number and duration of the reflux episodes recorded. The closer the electrode is to the LES, the more acid reflux episodes are detected.[6] Several methods have been proposed to determine the location of the electrode: fluoroscopy, calculating the esophageal length according to Strobel's formula, manometry, and endoscopy. Ideally, as in adults, the electrode should be situated in reference to the manometrically determined LES. However, this has at least two inconveniences: 1) manometry in infants and children is time-consuming, invasive, or at least unpleasant if only performed to locate the LES (in most clinical situations LES pressure will not affect patient management); and 2) the electrode is located at a fixed distance from the LES, while the length of the esophagus increases from less than 10 cm in an infant to over 25 cm in an adult. Moreover, manometry cannot be performed at all centers. The European Society for Pediatric Gastroenterology and Nutrition Working Group on GER, therefore, recommended the use of fluoroscopy to place the electrode.[3] The radiation involved is minimal and the method can be applied in each center. As the tip of the electrode moves with

TABLE 15.3 Comparison of Antimony Electrode* and Glass Micro-electrode** in 20 Patients		
	Antimony	**Glass**
Reflux index	3.94 + 3.68	3.61 + 3.25
Number episodes	15.15 + 11.09	17.45 + 10.41
Mean pH/24 h	5.46 + 0.39	5.33 + 0.25

* With internal reference electrode and Gastrograph Mark II device

** With external reference electrode and Gastrograph Mark II device

and during respiration, it should be positioned so that it overlies the third vertebral body above the diaphragm throughout the respiration cycle. Dislocation by a curled electrode is also prevented with fluoroscopy.

All companies that sell devices provide software, although some devices can be directly connected to a printer without a personal computer. These simple printouts provide sufficient information for routine clinical use, including a tracing, the reflux index (percentage of the total recording time with a pH < 4.0), the number of episodes with a pH less than 4.0, the number of reflux episodes with a pH less than 4.0 that last longer than 5 minutes, and the duration of the longest reflux episode. Although the information required for a valid interpretation of pH monitoring data is minimal, some commercial programs have been developed to meet the requirements of researchers around the world. These programs offer several ways to visualize the results of the investigation. The user should decide which system is best.

In addition to the parameters listed above, commercial software should at least provide the calculation of the area below pH 4.0 acidity of refluxate as related to incidence of esophagitis, and the oscillatory index (a parameter that considers risk for erroneous interpretation).[3]

The information brochures about the software should be read carefully by the users, since definitions might vary substantially between different programs. For example, in one software program, a reflux episode starts whenever the pH drops below 4.0 and stops when the pH rises above 4.0 (for the calculation of the % time with pH < 4.0, and for the calculation of the "area < 4.0"). If the pH has not risen above 5.0 before dropping again below 4.0, however, the second drop below 4.0 is considered a prolongation of the previous episode and not a new reflux. In version 5.60C4 of Synectics (Stockholm, Sweden) software, a reflux episode begins when the pH drops below a user-defined level (eg, pH 4.0) and conditionally ends when the pH rises above that level. The pH must remain above the set level for a user-defined period of time (eg, 30 sec) in order

for the reflux episode to be considered finished. According to the software and the device, a reflux episode might start at pH 4.0, 3.99, or 3.9 and stop at 3.9, 3.99, 4.0, or 4.1. No evidence in the literature demonstrates that one definition might be preferable to another, but it is clear that the user should know how his or her software works. The differences in definition add substantially to confusion regarding discussions on normal ranges and data interpretation.

Different areas of interest—feeding, postprandial, and sleeping periods, as well as symptoms, and medication—should be made apparent on the tracing by color printing or some other method.[3] The relevant parameters can be shown in one table, and the exact onset and duration of the reflux episodes should be listed.

In a comparison of data recorded with one device and three different software programs—two from the same company and a "copy-program" from another company—the results varied significantly (Table 15.4). It is difficult or impossible to prove which software provided the better reading, although the original program was probably more exact. Since the copy was designed to provide results identical to the original program, very subtle differences in software appear to greatly influence the quality of data.

Patient Preparation

No special patient preparation is required for pH monitoring. To avoid nausea and vomiting, however, it is preferable not to introduce the electrode during the immediate postprandial period. Anesthetic gel can be placed on the electrode or the nasal mucosa to facilitate insertion, although this is not necessary.

Histamine (H_2) receptor antagonists should be stopped at least 3 to 4 days before a diagnostic pH monitoring, if the investigation is not being performed to evaluate the acid-buffering effect of the drug. Prokinetics should be stopped at least 48 hours before the pH monitoring.[3] The continuation or cessation of drugs such as prokinetics will also depend on the aim of the pH study.

TABLE 15.4 Dependability of Esophageal pH Monitoring Data on the Software Program (37 recordings)			
	Program 1*	**Program 2****	**Program 3*****
Reflux Index (%<4.0)	4.85 + 3.84	4.86 + 3.90	5.02 + 4.15
Number episodes/24 h	87.38 + 149.14	16.05 + 10.38	19.05 + 9.85
N* Ep>5 min/24 h	2.32 + 2.42	2.27 + 2.25	2.92 + 2.78
Duration Lo Ep (min)	18.54 + 18.07	17.45 + 16.84	15.33 + 11.17

* MIC-program for Gastrograph Mark II: 4 measurements/s; calculates 43200 medians/24 h
** MIC-program for Gastrograph Mark II: 4 measurements/s; calculates 360 medians/24 h
*** Program for Gastrograph Mark II, developed by another company

PATIENT-RELATED INFLUENCES: RECORDING CONDITIONS

Patient-related factors that influence pH monitoring results constitute one of the most controversial topics.[3] Whether these factors should be minimized and standardized or not is a difficult and ambiguous question. If the pH monitoring is performed as part of the diagnostic workup of a patient, it is interesting to study the patient during normal daily life, with recording conditions that are as unrestricted as possible. If the pH monitoring is performed as part of a clinical research project, however, recording conditions should be standardized. Although less patient-specific information will be obtained, data from different patients will be comparable.

Feeding, position, and activity are examples of patient-related factors that greatly influence pH monitoring data. The rate of GER during sleep is low. Esophageal acid exposure increases substantially in the 3 hours after a meal. This effect is related to meal size, since gastric distention is a potent stimulus for GER. Physical exertion has also been shown to provoke reflux.

Duration of the Recording

The duration of the recording should be as near as possible to 24 hours, and at least 16 to 18 hours, including a day and a night evaluation period.[3,7,8] If the pH monitoring is performed for diagnostic purposes, there is no indication for short-duration pH tests such as Tuttle and Bernstein tests, 3-hour postprandial recording, etc. Nighttime recording has been proposed as optimal for diagnosing peptic esophagitis because healthy controls rarely reflux during sleep. Using the nocturnal period of recumbency only, however, 25% to 50% of refluxers may be misclassified as normal. There is now substantial evidence that esophageal acid exposure is highest during the day in the majority of patients, probably because food ingestion and physical activity provokes GER. Controls also have more reflux upright than supine and more reflux awake than asleep.[9] The relation between esophagitis and nocturnal reflux is far from clear.[10-12]

Feeding

Feeding during pH monitoring is still an area of controversy. Although it seems logical to forbid the intake of acidic foods and drinks, so many foods and beverages have a pH less than 5.0 (cola drinks, fruit juice, tea, soup, etc), that the result is a restricted diet. A restricted diet might alter the patient's normal daily habits in such a way that the investigation is no longer performed in physiologic conditions. Very hot beverages (eg, coffee or tea) or chilled food (eg, ice cream) should be forbidden because electrodes are temperature sensitive.[3] It is unclear if adults should be forbidden to smoke.

In infants, it is sometimes suggested that one or several feedings should be replaced with apple juice during pH monitoring.[13] This would certainly partially solve the problem of gastric anacidity after a milk feeding, but apple juice has a pH of about 4.0 and a very rapid gastric emptying rate. The best policy is to allow an unrestricted diet except for avoidance of very hot or chilled beverages and food. Although the ingestion of acidic beverages might simulate a reflux episode, the duration of ingestion is limited to a few minutes and most of the time it is irrelevant to the total 24-hour data. To minimize this negative influence on the data, these false reflux episodes can be eliminated from the data with the help of a precise diary. These standards apply only to diagnostic investigations. For research, all factors possibly influencing the pH data should be controlled and standardized as much as possible.

The influence of a particular food on the incidence of acid GER-episodes detected by pH monitoring might be opposite to its influence on the incidence of reflux episodes: a high-fat meal is known to provoke GER because of its delayed gastric emptying. The duration of postprandial gastric anacidity after a high-fat meal is prolonged, probably resulting in fewer acid reflux episodes detected by pH monitoring.[14] Some drugs influencing gastric emptying (eg, prokinetic agents) have a comparable effect on pH monitoring data. These drugs enhance gastric emptying, shorten the period of postprandial gastric anacidity, and prolong the periods during which acid GER can be detected.

Position

In asymptomatic adult volunteers, the gastroesophageal junction is more competent in the supine than in the upright position.[15] The recumbent posture fosters an increased duration of acid exposure if compared with the upright position, illustrating the importance of gravity.[16] The influence of an increased intra-abdominal pressure on the incidence of GER is illustrated by the detection of more acid reflux in the sitting position than lying down. Infants have up to four times more refluxes in a chalasia chair than when lying down.[17]

Contradictory opinions exist nowadays about the optimal position for infants. Orenstein et al[18] suggested that prone is the preferred position, since crying time is decreased when compared to the supine position. Different papers provide evidence that prone-anti-Trendelenburg 30° is effective in the treatment of GER, although this position is difficult to apply correctly because infants must be tied up in their beds. Current literature on sudden infant death syndrome (SIDS), however, suggests that infant mortality would decrease if all infants slept in the supine position.

Reproducibility

Different studies suggest that pH monitoring results are reproducible. Boesby[19] performed ten 12-hour registrations in one normal eupeptic volunteer with reproducible results. Bontempo et al[20] published data on duplicated recordings within 5 days in 20 subjects with reflux symptoms, showing a correlation in 16. In adults, the correlation coefficient for the reflux index on two consecutive days with antimony electrodes and in nonstandardized recording conditions is 0.87.[21] In 30 infants, a correlation coefficient of 0.95, ranging from 0.87 in pathologic to 0.98 in normal tracings, was obtained.[22]

PROVOCATIVE TESTING

The first reports on the clinical use of pH monitoring concerned esophageal tests of short duration. Tuttle and Grossman[23] developed the standard acid reflux test. This test was modified by Skinner and Booth[24] and Kantrowitz et al,[25] demonstrating that pH tests can contribute to define abnormal GER. The Tuttle test had a reported sensitivity of 70%.[26] After great initial enthusiasm for this test, criticism became more and more common. The test is unphysiologic because it requires intragastric instillation of acid and various artificial maneuvers to raise intragastric pressure. In the early 1980s it was reported that the false-positive rate might be as high as 4% to 20%, and the false-negative rate as high as 40%.[27-29]

Bernstein and Baker[30] demonstrated in 1958 that heartburn could be provoked by infusing diluted hydrochloric acid into the esophagus in susceptible individuals. This test was shown to be 100% positive in reflux patients.[31] A modified Bernstein test was used to illustrate the relation between GER, apnea, and stridor, and between nonspecific chest pain and GER.[32,33]

Short-term tests are not indicated in the diagnosis of GER disease, but provocative testing can be used in particular conditions to demonstrate the relation between GER and specific symptoms (eg, bradycardia in relation to the presence of esophageal acid). However, provocative testing is inconvenient because conditions are unphysiologic. The latter might be the cause of some discrepancies in the literature. Ramet et al[34] showed a prolongation of the R-R interval in infants during provocative testing with acid instillation in the esophagus, while others[35,36] could not reproduce these findings in 24-hour recordings under physiologic conditions.

DATA ANALYSIS

The analysis of a 24-hour recording depends partly on the indication of the investigation. The following parameters should be analyzed and printed:[3]

1. A pH tracing of the whole recording.

2. The percentage of time that pH is under the cut-off limit during the entire investigation. The number of episodes, the number of episodes lasting more than 5 minutes, and the duration of the longest episode all express the same phenomenon, and are therefore of limited value. If possible, the program should correct the data according to the drift of the electrode demonstrated by the calibration at the beginning and end of the pH monitoring.

3. The time and duration of reflux episodes for the entire investigation, including periods of sleep and wakefulness, fasting, postprandial (120 min after the end of a feeding), and feeding periods, as well as body position. An exact time relation should be provided to enable a time-related analysis of the diary. To facilitate this, a printout of actual pH data from any period of interest should be possible. It should also be possible

to mark any periods of interest for separate analysis.

4. The area under pH 4.0. This parameter provides additional information on acid exposure and thus the relative risk to the patient for peptic esophagitis.

5. The oscillatory index. This gives some idea of errors that result from a fixed pH cut-off.

6. Alkaline shifts. Shifts with a pH above 7.5 should be counted. If these episodes exceed normal limits, alkaline reflux should be investigated further.[37]

Normal Ranges

Although pH monitoring has recently been reported as the gold standard of reflux investigations, its limitations should not be forgotten. It only measures the pH in the esophagus, and not GER. Since no GER investigation consistently provides a clear-cut discrimination between normal and abnormal, there is no reason why pH monitoring results should do so. Various complex reflux scoring systems (eg, Jolley, De-Meester, Branicki, Boix-Ochoa, and Kaye) have been developed, most of which—together with the parameters usually measured or calculated—have been developed for assessing reflux esophagitis in adults. In marked contrast to these complex scoring systems is the simple recommendation by some investigators that total acid exposure time (ie, reflux index) should be regarded as the most important, if not the only, variable in clinical practice.[33]

A correct interpretation starts with a visual appreciation of the entire pH tracing, which is certainly subjective and difficult to standardize. Nevertheless, it is of utmost importance. From all classic parameters, the acid exposure time is the most relevant. The other classic parameters are closely related to the acid exposure time, which is logical because they are based on the same boundaries (ie, the number of reflux episodes with pH < 4.0, the number of episodes lasting more than 5 min, and the duration of the longest episode). There is a good correlation between all four parameters.[38]

The parameters should also be automatically calculated for different periods of interest: sleep, wakefulness, feeding, postprandial, fasting, and body position. An exact time relation between atypical manifestations (eg, cough) and changes in pH—not necessarily a drop in pH below 4.0—should be established. The response time that an electrode takes to reach 95% of the exact pH is about 5 seconds.

The area below pH 4.0,[39] a parameter that considers the acidity of reflux episodes,[38] correlates better than the reflux index with the presence of reflux esophagitis. A major factor that interferes with a correct interpretation of pH monitoring results is the "yes" or "no" interpretation of the data by computer software. A pH of 4.01 will be regarded as normal, whereas a pH of 3.99 will be considered as evidence of acid in the esophagus. Minimal changes of esophageal pH thus result in totally different interpretations, although there is no difference in clinical meaning. Therefore, we developed the oscillatory index, a parameter that measures the time the pH oscillates around 4.0.[40]

Normal ranges proposed by one group can be used by another only if the investigations are performed and interpreted in a comparable manner; the materials and methodology must be identical. There will inevitably be an overlap between normal and abnormal data. However, for some individuals and for some clinical situations, it is more important to relate events such as coughing, wheezing, or apnea to pH changes than to know if global results are within the normal range or not. It should be borne in mind that normal ranges for a group are not always applicable to an individual.

Alkaline GER

Single esophageal pH monitoring cannot detect alkaline reflux, although cut-off limits have been published that are comparable to the normal ranges for acid GER, above which alkaline GER should be suspected.[37] There is no agreement on the incidence of alkaline GER. Some investigators suggest double recordings (ie, one electrode in the stomach and one in the esophagus, or both electrodes in the esophagus) or the aspiration and analysis of the material that refluxed into the esophagus for the presence of bile salts. The newly developed Bilitec 2000 ambulatory bile reflux recording system from Synectics might provide an answer to this question.

CONTRIBUTION OF RESULTS TO PATIENT MANAGEMENT

Esophageal pH monitoring results will affect management of patients with unusual presentations, since the latter is the main indication to perform the investigation.[3] In other situations, pH monitoring results will not often directly lead to a different patient approach, but abnormal results provide reasons to perform other procedures, such as upper gastrointestinal endoscopy or contrast radiography.

If the purpose of pH monitoring is to evaluate treatment, the results—if not improved with treatment—will contribute to a change in the therapeutic approach.

COMBINED PRESSURE-pH RECORDING: APPLICATIONS IN PEDIATRICS

Esophageal pH monitoring is often considered an investigational technique for studying esophageal motility, although it does not actually measure motility. Esophageal pH monitoring only measures the pH in the esophagus.

That the information from pH monitoring is indirectly related to GER and esophageal motility is far too often overlooked. For a practical patient-related diagnostic approach, pH monitoring is sufficient in most situations. However, if the goal is understanding the pathophysiologic mechanisms causing GER and/or clearing the reflux out of the esophagus, combined pressure and pH recording could be a more appropriate technique. The relation between reflux and esophageal peristalsis before, during, and after a reflux episode might provide the answer to why some patients with GER pathology vomit and others develop chronic asthma or apnea (Fig. 15.1).

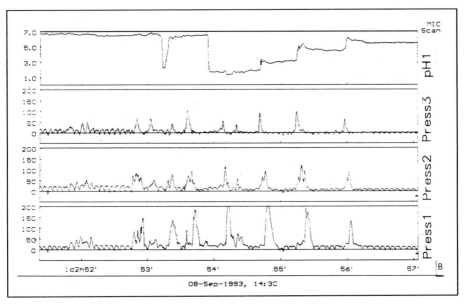

Fig. 15.1 Combined pressure (three-level recording) and pH monitoring.

CONCLUSION

In clinical diagnostic situations, the indication for pH monitoring is often a decision of common sense; the investigation is of interest when the result will change the management of the patient with regurgitations and emesis. Esophageal pH monitoring is also of interest in patients whose symptoms suggest occult GER. The duration of the investigation should be between 18 and 24 hours, and the recording conditions should be as unrestricted as possible, on condition that a diary is scrupulously kept. In research, the recording conditions should be standardized.

The contributions of Saskia de Pont, Wim Mertens, and the Nursery staff of the Academic Children's Hospital in Brussels, Belgium were very much appreciated.

REFERENCES

1. Vandenplas Y, Ashkenazi A, Belli D, et al. A proposition for the diagnosis and treatment of gastro-oesophageal reflux disease in children: a report from a working group on gastro-oesophageal reflux disease. *Eur J Pediatr* 1993;152:704-11.

2. Vandenplas Y, DeWolf D, Sacre L. Influence of xanthines on gastroesophageal reflux in infants at

risk for SIDS. *Pediatrics* 1986;77:807-10.

3. Vandenplas Y, Belli D, Boige N, et al. A standardized protocol for the methodology of esophageal pH monitoring and interpretation of the data for the diagnosis of gastro-esophageal reflux. *J Pediatr Gastroenterol Nutr* 1992;14:467-71.

4. Emde C, Hopert R, Riecken ED. Basic principles of pH registration. *Neth J Med* 1989;34:S3-9.

5. Vandenplas Y, ed. *Oesophageal pH Monitoring for Gastro-oesophageal Reflux in Infants and Children.* Chichester, England: J Wiley & Sons, 1992.

6. Cravens E, Lehman G, O'Connor K, Flueckiger J, Kopecky K. Placement of esophageal pH probes 5 cm above the lower esophageal sphincter: can we get closer? *Gastroenterology* 1987;92:1357.

7. Vandenplas Y, Casteels A, Naert M, Derde MP, Blecker U. Abbreviated oesophageal pH monitoring in infants. *Eur J Pediatr* (In press).

8. Belli DC, Le Coultre D. Comparison in a same patient of short-, middle-, and long-term pH metry recordings in the presence or absence of gastro-esophageal reflux. *Pediatr Res* 1989;26:269.

9. Vandenplas Y, DeWolf D, Deneyer M, Sacré L. Incidence of gastro-esophageal reflux in sleep, awake, fasted, and postcibal periods in asymptom-

atic and symptomatic infants. *J Pediatr Gastroenterol Nutr* 1988;7:177-81.

10. Schindbeck NE, Heinrich C, Konig A, Demdorfer A, Page F, Müller-Lissner SA. Optimal thresholds, sensitivity, and specificity of long-term pH metry for the detection of gastroesophageal reflux disease. *Gastroenterology* 1985;93:85-90.

11. Robertson D. Patterns of reflux in complicated oesophagitis. *Gut* 1987;2B:1484-8.

12. De Caestecker JS, Blackwell JN, Pryde A, Heading RC. Daytime gastro-oesophageal reflux is important in oesophagitis. *Gut* 1987;28:519-26.

13. Tolia V, Kaufmann RE. Comparison of evaluation of gastroesophageal reflux in infants using different feedings during intraesophageal pH monitoring. *J Pediatr Gastroenterol Nutr* 1990;10:426-9.

14. Vandenplas Y, Sacre L, Loeb H. Effects of formula feeding on gastric acidity time and oesophageal pH monitoring data. *Eur J Pediatr* 1988;148:152-4.

15. DeMeester TR, Johnson LF, Joseph GJ, Toscano MS, Hall AW, Skinner DB. Patterns of gastroesophageal reflux in health and disease. *Ann Surg* 1976;184:459-66.

16. Orenstein SR, Whitington PF. Positioning for prevention of infant gastroesophageal reflux. *Pediatrics* 1982;69:768-72.

17. Orenstein SR, Whitington PF, Orenstein DM. The infant seat as treatment for gastroesophageal reflux. *N Engl J Med* 1983;309:709-12.

18. Orenstein SR. Effects on behavior state of prone versus seated positioning for infants with gastroesophageal reflux. *Pediatrics* 1990;85:765-7.

19. Boesby S. Continuous oesophageal pH recording and acid-clearing test: study of reproducibility. *Scand J Gastroenterol* 1977;12:245-7.

20. Bontempo I, Corriazziari E, Cugini P, Tesoni M, Torsoli A. Time-related variability of gastroesophageal reflux episodes. Presented at Third European Symposium on Gastrointestinal Motility. A14;1986. Abstract.

21. Johnsson F, Joelsson B. Reproducibility of ambulatory oesophageal pH monitoring. *Gut* 1988;29:886-9.

22. Vandenplas Y, Goyvaerts H, Helven R, Sacre L. Reproducibility of continuous 24-hour oesophageal pH monitoring in infants and children. *Gut* 1990;31:374-7.

23. Tuttle SG, Grossman MI. Detection of gastroesophageal reflux by simultaneous measurement of intraluminal pressure and pH. *Proc Soc Exp Biol Med* 1958;98:225-30.

24. Skinner DB, Booth DJ. Assessment of distal esophageal function in patients with hiatal hernia and/or gastroesophageal reflux. *Ann Surg* 1970;172:627-36.

25. Kantrowitz PA, Corson JG, Fleischer DJ, Skinner DB. Measurement of gastroesophageal reflux. *Gastroenterology* 1969;56:666-74.

26. Kaul B, Petersen H, Grette K, Myrvold HE. Scintigraphy, pH measurements, and radiography in the evaluation of gastroesophageal reflux. *Scand J Gastroenterol* 1985;20:289-94.

27. Arasu TS, Wyllie R, Fitzgerald JF, et al. Gastroesophageal reflux in infants and children: comparative accuracy of diagnostic methods. *J Pediatr* 1980;96:798-803.

28. Holloway RH, McCallum RW. New diagnostic techniques in esophageal disease. In: Cohen S, Soloway RD, eds. *Diseases of the Esophagus.* New York, NY: Churchill Livingstone 1982;75-95.

29. Richter JE, Castell DO. Gastroesophageal reflux disease: pathogenesis, diagnosis, and therapy. *Ann Intern Med* 1982;97:93-103.

30. Bernstein IM, Baker IA. A clinical test for esophagitis. *Gastroenterology* 1958;34:760-81.

31. Benz LJ. A comparison of clinical measurements of gastroesophageal reflux. *Gastroenterology* 1972;62:1-3.

32. Herbst JJ, Minton SD, Book LS. Gastroesophageal reflux causing respiratory distress and apnea in newborn infants. *J Pediatr* 1979;95:763-8.

33. Berezin S. Use of the intraesophageal acid perfusion test in provoking non-specific chest pain in children. *J Pediatr* 1989;115:709-12.

34. Ramet J, Egreteau L, Curzi-Dascalova L, Escourrau P, Dehan M, Gaultier C. Cardia, respiratory, and arousal responses to an esophageal acid infusion test

in near-term infants during active sleep. *J Pediatr Gastroenterol Nutr* 1992;15:135-40.

35. Kahn A, Rebuffat E, Sottiaux M, Dufour D, Cadranel S, Reitere F. Lack of temporal relation between acid reflux in the proximal oesophagus and cardiorespiratory events in sleeping infants. *Eur J Pediatr* 1992;151:208-12.

36. Suys B, DeWolf D, Hauser B, Blecker U, Vandenplas Y. Bradycardia and gastroesophageal reflux in term and preterm infants: is there any relation? *J Pediatr Gastroenterol Nutr* (In press).

37. Vandenplas Y, Loeb H. Alkaline gastroesophageal reflux in infants. *J Pediatr Gastroenterol Nutr* 1991:12:448-52.

38. Vandenplas Y, Goyvaerts H, Helven R, Sacre L. Gastroesophageal reflux, as assessed by 24-hour pH monitoring, in 509 health infants screened for SIDS-risk. *Pediatrics* 1991;88:834-40.

39. Vandenplas Y, Franckx-Goossens A, Pipeleers-Marichal M, Derde MP, Sacre L. "Area under pH 4.0": advantages of a new parameter in the interpretation of esophageal pH monitoring data in infants. *J Pediatr Gastroenterol Nutr* 1989;9:34-9.

40. Vandenplas Y, Lepoudre R, Helven R. Dependability of esophageal pH monitoring data in infants on cut-off limits: the oscillatory index. *J Pediatr Gastroenterol Nutr* 1990;11:304-9.

CHAPTER
16
Transit Tests

MICHELE SCAILLON, SAMY CADRANEL

Normal gastrointestinal transit is characterized by an appropriately paced movement of material from one point to another. The final state of the material depends on the speed as well as the mechanical and chemical conditions encountered at each segment of the gastrointestinal tract. Transit disorders can cause severe diseases that lead to life-threatening complications, but more often they are responsible for individual or social discomfort. Transit disorders are usually underrated, misunderstood, or not recognized by the physician. The patient is left alone with no proper solution to his problem.

Abnormal transit can lead to retrosternal pain, pyrosis, belching, vomiting, bloating, abdominal pain, diarrhea, and constipation. These symptoms point to different levels of the gastrointestinal tract where a disturbed segmental transit can occur. They can be originated either by an organic obstacle (intrinsic, extrinsic, or intramural), neuromuscular disease, functional disorders following dietetic errors, or emotional stress. All the segments of the digestive tract can be involved. The influence on the total transit time is usually proportional to the duration of the normal transit time in the affected segment.

The success of the different methods of investigation that are available depends on the accuracy, reliability, and reproducibility of the technique, the availability and cost of the procedure, as well as respect of the physiology and comfort of the patient. The ideal transit study should be easily interpretable and properly standardized. In reality, however, too many parameters are involved and the ideal protocol for transit study has yet to be designed. Among the techniques used to evaluate motility disorders, some are designed to directly study the transit time of different segments (eg, esophageal, gastric, orocecal, colon, and total). Other tests measure motor patterns or electrical activities, thereby indirectly assessing the quality of transit in a particular segment.

INVESTIGATIONAL TECHNIQUES
Radiology

Plain radiologic films of the abdomen, widely used in pediatrics, can help to illuminate the quality of transit by the distribution pattern of such natural contrast media as air, liquids, or solids (eg, food or feces). Contrast media, such as barium and hydrosoluble molecules, are generally used to explore anatomic features of the gastrointestinal tract and can also give an idea of the transit time. Radiopaque pellets of different shapes mixed with the food progress along the alimentary canal, acting as markers that are easily detected by plain radiologic film of the abdomen. Cineradiography dynamically records the progression of any contrast medium.

Advantages. Radiologic techniques are widely available and provide mainly topographic anatomic data, which are almost impossible to obtain by other techniques.

Disadvantages. Radiology carries the risk of radiation exposure, although the new digitalized facilities have considerably reduced the doses. Only a few short motor events can be observed. Radiology describes motor events elicited by intraluminal distention due to contrast medium, which are not always comparable to those induced by food. Radiology detects wall movements caused by contraction of the circular muscle layer, but is inadequate in the investigation of longitudinal muscle-layer contractions.[1] Finally, radiologic observations are essentially qualitative and do not usually allow quantification of data.

Ultrasonography

Real-time ultrasonography follows the motion of liquids or solid particles leaving the stomach or spilling over the gastroesophageal junction.[2] Measuring the changes in the dimensions of the antrum after a standardized meal reliably assesses transit time through the stomach.

Advantages. Ultrasound is a noninvasive, painless procedure in which standard meals very similar to the patient's usual food are used. Physiologic conditions are therefore closely mimicked.

Disadvantages. Ultrasound is time-consuming, and requires a motivated, skilled radiologist. It is not always feasible because air bubbles, which are frequent in the stomach, represent an obstacle to the ultrasound. This technique is described in Chapter 20.

Radioactive Isotopes

A radioactive isotope is incorporated into a compound mixed in a solid or liquid meal, and travels through the digestive tract with the food. Its activity is detected with a gamma camera and the results are given after processing the computer-generated time-activity curves for the different regions of interest. The isotope can also be used to label nondigestible bran particles or pellets that act as markers.

Advantages. Radiation exposure is minimal compared with cineradiography. This technique is suitable for the study of the different segments considered as separate regions of interest. The radioisotope in standardized meals does not interfere with the natural digestion of the food.

Disadvantages. In some cases, it may be difficult to ascribe radioactivity to a specific organ because of overlap between different segments of the gastrointestinal tract. The patient is also required to lie motionless under a gamma camera. Scintigraphy is described in detail in Chapter 18.

Nonabsorbable Markers

Carmine red and other colored markers have been used for many years to indicate the beginning and end of stool collections, such as in balance studies of fat and nitrogen.[3] These markers are assumed to travel along the digestive tract with the food and indicate the appropriate fecal material to collect for metabolic studies. Carmine red and other color-based markers, such as brilliant blue and charcoal, are still used[4] for evaluation of total, or "mouth-to-anus," transit time, especially in developing countries where other techniques requiring costly equipment are not available. Though helpful in this particular context, these markers are not precise and cannot provide information on segmental transit time. Intubation of a specific organ—usually the stomach—to collect residual fluids has been widely used for evaluating gastric emptying disorders in premature, newborn, and sick infants.

Advantages. Tests with nonabsorbable markers are simple to perform and require little or no costly equipment.

Disadvantages. These are imprecise methods and must be considered only as rough estimations of total transit time. The assessment of gastric emptying by nasogastric intubation and collection of gastric residual fluid is an invasive technique that may interfere with the normal motility of the upper gastrointestinal tract.

Blood and Breath Analysis

A marker is given orally to the patient either in a water solution or mixed in a test meal. It is then assayed in the blood or expired breath at a predetermined time, which is chosen based on the expectation of arrival at its absorption site. Acetaminophen, absorbed in the duodenum, marks the gastric emptying time. Salazopyrine, split into its two components by the colic flora, can be used as a marker of the orocecal transit time. Another application of this principle is the widely used hydrogen breath test. The non-absorbed portion of the tested carbohydrate reaches the colon, where it is metabolized by resident bacterial flora. The subsequent excretion of hydrogen is assayed in the expired breath. Instead of assaying H_2 excretion for orocecal transit time, other techniques use the stable isotope labeling of carbohydrates and ^{13}C mass spectrometric assay in the expired breath for assessing gastric emptying.

Advantages. The simplicity of collecting samples (painless for breath) makes these noninvasive techniques appropriate for pediatric clinical gastroenterology.

Disadvantages. Reproducibility is influenced by mucosal integrity, motility, bacterial flora, and use of antibiotics. Mass spectrometric assay of stable isotopes is not widely available because of cost.

Electrical Signals

Impedance epigastrography (IE) and applied potential tomography (APT) are used to follow gastric emptying after a meal (usually liquid or semisolid) by means of skin electrodes that measure the changes in electrical resistivity or impedance. Impedance epigastrography uses only four electrodes and gives a simple curve, but APT requires many circumferential electrodes on the abdomen and more complicated equipment. Applied potential tomography, however, is less vulnerable to artefacts produced by movement.

Intraluminal electrical impedance is a novel method that uses several electrodes attached by a thin, flexible plastic tube to an impedance voltage transducer outside the body. The transit of a bolus through the different segments can then be studied by the change in electrical impedance between the electrodes.[5]

Advantages. These relatively inexpensive, noninvasive techniques assess the effect of drugs[6] in volunteers as well as in diabetic neuropathy.[7] Validated results seem comparable to those of isotopic techniques.[8]

Disadvantages. The type of test meal is a limitation because solids are not suitable for this investigation.[9] The accuracy of the method is susceptible to changes in gastric acid secretion. For this reason, subjects are usually given a histamine-H_2 antagonist before the test.[10]

SEGMENTARY TRANSIT TIMES
Esophagus

Radiologic, endoscopic, and manometric studies are the traditional means of evaluating symptoms suggestive of esophageal dysfunction. Endoscopy, however, is mainly aimed at investigating the mucosa and provides no information about transit. Manometry mainly gives information about sphincters and measures the amplitude, duration, and velocity of contractions. In children, 24-hour esophageal manometry is a promising tool that can best study peristaltic movements in correlation with swallows and symptoms (See Chapter 11).[11]

Barium radiography is the most widely used method to examine esophageal structure and function. Cinefluorography is the preferred radiologic method for evaluating function, because it provides a qualitative or semiquantitative assessment. Barium radiographs may show the characteristic "beak deformity" of the lower esophageal sphincter in achalasia, or demonstrate tertiary contractions associated with diffuse esophageal spasm. The assessment of swallowing by administering barium mixed with solid foods is difficult to interpret and is too reliant on subjective evaluation to be of clinical value.

Because of its universal availability, barium radiographs are still considered the first test in the evaluation of gastroesophageal reflux, even if other techniques (eg, 24-h pH monitoring) are more sensitive and specific.

Esophageal Transit Scintigraphy. Since 1972,[11] [99mTc] pertechnetate has been used to monitor swallowing. Several radioisotopes can assess the presence of gastroesophageal reflux, demonstrate pulmonary aspiration, and evaluate esophageal contractility as well as gastric emptying. The major advantage of esophageal scintigraphy compared with continuous pH-metry is the detection of nonacid reflux.[12] The only risk of esophageal transit scintigraphy is the radiation dose, although it compares favorably with the radiation dose for fluoroscopy.[13] Calculations for swallowed [99mTc] sulfur colloid in the pediatric population show significant increases in the number of rads per μCi-h transmitted between source and target organs. With [99mTc], the radiation dose for newborns is more than ten times that for adults, although these are results obtained with 300 μCi doses in adults, whereas only a half-dose is used in infants.[14]

Because of its ultrashort half-life, the radiation dose is much lower with [31mKrypton]. Although it is expensive, it is the most suitable tracer for detecting esophageal transit impairment due to negligible irradiation and high-quality images that allow any swallowing artefact to be recognized. The technique is useful for detecting transit delay in the follow-up of peptic and caustic esophagitis[15] and after surgical procedures involving the gastroesophageal area. Asynchronous peristaltic movements occurring in neuromuscular disease can best be examined with esophageal transit scintigraphy.[12] Because the esophageal transit time of a single bolus may not be comparable to that of multiple swallows for the detection of transit abnormality, radionuclide esophageal transit tests should be performed using a single, swallowed bolus.[14] The child is asked to ingest 10 ml of a 5% glucose solution containing [81mKr] (total activity of 6 to 8 μCu) in a single swallow.

The progression of the bolus through the esophagus is monitored with a gamma-camera and computer system. The data processing allows the determination of a mean transit time and also of regional transit time that corresponds to the upper, middle, and inferior thirds of the esophagus. Esophageal transit is considered normal when the entire radioactive bolus passes through the esophagus after swallowing and enters the stomach in less than 8 seconds, leaving no residual activity in the esophageal area. Table 16.1 demonstrates the three scores that can be defined in the presence of residual activity.[15]

Stomach

Delayed gastric emptying is more frequently suspected than acceleration (ie, dumping) and can be the cause of such common symptoms as epigastric pain, pyrosis, early satiety, bloating, and nausea. Many of these symptoms are part of "nonulcer dyspepsia." Gastroparesis in the premature newborn, or immediately following GI surgery, leads to transitory delays in the gastric emptying of liquids. In the diabetic patient, gastroparesis due to intestinal neuropathy may induce digestive discomfort and instability of glycemic control.[16] Delayed gastric emptying of solids has been reported in adults

TABLE 16.1 Delayed Esophageal Transit (ET)

	Residual Activity (%)	Duration (seconds)
Light ET delay	<5	>8 - <15
Moderate	<5	>15
	>5	<20
Severe	>5	>20

with gastroesophageal reflux and dyspepsia.[17]

Gastric transit time is influenced by the volume and nature of the test meal, including its osmolality, lipid and protein contents, caloric density,[18] and physical properties (ie, liquids, solid food, or nondigestible solids, which leave the stomach during phase III of the migrating motor complex [MMC]).[19]

To minimize variability, the test meal should be standardized according to the patient's age and the feeding habits of the population to which he or she belongs. Details about the milk composition are often lacking in studies dealing with gastric emptying in infants. In a recent study, we found differences in the gastric emptying rate of the same infants, studied echographically on two subsequent days, first with the usual and then with a modified, low-fat, fiber-enriched, thickened formula. Detailed composition of volume, fat, carbohydrates, nitrogen, fiber, osmolality, and degree of protein hydrolyzation should be stated in any study related to gastric emptying in infants. However, factors such as stress, physical activity, and body position can be difficult to control and will influence gastric transit. Therefore, noninvasive methods are preferred. A local, age-matched control population should be included in any clinical study unless the patients can be used as their own controls.

TESTS OF GASTRIC TRANSIT

More than any other technique, scintigraphy with radioactive isotopes is considered the gold standard for studying the gastric transit of solids and liquids. Echography of the antrum is noninvasive and is becoming more popular in pediatrics. These two techniques are described in Chapters 18 and 20.

Radiology

Gastric dilation, residual food or bezoars, and barium retention strongly suggest gastric emptying delay, whereas the passage of the contrast medium proves the absence of an anatomic obstacle. Normal evacuation of the contrast medium, however, does not rule out functional abnormalities of the transit time for digestible solids or liquids.

The presence of a gastric phase 3 of the MMC can be assessed by following up the gastric emptying of indigestible solid particles of more than 2-mm diameter.[20]

Colored Markers

Colored markers such as phenol red, given orally, are collected in the duodenum by means of a nasojejunal tube.[21] The color of the aspirated fluid indicates the gastric transit time. This is an invasive technique that influences the motor activity of the stomach and is not suitable for the study of solids.[22]

Absorbable Markers

Acetaminophen. A dose of 1.5 g of acetaminophen included in a 200-ml, high caloric, pasty meal is absorbed in the duodenum and assayed in the plasma at 45 minutes. In the normal adult, the plasma concentration is 9.4 ± 3.6 mcg/ml.[23] In one study, plasma samples were taken at 20, 40, and 60 minutes with a plasma peak at 40 minutes.[24]

Labeled Bicarbonate. ^{13}C-labeled bicarbonate converted to $^{13}CO_2$ through the action of gastric acid is rapidly absorbed by the gastrointestinal tract, excreted in the lungs, and assayed by mass spectrometry. Unfortunately this noninvasive method is expensive and seems unreliable.[25]

Labeled Octanoic Acid. Octanoic acid is readily absorbed in the proximal small intestine as a medium-chain fatty acid and transported via the portal vein to the liver, where it preferentially undergoes hepatic oxidation to CO_2. The ^{13}C-octanoic acid breath test is based on the solubility of the labeled fatty-acid isotope in the yolk of an egg. Since gastric emptying of the meal limits the rate in the whole process, the rate of labeled CO_2 excretion in breath is correlated with the emptying rate of the solid phase of the meal.[26] With the same caloric intake of 250 kcal, children showed a prolonged half emptying time ($T_{1/2}$) compared with adults (122 ± 65 min vs 76 ± 26 min). When the same children were given a 150-kcal feed,[27] their $T_{1/2}$ was similar to that of adults (65 ± 25 min).

Ambulatory Radioisotopic Study

The use of radioisotopes such as ^{99m}Tc-labeled is convenient in children because the absorbed radiation doses are lower than those in radiographic procedures. Immobilizing a child in a supine position, however, is often difficult. The possibility of performing adulatory radioisotopic studies using a cadmium tellurite crystal as sensor of the radioisotopic activity coupled with a recording device (Memolog 400, Simonsen Medical, Randers, Denmark) is currently under evaluation and has shown promising results. Since this device allows a 2-channel recording, two CdTe sensors can be attached to the child's abdominal skin in front of the stomach and the terminal ileum. After ingesting a ^{99m}Tc-labeled standard meal (either the usual formula in infants or a hamburger with mashed potatoes in children), the child is allowed normal activity during the 2 hours' recording of the activity curve (Cadranel, unpublished data). Newer, smaller CdTe sensors are currently under development.

SMALL INTESTINE

Abnormal transit time can be either too rapid, such as that in thyrotoxicosis, toddler's diarrhea, and intestinal infections, or too slow, as is found in some idiopathic constipation, neuro- or myopathic pseudo-obstructions, and cystic fibrosis.[28] These disturbances can lead to absorptive defects.

Hydrogen Breath Test

Hydrogen breath tests are routinely used in pediatrics because of their innocuousness and simplicity. For transit-time studies, lactulose is the nonabsorbable carbohydrate substrate more frequently used. Its excretion in breath samples corresponds to mouth to cecum transit time. The procedure is simple: 30 ml of end-expiratory-air samples are collected through an adapted mouthpiece into a syringe and assayed for hydrogen content by gas chromatography. Currently, commercially available devices using an electrochemical cell provide immediately readable, accurate results comparable to those obtained by gas chromatography. In infants, proper collection of breath samples is often difficult. A

technique in which the child is allowed a few expirations or crying into a mask with a unidirectional valve attached to the syringe is preferable. Others have used a perspex hood.[29]

To avoid transit time acceleration by the osmotic laxative effect of lactulose, only trace doses are given. Crystalline lactulose powder 2.0 mg/kg body weight, or 0.3 ml/kg of the commercial solution Duphalac, which also contains small amounts of galactose (<11%) and lactose (<6%) can be used.

Other substrates can also be given. Lactitol, an alcohol derived from lactose, is less sweet than lactulose and its fermentation produces higher amounts of H_2.[30] Baked beans can be used in standardized meals. Although more physiologic, they are rarely given to children. In the adult, orocecal transit time averages between 4 and 4½ hours.[31]

Many attempts at standardization of the lactulose-hydrogen breath have been reported, but because of the many factors involved, it still remains difficult. Variables to consider include:

1. *Quality of colonic flora:* This can be easily altered by laxatives or antibiotics.[32] For the same reason, small-bowel transit times are not possible in patients with suspected bacterial overgrowth such as that found in blind-loop syndromes or pseudo-obstruction.

2. *Fasting state:* To standardize the test, patients are often studied in a fasting state because the previous meal can influence the breath-H_2-excretion baseline and GI motility. Avoiding nonabsorbable carbohydrates (including lactose in suspected lactose-intolerant children) on the day preceding the test is advised.

3. *Meal:* Fasting activity of the gastrointestinal tract is not interrupted by oral or duodenal administration of lactulose diluted in water. This explains the variability of the test in the fasting condition (155 ± 26 min in MMC phase 1, compared with 94 ± 14 min in phase 3), and the more constant results when a meal which interrupts the fasting pattern is given.[33]

4. *Presentation:* Introducing the substrate

in a solid or liquid form can modify the transit time, probably because of the differences in gastric emptying time. In a study of adults by G. Vantrappen, MD, (personal communication), the results varied considerably when the substrate was introduced in cakes (Table 16.2).

5. *Dilution:* The volume and concentration of the substrate are important (see stomach) as shown in studies[34] measuring transit times with different dilutions of a fixed dose of 10 g lactulose in children from 5 to 17 years of age (Table 16.3).

When lactulose doses are adapted to the child's weight, transit time decreases with age, but this seems to be biased by the fact that small-bowel length is not perfectly correlated with body weight or age.[35]

6. *Partial lactose malabsorption:* In infants, this condition can also modify the lactulose hydrogen breath test.[36] However, small-intestine transit time studies are rarely relevant for clinical purposes in infants.

Procedure. Recommendations include:

1. a baseline breath sample;

2. a fasting period of 4 hours minimum in infants to 12 hours in older children and adolescents;

3. the test should be carried out in the morning;

4. lactulose (0.25 mg/kg) is given in 100 ml water associated with a low-fiber, no-sugar breakfast (or the usual formula in infants);

5. a rise of 20 ppm above the baseline is considered a positive response;

6. a sampling timing of every 15 minutes during the first hour to avoid misinterpretation because of early rise due to bacterial overgrowth, and every 30 minutes thereafter.

COLON

Mouth to anus transit time can be measured by the recovery of colored radioactive or radiopaque markers in stool,[37, 38] as well as by the radiopaque marker method of Arhan, which measures transit time through individual colonic segments.[39] The subjects swallow N radiopaque markers and undergo plain abdominal radiographs daily until all markers have been evacuated. In a simplified version proposed by Metcalf,[40] the subjects swallow differently shaped markers on three successive days and a single radiograph is taken on the fourth day. Mean colonic transit time (MCT) is calculated according to the equation:

$$MCT = 1.2(N1 + N2 + N3)$$

N1, N2, and N3 are the number of, respectively, the first, second, and third types of markers present on a single radiograph taken on the fourth day.

Normal values for transit time—calculated in hours—exhibit a wide range, de-

TABLE 16.2 **Solids and Liquids in Transit**		
	Liquid	*Solid*
Lactulose 15 g	118 ± 29 min	197 ± 29 min
Lactitol 15 g	100 ± 47 min	172 ± 36 min

TABLE 16.3 **Volume and Concentration**		
Lactulose (g)	*Water (ml)*	*Transit Time (min)*
10	150	45 - 90
10	15	58 - 153

pending on age and on the country where the study was performed (Table 16.4).[41]

In addition to physiologic studies, the main indication for studying colonic transit times is constipation. In a group of 176 children aged 2 to 15 years who were investigated for idiopathic disorders, 70 were constipated before the end of the first month of life and 50% had symptoms before the training period.[42] Spina bifida was a significant cause of delayed transit (Table 16.5).

In Spanish children with constipation secondary to meningomyelocele, total colonic transit time was delayed but a slow transit occurred in each segment of the colon (Table 16.6).[42]

In the majority of children with nonorganic constipation, the main alteration is retention and accumulation of feces in the rectal ampulla, without slowing of colonic segmental transit time.[43] However, there have been reports of slow transit in constipated children.[44] The discrepancies in the literature may be due to several factors:

TABLE 16.4 Variance of Normal Colonic Transit Times by Age and Region

	Patients (n)	Right Colon	Left Colon	Rectosigmoid Colon	Total
French adults	22	24 h	30 h	44 h	67 h
Canadian adults	37	38 h	37 h	34 h	93 h
French children	23	18 h	20 h	34 h	62 h
Spanish children	10	18 h	17 h	19 h	50 h

TABLE 16.5 Idiopathic Disorders

	Normal Transit	Constipated	Constipated with Spina Bifida
Stomach and small intestine	6 h 24 min	4 h 50 min	5 h 37 min
Ascending colon	7 h 10 min	13 h 24 min	12 h 15 min
Descending colon	7 h 37 min	13 h 49 min	14 h 30 min
Rectum	11 h 4 min	30 h 22 min	25 h 8 min

TABLE 16.6 Constipation in Spanish Children

	Right Colon	Left Colon	Rectosigmoid	Total
Normal	10.8 ± 3.5 h	12.2 ± 2.7 h	14.7 ± 2.1 h	37.8 ± 6.2 h
Meningo- myelocele	15.9 ± 2.3 h	18.9 ± 2.3 h	25.0 ± 2.6 h	59.9 ± 5.4 h

1. differences in local and national food habits;

2. previous treatments;

3. widely varying degree of individual fecal impaction;

4. unstandardized nutritional intakes during the investigation.

Any study of transit time in constipated children should be compared with a local normal control population. Food intake should be standardized for both populations, as is done in balance studies. Furthermore, a delayed transit time when the colon is full of feces does not seem very reproducible. The so-called slowing of segmental transit time should not be accepted unless the study has been performed after proper bowel cleansing.

Delayed gastrointestinal transit time has also been reported in anorexia nervosa and bulimia (Table 16.7).[45]

Delayed transit could contribute to eating disorders by causing the patient to feel bloated, exacerbating fear of fatness, or by causing rectal distention that reflexively inhibits gastric emptying.

For physiologic studies, more sophisticated methods using scintigraphic techniques have been validated in healthy volunteers, combining measurement of gastric emptying, intestinal transit time, and colonic filling[46] in a single test. However, for clinical purposes in children we recommend the radiopaque markers technique. In our unit we use differently shaped markers (Portex radiopaque polythene pellets, Portex Ltd, Hythe Kent, England) given with standardized lunch meals on three successive days with a plain abdominal radiograph on the fourth day. In case all the markers have not been evacuated, a second film is taken on the seventh day.[41] To avoid unnecessary radiation, the stools can be collected each day during 1 week and the number of markers counted in the radiography of the stools.

On the basis of radiopaque marker studies, patients with constipation may be divided into three different groups. In the first, there is delay in the entire colon. Various labels have been used for this condition, such as slow-transit constipation and colonic inertia. Colonic pseudo-obstruction is an example of this condition. In the second group, feces pass normally along the right colon but are stored too long in the distal colon. Patients with this pattern have been labeled as having hindgut dysfunction. In the third and largest group, the radiopaque markers are retained for a long time only in the rectum. This is typical of children with functional fecal retention and outlet obstruction.

TABLE 16.7 Delayed Transit and Eating Disorders

	Whole Gut	Mouth to Cecum
Controls	38 ± 19 h	84 ± 27 min
Anorexia nervosa	66 ± 29 h	109 ± 33 min
Bulimia	70 ± 32 h	106 ± 24 min

REFERENCES

1. Corazziari E, Torsoli A. *Radiology* In: Kumar D, Gustavssons, eds. *An Illustrated Guide to Gastrointestinal Motility*. Chichester, England: J Wiley & Sons, 1988.

2. King PM, Pryde A, Heading RC. Transpyloric fluid movement and antroduodenal motility in patients with gastro-oesophageal reflux. *Gut* 1987;28:545-8.

3. Roy CC, Sliverman A, Cozzetto FJ. In: *Pediatric Clinical Gastroenterology,* 2nd ed. St Louis, MO: 1975;692-3.

4. Roy SK, Akramuzzaman SM, Akbar MS. Persistent diarrhea: total gut transit time and its relationship with nutrient absorption and clinical response. *J Pediatr Gastroenterol Nutr* 1991;13:409-14.

5. Silny J, Knigge KP, Fass J, Rau G, Materne S, Schumpelick V. Verification of the intraluminal multiple electrical impedance measurement for the recording of GI motility. *J Gastrointest Motil* 1993;5:107-22.

6. McClelland GR, Sutton JA. A comparison of the gastric and central nervous system effects of two substituted benzamides in normal volunteers. *Br J Clin Pharmacol* 1986;21:503-9.

7. Gilbey SG, Watkins PJ. Measurement by epigastric impedance of gastric emptying in diabetic autonomic neuropathy. *Diabetic Med* 1987;4:122-6.

8. Mangnall YF, Barnish C, Brown BH, Barber DC, Johnson AG, Read MW. Comparison of applied potential tomography and impedance epigastrography as methods of measuring gastric emptying. *Clin Phys Physiol Meas* 1988;9:499-507.

9. Sutton JA, Thompson S. Measurement of gastric emptying rate by isotope scanning and epigastric impedance. *Lancet* 1985;1:888-90.

10. Smith HL, Hollins GW, Booth IW. Epigastric impedance recording for measuring gastric emptying in children: how useful is it? *J Pediatr Gastroenterol Nutr* 1993;17:201-6.

11. Kazem I. A new scintigraphic technique for the study of the esophagus. *AJR* 1972;115:681-8.

12. Piepsz A. Gastro-esophageal radionuclide methods. Proceedings of the First International Symposium on Gastroesophageal Reflux and Respiratory disorders. Brussels, Belgium: 1988. Abstract.

13. Siegel JA, Wu RK, Knight LC, Zelac RE, Stern HS, Malmud LS. Radiation dose estimates for oral agents used in upper gastrointestinal disease. *J Nucl Med* 1983;24:835-7.

14. Ham HR, Georges B, Froideville JL, Piepsz A. Oesophageal transit of liquid: effects of single or multiple swallows. *Nucl Med Commun* 1985;6:263-7.

15. Cadranel S, Di Lorenzo C, Rodesch P, Piepsz A, Ham HR. Caustic ingestion and esophageal function. *J Pediatr Gastroenterol Nutr* 1990;10:164-8.

16. Reid B, Di Lorenzo C, Travis L, Flores AF, Rill BB, Hyman PE. Diabetic gastroparesis due to postprandial antral hypomotility in childhood. *Pediatrics* 1992;90:43-6.

17. Corinaldesi R, Stanghellini V, Tosetti C, Cecchini D, et al. Gastric emptying of solids in subpopulations of patients with idiopathic dyspepsia. *J Gastrointest Motil* 1992;4:A215.

18. Billeaud C, Guillet J, Sandler B. Gastric emptying in infants with or without gastro-oesophageal reflux according to the type of milk. *Eur J Clin Nutr* 1990;44:570-83.

19. Ewe K, Press AG, Bollem S, Schuhn I. Gastric emptying of indigestible tablets in relation to composition and time of ingestion of meals studied by metal detectors. *Dig Dis Sci* 1991;36:146-52.

20. Feldman M, Smith HJ, Simon JR. Gastric emptying of solid radio-opaque markers: studies in healthy subjects and diabetic patients. *Gastroenterology* 1984;87:895-904.

21. Hyman PE, Abrams C, Dubois A. Effect of metoclopramide and bethanechol on gastric emptying in infants. *Pediatr Res* 1985;19:1029-32.

22. Read NW, Janabim N, Bates TE, Barber DC. Effect of gastro-intestinal intubation on the passage of a solid meal through the stomach and small intestine in humans. *Gastroenterology* 1983;84:1568-72.

23. Harasawa S, Tani N, Suzuki S, et al. Gastric

emptying in normal subjects and patients with peptic ulcer: a study using the acetaminophen method. *Gastroenterol Jpn* 1979;14:1-10.

24. Palmas F, Brazioli D, Guerra P, et al. Gastric emptying with paracetamol. *Ital J Med* 1986;2:37-41.

25. Bjorkman DJ, Moore JG, Klein PD, Graham DY. ^{13}C-bicarbonate, breath test as measure of gastric emptying. *Am J Gastroenterol* 1991;86:821-3.

26. Ghoos Y, Maes B, Geypens B, et al. Measurement of gastric emptying rates of solids by means of a carbon-labelled octanoic acid breath test. *Gastroenterology* 1993;104:1640-7.

27. Ghoos Y, Maes B, Hiele M, et al. Gastric emptying rate of solids is slower in children than in adults as demonstrated by the ^{13}C-octanoic acid breath test. *Gastroenterology* 1993;104:A511.

28. Dalzell AM, Freestone NS, Billingtone D, Heaf DP. Small intestinal permeability and orocaecal transit time in cystic fibrosis. *Arch Dis Child* 1990;65:585-8.

29. Tadesse K, Leung DTY, Lau SP. A new method of expired gas collection for measurement of breath hydrogen in infants and small children. *Acta Pediatr Scand* 1988;77:55-9.

30. Greissen M, Bergoz R, Balant L, Loizeau E. Effet du lactitol sur la production d'hydrogene expire chez l'homme normal. *Schweiz Med Wochenschr* 1986;116:469-72.

31. Read NW, Miles CA, Fisher D, et al. Transit of a meal through the stomach, small intestine, and colon in normal subjects and its role in the pathogenesis of diarrhea. *Gastroenterology* 1980;79:1276-82.

32. Permans JA, Molder S, Olson AC. Role of pH in production of hydrogen from carbohydrates by colonic bacterial flora. *J Clin Invest* 1981;67:643-50.

33. Di Lorenzo C, Dooley CP, Valenzuela JE. Role of fasting gastrointestinal motility in the variability of gastrointestinal transit time assessed by hydrogen breath test. *Gut* 1991;32:1127-30.

34. Murphy MS, Nelson R, Eastham EJ. Measurement of small intestinal transit time in children. *Acta Paediatr Scand* 1988;77:802-6.

35. Vreugdenhil G, Sinaasappel M, Bouquet J. A comparative study of the mouth to caecum transit time in children and adults using a weight adapted lactulose dose. *Acta Paediatr Scand* 1986;75:483-8.

36. Stevenson DK, Cohen RS, Ostrander CR, et al. A sensitive analytical apparatus for measuring hydrogen production rate: application to studies in human infants. *J Pediatr Gastroenterol Nutr* 1982;1:233-7.

37. Hinton JM, Lennard-Jones JE, Young AC. A new method for studying gut transit times using radioopaque markers. *Gut* 1969;10:842-7.

38. Cummings JH, Wiggins HS. Transit through the gut measured by analysis of a single stool. *Gut* 1976;17:219-23.

39. Arhan P, Devroede G, Jehannin B, et al. Segmental colonic transit time. *Dis Colon Rectum* 1981;24:625-9.

40. Metcalf AM, Phillips SF, Zinsmeister AR, MacCarty R, Beart RW, Wolff BG. Simplified assessment of segmental colonic transit. *Gastroenterology* 1987;92:40-7.

41. Arhan P, Devroede G, Jehannin B, et al. Idiopathic disorders of fecal continence in children. *Pediatrics* 1983;71:774-9.

42. Bautista Casasnovas A, Varela Cives R, Jeremias AV, Castro-Gago M, Cadranel S, Tojo RS. Measurement of colonic transit time in children. *J Pediatr Gastroenterol Nutr* 1991;13:42-5.

43. Corazziari E, Cucchiara S, Staiano A, et al. Gastrointestinal transit time, frequency of defecation, and anorectal manometry in healthy and constipated children. *J Pediatr* 1985;106:379-82.

44. Benninga MA, Buller HA, Akkermans LM, Taminiau JA. Does slow transit constipation exist in children? *Gastroenterology* 1993;104:A475.

45. Kamal N, Chami T, Andersen A, Rosell FA, Schuster MM, Whitehead WE. Delayed gastrointestinal transit times in anorexia nervosa and bulimia nervosa. *Gastroenterology* 1991;101:1320-4.

46. Lartigue S, Bizai Y, Bruley S, Clarec D, Galmiche JP. Mesure de vidange gastrique, du temps de transit intestinal, du remplissage colique par scintigraphie chez le sujet sain. *Gastroenterol Clin Biol* 1991;15:379-85.

17

Marker Dilution Tests

VICTOR M. PIÑEIRO-CARRERO, ANDRE DUBOIS

The opinions and assertions contained herein are the private ones of the authors and are not to be construed as official or reflecting the views of the Department of Defense or the Uniformed Services University of the Health Sciences.

The electrical and motor activity of the gastrointestinal tract is primarily directed towards transporting nutrients to areas where they can be digested and/or absorbed. This mechanical activity may be an aborad propulsion of intestinal contents or a retropulsion of gastrointestinal contents in an orad direction. The end result of gastric muscular activity is to empty the stomach contents into the duodenum in a form appropriate for continued digestion and absorption. Since the small intestine is the main absorbing organ, the limit to absorption from the lumen of the intestinal tract is controlled by the rate of gastric emptying into the intestine and by the maximal absorption rate of the mucosa. Normally, transfer of substances from the stomach to the duodenum is timely, and serves as the rate-limiting step in intestinal digestion and absorption. Disturbances in the control mechanisms of gastric emptying may result in stasis (gastroparesis), leading to nausea, vomiting, and possibly malnutrition. Excessively fast gastric emptying (eg, dumping), in contrast, may cause osmotic diarrhea if the amount delivered to the small bowel exceeds its absorptive capacity. Determining the rate of gastric emptying in patients with symptoms of the upper gastrointestinal tract and no evidence of mucosal disease or anatomic anomalies is therefore essential.

The methods available to study gastrointestinal motility often provide information about the electromechanical events produced by intestinal contraction. Although tests such as manometry and electrogastrography provide useful clinical information, they do not describe the end result of electromechanical activity (ie, gastric emptying and intestinal transit). Gastric emptying tests in children were initially limited to radiographic studies with a barium meal.[1] This technique has been widely criticized due to its 2-dimensional character and the nonphysiologic nature of the meal. In this chapter, marker-dilution tests will be discussed with specific reference to their use in studying gastric emptying and intestinal transit. Their role in the study of colonic transit will be covered briefly.

GASTRIC EMPTYING METHODS
Aspiration

The earliest methods developed to study gastric emptying and gastric secretion involved aspiration of gastric contents. The Ewald-Boas test meal, or single aspiration method,[2] consists of administering a mixed solid and liquid meal at time 0. Thirty to 60 minutes later, a nasogastric tube is passed and the gastric contents are completely aspirated. The Ewald-Boas test meal has undergone many modifications, including the use of liquid meals to explore the emptying of liquids (eg, 750-ml saline load).[3] These techniques suffer from limitations: 1) the volume in the stomach may not be totally reaspirated; and 2) the total gastric volume is measured without determining the volume of fluids secreted into the stomach, which can represent a large percentage of gastric volume. Therefore, these tests do not differentiate between large residual gastric volumes due to delayed gastric emptying versus gastric hypersecretion in the presence of normal gastric emptying.

Serial Test Meal

Nonabsorbable markers were introduced in the pioneer studies of Mathieu and Rémond[4] with their modification of the Ewald-Boas test meal to measure gastric secretion. In an attempt to estimate the dilution of the gastric secretion by the ingested meal, they added 10 g of almond oil to the Ewald-Boas meal. After determining the total gastric volume aspirated at 60 minutes, they measured the concentration of oil and thereafter calculated the volume of the meal and the volume of gastric secretion retained in the stomach at that time. Phenol red (phenolsulfonphthalein) was first used as the nonabsorbable marker by Gorham,[5] who added 6 mg of phenol red to 400 ml of distilled water as the test meal. He performed both fractional gastric analysis (6-15 ml of gastric contents obtained every 15 min for a defined period of time) and the single aspiration method. He then calculated the percent of meal remaining in the stomach, the gastric juice secreted, and the corrected total acidity of the gastric juice from the volume aspirated as well as the concentration of phenol red in the gastric contents and the original meal.

Nonabsorbable markers were used extensively by Enríquez de Salamanca[6] in Madrid from 1935 to the late 1950s and by Hunt[7] in England with their so-called serial test meal technique. This technique involves administering a series of standard meals on several days, after washing out the stomach, and recovering the gastric contents after different digestive periods. At each of these times, the total volume of the gastric contents (V_G) is reaspirated to determine the concentration of the marker in the gastric aspirate (C_G) and the original meal (C_M). The volume of meal (V_M) remaining in the stomach at the time of aspiration can then be calculated:

$$V_M = V_G(C_G/C_M)$$

If standard conditions are maintained and a slow-emptying meal is used, gastric emptying is reproducible from day to day. Therefore, the percent of meal remaining in the stomach at different times on different days can be calculated to determine the overall rate of gastric emptying of the meal.

The problem with this technique is that it does not allow repeated measurements of gastric emptying over the entire course of emptying the meal on any given day. Rigid control of the test meal's composition and of the duration of fasting before testing are needed to ensure minimal day-to-day variability in the serial test meal technique. Multiple gastric intubations are also required, which is why most studies relied on only one postprandial time.

Gastric Marker Dilution

Principles. Repeated samplings of the gastric contents are taken without completely emptying the stomach, thereby allowing calculation of the volume present in the stomach at various intervals during a single session. The calculation is performed using the dye dilution principle[4,8-10] initially developed by Hildes and Dunlop.[8] Rediscovered by George[9] in 1968, it was termed the double sampling test meal (Fig. 17.1).

The resulting intragastric volume, however, reflects not only the meal, but also the additional secreted juice. If emptying is to be expressed independently from gastric secretion, the intragastric marker concentration must be used to correct for the secretory participation in the buildup of intragastric volume.[8,11-14] Therefore, a decrease in *concentration* of the indicator marker is effected by gastric secretion, whereas a decrease in *quantity* of marker present in the stomach is effected by emptying through the pylorus. Moreover, the calculated intragastric volume is an approximation that neglects the emptying and secretion during the 1-minute dye dilution procedure. Correction for this error can be performed after emptying and secretion has been determined, as indicated below.[13,14]

If the marker is not absorbed or secreted by the stomach, and if gastric volume is determined twice at a 1-minute interval (V_2 and V_1'), the amount of marker in the stomach at time t is ($= V_1' \cdot C_1'$). If the amount of marker in the stomach at time 0 is M_2 ($= C_2 \cdot V_2$), the amount of marker, M_E, which was emptied over the interval is

$$M_E = V_2 \cdot C_2 - V_1' \cdot C_1'$$

However, the emptying of the marker is not what should be calculated. The relevant information is the emptying rate for any fluid or electrolyte that is present in the stomach, mixed with the marker. This can be determined by assuming that emptying is a first-order process (exponential emptying), as described by Enríquez de Salamanca and Tamarit,[6] and Hunt.[7] A number of studies in children have confirmed the exponential nature of liquid emptying.[15,16] The volume of meal remaining in the stomach at time t (V_t) can be expressed as a function of the volume at time 0 (V_0) multiplied by a function of the time:

$$V_1' = V_2 \cdot e^{kt}$$
and
$$M_1' = M_2 \cdot e^{-kt}$$

In these equations, e is the base of natural (Neperian) logarithms and it is equal to 2.718; k is the rate constant for emptying, which has been termed the fractional emptying rate (FER).[13,14] Solving this equation for k, now termed FER, gives:

$$FER = -\log_e(M_1'/M_2)/t$$
and
$$FER = -\log_e[(V_1' \cdot C_1')/(V_1 \cdot C_2)]/t$$

When $M_1' = M_2/2, t = T_{1/2}$, which gives the following relation between FER and $T_{1/2}$:

$$FER = -\log_e(0.5)/T_{1/2} = 0.69/T_{1/2}$$

This relation can be used to calculate one of two parameters when the other is known.

The emptying rate of fluid (F_E in ml/min) is then equal to the volume of fluid in the stomach multiplied by FER. However, since the intragastric volume fluctuates constantly as a function of both gastric secretion and emptying, the rate of fluid secretion (F_s in ml/min) must first be calculated:

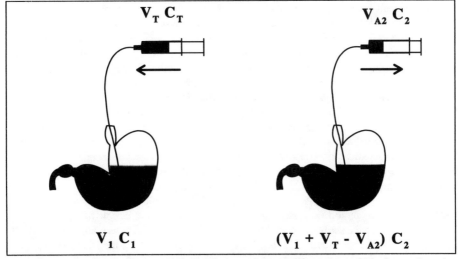

Fig. 17.1 Principle of the marker dilution technique. A known test volume (V_T) of a marker at a concentration (C_T) is added to an unknown volume (V_1) containing a known concentration of the marker (C_1). Mixing the two volumes will result in a concentration (C_2), which is measured in an aspirated aliquot (V_{A2}). This can be expressed as $V_1C_1 + V_TC_T = (V_1 + V_T)C_2$. Since the only unknown is V_1, one can solve the equation $V_1 = V_T(C_T - C_2)/(C_2 - C_1)$ to calculate V_1, the original volume of the gastric contents.

$$F_s = [V_1' - V_2 \cdot \exp(-FER \cdot t)] \cdot [FER/(1 - \exp(-FER \cdot t))]$$

Then, the rate of fluid emptying (F_E) is

$$F_E = V_2 \cdot [1 - \exp(-FER \cdot t)] + F_s \cdot t - F_s \cdot [1 - \exp(-FER \cdot t)]/FER$$

Knowing these initial estimates of FER and F_s, V_1 and V_1' can be recalculated, as can a second approximation of FER and F_s.[13,14] This iterative process procures new estimates of intragastric volumes, FER, and F_s. A good estimate is reached when the last iteration modifies all the values by less than 1%. This method allows correction for emptying and fluid output occurring during the 1-minute dye dilution interval.

Similar equations may be used to calculate the rate of acid secretion and emptying if acid concentration is determined in the gastric samples.[13,14] The same calculations may be applied to any ion or element that is measured in the gastric contents. The fraction of the meal remaining in the stomach over time can also be calculated. Slightly modified equations are used for the interval corresponding to the liquid test meal to account for its intragastric administration.[13]

An important advantage of the technique is that it allows for variations of the FER from one interval to another and does not require curve fitting of the entire emptying curve. This is relevant because some investigators have shown that the emptying of formula follows a biphasic pattern in some infants, with an initial rapid phase lasting 20 minutes followed by a slower phase.[17,18] In this situation, the values for FER during the first 20 minutes will be greater than later, while all the values may be averaged to calculate the mean FER.

Method. Infants should be fasted for at least 4 hours before the study; older children for 6 to 8 hours. Since sedation cannot be used, the patient should be made as comfortable as possible. Infants can be studied while lying in a crib or cradled in the arms of a nurse. Older infants can sit in the nurse's lap; children can sit in a recliner. Whatever the position, it should be consistent in all studies, as it may affect gastric emptying.[19,20] A 10- or 12-Fr double lumen sump tube is placed through the naso- or oropharynx into the stomach, and the stomach is emptied of residual contents. Proper position of the tube in the most dependent portion of the stomach is verified by immediate recovery of 90% to 100% of an injection of 5 to 10 ml of water (80% recovery of an injection of 20 ml water is acceptable in older children). Following a 30-minute stabilization period, a 2.5-ml sample (V_{A1}) of mixed gastric contents is aspirated (Fig. 17.2). Immediately thereafter, 5.0 ml (V_T) of water with phenol red 50 mg/dl (C_T) is introduced into the stomach (see Figs. 17.1, 17.2). After mixing the added volume with gastric contents for 1 minute, a second 2.5 ml (V_{A2}) sample of gastric fluid is aspirated. These procedures are repeated every 10 minutes during a 40-minute fasting period. A meal of 15 ml/kg 5% dextrose adjusted to pH 7.0 at 37° C and containing phenol red 5 mg/dl is instilled into the stomach with a constant-infusion pump for 2.5 minutes. The dilution procedure is then repeated at 5, 10, 20, 30, 40, 50, and 60 minutes after the test meal.

The test is usually performed by a physician or gastrointestinal assistant experienced in the technique. A nurse should be present if the patient is an infant or young child. The procedure lasts approximately 2 hours. Another 3 hours are required to prepare the solutions and analyze the samples. Potential complications related to gastric intubation include nasopharyngeal bleeding and, less frequently, trauma to the esophagus or stomach. In addition, vomiting that causes pulmonary aspiration may occur. However, the procedure is generally well tolerated and complications are rare.

Each sample of gastric juice and the phenol red solutions are centrifuged. Samples of the clear supernatant are adjusted to pH 10 with 0.25% Na_3PO_4, then analyzed for phenol red concentration with a visible light spectrophotometer at 560 nm. The concentration of acid in each sample is determined by endpoint titration to pH 7.4 with a titrator and autoburette. Intragastric volumes of flu-

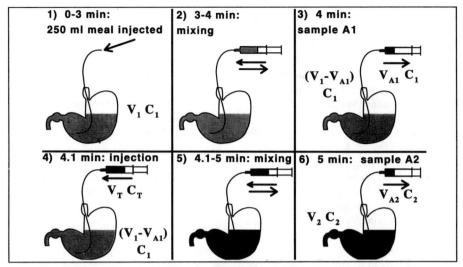

Fig. 17.2 Double sampling test meal. 1) At time 0 to 3 min, a 250-ml test meal is injected (15-20 ml/kg in infants and children); 2) the gastric contents are mixed for 1 min; 3) a 2.5-ml sample (A_1) is aspirated; 4) 5.0 ml of water with phenol red is introduced into the stomach; 5) gastric contents are mixed again for 1 minute; 6) a second 2.5-ml sample of gastric fluid is aspirated (A_2).

id (V_1, V_1'...) and masses of phenol red (P_1, P_1'...) are calculated at each sampling using the marker dilution principle.[13] Fractional emptying rate and net rate of fluid output are determined for each 5- or 10-minute interval between two dilutions, using the assumptions listed below. Similar calculations determine the amounts of intragastric H^+ at the time of each sampling and the net H^+ secretory rates between any two samplings. In addition to determining the fractional emptying rate, this method permits simultaneous measurement of net fluid output (expressed as the volume secreted in ml) and of net H^+ secretion (in µeq/min). It can be applied during fasting and after a liquid meal.

Assumptions. Several assumptions must be met to calculate intragastric volume at the time of the dilution procedure as well as the rates of emptying and secretion during the intervals between these procedures.

1. The marker used as a dilution indicator should not be absorbed, adsorbed, secreted, or degraded by the stomach. Phenol red and polyethylene glycol (PEG) are the most popular nonradioactive markers. Many studies in human and animal models have validated their suitability.[21-24] Phenol red is readily

and reproducibly measured with a spectrophotometer. Its major disadvantage is that it can only be used with clear test meals; bile or blood in the samples may interfere with measurement. In contrast, PEG can be used with opaque meals but its measurement is long and tedious, increasing the possibility of operator error. A better nonabsorbable marker is diethylene triamine pentacetic acid, to which technetium 99m has been attached (^{99m}Tc-DTPA). A dose of 100 µCi gives accurate results while the 6-hour half life of the isotope ensures very low radiation exposure.[25] ^{99m}Tc-sulphur colloid was studied in premature infants using the single aspiration method.[26] However, sulphur colloid (but not DTPA) is subject to layering upon centrifugation, which introduces systematic errors in concentration determinations when used with the double sampling technique. Radionuclides are not influenced by the turbidity of the feeding, and measurements can be automated. They do not interfere with colorimetric assays of components of the gastric contents. However, radionuclides are infrequently administered to pediatric patients because healthy controls cannot be exposed to radiation.

2. To accurately determine the concen-

tration of ions in the gastric juice, water absorption across the gastric mucosa must be negligible. With a test meal of 750 ml, Hunt[27] calculated that the percentage of water absorbed was 1% to 2% of the volume of gastric contents in the first 60 minutes. Other investigators have found evidence of more rapid water absorption, especially with hypotonic meals while absorption is minimized with isotonic meals.[28] Also, all results should be expressed as *net* secretion (ie, the difference between secretion and absorption).

3. A 5- to 20-ml marker solution injected into the stomach can be mixed completely with the gastric contents by aspirating and reinjecting 5- to 20-ml aliquots 4 times during a 1-minute period.[8,9,13]

4. Over 5- to 10-minute intervals, the rate of decline of intragastric marker is proportional to the marker's intragastric mass.

5. The marker remains homogenously mixed with the gastric contents during the intervals between samplings,[29] which implies that this technique cannot be used to study emptying of solids or nonhomogenous liquids (eg, fats). A corollary of this assumption is that any element in the stomach (eg, water or ions) is emptied at a fractional rate identical to that for the marker.

6. The fractional rates of emptying and secretion are constant during each 5- or 10-minute interval but can vary between intervals.

7. Net rate of fluid output remains constant over the given interval.

8. Gastroesophageal and duodenogastric reflux are assumed to be negligible during the procedure. Therefore, any vomiting during the procedure can lead to errors in the calculated fractional emptying rate and gastric volume.

This technique is simple, requiring only gastric intubation and determination of the concentration of the marker, acid, and other elements in the gastric juice for which the rate of secretion will be measured. Hurwitz[30] analyzed the double sampling method and demonstrated that random errors in the calculated gastric volume are magnified due to the accumulation of dye in the stomach. However, this cause of error is minimal if

gastric secretion is present, thus causing problems only in atrophic gastritis, if acid output is suppressed by antisecretory agents, or if measurements are performed for more than 1 hour after the meal. Hurwitz proposed to reduce the error by using dye-free water and doubling the concentration of dye added at the time of each successive dilution. Despite elegant mathematical analysis and in vitro demonstration of his modification, these changes have not been widely adopted, possibly because they complicate the experiment's design and practically double the number of samples to be analyzed.

Data analysis and interpretation. The gastric fractional emptying rate (percentage of meal leaving the stomach per min), percentage of meal remaining in the stomach, gastric fluid output (ml/kg/h), and gastric acid output (μmol/kg/h) are determined using the marker dilution principle as described above. These calculations are easily performed with a computer program that can be used with any IBM or compatible personal computer.[31]

The interpretation of results in the clinical setting is difficult due to the lack of data for healthy controls. Most studies of gastric emptying of liquids in the pediatric population have used different modifications of the dye dilution principle. In addition, the composition and volume of the meal have been inconsistent. A large amount of information has been obtained, as indicated in the summary of selected studies[15,17-19,26,32-36] in children depicted in Tables 17.1 and 17.2.

Indications. Vendel[37] studied the gastric emptying pattern of infants by repeatedly measuring aspirated gastric contents, returning the meal to the stomach after each measurement. Despite the potential artefacts produced by multiple intubations and the abrupt changes in gastric volume, the method gave consistent results. He described delayed gastric emptying in premature infants when compared to term infants. In 1945, Enríquez de Salamanca et al[36] published their studies in normal children using the serial test meal.

TABLE 17.1 Gastric Emptying of Liquids in Infants and Children: Marker Dilution Technique

Author	Age Studied	No. of Patients	Diagnosis	Meal Type	Meal Volume	$T_{1/2}$ (min)
Enríquez de Salamanca[36]	Unknown	13	Normal	Tea	250 ml	28.2
Pérez Delgado[35]	5-38 mo	50	Normal	Tea	250 ml	32.67*
Bardhan[15]	6-12 mo	10	S/P rotavirus infection	5% glucose	20 ml/kg	13.1
Hyman[33, 34]	4-12 mo	9	Recurrent vomiting	5% glucose	15 ml/kg	11.9**
	0.5-4 mo	7	Gastroparesis prematurity			14.4
	0.75-4 mo	6	Postoperative gastroparesis			21.6

* Values estimated from the percent meal retained at 60 min
** Values estimated from the mean fractional emptying rate

TABLE 17.2 Gastric Emptying of Liquids in Neonates and Young Infants: Marker Dilution Technique

Author	Age Studied	No. of Patients	Diagnosis	Meal Type	Meal Volume	$T_{1/2}$ (min)
Husband[32]	1-8 wk	13	Normal term and preterm (32-41 wk)	Water 5% glucose 10% glucose	22 ml/kg	10.5* 19 29
Yu[19]	1-2 wk	12 12	Normal term Normal preterm (33-37 wk)	10% glucose	7 ml/kg	23.64** 22.80
Cavell[17]	1-9 wk	11	Normal preterm (29-34 wk)	Human milk Formula	22 ml/kg	25.1 51.9
Siegel[18]	1-9 wk	10	Normal preterm (26-34 wk)	Iso-osmolar formula Hyperosmolar formula	22 ml/kg	29.66** 34.47
Sidebottom[26]	1-4 wk	16	Normal preterm (30-35 wk)	Formula (14% MCT) Formula (50% MCT)	20 ml/kg	28.81** 34.47

* Values estimated from figure 1 in Husband and Husband[32]
** Values estimated from the percent meal at 30 min

They were the first to use the marker dilution technique in children, demonstrating that the emptying of a liquid meal is exponential and similar to that of normal adults. This technique was subsequently used to compare the gastric emptying rate of water, 5% glucose, and 10% glucose test meals in the newborn.[32] Pediatric studies using the double sampling technique (PEG as the nonabsorbable marker) have initially focused on the gastric emptying response to different formulas in premature infants.[17,18,38] The response to prokinetic agents in infants with upper gastrointestinal motor disorders was studied by Hyman et al [33,34] using the phenol red marker dilution technique.[13,14] Most recently, gastric emptying was studied in 10 infants with acute rotaviral gastroenteritis.[15]

The pediatric use of the gastric marker dilution method has been limited to newborns and infants. In this age group, the technique can be valuable in patients with suspected gastric motor disorders (ie, severe gastroesophageal reflux, suspected gastroparesis of prematurity, intestinal pseudo-obstruction, or postoperative gastroparesis). Older children and adolescents with gastric stasis associated with severe gastroesophageal reflux, suspected pseudo-obstruction, or diabetes mellitus may also benefit. A major advantage of the marker dilution method is that it allows simultaneous determination of gastric emptying, volume of secretions, and rate of acid secretion. Therefore, suspected gastric hypersecretion (eg, intractable peptic ulcer disease or suspected Zollinger-Ellison syndrome) is another indication for this method. Acid output may also be determined with the intragastric titration method,[39] but the unphysiologic neutralization of the intragastric contents this technique requires has the disadvantage of stimulating gastric secretion.[40]

INTRADUODENAL MARKER DILUTION

Principles. This technique was developed almost simultaneously in the United States,[41,42] Sweden,[43] and France.[44] It is based on dilution techniques previously developed to measure propulsion of fluids in the jejunum[45-47] and has been extensively described by Malagelada et al.[48] In brief, a meal containing marker 1 is eaten or directly placed into the stomach, while marker 2 is continuously infused into the proximal duodenum (Fig. 17.3). At the same time, continuous suction is applied to the distal duodenum, permitting collection every 10 minutes of duodenal samples that contain marker 1 from the stomach, and marker 2 as it perfuses into the duodenum.

Gastric samples are taken at 10-minute intervals to determine intragastric concentration of marker 1 (m_t, m_{t+10}, m_{t+20}...). During a given 10-minute interval from t to t+10, the average concentration of marker 1 present in the stomach (g) is calculated:

$$g=(m_t + m_{t+10})/2$$

The concentration of marker 2 in the 10-minute duodenal aspirate (d) is also measured. Knowing the rate of infusion of duodenal marker (ΔD), allows calculation of the emptying rate of the gastric marker (ΔM) over the 10-minute interval:

$$\Delta M = \Delta D(g/d)$$

When the amount of marker originally present in the meal (M_o^*) is known, ΔM can be subtracted from M_o^* and the amount of marker remaining in the stomach at time 10 can be calculated. However, unaccountable marker losses may make this M_o^* greater than the sum of all the ΔMs calculated over the entire study.[48] Therefore, $M_o (=\Sigma\Delta m)$ was calculated as the amount of marker calculated as orginally present in the stomach, instead of the known amount M_o^*. By dividing the calculated M_o by the measured volume of the meal V_o, an "effective concentration of gastric marker at time 0 (m_o)" was computed. An estimate of the precision of the study would be provided by comparing this calculated m_o with the measured concentration of marker 1 in the meal, although such data are not available in the literature.

The amount of marker in the stomach at time 10, M_1 ($=M_o - \Delta M_{0-10}$), in the meal was then calculated. Knowing the concentration

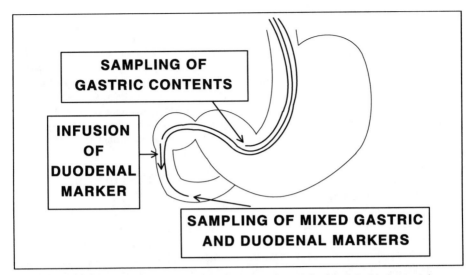

SAMPLING OF
GASTRIC CONTENTS

INFUSION
OF
DUODENAL
MARKER

SAMPLING OF MIXED GASTRIC
AND DUODENAL MARKERS

Fig. 17.3 Intraduodenal marker dilution technique. Gastric and duodenal double-lumen tubes are depicted. A meal containing marker 1 is eaten or infused into the stomach while marker 2 is continuously infused into the proximal duodenum. Sampling the mixed gastric and duodenal markers allows for calculation of gastric emptying and duodenal transit time.

of marker m_{10} and the amount of marker (M_{10},) the volume present in the stomach (V_{10}), was calculated. The volume of gastric contents emptied into the duodenum (ΔV), ie, the rate of fluid emptying, was also calculated:

$$\Delta V = \Delta M/g$$

The volume of fluids secreted by the stomach plus the flow of bile and pancreatic juice (F_s) was then calculated as

$$F_s = V_0 - V_{10} + \Delta V_{0\text{-}10}$$

Knowing the acid concentration in the stomach at any sampling time t (a_t), the amount of acid in the stomach ($A_t = a_t \cdot V_t$), the rate of acid emptying and, by difference, the rate of acid secretion were calculated.

Similar calculations were used to determine the rates of secretion of bile acids, bilirubin, and pancreatic enzymes after measuring the concentration of these elements in the duodenal aspirates.[41]

Several variations have been reported. Johansson[43] and MacGregor et al[42] positioned the duodenal perfusion site more distally at the level of the ligament of Treitz

with the reaspiration site 25 to 65 cm below. This modification allows more homogeneous mixing of food with duodenal secretions and marker, and prevents reflux of the duodenal marker into the stomach. It also permits the calculation of mean transit time of the infused marker in the proximal jejunum.[43] However, this method creates a larger dead space—the entire duodenum—for which the volume and delay between gastric and jejunal sampling are difficult to control. Johansson[43] also used three different duodenal markers in successive sequence, thus ensuring that a duodenal steady state was established by perfusion.

Assumptions. The method is based on a number of assumptions. Some errors may be magnified because each equation uses values calculated in the previous one.

1. The time necessary to administer or consume the meal was assumed to be negligible and was not recorded or used in any equation.

2. The time necessary for marker 1 to reach the duodenal aspiration site was assumed to be 5 minutes. Therefore, the time for duodenal sampling was equal to the time for gastric sampling plus 5 minutes. This 5-

minute delay, however, is only a mean transit time which may vary under different physiologic and pathologic conditions.

3. The concentration of marker is assumed to vary linearly over a 10-minute interval, as the equations used an average intragastric concentration of marker 1, g $(= m_1 + m_{t+10})$. However, this assumption may be a source of error as the marker concentration depends on gastric secretion of fluids and gastric emptying.

4. The gastric and duodenal markers were assumed to be homogenously mixed with the gastric and duodenal contents, which may be difficult in the presence of solid particles. Furthermore, the gastric marker is drunk with water when the solid meal is consumed. Thus, emptying of solids cannot be measured directly. Subsequent attempts at measuring solid emptying by incubating ^{51}Cr with uncooked ground meat[49] did not appear to provide worthwhile information as subsequent use of this tagging method was not reported.

5. Perfusion of the duodenum with physiologic saline at 2 ml/min[48] to 10 ml/min[41] did not affect gastric and duodenal secretory and motor functions. This assumption was based on the observation that the position of the duodenal tube in the stomach or its passage through the pylorus did not influence either the total gastric volume remaining from 1 to 3 hours postcibal, intragastric concentration of marker, intragastric acidity, or serum gastrin.[50] However, perfusion of fluid was not performed in those validation studies.

Despite theoretic uncertainties, these calculations have provided considerable physiologic information about the rates of gastric emptying for liquids and solids, thus clarifying a number of questions regarding the pathophysiology of gastric emptying.

Indications. The general indications for the intraduodenal marker dilution technique are similar to those described for the gastric marker dilution technique. Since biliary and pancreatic secretions can be measured,[41] this method also could be valuable for patients with suspected pancreatic insufficiency or chronic cholestasis. The ability to measure transit time in the proximal jejunum[43] would favor its use over other gastric marker dilution methods in patients with suspected pseudo-obstruction with gastric and small-bowel involvement. Nevertheless, this technique has not been widely applied to the pediatric population, possibly because emptying of solids is not as important in infants as in adults.

SMALL INTESTINE AND COLON

In the small bowel, marker dilution methods were initially devised to measure absorption, but they also provide information concerning the progression of fluids within 15 cm of an intestinal loop.[45] They require intubation with multiple lumen tubes and the establishment of a steady-state flow of fluids from the proximal lumen, placed 235 cm from the teeth. A second lumen, placed 25 cm distally, is used to inject boluses of nonabsorbable markers into the steady-state flow. Continuous aspiration is performed 15 cm below and the concentration of dye and volume recovered are measured during 1-minute periods, allowing the calculation of a mean transit time for the segment of intestine that was intubated.[46,47] This method, however, is limited to measuring propulsion of fluids instilled into the intestinal lumen and does not permit the study of the entire small intestine. Furthermore, it may yield inaccurate estimates of the integrated intestinal flow.[51]

Devroede and Phillips[52] modified the technique of small-bowel perfusion[45] to study colonic transit, volume, and absorption. A four-lumen polyvinyl catheter is introduced through the mouth. Fluoroscopy is used to position the distal opening in the cecum. After cleansing the colon with 1 to 2 l of normal saline, the colon is perfused at 10 ml/min with a solution containing PEG as the marker, and a rectal tube is utilized to recover samples of colonic effluent. Aliquots of the fluid recovered from the rectum are analyzed every 10 minutes; the PEG concentration is measured to determine the time at which steady state conditions are attained. Phenol red is then infused into the cecum and measured in subsequent samples, collected in 5- to 10-minute intervals from the rectal tube. Marker dilution curves are determined from the concentration of the phenol red collected at the rectum. Mean total colonic transit time for the phenol red is then calculated. The technique's main limitation is that it measures transit of liquids in the colon under conditions that do not exist in normal subjects.

Brigham et al[53] measured intestinal transit time in adult patients with acute and convalescent cholera diarrhea. Colonic transit studies have been used in adults with chronic constipation.[54] The use of these two methods in children with intestinal pseudo-obstruction syndromes, severe chronic diarrhea, and chronic constipation may provide valuable information, although they have not been used in the pediatric population. This may be due to their invasiveness. Fluoroscopy is required to position the tubes, and prolonged periods of intubation are necessary.

REFERENCES

1. Bouslog JS, Cunningham TD, Hanner JP, Walton JB, Waltz HD. Roentgenologic studies of the infant's gastrointestinal tract. *J Pediatr* 1935;6:234-48.

2. Ewald CA, Boas J. Beitrage zur physiologie und pathologie der verdauung. *Virchows Arch[A]* 1885;101:325-75.

3. Goldstein H, Boyle JD. The saline load test: a bedside evaluation of gastric retention. *Gastroenterology* 1965;49:375-80.

4. Mathieu A, Rémond A. Note sur un moyen de determiner la quantite de liquide contenu dans l'estomac et al quantite travail chlorhydropeptique effectue par cet organe. *C.R. Soc Biol (Paris)* 1890;96:591-3.

5. Gorham FD. The factor of dilution in gastric analysis. *JAMA* 1923;81:1738-42.

6. Enríquez de Salamanca F, Tamarit Torres J. Estudios de Fisiologia Gástrica. Consejo Superior de Investigaciones Científicas. Madrid: Instituto de Medicina Experimental, 1956.

7. Hunt JN. Gastric emptying and secretion in man. *Physiol Rev* 1959;39:491-533.

8. Hildes JA, Dunlop DL. A method for estimating the rates of gastric secretion and emptying. *Can J Med Sci* 1951;29:83-9.

9. George JD. New clinical method for measuring the rate of gastric emptying: the double sampling test meal. *Gut* 1968;29:237-42.

10. Dubois A, Watanabe A, Kopin IJ. Postoperative gastric retention in the dog. *Am J Dig Dis* 1973;18:39-42.

11. Schoen AM, Knoefel PK. The measurement of human gastric function. *J Lab Clin Med* 1947;32:345-6.

12. Hunt JN. Modification to the method of George for evaluation of gastric emptying. *Gut* 1974;17:812-3.

13. Dubois A, Natelson BH, Van Eerdewegh P, Gardner JD. Gastric emptying and secretion in the rhesus monkey. *Am J Physiol* 1977;232:E186-92.

14. Dubois A, Van Eerdewegh P, Gardner JD. Gastric emptying and secretion in Zollinger-Ellison syndrome. *J Clin Invest* 1977;59:255-63.

15. Bardhan PK, Salam MA, Molla AM. Gastric emptying of liquid in children suffering from acute rotaviral gastroenteritis. *Gut* 1992;33:26-9.

16. Signer E, Fridrich R. Gastric emptying in newborns and young infants. *Acta Paediatr Scand* 1975;64:525-30.

17. Cavell B. Gastric emptying in preterm infants. *Acta Paediatr Scand* 1979;68:725-30.

18. Siegel M, Lebenthal E, Topper W, Krantz B, Li PK. Gastric emptying in prematures of isocaloric feedings with differing osmolalities. *Pediatr Res* 1982;16:141-7.

19. Yu VYH. Effect of body position on gastric emptying in the neonate. *Arch Dis Child* 1975;50:500-4.

20. Burn-Murdoch R, Fisher MA, Hunt JN. Does lying on the right side increase the rate of gastric emptying? *J Physiol (Lond)* 1980;302:395-8.

21. Penner A, Hollander F, Saltzman M. Gastric absorption of phenol red in humans. *Am J Dig Dis* 1938;5:657-61.

22. Bloom DS, Jacobson ED, Grossman MI. Vali-

dation of dilution indicators in the stomach. *Gastroenterology* 1967;52:205-10.

23. Ivey KJ, Schedl HP. Gastric nonabsorbable indicators for studies in man. *Gastroenterology* 1970;59:234-9.

24. Domschke S, Demling J, Domschke W, Hacker J, Clasen M, Demling L. Gastric nonabsorbable indicators in man: a comparison of phenol red and Polyethylene-^{14}C glycol. *Scand J Gastroenterol* 1973;8:17-9.

25. Dorval ED, Mueller GP, Eng RR, Durakovic A, Conklin JJ, Dubois A. Effect of ionizing radiation on gastric secretion and gastric motility in monkeys. *Gastroenterology* 1985;89:374-80.

26. Sidebottom R, Curran JS, Williams PR, Kanarek KS, Bramson RT. Effects of long-chain vs medium-chain triglycerides on gastric emptying in premature infants. *J Pediatr* 1983;102:448-50.

27. Hunt JN. The simultaneous estimation of the absorption of water and sulphaguanidine from the stomach of man. *J Physiol (Lon)* 1949;109:134-41.

28. Bandes J, Hollander F, Glickstein J. The effect of fluid absorption on the dilution indicator technique of gastric analysis. *Am J Physiol* 1940;131:470-82.

29. McLeod GM, French AB, Good CJ, Wright FS. Gastrointestinal absorption and biliary excretion of phenolsulfonphthalein (phenol red) in man. *J Lab Clin Med* 1968;71:192-200.

30. Hurwitz A. Measuring gastric volumes by dye dilution. *Gut* 1981;22:85-93.

31. Dubois A, Mizrahi M. New PC-based program to calculate gastric secretion and emptying using a marker dilution technique. *Dig Dis Sci* 1992;37:1302-4.

32. Husband J, Husband P. Gastric emptying of water and glucose solutions in the newborn. *Lancet* 1969;2:409-11.

33. Hyman PE, Abrams CE, Dubois A. Effect of metoclopramide and bethanechol on gastric emptying in infants. *Pediatr Res* 1985;19:1029-32.

34. Hyman PE, Abrams CE, Dubois A. Gastric emptying in infants: response to metoclopramide depends on the underlying condition. *J Pediatr*

Gastroenterol Nutr 1987;7:181-4.

35. Pérez Delgado C, García-Morato V. Estudios de fisiologia gástrica infantil. *Medicina (Spain)* 1946;14:408-27.

36. Enríquez de Salamanca F, García-Morato V, Pérez Delgado C. Extraciones seriadas del té de prueba en la infancia. *Trab Inst Nac Ciencias Med* 1945;4:29-42.

37. Vendel S. The principle of evacuation of the stomach in infants and prematures. *Acta Physiol Scand* 1946;11:380-5.

38. Cavell B. Gastric emptying in infants. *Lancet* 1969;2:904-5.

39. Hogan DL, Turken D, Stern AI, Isenberg JL. Comparison of the serial dilution indicator and intragastric titration methods for measurement of meal-stimulated gastric acid secretion in man. *Dig Dis Sci* 1983;28:1001-4.

40. Feldman M. Comparison of acid secretion rates measured by gastric aspiration and by in vivo intragastric titration in healthy human subjects. *Gastroenterology* 1979;76:954-7.

41. Go VLW, Hofmann AF, Summerskill WHJ. Simultaneous measurements of total pancreatic, biliary, and gastric outputs in man using a perfusion technique. *Gastroenterology* 1970;58:321-8.

42. MacGregor IL, Gueller R, Watts HD, Meyer JH. The effect of acute hyperglycemia on gastric emptying in man. *Gastroenterology* 1976;70:190-6.

43. Johansson C. Studies of gastrointestinal interactions. *Scand J Gastroenterol* 1974;9 (Suppl 28):1-60.

44. Bernier JJ, Lebert A, Vitesse de l'evacuation de l'estomac et du duodenum au cours de l'hyperglycemie provoquee per os. Biol Gastroenterol 1971;4:351-2.

45. Dillard RL, Eastman H, Fordtran JS. Volume-flow relationship during the transport of fluid through the human small intestine. *Gastroenterology* 1965;49:58-66.

46. Barreiro MA, McKenna RD, Beck IT. Determination of transit time in the human jejunum by the single-injection indicator-dilution technique. *Am J Dig Dis* 1968;13:222-3.

47. Barreiro MA, McKenna RD, Beck IT. The physiologic significance of intraluminal pressure changes in relation to propulsion and absorption in the human jejunum. *Am J Dig Dis* 1968;13:234-51.

48. Malagelada J-R, Longstreth GF, Summerskill WHJ, Go VLW. Measurement of gastric functions during digestion of ordinary meals in man. *Gastroenterology* 1976;70:203-10.

49. Malagelada J-R. Quantification of gastric solid-liquid discrimination during digestion of ordinary meals. *Gastroenterology* 1977;72:1264-7.

50. Longstreth GF, Malagelada J-R, Go VLW. The gastric response to a transpyloric duodenal tube. *Gut* 1975;16:777-80.

51. Worning H, Amdrup E, Henriksen FW. Experimental studies on the intestinal flow using ^{51}Cr as indicator. *Scand J Gastroenterol* 1966;1:111-20.

52. Devroede GJ, Phillips SF. Studies of the perfusion technqiue for colonic absorption. *Gastroenterology* 1969;56:92-100.

53. Brigham KL, Banwell JG, Pierce NF, Mitra RC, Fedson DS, Mondal A. Indicator dilution studies in the small bowel of patients with cholera diarrhea: comparisons of absorbable and poorly absorbable substances. *Hopkins Med J* 1970;127:107-18.

54. Devroede G, Soffie M. Colonic absorption in idiopathic constipation. *Gastroenterology* 1973;64:552-61.

18

Radionuclide Transit Studies

SYDNEY HEYMAN

Radionuclide studies are utilized for the noninvasive evaluation of gastrointestinal transit. Techniques introduced for studying adults have usually been modified for pediatric patients. This chapter will discuss esophageal transit, gastroesophageal reflux, and gastric emptying. The use of radionuclides for measuring small- and large-bowel transit in children has been limited, and will be briefly reviewed.

ESOPHAGEAL TRANSIT

The transit time of a swallowed bolus is determined by the forces generated during the act of swallowing, the effect of gravity, and esophageal peristalsis. Primary motor disorders have been noted in children with tracheoesophageal fistula, Down syndrome, and psychomotor retardation.[1,2] Abnormal motility may occur secondary to esophagitis[3] or scleroderma.[4] Esophageal motor function may be studied by cine-esophagography or manometry. The former results in a high dose of radiation. Esophageal manometry, therefore, is regarded as the investigation of choice, and recording intraluminal pressures gives a measure of esophageal motility. Although the evidence is not yet conclusive, there appears to be a correlation between esophageal motor activity and transit[5] when manometry is performed concurrently with an analysis of liquid transit.[6]

A scintigraphic technique for evaluating esophageal function was first proposed by Kazem.[7] Since then several protocols have been described to quantitate the transit of both solids and liquids.[8-15] These may be used in older children who can cooperate,

since they all require a bolus to be swallowed on command. This technique has also been adapted for infants and small children.

When using a single liquid bolus, 100 to 150 uCi of ^{99m}Tc sulfur colloid is added to 10 ml of water or milk feeding. Patients are placed in the supine position with the low-energy, high-sensitivity collimator of the gamma camera positioned posteriorly. The mouth and stomach are included in the field of view. The computer is programmed to obtain 150 frames per 0.4 seconds. After a practice run with unlabeled liquid, the labeled bolus is sucked into the mouth through a straw. The computer is started and the patient swallows the bolus on command. A second "dry" swallow is requested after 30 seconds. If the transit is abnormal, the procedure is repeated with the patient sitting or standing upright to enhance the effect of gravity. The study is played back in the dynamic mode to identify the cricoid region and the gastroesophageal junction. A small radioactive marker may be placed alongside the cricoid cartilage to aid the localization. Equal regions of interest are placed over the upper, middle, and lower thirds of the esophagus, with a fourth region around the stomach. The time-activity curves that are generated from these regions may be used to make a qualitative or quantitative assessment. The normal transit of the swallowed bolus is characterized by a sharp peak in the upper esophagus, which can be followed through the middle and lower thirds (Fig. 18.1). There is no delay in the detection of gastric activity. The transit time is expressed as the time of initial entry into the esophagus to total

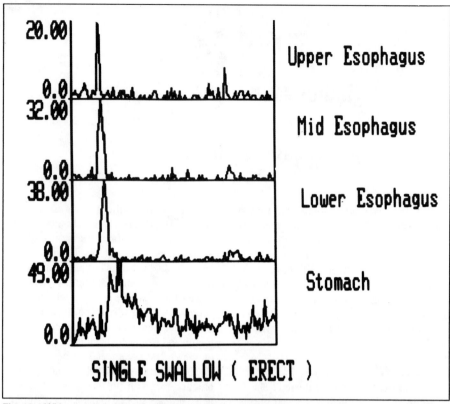

Fig. 18.1 With a normal single swallow in the supine position, the time-activity curves reveal a sharp peak in the upper third of the esophagus, which remains intact and can be followed into the middle and lower thirds. Transit times may be determined as described in the text.

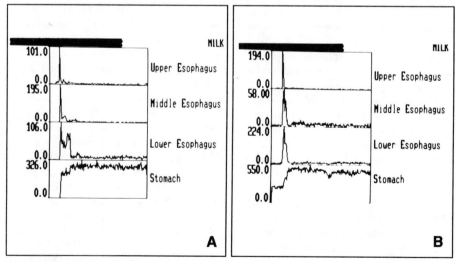

Fig. 18.2 **A,** Transit study of a young boy with esophagitis shows a normal curve in the upper third of the esophagus in the supine position, but a delay in the middle third that is even more marked in the lower third. **B,** A repeat swallow in the upright position shows the transit to be significantly improved with the aid of gravity.

clearance. Normal values have been reported in adults.[12] Deviations from the normal pattern are usually obvious from a qualitative assessment of the curves. Abnormal transit has been observed in several conditions, including achalasia, scleroderma, esophageal stricture, and esophagitis (Fig. 18.2). When the transit disorder is severe, "to and fro" movement of the bolus may be seen in the supine position, but this improves when the test is repeated in the upright position. This pattern has been observed with scleroderma and esophagitis.

A functional display, known as the bolus-transport diagram, has been applied to esophageal studies. After swallowing a single bolus, the transit is recorded on the computer in list mode. On completion of the study, a sequence of images is obtained in which each picture displays the bolus position during a fixed time interval that is not less than the interval between two time markers. By combining a number of such strips into one picture, a representation of the bolus position relative to time is obtained (Fig. 18.3). This method provides a good visual display of the bolus transit, and reveals any episodes of reflux during the study.[14] With the condensed image, the end point for determining the mean transit time may be more clearly defined when compared with a more detailed analysis of the single swallow.[15]

Another approach in both adults and children has been to use ^{81m}Kr labeled glucose. Glucose in water (5%) infused through a 15 mCi ^{81}Rb - ^{81m}Kr generator results in several mCi of ^{81m}Kr solution. Due to its short physical half-life (13 seconds), relatively large doses may be administered. In children, 2 ml is delivered into the mouth by syringe. The patient then swallows as before. Computer acquisition is at 1-second intervals for 60 seconds. These images are first corrected for decay. A mean time for each pixel is calcu-

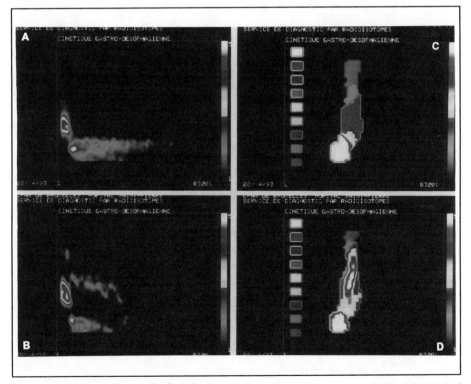

Fig. 18.3 **A,** Normal condensed image. **B,** Abnormal condensed image shows stasis at the level of the upper esophagus. **C,** Normal mean time image. **D,** This mean time image depicts the same transit abnormality, and demonstrates the time taken to traverse different levels of the esophagus. (Courtesy of Amnon Piepsz, MD, Hôpital Saint Pierre, Brussels)

lated from the time activity curve, which is represented by

$$\frac{\Sigma An(t) \cdot t}{\Sigma An(t)}$$

An(t) is the activity at the nth pixel at time (t). A time image may be constructed using the mean time as a parameter. When presented as a color display, each color corresponds to a specific value of mean time (see Fig. 18.3). The mean transit time for adults is less than 5 seconds in the erect position, and about 8 seconds when supine.[16]

This study can be modified for evaluating esophageal transit in infants. The patient is positioned with his or her back to the collimator, which is inclined at about 45.° To avoid facilitating aspiration, horizontal positioning should not be used. Esophageal transit is usually studied during a scan for gastroesophageal reflux. The bottle containing the labeled milk is placed in a lead shield

to reduce scatter. It may contain 200 to 1000 uCi of ^{99m}Tc sulfur colloid, depending on the size of the meal. While the patient sucks normally, sequential 0.5-second images are collected for 120 seconds on the computer for later playback and analysis.[17] A similar technique has been described for infants, but the erect position[18] is used for greater gravitational effect. Time-activity curves are obtained from regions of interest drawn over the upper, middle, and lower esophagus, as well as the stomach. These normally show a series of waves associated with the multiple swallows that progress down the esophagus, without the buildup of activity within any one region. There is an early appearance of activity in the stomach (Fig. 18.4). Abnormal patterns have been recognized in several conditions, including tracheoesophageal fistula, scleroderma, stricture, esophagitis, and achalasia (Fig. 18.5).[17]

The qualitative assessment of the curves

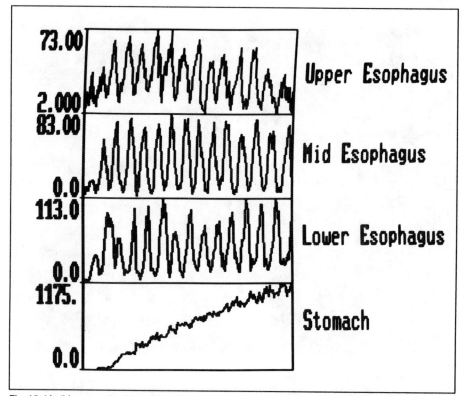

Fig. 18.4 In this example of normal multiple swallows in an infant, the sequential boluses are depicted as sharp waves which progress uniformly down the esophagus. The early appearance of activity in the stomach is also shown. (Reprinted with permission from Heyman S, 1985[68])

are reliable. Quantitative data in one study showed an overlap between normals and abnormals, possibly due to the upright position and the effect of gravity on transit.[18]

GASTROESOPHAGEAL REFLUX

Gastroesophageal scintigraphy has been adapted for use in children.[19-21] When ^{99m}Tc sulfur colloid is mixed with milk or formula, the radioactive tag remains stable as it mixes with gastric secretions. It is important that the radioactive marker is not absorbed from the gastrointestinal tract since this increases the background interference and decreases the sensitivity for detecting reflux and aspiration. The radiation exposure has been estimated at a whole-body dose ranging from 0.0200 rad/100 uCi in the newborn to 0.00026 rad/100 uCi at the age of 15 years. The critical organ is the lower large bowel, where the absorbed dose ranges from 0.927 rad/100 uCi to 0.072 rad/100 uCi over the same age range.[22]

Gastroesophageal scintigraphy is best performed at the time of a scheduled feeding. The reported administered doses vary between 100 uCi and 1 mCi. To ensure a high sensitivity, a concentration of about 5 uCi/ml is preferred, with a minimum dose of 200 uCi. Older children should receive the maximum dose of 1 mCi. Ideally, the size of the feeding should be standardized according to age, especially because most studies are performed in conjunction with gastric emptying rates. Many infants are on modified schedules, so the feeding the patient currently receives can be used. If the child is allergic to milk, another medium such as fruit juice is used. The radioactive tracer is placed in about two thirds of the volume to be fed. The initial swallowing can be recorded and the esophageal transit evaluated at

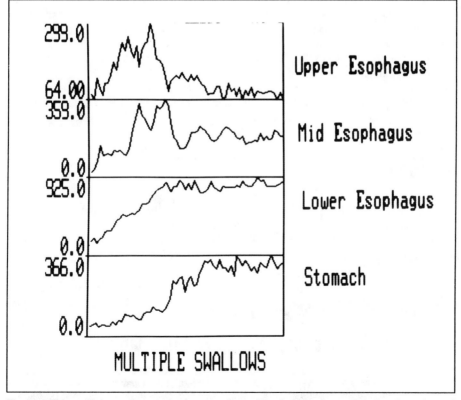

Fig. 18.5 This multiple swallow study of a young boy with achalasia shows disordered esophageal motility. Activity builds up in the lower esophagus. Activity in the stomach is delayed.

this stage, as previously described. After consuming the radioactive portion of the feeding, the unlabeled milk or formula is given to wash out residue in the mouth and esophagus. After burping, the patient is placed supine under the gamma camera, using a low-energy, high-sensitivity collimator. Both the stomach and the thorax must be in the field of view. In infants, reflux appears to occur more readily in the supine than in the prone position.[23] It is possible to image posteriorly, but the spine may attenuate smaller reflux episodes.

Imaging is commenced as soon after the feeding as possible. When the feeding has been delivered by nasogastric tube, the tube should be removed, if possible, before beginning the study. Although the role of the nasogastric tube in precipitating reflux may be questioned, it is usually blamed when reflux is present. Most patients lie quietly at this time, but swaddling and sandbags may be required for restraint.

Computer acquisition is essential if quantitation is to be performed. The playback of enhanced images may reveal reflux that is not evident on analog images. Data acquisition should continue for at least 60 minutes. By limiting the study to 30 minutes, at least 25% of the reflux may be missed.[24] Analog images are obtained at 30- or 60-second intervals; the intensity is maximized to increase the sensitivity of the study. While the dynamic data are usually acquired at 20, 30, or even 60 seconds per frame, there is an advantage to more rapid framing. Reflux episodes are usually brief, so that a 5-second framing rate gives more information about the number of episodes and the clearance rate from the esophagus (Fig. 18.6).

When reviewing the study, the analog images usually reveal episodes of reflux. With the newer gamma cameras it is more usual to have only digital data. When reflux is brief and of minimal volume, the low count abnormality may be better visualized using a 5-second rate rather than a longer framing rate. This does not apply when reflux persists in three or more 5-second frames. Separate regions of interest are placed over the entire esophagus, with a second region over the upper half. Time-activity curves are generated which will demonstrate the number of reflux episodes, delineate those reaching the upper esophagus, and exhibit the clearance rate. Since patient movement may produce a spike in the curves, it is important to exclude this possibility during the dynamic playback of the study.

Reflux indices have been described to quantitate reflux. These all depend on the number of episodes, the volume (activity)

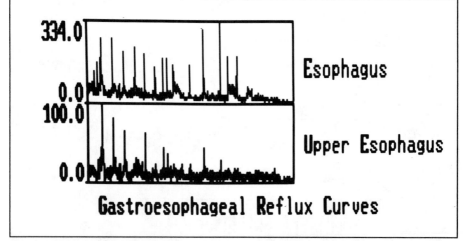

Fig. 18.6 These curves are derived from 5 s/frame images and demonstrate multiple episodes of reflux, many reaching the upper esophagus. In this instance, the refluxate appears to be cleared rapidly from the esophagus between events. (Reprinted with permission from Gelfand M, Thomas SR, 1988[69])

refluxed, and the clearance rate from the esophagus. Fisher et al[25] acquired 30-second images, which were repeated with increasing abdominal pressure. They determined the ratio of esophageal activity—corrected for background interference—to the initial gastric activity. In adults, this clearly distinguished patients (11.7 ± 1.8%) from controls (2.7 ± 0.3%). Devos et al[26] expressed the mean value of the esophageal time-activity curve as a percentage of the initial gastric activity. There was a significant difference between normals (0.66 ± 0.12%) and those with peptic esophagitis (3.66 ± 0.81%). Using a frame rate of 20 seconds, Piepsz et al[24] determined the activity in each episode as a percentage of the gastric activity at that time, and summed for the 60-minute study. Peaks greater than 5% usually corresponded to reflux episodes, but quantitation could not predict the presence of esophagitis. The reflux index can be derived by first reformatting the data to give 30-second frames. The esophageal time-activity curve is background corrected, then integrated over the 60 minutes. The area under the curve is expressed as a fraction of the initial gastric activity. Values range from 0.085 ± 0.032 without reflux to 1.087 ± 0.455 when reflux is severe. These values have not been correlated with the presence of esophagitis, but are useful in follow-up studies.

A comparison of the various techniques has been difficult because methodology is not uniform. Scintigraphy is usually compared to intraesophageal pH monitoring. A review of the earlier studies reveals a sensitivity between 75% and 100%, with a low value of 56% when computer enhancement was not used.[21, 25-29] All showed a sensitivity greater than that of barium studies or manometry. In a group of patients selected for surgery, the radionuclide study was abnormal in 69%. Assuming a similar sensitivity in the nonoperated group, the specificity of the test was 95%. The best sensitivity, 87%, was achieved with a combination of scintigraphy, pH probe, and manometry. A definite role was found for the radionuclide study as a screening procedure.[30] Simultaneous intraesophageal pH monitoring and scintigraphy revealed a sensitivity of 79% and a specificity of 93%.[27] It should be stressed that the sensitivity of the scintigraphic study depends on the concentration of the isotope, the gamma camera sensitivity, attenuation, as well as the volume and esophageal residence time of the refluxate.

There are differences between scintigraphy and pH monitoring when the studies are performed concurrently. Scintigraphy integrates counts during the collection frame, while the pH probe records instantaneous events approximately every 7.5 seconds, thereby missing very short episodes. Furthermore, if milk is used as a feeding there will be a buffering effect so that more events will be evident early in the scintigraphic study.[31] The sensitivity of the radionuclide reflux study has also been questioned as the result of an in vitro simulation test. Vomiting has been observed without an obvious change in esophageal activity in the contrasted images.[32] Using the milk concentration and collection parameters described seems to bypass this phenomenon, making scintigraphy a good screening procedure.

GASTRIC EMPTYING

Symptoms associated with delayed gastric emptying include nausea, vomiting, abdominal discomfort, and early satiety. Gastric emptying studies are indicated when the symptoms are consistent with an altered rate of gastric emptying. Follow-up examinations document the effect of interventions such as surgery or prokinetic drugs.

The tone of the gastric fundus is believed to be important in the emptying of liquids through volume displacement, though antral contractions initiated by solids may also play a role.[33] Antral hypomotility is assumed to be the major cause of delayed gastric emptying, but it may also be due to impaired coordination of contractions. The motor functions of the antrum, pylorus, and duodenum are not independent and are closely integrated.[34] Liquids, solids, and indigestible solids all have different rates of emptying.[35] Several factors influence the emptying rate. The caloric content of the meal, rather than its size, has been shown to delay emptying.[36] In adults, increasing the osmolality of the meal prolongs the emptying time[37-39] but, within limits, osmolar loads were not found to exert a significant effect in premature infants and normal newborns.[40,41] Feeding with cow's milk results in slower emptying than with human milk, even though the feedings are isocaloric. This difference is most likely due to the different compositions of the milks.[42] Emptying is more rapid with whey-based than casein-based milk formulae, even when there are no differences in osmolality, caloric value, or fat content.[43] A possible exception is acidified cow's milk formula, which was also shown to empty rapidly.[44] Fatty acids with carbon chain lengths between 2 and 8, or 14 and 18,[45] as well as physiologic concentrations of L-tryptophan,[37] and increasing concentrations of acid solutions[46] have all been found to delay the emptying process. It is thus clear that quantitation of gastric emptying should be peformed using a meal of standard size and composition.

In infants, the meal used to assess gastric emptying is usually milk or formula. Ideally, the type and volume of milk should be standardized according to age. In practice, many children are on modified feeding regimens, and standardization is difficult in this group of patients. It is usually best to administer the patient's usual feeding or institute a modification as requested by the referring physician. The study is often performed in conjunction with one for gastroesophageal reflux, in which case the administered dose of ^{99m}Tc sulfur colloid is 200 to 1000 uCi. If the focus is only on gastric emptying, then 100 uCi is adequate.

The patient receives the meal at the time of a usual feeding, having fasted since the previous meal. After consuming the milk, the infant is burped and placed supine beneath the gamma camera using a low-energy, high-sensitivity collimator. Computer acquisition is at 30 seconds per frame. If a more rapid framing rate is employed, as in a gastroesophageal reflux study, the data can be reformatted prior to analysis. The study is continued for at least 1 hour. If the number of radionuclide markers remaining in the stomach is abnormally high at this time, it is advisable to extend the study for a further hour. Patients who show slightly delayed emptying at 1 hour are frequently in the normal range by 2 hours, in which case they are regarded as normal, provided that the pattern of the emptying curve is acceptable, as discussed below.

A time-activity curve is obtained from a region of interest drawn around the stomach in the initial frame. The curve is corrected for decay. Gastric emptying has been expressed as the time taken for the gastric activity to decrease to half the original value ($T^{1/2}$), the percentage of the peak activity remaining after a specific time (R%), or the percentage emptied (100-R%). If the patient has moved, the images need to be reregistered or separate regions should be drawn at various time points (eg, every 15 min). Milk usually empties in a monoexponential or biexponential fashion, but emptying patterns may vary so widely that the $T^{1/2}$ measurement may not always separate normals from abnormals. It is usual to express gastric emptying as the residual or amount emptied over a specific period. The graphic representation will suggest any abnormal emptying pattern.

Since healthy children are not usually studied, the normal range for gastric emptying has been difficult to establish. An early study of normal infants using ^{113m}In microcolloid in milk showed that milk emptied monoexponentially with a $T^{1/2}$ of 87$\pm$29 minutes and a diphasic pattern with a smaller number that was attributed to swallowed air.[47] Extrapolating from these data, the residual activity at 60 minutes was between 48% and 70%; at 120 minutes it was 24% and 48%. This range can be used as a guide. More recently, values have been reported in children who were in retrospect thought to be normal. Using ^{99m}Tc sulfur colloid in milk, a residual of 36% to 68% at 60 minutes was reported in infants, and 42% to 56% in a small number of older children. The emptying pattern is also important. For example, the plateau pattern (periods of long delay in emptying followed by sharp falls in gastric activity) has been associated with pylorospasm as well as antral membrane.[48] Dextrose labeled with the same radiopharmaceutical was shown to have a residual of 27% to 81% at 60 minutes in children under 2 years, and 11% to 47% in older children.[49] This age-related difference in the rate of gastric emptying has also been suggested by others,[50] although the composition of the meal may play a role in older children. It is thus clear that while guidelines exist for evaluating gastric emptying in infants using radionuclide techniques, the values adopted for the normal range should be determined by individual laboratories.

In older children, techniques used for measuring solid, liquid, or combined emptying in adults are applicable. It is essential that the radio-label remains firmly attached to the test meal. In the clinical setting, the solid meal may consist of eggs labeled with ^{99m}Tc sulfur colloid. The egg white is separated, the measured dose of the radiopharmaceutical is mixed in (approximately 250-300 uCi), and then fried. The meal size is based on four egg whites for an adult patient, and scaled down by body surface area. The whole egg may also be used. Radiopharmaceutical in a volume not exceeding 0.1 ml is carefully injected into the yolk so that it does not rupture. After an incubation period of 5 minutes, the egg(s) are scrambled and fried. The meal is then presented as a sandwich.[51] The number of eggs is two for a patient over 7 years of age, and one if younger. Although the label is not as firm as that in chicken liver labeled in vivo,[52] the labeling method is more practical clinically and quantitation has been satisfactory. Other solid meals which have been satisfactorily labeled include iodinated fiber,[53] ^{99m}Tc labeled bran,[54] or pudding.[50] If liquid emptying is to be evaluated simultaneously, water in a volume scaled down from 500 ml and containing 50 uCi of ^{111}In DTPA (diethylenetriaminepentaacetic acid) is offered after the solid meal. Since solid emptying is usually a more sensitive indicator of abnormal gastric emptying, in children solid emptying alone should be quantitated to limit the radiation exposure. The standard unlabeled liquid volume is also given, since liquids influence the rate of solid emptying. Occasionally, simultaneous solid and liquid emptying is requested. The ^{99m}Tc:^{111}In activity ratio should be at least 6:1 to minimize the down-scatter from the ^{111}In channel down to the ^{99m}Tc channel.

Patient position needs to be standardized, since differences in the emptying rate can be demonstrated between upright and supine positions.[55,56] Ideally, patients are placed supine. The gamma camera, which has been fitted with a high-sensitivity collimator, is positioned anteriorly. Thirty-second images are obtained every 10 minutes for 120 minutes. Between images, patients sit up or stand.

For measuring gastric emptying, regions of interest are placed around the stomach at each time point. The counts are decay-corrected and the percentage of residual activity is plotted against time. If two isotopes have been used for simultaneous solid/liquid quantitation, it is necessary to determine the percentage of down-scatter from the ^{111}In into the ^{99m}Tc channel, and also the scattered ^{99m}Tc counts appearing in the ^{111}In channel. In the latter instance, a medium-energy collimator must be used. The actual numbers for the cross-over will depend on the camera-collimator system and the window settings, but typical values would be 20% for ^{111}In to ^{99m}Tc and 3% in the reverse direction. As mentioned, the effect can be minimized by having a suitable ratio of activity. Only after this correction are the ^{99m}Tc counts decay-corrected. It is not necessary to decay the ^{111}In counts. Software is available to reregister images to account for movement, so that a computer-generated curve may be obtained. As in the case of infants, the normal rate of gastric emptying using these standard meals has not been established in children. As a guide, values reported for young adults using anterior imaging can be utilized by converting them to percentage residuals at 10-minute intervals for up to 2 hours (Fig. 18.7).

Potential errors with radionuclide technique include overlapping gastric and duodenal activity, scatter from adjacent bowel into the stomach region of interest, scattered activity when two isotopes are used, and posteroanterior movement within the stomach. Blurring of the gastric outline is more of a problem in delayed images. When this occurs, it is useful to either truncate the study somewhat, or to extend it for a further 10 to 15 minutes until a clearer distinction between the stomach and small bowel is

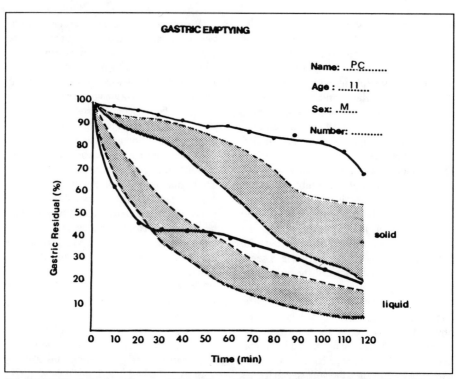

Fig. 18.7 In this study of an 11-year-old boy with gastric outlet obstruction, emptying of the solid phase is markedly delayed. The liquid phase empties at a normal rate for about 20 minutes, but is abnormally slow thereafter. The curves are superimposed on the normal range for solids and liquids in young adults, as described by the literature.

evident. Scattered activity from the small bowel into the gastric region has been found to be insignificant.[57] The "cross-talk" when two isotopes are used may need correcting, as described above. Posteroanterior movement of gastric contents with passage from the fundus to the antrum has been reported to cause a significant error when using a low-energy radionuclide such as ^{99m}Tc. As the radionuclide is positioned more anteriorly with time, there is less attenuation of photons. The effect suggests a slower than actual rate of emptying, with a prolonged lag phase. One way to compensate for this is to obtain conjugate views of the stomach. Anterior and posterior images are obtained at each time point. The gastric counts are determined from regions of interest and the geometric mean is calculated (ie, anterior counts x posterior counts).[1/2] The geometric mean is insensitive to the changing source depth. Acquisition of the images is especially easy

if a gamma camera is available with two opposing heads. Several small children have been studied in this manner; with a thin abdominal wall the attenuation effect is small, so that conjugate counting is unnecessary and anterior imaging is sufficient. Attenuation correction is probably necessary with obese or older patients, or if the standard meal is particularly large.

SMALL- AND LARGE-BOWEL TRANSIT

Several techniques can measure gastrointestinal transit times, including manometry, electromyography, radiography, indicator dilution studies, and the hydrogen breath test.[58] Scintigraphy was introduced as a physiologic test, and has gained acceptance in adult patients both as a research tool and in clinical practice. There are no published data of the application in pediatric patients. Small-bowel transit has been evaluated using radio-labeled solid meals, liquids, and insoluble solids.[59,60] The radioactive labels have been either ^{99m}Tc sulfur colloid, ^{99m}Tc DTPA, ^{99m}Tc, or ^{111}InCl$_3$ tagged particles. From regions of interest drawn over the stomach, cecum, or ascending colon, total counts are determined at suitable time points, then corrected for attenuation and decay. As described for gastric emptying, conjugate counting will allow for attenuation. The results are expressed as a mean small-bowel transit time, a mean orocecal transit time, or a colonic appearance time. Since small-bowel transit is influenced by oral intake, it is necessary to standardize the initial meal. The low-resolution images may present problems in selecting the regions of interest, since ileal loops are superimposed on the cecum and ascending colon. For studying large-bowel transit, the tracer may be delivered orally via a delayed-release capsule containing radio-labeled pellets,[61] by passing a tube orally to deliver the radioactive test solution into the cecum,[62] or by passing a colonoscope for delivery into the colon.[63] Methods requiring intubation are applicable for research purposes but are unacceptable for routine clinical studies. Again, patients must be prepared with a standard meal. Regions of interest are drawn over the cecum, segments of the colon, and the rectosigmoid. The data may be represented as an emptying rate or the geometric center,[64] which is a weighted average of counts in the colon, and may be used to summarize overall transit in the colon. This value is calculated by drawing five regions of interest: 1) cecum, ascending colon, and hepatic flexure; 2) transverse colon; 3) splenic flexure; 4) descending colon; and 5) sigmoid and rectum. The proportion of activity in each region at a given time (including a percentage for the defecated material) is multiplied by the regional number, and the results are added together. The resulting value represents the location of the geometric center of activity. Yet another technique is to determine the geometric mean counts in each region with time, and to display the result as a condensed image, similar to that described for esophageal transit.[65] Transit studies of the bowel are often extremely long and demanding of gamma camera time. Attempts have been made to limit data collection while preserving accuracy, increasing the practicality of these studies. Simplified data analysis from scans taken at 2, 4, and 6 hours after ingestion of a radio-labeled meal identified motility disorders of the stomach and small bowel.[66] For the large bowel, activity measured in colonic regions at 4 and 24 hours after ingestion of a delayed-release capsule containing radio-labeled pellets provided a high degree of sensitivity for identifying disordered transit. The radiation dose from 0.25 mCi ^{111}InCl$_3$ results in the same total body exposure as a single abdominal x-ray (80 mrads).[61] The doses used in children could be scaled down proportionately. With standardization of the technique and simplification of the analysis, radionuclide transit studies of the small and large bowel are feasible in pediatric patients and merit further consideration.

CONCLUSION

Radionuclide studies to evaluate transit through the esophagus and stomach are well established in pediatric patients. They can be performed individually or in conjunction with a scan for gastroesophageal reflux. These studies are physiologic in nature and are easy to perform, requiring only a standard gamma camera interfaced with a computer. While the gastroesophageal reflux study is largely regarded as a screening procedure, its sensitivity and specificity when compared to a simultaneous pH probe study is acceptably high. The gastric emptying study is widely used and provides an accurate measure of gastric function. Comparison of the data requires that the methodology be standardized, especially with regard to the test meal. Esophageal transit studies are not extensively used in pediatrics, but they do have the potential to document abnormalities in transit and to evaluate the response to treatment, as with reflux esophagitis. Transit studies of the small and large bowel have not been addressed to any great extent in children. Noninvasive techniques for delivering the isotope appear to provide meaningful results; therefore, the application of these tests in this population should be feasible.

REFERENCES

1. Hillemeier C, Buchin P, Gryboski J. Esophageal dysfunction in Down's syndrome. *J Pediatr Gastroenterol Nutr* 1983;1:101-4.

2. Staiano A, Cucchiara S, Del Giudice E, Andreotti MR, Minella R. Disorders of oesophageal motility in children with psychomotor retardation and gastro-oesophageal reflux. *Eur J Pediatr* 1991;150:638-41.

3. Little AG, DeMeester TR, Kirchner PT, O'Sullivan GC, Skinner DB. Pathogenesis of esophagitis in patients with gastroesophageal reflux. *Surgery* 1980;77:101-7.

4. Davidson A, Russel C, Littlejohn GO. Assessment of esophageal abnormalities in progressive systemic sclerosis (scleroderma). *Arthritis Rheum* 1980;23:581-90.

5. Holloway RH, Orenstein SR. Gastroesophageal reflux disease in adults and children. *Baillieres Clin Gastroenterol* 1991;5:337-70.

6. Richter JE, Blackwell JN, Wu WC, Johns DN, Cowan RJ, Castell DO. Relationship of radionuclide liquid bolus transport and esophageal manometry. *J Lab Clin Med* 1987;217-24.

7. Kazem I. A new scintigraphic technique for the study of the esophagus. *AJR* 1972;115:681-8.

8. Holloway RH, Krosin G, Lange RC, Baue AE, McCallum RW. Radionuclide esophageal emptying of a solid meal to quantitate results of therapy in achalasia. *Gastroenterology* 1983;84:771-6.

9. Bosch A, Dietrich R, Lanaro A, Frias Z. Modified scintigraphic technique for the dynamic study of the esophagus. *Int J Nucl Med Biol* 1977;4:195-9.

10. Mayron LW, Kaplan E. The use of [81m]Kr in deglutition kinetic studies. *Int J Nucl Med Biol* 1975;2:42-3.

11. Tolin RD, Malmud LS, Reilley J, Fisher RS. Esophageal scintigraphy to quantitate esophageal transit (quantitation of esophageal transit). *Gastroenterology* 1979;76;1402-8.

12. Russell COH, Hill LD, Holmes ER III, Hull DA, Gannon R, Pope CD II. Radionuclide transit: a sensitive screening test for esophageal dysfunction. *Gastroenterology* 1981;80:837-92.

13. Blackwell JN, Hannan WJ, Adam RD, Heading RC. Radionuclide transit studies in the detection of esophageal dysmotility. *Gut* 1983;24:421-6.

14. Svedburg JB. The bolus transport diagram: a functional display method applied to oesophageal studies. *Clin Phys Physiol Meas* 1982;3:267-72.

15. Klein HA, Wald A. Computer analysis of radionuclide esophageal transit studies. *J Nucl Med* 1984;25:957-64.

16. Ham HR, Piepsz A, Georges B, Verelst J, Guillaume M, Cadranel S. Quantitation of esophageal transit by means of [81m]Kr. *Eur J Nucl Med* 1984;9:362-5.

17. Heyman S. Esophageal scintigraphy (milk scans) in infants and children with gastroesophageal reflux. *Radiology* 1982;144:891-3.

18. Guillet J, Wynchank S, Basse-Cathalinat B, Christophe E, Ducassou D, Planquet P. Pediatric esophageal scintigraphy: results of 200 studies. *Clin Nucl Med* 1983;8:427-33.

19. Heyman S, Kirkpatrick JA, Winter HS, Treves S. An improved method for the diagnosis of gastroesophageal reflux and aspiration in children (milk scan). *Radiology* 1979;131:479-82.

20. Rudd TG, Christie DL. Demonstration of gastroesophageal reflux in children by radionuclide gastroesophagography. *Radiology* 1979;131:483-6.

21. Blumhagen JD, Rudd TG, Christie DL. Gastroesophageal reflux in children: radionuclide gastroesophagography. *AJR* 1980;135:1001-4.

22. Castronovo FP. Gastroesophageal scintigraphy in a pediatric population: dosimetry. *J Nucl Med* 1986;27:1212-14.

23. Blumenthal I, Lealman GT. Effect of posture on gastroesophageal reflux in the newborn. *Arch Dis Child* 1982;47:555-6.

24. Piepsz A, Georges B, Perlmütter N, Rodesch P, Cadranel S. Gastroesophageal scintiscanning in children. *Pediatr Radiol* 1981;11:71-4.

25. Fisher RS, Malmud LS, Roberts GS, Lobis IF.

Gastroesophageal (GE) scintiscanning to detect and quantitate GE reflux. *Gastroenterology* 1976;70:301-8.

26. Devos PG, Forget P, DeRoo M, Eggermont E. Scintigraphic evaluation of gastrointestinal reflux (GER) in children. *J Nucl Med* 1979;20:636. Abstract.

27. Seibert JJ, Byrne WJ, Euler AR, Lature T, Leach M, Campbell M. Gastroesophageal reflux— the acid test: scintigraphy or pH probe? *AJR* 1983;140:1087-90.

28. Heyman S. Gastric emptying, gastroesophageal reflux and esophageal motility. In: Gelfand MJ, Thomas SR, eds. *Effective Use of Computers in Nuclear Medicine.* New York: McGraw Hill 1988;412-37.

29. Arasu TS, Wyllie R, Fitzgerald JF, et al. Gastroesophageal reflux in infants and children: comparative accuracy of diagnostic methods. *J Pediatr* 1980;96:798-803.

30. Davies RP, Morris LL, Savage JP, Davidson GP. Gastro-oesophageal reflux: the role of imaging in the diagnosis and management. *Australas Radiol* 1987;31:157-63.

31. Vandenplas Y, Derde MP, Piepsz A. Evaluation of reflux episodes during simultaneous esophageal pH monitoring and gastroesophageal reflux scintigraphy in children. *J Pediatr Gastroenterol Nutr* 1992;14:256-60.

32. Payton JY, Cosgriff PS, Nanagakkra CS. The analytical sensitivity of Tc^{99m} radionuclide "milk" scanning in the detection of gastro-esophageal reflux. *Pediatr Radiol* 1985;15:381-3.

33. Kelly KA. Gastric emptying of liquids and solids: roles of proximal and distal stomach. *Am J Physiol* 1980;239:G71-6.

34. Horowitz M, Dent J. Disordered gastric emptying: mechanical basis, assessment, and treatment. *Basillieres Clin Gastroenterol* 1991;5:371-407.

35. Hinder RA, Kelly KA. Canine gastric emptying of solids and liquids. *Am J Physiol* 1977;233:E335-40.

36. Christian PE, Moore JG, Brown F, et al. Effect of caloric content and meal size in gastric emptying (abstract). *J Nucl Med* 1982;23:P20.

37. Cooke AR, Mouland J. Control of gastric emptying by amino acids. *Gastroenterology* 1972;62:528-32.

38. Elias E, Gibson GJ, Greenwood LF, Hunt JN, Tripp OH. The slowing of gastric emptying by monosaccharides and disaccharides in test meals. *J Physiol* 1986;194:317-28.

39. Hunt JN, Pathak JD. The osmotic effects of some simple molecules and ions on gastric emptying. *J Physiol (Lond)* 1960;154:254-69.

40. Siegel M, Lebenthal E, Topper W, Krantz B, Li PK. Gastric emptying in prematures of isocaloric feedings with differing osmolalities. *Pediatr Res* 1982;16:141-7.

41. Hunt LI, Antonson DL, Paxson CL, Vanderhoof JA. Osmolality of carbohydrate solutions and gastric emptying in the newborn. *Am J Dis Child* 1982;136:448-51.

42. Cavell B. Gastric emptying in preterm infants. *Acta Paediatr Scan* 1979;68:725-30.

43. Friad MD, Khoshoo V, Secker DJ, Gilday DL, Ash JM, Pencharz PB. Decrease in gastric emptying time and episodes of regurgitation in children with spastic quadriplegia fed a whey based formula. *J Pediatr* 1992;120:569-72.

44. Billeaud C, Gillet J, Sandler B. Gastric emptying in infants with or without gastro-esophageal reflux according to the type of milk. *Eur J Clin Nutr* 1990;44:577-83.

45. Hunt JN, Knox MT. A relation between the chain length of fatty acids and the slowing of gastric emptying. *J Physiol (Lond)* 1968;194:327-36.

46. Hunt JN, Knox MT. The slowing of gastric emptying by four strong acids and three weak acids. *J Physiol (Lond)* 1972;222:187-208.

47. Signer E, Fredrich R. Gastric emptying in newborns and young infants. *Acta Paediatr Scan* 1975;64:525-30.

48. Seibert JJ, Byrne WJ, Euler AR. Gastric emptying in children: unusual patterns detected by scintigraphy. *AJR* 1983;141:49-51.

49. Rosen PR, Treves S. The relationship of gastroesophageal reflux and gastric emptying in infants and children: concise communication. *J Nucl Med* 1984;25:571-4.

50. Di Lorenzo C, Piepsz A, Ham H, Cadranel S. Gastric emptying with gastro-oesophageal reflux. *Arch Dis Child* 1987;62:449-53.

51. Malmud LS, Fisher RS, Knight LC, Rock E. Scintigraphic evaluation of gastric emptying. *Semin Nucl Med* 1982;12:116-25.

52. Sheiner HJ. Progress report: gastric emptying tests in man. *Gut* 1975;16:235-47.

53. Malagelada J-R, Carter SE, Brown ML, Carlson GL. Radiolabeled fiber: a physiologic marker for gastric emptying and intestinal transport of solids. *Dig Dis Sci* 1980;25:81-7.

54. Sagar S, Grime JS, Little W, et al. Technetium[99m] labeled bran: a new agent for measuring gastric emptying. *Clin Radiol* 1983;34:275-8.

55. Tothill P, McLoughlin GP, Heading RC. Techniques and errors in scintigraphic measurements of gastric emptying. *J Nucl Med* 1978;19:256-61.

56. Tothill P, McLoughlin GP, Holt S, Heading RC. The effect of posture on errors in gastric emptying measurements. *Phys Med Biol* 1980;25:1071-8.

57. VanDeventer G, Thomson J, Graham LS, Thomasson D, Meyer JH. Validation of corrections for errors in collimation during measurements of gastric emptying of nuclide labeled meals. *J Nucl Med* 1983;24:187-96.

58. Hellstrom PM, Hosebye E, Kraglund K. Methodology for motility studies on the small intestine: a Scandinavian consensus. *Eur J Surg Suppl* 1991;564:51-61.

59. Nielson OH, Gjorup T, Christensen FN. Gastric emptying rate and small bowel transit time in patients with irritable bowel syndrome determined with ^{99m}Tc-labeled pellets and scintigraphy. *Dig Dis Sci* 1986;31:1287-91.

60. Madsen JL, Larsen NE, Hilsted J, Worning H.
Scintigraphic determination of gastrointestinal transit times: a comparison with breath hydrogen and radiologic methods. *Scand J Gastroenterol* 1991;26:1263-71.

61. Camilleri M, Zinsmeister AR. Towards a relatively inexpensive, noninvasive, accurate test for colonic motility disorders. *Gastroenterology* 1992;103:36-42.

62. Krevsky B, Malmud LS, D'Ercole F, Maurer AH, Fisher RS. Colonic transit scintigraphy: a physiologic approach to the quantitative measurement of colonic transit in humans. *Gastroenterology* 1986;91:1102-12.

63. Moreno-Osset E, Bazzocchi G, Lo S, et al. Association between postprandial changes in colonic intraluminal pressure and transit. *Gastroenterology* 1989;96:1265-73.

64. Miller M, Galligan J, Burks T. Accurate measurement of intestinal transit in the rat. *J Pharmacol Methods* 1981;6:211-17.

65. Notghi A, Kumar D, Panagamuwa B, Tulley NJ, Hesslewood SR, Harding LK. Measurement of colonic transit time using radionuclide imaging: analysis by condensed images. *Nucl Med Commun* 1993;14:204-11.

66. Camilleri M, Zinsmeister AR, Greydanus MP, Brown ML, Proano M. Towards a less costly but accurate test of gastric emptying and small bowel transit. *Dig Dis Sci* 1991;36:609-15.

67. Orenstein SR. Controversies in pediatric gastroesophageal reflux. *J Pediatr Gastroenterol Nutr* 1992;14:338-48.

68. Heyman S. Pediatric nuclear gastroenterology. *Nucl Med Ann* 1985;142.

69. Gelfand M; Thomas Sr. *Effective Use of Computers in Nuclear Medicine.* New York, NY; McGraw Hill, 1988:421.

19

Electrogastrography

SALVATORE CUCCHIARA

The smooth-muscle cells of the distal two thirds of the stomach exhibit a cyclic recurrent electrical activity that is characterized by regular depolarization of the cellular membranes.[1] This cyclic electrical activity, known as slow waves or electrical control activity (ECA),[1] continues whether mechanical contractions occur or not.

Slow waves are caused by cyclic changes of the myocyte resting membrane potential, which varies from approximately - 40 mV to -80 mV. This potential is derived from several factors: 1) diffusion of K^+ out of the cells through K^+ channels; 2) the Na^+/K^+ pump that transports three Na^+ ions out of the cells for every two K^+ ions that enter the cells (the net outward flow of positive charge accounts for about 30 mV of the resting membrane potential); and 3) a Cl^- pump that transports Cl^- into the cells. The smooth-muscle cell membrane is depolarized due to an inward Na^+ current, but the generation of an outward Na^+ current by the Na^+/K^+ pump repolarizes cell membranes to their resting potential.[2]

During muscle contraction, the slow waves are accompanied by a second type of electrical activity, which is referred to as spikes, or electrical response activity (ERA). Electrophysiologic studies suggest, however, that mechanical contractions can also be triggered in the stomach by changes in the amplitude or duration of the slow waves.[3]

Spikes appear if the membrane potential depolarizes beyond a threshold level. Depolarization is usually prompted by the delivery of hormones, neurotransmission from enteric nerves, or local paracrine secretion. Spikes are produced by the rush of Ca^{2+} into

the cells that occurs when depolarization causes the Ca^{2+} channels to open.[4]

The frequency of slow waves varies among the regions of the gut. In the human stomach, slow waves recur at about 0.05 Hz (3 cpm). They originate from a pacemaker region that is located in the greater curvature, near the orad one third of the corpus, and propagate in an orderly aboral fashion at an increasing velocity. It was recently suggested that slow waves are generated in a pacemaker region within a population of nonneural, nonmuscle cells that compose an extensive plexus between the main muscle layers, as well as at the level of the deep muscular plexus. These interstitial Cajal cells are spontaneously active and give rise to wavelike depolarization. They also contact muscle cells and nerve terminals.[5]

The maximum rate of mechanical contractions in a given segment of the intestine will never exceed the frequency of slow waves in that segment; the propagation of contractions follows that of slow waves. Slow waves determine the spatial and temporal organization of all mechanical activity.[1] Disorders of either gastric electrical rhythms or spatial arrangement of slow waves might result in disturbed gastric motility.

Myoelectric activity in the stomach can be measured by serosal electrodes that are surgically implanted on the serosa, electrodes mounted on intraluminal probes, or cutaneous electrodes attached to the epigastric skin.[6] The latter technique is known as cutaneous electrogastrography (EGG). Recent evidence suggests that cutaneous EGG accurately reflects the electrical activity of the stomach and is an interesting alternative

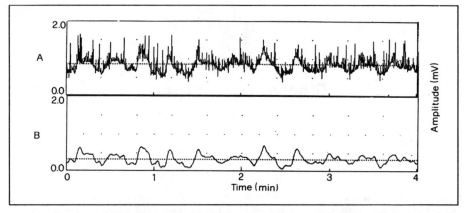

Fig. 19.1 Example of EGG signal recorded from a normal subject before (**A**) and after (**B**) digital filtering (0.6-30.0 cpm). The figure shows a typical EGG with slow waves at about 3.0 cpm. The smaller but higher frequency signals superimposed on the EGG are the EKG and the respiratory signal (**A**). Only EGG and EKG are of sufficiently different frequency (3 cpm v. 60 cpm) that the EKG can be virtually eliminated by filtering (**B**).

to serosal and intraluminal recording of gastric electrical activity.[7] Several points remain unsettled, including how the EGG correlates with gastric motility and emptying, which myoelectric variables can reliably be recorded by EGG, and the role that EGG plays in the diagnosis of patients with symptoms of upper gastrointestinal dysfunction.

RECORDING AND ANALYSIS

Gastric myoelectric signals are distorted by electrocardiogram (EKG), respiratory movement, and body motion. The EGG therefore requires filtration to block unwanted signals without removing potentially useful information. When choosing a filter system, the benefits of an enhanced signal must be weighed against the possibility of losing pertinent data in the filtered signals. The normal frequency of gastric slow waves is about 3 cpm. Abnormal gastric electrical rhythms can be as low as 1 cpm and as high as 9 cpm. Interference by high-frequency signals such as those emitted by the heart (60 cpm, 1 Hz) is eliminated by setting the high-cutoff frequency at 18 cpm (0.3 Hz). A high-frequency filter should remove the respiratory signal (0.2 Hz), but should not be low enough to eradicate the harmonics of the fundamental frequency or distort the gastric electrical signal. The low-frequency filter should be set at 1 cpm (0.16 Hz) to eliminate

electrode baseline drifts caused by a low-frequency electrical signal, which is produced when the skin and electrodes make contact. Conventional filters do not always completely remove unwanted signals. Undesired frequencies may be present on the "filtered" EGG signal.

Signals from the EGG can be recorded and amplified through a commercial physiograph that records other bioelectric signals. It can also be displayed on a recording chart. The amplified EGG signal, stored on an FM tape recorder, is subsequently digitized by an analog/digital converter, which is usually installed on a personal computer. Special EGG equipment (Hewlitt Packard, HP vectra R620, Milano, Italy) can also be used. The amplified EGG signals are digitized on-line by an HP 3852A A/D converter with a sampling frequency set at 1 Hz.

Visual analysis of the EGG is difficult and unreliable because of variable interference from other signals (Fig. 19.1). Computer analysis speeds data analysis, increases accuracy, and extracts frequency information from tracings that are unsuitable for visual analysis. The most common computer-assisted technique for analyzing EGG includes a frequency spectral analysis.[8] One popular choice is the fast Fourier transform (FFT) process, which separates the waveform data into different frequency components, and determines the relative power of a certain frequency range to the whole signal. The power spectral analysis uses the FFT to extract the frequency components of the signal and the strength or power of the different frequency components.

Running spectral analysis can acquire information about time variation of the frequencies. A Hamming window is first applied to reduce signal leakage. Every 64 seconds, a power spectrum from the preceding 256 seconds of the EGG signals is computed. A series of overlapping spectra is thus generated, and both frequency and time analysis are possible (Fig. 19.2). If in addition to time and frequency ranges the power of frequencies is reported, a "pseudo-three-dimensional plot" can illustrate both the frequency spectrum and the frequency power over time. The running spectral analysis can also be represented as gray-scale plots where the blackness is proportional to the magnitude of power of the EGG signal, divided into several distinct gray levels.[9]

Autocorrelation is another technique for analyzing the EGG signal. Unlike spectral analysis, it does not provide information about amplitude. With this technique, a correlation between the digitized record and the signal is made. The original and the digitized records are lagged by one point. Computing is repeated for a number of lag durations to obtain a superposition of the two signals and their highest product. The results are represented as a graphic that relates the correlation to the lag at which it was computed. Autocorrelation is most useful for detecting periodicity and in eliminating side electrical noises.[10]

The EGG signal is normally recorded bipolarly with adhesive silver/silver chloride electrocardiograph (EKG) electrodes placed on the epigastric area, which has been cleansed with alcohol. Applying a thin coating of electrode paste to the electrodes before they are placed on the abdominal surface lowers skin impedance. In adolescents and adults, the skin is lightly abraded with fine sandpaper to lower the skin-to-electrode impedance to less than 5000 ohm, and to avoid skin-potential responses that could confound the EGG. Cutaneous EGG can be recorded with monopolar electrodes (one electrode on the abdomen and another on the limb), but bipolar recordings provide better signal-to-noise ratio.

Interindividual

Fig. 19.2 Running spectra obtained from the same recording session shown in Fig. 19.1 The spectral analysis shows approximately 78 min of EGG data (preprandial 16 min, postprandial 62 min). Running spectra were obtained as follows: Every 64 sec, a power spectrum was computed from the preceding 256 sec of the EGG time signal. This procedure generates a series of partially overlapping spectra graphed as a pseudo-three-dimensional display and makes both frequency and time analysis possible. Note the consistent spectral peak at 3.0 cpm and the power increase following the test meal. The peaks near 6 cpm are second harmonics of the first harmonic, which is 3.0 cpm, the normal EGG frequency. Harmonics are seen in the spectra when a periodic signal deviates from a sinusoidal wave.

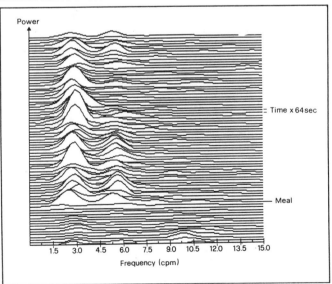

differences in gastric anatomy preclude a standard electrode position. Most investigators use two pairs of electrodes placed along the antral axis of the stomach, which is the imaginary line along the proximal to distal portion. The lead with the best signal-to-noise ratio is then selected for computer analysis. The electrodes are positioned equidistant from the xiphoid and umbilicus. A reference electrode is placed on the right ankle. The respiratory rate can be recorded with a belt pneumograph. Because of the interindividual variability in the gastric position and shape, a supine ultrasonography may be used to mark the longitudinal axis of the distal stomach on the abdomen, before placing the electrodes on the abdomen. The patient should fast for at least 4 to 6 hours before the study. The EGG study must be performed without sedation, while the patient is awake. The study should not be performed on a patient who has eaten within the past 4 hours or has just had an endoscopy with sedative drugs or a barium upper gastrointestinal x-ray.

Promotility agents, anticholinergics, sedatives, nitrates, calcium channel blocking agents, or other medications that can interfere with gastric functions should be discontinued 48 hours before the study. The patients typically lie supine except when sitting up to eat. Patients should maintain the same posture throughout the recording period because changes in body position will alter the position of the stomach. In order to make useful comparisons with other gastric motility tests, the patient's position during EGG should be the same as during gastrointestinal manometry or gastric emptying studies. Usually, four ordinary Ag/AgCl electrocardiography electrodes are placed on the skin of the epigastric region to form two pairs of bipolar recording electrodes. The EGG is recorded for 1 hour during fasting and for 60 to 90 minutes after a test meal. See Table 20.1 for the standard meals that can be administered for EGG and ultrasonographic measurement of gastric emptying.

PARAMETERS

There is no standardized definition for gastric electrical dysrhythmias. Most investigators have proposed both rate and duration criteria. A frequency between 2.5 and 3.5 cpm is normal. Tachygastria is defined as a frequency between 5 and 9 cpm occurring at a regular rhythm and lasting at least 1 minute. Bradygastria is defined as a basal rate of less than 2 cpm for at least 1 minute. Periods of absent electrical signal are designated as flat-line patterns. An irregular rhythm resulting from a combination of tachygastria and bradygastria is called mixed dysrhythmias or tachybradyarrhythmia.

Different EGG parameters can be obtained with spectral analysis:

1) *Prevailing frequency of the EGG and its power.* The contribution of a given frequency band to the entire signal is called its power. Three major frequency ranges are identified: 1 to 2 cpm, 2.5 to 3.5 cpm, and 4 to 9 cpm. The percentage of power distribution is defined as the ratio between power within one of the three major frequency ranges and total power in all three bands.

2) *Relative EGG power changes of the dominant frequency.* The change in the relative power of the dominant frequency is related to changes in the EGG amplitude signal and to the regularity of the signal. It is commonly believed that EGG power changes parallel those in the contractile strength of gastric contractions.

3) *Percentage of normal electrical rhythm (2-4 cpm) in the EGG recording.* This variable relates to the regularity of the EGG or gastric slow waves.

4) *Dysrhythmic index.* This is the percentage of dysrhythmic time during the evaluation. Values for the dysrhythmic index (as median and ranges) for 1-hour recording both in fasting and fed states have recently been reported in ten asymptomatic children and in 14 children with dyspepsia.[11] Mean (SD) age for these two groups was 7.5 (2) and 7.0 (3) years, respectively. Fasting dysrhythmic index was 1.6% (range: 1.6-33.3) in the controls and 33.3% (10.0-48.3) in the dyspeptic patients. Fed dysrhythmic index was 2.7% (1.6-5.5) in the controls and 15.0% (11.6-66.6) in the patients.

The value of EGG in detecting gastric slow-wave propagation is still unsettled.

Detection of this parameter would provide important information about gastric contractions. Preliminary data indicate that detection of slow-wave propagation with the EGG is possible.[12] Cutaneous multielectrodes should be placed along the antral axis and each of them must be connected to a common reference electrode, yielding multichannel EGG recordings. Normal aboral propagation has been observed in normal volunteers and in diabetic patients for more than 80% of the entire recording time. Episodes of tachygastria and retrograde propagation of tachygastria have been detected in individual cases.[7] The ability of EGG to detect the direction of spread of gastric electrical activity over the stomach has not been confirmed in recent studies that have been performed with different cutaneous electrode sites.[13]

VALIDATION

Simultaneous recordings in animals and humans by serosal and surface cutaneous electrodes have shown that gastric electrical frequency is the same with both methods.[14-16] It was also shown that the amplitude of the EGG signal was related to the occurrence of spikes, as detected by serosal electrodes. Recent data, however, suggest that some parameters of gastric electrical activity (eg, propagation and coupling of slow waves) might not be successfully detected by cutaneous EGG.[13,17]

It is generally agreed that a relative EGG amplitude increase is related to increased amplitude of gastric contractions. Yet the amplitude of cutaneous EGG signals also increases when neither antral contractions nor spikes occur, as a consequence of mechanical distention of the stomach.[13] It is likely that both gastric distention and gastric contractions contribute to postprandial increases in EGG amplitude. Whether postprandial EGG power represents a reliable index of postprandial gastric motility is still unknown.

INDICATIONS

Although EGG is considered a reliable tool for recording gastric myoelectrical ac-

tivity and great progress has recently been made in measurement, analysis, and validation, this technique appears to be of clinical relevance only in selected patient groups.

The EGG has been proposed as one of the initial tests for children with suspected enteric neuromuscular disease causing persistent vomiting and episodes of functional obstruction. In these patients, the test may provide useful pathophysiologic information. Persistent tachygastria seems to be highly suggestive of a neuropathic dysmotility. In cases with no dominant frequency, the gut motor disorder is frequently myopathic.[18]

The EGG can be used in the diagnostic evaluation of children with persistent symptoms such as recurrent vomiting, nausea, epigastric distention and/or pain, regurgitation, and early satiety. In the absence of endoscopic and radiographic abnormalities, this clinical picture is commonly referred to as functional or nonulcer dyspepsia. Abnormalities of the EGG have been reported in several patient populations with symptoms due to functional disorders of the upper gut (Figs. 19.3, 19.4).[11,19-23]

The EGG has been shown to be an objective measure of the effects of putative therapeutic agents in selected patients. Domperidone induces a normal 3-cpm gastric myoelectrical activity and improvement in upper-gastrointestinal symptoms in diabetic patients.[24] Erythromycin decreased the percentage of normal slow waves, and increased the amplitude (overall power) of the EGG.[25] Cisapride reversed gastric electrical dysrhythmias in some patients with functional dyspepsia and gastroparesis.[26,27] Recently, a low-frequency component superimposed on the normal 3 cpm was shown to occur after administration of cisapride.[26,28]

Several studies have reported on the clinical application of the EGG. The diagnostic value of EGG remains in question, though, because it is difficult to interpret its signals and correlate them with other variables of gastric motor activity and clinical symptoms. Electrogastrographic abnormalities, however, have been shown to differentiate patients with gastroparesis from healthy adults and children.[11,19-21] The most commonly reported EGG abnormalities in gas-

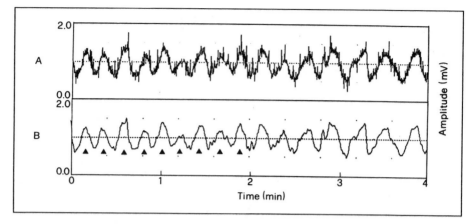

Fig. 19.3 Example of raw (**A**) and filtered (**B**) EGG signals recorded in a patient with nonulcer dyspepsia. A clear episode of tachygastria at approximately 5.0 cpm can be seen (arrowheads), followed by a normal 3-cpm rhythm. The smaller but higher frequency signal superimposed on the EGG signal is the EKG (**A**). After filtering (**B**), a superimposed respiratory signal is still present.

troparesis are preprandial and postprandial dysrhythmias, and decreased EGG amplitude after a test meal. Significantly higher gastric dysrhythmic indices are usually recorded in gastroparetic patients as compared with normal subjects. The EGG abnormalities may occur in both the fasting and fed states. Therefore, recordings should always be performed under both conditions. Furthermore, because meals with different composition may have different effects on gastric motility, a uniform test meal should be administered during the EGG so that results from different centers can be compared. Since gastric electrical activity is one of the factors regulating gastric emptying (in addition to antroduodenal coordination, and pyloric as well as duodenal motor activity), establishing a strong correlation between the EGG and gastric emptying might be difficult. This correlation is not a one-to-one phenomenon. A normal EGG recording is not necessarily associated with normal gastric emptying, whereas abnormal EGG strongly predicts gastroparesis. Dysrhythmias, however, do not appear to play a major role in the development of postsurgical gastroparesis.

Fig. 19.4. Running spectra obtained from the same recording session shown in Fig. 19.3. The spectral analysis shows approximately 78 min of EGG data. The gastric spectral peak shows a wide frequency variability and a period of tachygastria that lasts 6 min.

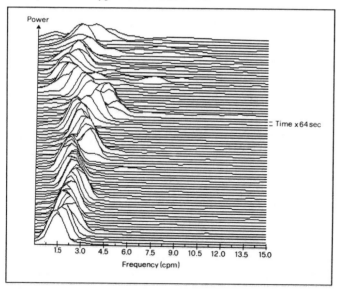

ELECTROGASTROGRAPHY AND GASTRIC MOTILITY

The correlation between the EGG frequency and gastric motility has also been investigated. During fasting, both EGG power and frequency are significantly lower and less stable throughout periods of motor activity than they are during motor quiescence. After eating, the EGG frequency tends to decrease from the baseline for a short period, subsequently rising gradually above the baseline.[22,29]

The presence of gastric dysrhythmias is believed to be associated with gastric dysmotility. The latter has been observed in patients with defective antral motor function.[22,29] However, the relationship between gastric dysrhythmias and gastric motility is variable. In one study, bradygastria in dogs correlated with strong antral contractions.[30] More recently, however, both spontaneous or induced bradygastrias were associated with antral hypomotility.[15,31] An association between tachygastria and gastric motor disorders has been substantiated by several studies that have demonstrated the presence of tachygastria in patients with impaired antral motor function.[7] Recent data indicate an association between tachygastria and gastric motor quiescence.[28]

OTHER STUDIES

Gastric dysrhythmias of various types (tachygastria, bradygastria, and mixed arrhythmias) have been found in pregnant women with nausea and vomiting. Pregnant women without symptoms usually exhibit normal gastric slow-wave activity.[31,32] Abnormalities in the EGG and nausea disappear after delivery or interruption of pregnancy. Other abnormalities in this group were instability of the EGG and reduced responsiveness to the test meal.

Electrogastrography has contributed to the understanding of motion sickness. Tachygastria was recorded in patients developing symptoms of motion sickness during experimental rotation, but a persistent 3-cpm gastric electrical signal was noted in subjects without motor sickness during rotation.[23,33]

REFERENCES

1. Bortoff A. Myogenic control of intestinal motility. *Physiol Rev* 1976;56:418-34.

2. Szurszewski JH. Electrical basis for gastrointestinal motility. In: Johnson LA, ed. *Physiology of the Gastrointestinal Tract.* New York, NY: Raven Press, 1987;383-422.

3. Makhlouf GM. Smooth muscle of the gut. In: Yamada T, ed. *Textbook of Gastroenterology.* Philadelphia, PA: Lippincott, 1991;61-84.

4. Bauer AJ, Publicover MJ, Sanders KM. Origin and spread of slow waves in canine gastric antral circular muscle. *Am J Physiol* 1985;249:4800-6.

5. Rumessen JJ, Mikkelsen HB, Qvorttrup K, Thuneberg L. Ultrastructure of interstitial cells of Cajal in circular muscle of human small intestine. *Gastroenterology* 1993;104:343-50.

6. Abell TL, Malagelada J-R. Electrogastrography: current assessment and future perspective. *Dig Dis Sci* 1988;83:806-11.

7. Chen J, McCallum RW. Electrogastrogram: measurement, analysis, and prospective applications. *Med Biol Eng Comput* 1991;29:339-50.

8. Kingma YJ. The electrogastrogram and its analysis. *Crit Rev Biomed Eng* 1989;17:103-32.

9. Van der Schee EJ, Grashuis JT. Running spectrum analysis as an aid in the representation and interpretation of electrogastrographic signals. *Med Biol Eng Comput* 1987;25:57-62.

10. Stern RM. Recording the electrogastrogram. In: Stern RM, Koch KL, eds. *Electrogastrography: Methodology, Validation, and Applications.* New York, NY: Prager, 1985;19-28.

11. Cucchiara S, Riezzo G, Minella R, Pezzolla F, Giorgic I, Auricchio S. Electrogastrography in non-ulcer dyspepsia. *Arch Dis Child* 1992;67:613-7.

12. Chen J, Vandewalle J, Sansen W, Van Cutsen E, Vantrappen G, Janssens J. Observation of the propagation direction of human electrogastric activity from cutaneous recordings. *Med Biol Eng Comput* 1989;27:538-42.

13. Mintchev MP, Kingma YJ, Bowes KL. Accu-

racy of cutaneous recordings of gastric electrical activity. *Gastroenterology* 1993;104:1273-80.

14. Smout AJPM, Van de Schee EJ, Grashuis JL. What is measured in electrogastrography? *Dig Dis Sci* 1980;25:179-87.

15. Abell TL, Malagelada J-R. Glucagon-evoked gastric dysrhythmias in humans shown by an improved electrogastrographic technique. *Gastroenterology* 1985;88:1932-40.

16. Hamilton JW, Bellahsene B, Reichelderfer M, Webster JG, Bass P. Human electrogastrogram; comparison of surface and mucosal recordings. *Dig Dis Sci* 1986;31:33-9.

17. Familoni BO, Bowes KL, Kingma YJ, Cote KR. Can transcutaneous recordings detect gastric electrical abnormalities? *Gut* 1991;32:141-6.

18. Devane SP, Ravelli AM, Bisset WM, Smith VV, Lake BD, Milla JP. Gastric antral dysrhythmias in children with chronic idiopathic intestinal pseudoobstruction. *Gut* 1992;33:1477-81.

19. Chen J, McCallum RW. Gastric slow wave abnormalities in patients with gastroparesis. *Am J Gastroenterol* 1992;87:477-82.

20. Geldof H, Van der Schee EJ, Van Blankenstein M, Grashuis JL. Electrogastrographic study of gastric myoelectrical activity in patients with unexplained nausea and vomiting. *Gut* 1986;26:799-808.

21. Abell TL, Camilleri M, Hench VS, Malagelada J-R. Gastric electromechanical function and gastric emptying in diabetic gastroparesis. *Eur J Gastroenterol Hepatol* 1991;3:163-7.

22. You CH, Chey WY, Lee KY, Menguy Y, Bortoff A. Gastric and small intestinal myoelectrical dysrhythmias associated with chronic intractable nausea and vomiting. *Ann Intern Med* 1981;95:449-51.

23. Stern MR, Koch KL, Stewart WR. Spectral analysis of tachygastria recorded during motion sickness. *Gastroenterology* 1987;92:92-7.

24. Koch KL, Stern RM, Stewart WR, Vasey MW. Gastric emptying and gastric myoelectrical activity in patients with diabetic gastroparesis: effect of long-term domperidone treatment. *Am J Gastroenterol* 1989;84:1069-75.

25. Chen J, Yeaton P, McCallum RW. Effect of erythromycin on gastric myoelectrical activity in normal human subjects. *Am J Physiol* 1992;263;G24-8.

26. Koch KL, Bingaman S, Sperry N, Stern RM. Effect of cisapride on gastric electromechanical activity in healthy volunteers: a double-blind, placebo-controlled study. *Gastroenterology* 1991;100:A459. Abstract.

27. Cucchiara S, Minella R, Riezzo G, et al. Reversal of gastric electrical dysrhythmias by cisapride in children with functional dyspepsia. *Dig Dis Sci* 1992;37:1136-40.

28. Chen J, Richards R, McCallum RW. Frequency components of the electrogastrogram and their correlations with gastrointestinal motility. *Med Biol Eng Comput* 1993;31:60-6.

29. Telander RL, Morgan KG, Kreulen DL, Schemalz PF, Kelly KA, Szurszewsky JH. Human gastric atony with tachygastria and gastric retention. *Gastroenterology* 1978;75:495-501.

30. Van der Schee ET, Grashuis JL. Contraction-related, low- frequency components in canine electrogastrographic signals. *Am J Physiol* 1983;245:G470-5.

31. Koch KL, Stern RM, Vasey M. Gastric dysrhythmias and nausea of pregnancy. *Dig Dis Sci* 1990;35:961-8.

32. Riezzo G, Pezzolla F, Darconza G, Giorgio I. Gastric myoelectrical activity in the first trimester of pregnancy: a cutaneous electrogastrographic study. *Am J Gastroenterol* 1992;87:702-7.

33. Hu S, Stern RM, Koch KL. Electrical acustimulation relieves vection-induced motion sickness. *Gastroenterology* 1992;102:1854-8.

CHAPTER

20

Ultrasound

SALVATORE CUCCHIARA

Real-time ultrasonography has recently been employed to estimate gastric volume and gastric motor activity. The ultrasound probe is positioned over the epigastrium of seated or supine subjects both during fasting and following ingestion of a meal. Ultrasound scanning with high-resolution, real-time equipment provides a tool for visualizing moving structures inside the body. When a beam of high-frequency impulses (1.5-10 MHz) is sent into the human body, the rate at which it is reflected back is determined by the density of the medium through which it is traveling. The returning echoes generate a series of dots on the screen. Their brightness is related to the density of the reflecting medium. Echoes of strong intensity appear white on the screen, whereas feeble echoes appear dark gray.

Adequate ultrasonographic assessment of the stomach is not possible in the presence of intragastric gas. Filling the stomach with liquids or solid/liquid meals, however, displaces the intragastric gas and distends the gastric walls, allowing identification of the stomach walls.[1]

The main advantages of ultrasonography for measuring gastric emptying time are that it is noninvasive and equipment is readily available. Ultrasonography is safe and repeatable. These are important considerations because some subjects require several studies to assess changes under different experimental conditions, or to determine the effects of drug therapy. Furthermore, whereas radioscintigraphy measures the amount of meal components in the stomach but does not account for intragastric secretions, ultrasonography measures total (ie, ingested plus secreted) intragastric volume. Duodenogastric reflux cannot be measured by the radioisotope method, but can be assessed with the ultrasound study of gastric emptying. Studies repeated on different days in the same subjects have also shown that the technique is highly reproducible.[2] The main disadvantage is that standardization is difficult because results are highly dependent on the operator's technique. In addition, ultrasound measurement of gastric emptying is cumbersome and time-consuming.

Different test meals have been used to distend and visualize the stomach. Generally, the quality of the data is lessened by denser, more echogenic meals. By administering a meal of orange juice, the gastric volume can be calculated by adding a series of parallel, two-dimensional, cross-sectional areas of the liquid-filled stomach along the long axis of the organ. Nevertheless, assessment of gastric emptying by serial quantitation of total gastric volume can be difficult and unreliable. Ultrasound scanning of the fundus is hampered by the presence of gas and inaccessibility of the fundus behind the coastal margin. This method has not, therefore, received widespread application in current clinical practice. Most authors assess gastric emptying time by measuring the width of the gastric antrum at selected levels before and after a mixed solid/liquid meal. The relationship between this measurement and the total gastric volume, however, is uncertain.[3-5]

The standard meal should be administered over a period of no more than 15 minutes. Table 20.1 illustrates the meals given to different age groups. Ingestion of

Age*	Bread	Parma Ham	Butter	Fruit Juice
(years)	(grams)	(grams)	(grams)	(ml)
2-3	60	30	5	85
3-6	75	30	5	175
6-9	60	45	7.5	120
9-12	100	50	8	125
> 12	120	45	12	125

TABLE 20.1 Meals Administered for Ultrasonographic Measurement of Gastric Emptying Time

*In children younger than 2 years, the standard meal is the usual milk formula, 300ml/m² body surface area.

these meals has been shown to interrupt the interdigestive cycle of fasting children, resulting in a pattern of gastroduodenal motor activity which resembles that of the postprandial period.[6]

Subjects are preferably examined in the morning, after 6 to 8 hours of fasting. A real-time scanner that uses a 5 MHz linear array transducer should be applied with minimal abdominal compression. The examination is performed with the child sitting at 30° to the horizontal plane of the examination couch. Measurements are taken 30 minutes after the start of the meal and subsequently at regular 15-minute intervals. During the first 90 minutes, measurements can be taken at longer intervals. After the meal, changes in the shape and position of the antrum are easily recognizable. Contractions of the antral walls are often noted. The images can be continuously recorded on videotape for later review.

To obtain the same scanning level consistently, gastric emptying time can be calculated by measuring the cross section of the gastric antrum that corresponds to the sagittal plane, passing through the superior mesenteric vein as point of reference. The cross-section of the gastric antrum at this level is elliptical. Its area (cm²) can be calculated by the following formula: $\pi \times A \times B/4$, where A is the longitudinal and B the anteroposterior diameters (Figs. 20.1, 20.2). Since the orientation of the antrum differs among individuals, various degrees of slope are used with

the probe to make correct scans.

Another method consists of measuring the volume of the whole antropyloric region by determining the longitudinal and anteroposterior diameters at three different levels: 1) the angle region, 2) the pylorus, and 3) an intermediate level that corresponds to the scanning plane passing through the superior mesenteric vein. The angle region can be recognized by real-time ultrasound at that

Fig. 20.1 Cross-sectional area of the gastric antrum corresponding to the sagittal plane passing through the superior mesenteric vein. This area is elliptical, and can be calculated using the formula π AB/4, where A is the longitudinal and B the anteroposterior diameters.

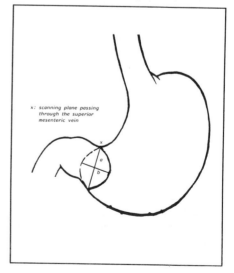

x: scanning plane passing through the superior mesenteric vein

Fig. 20.2 Cross-sectional image of the antrum at three different levels: angle region (x), pylorus (z), and intermediate level (y).

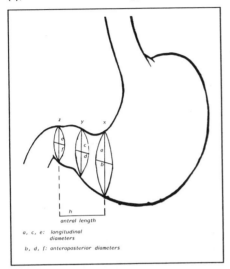

a, c, e: longitudinal diameters

b, d, f: anteroposterior diameters

level because the wall of the lower curvature changes direction from a transverse to a longitudinal plane. The antral length (H), which runs from the pylorus to the angle region, is measured by a transverse scan at the epigastrium (Fig. 20.3). The volume of the antropyloric region is determined according to the formula: volume = 0.065 x h x (2 ab + ef + 4 cd + ad + bc + cf). H is the antral length; a, c and e are the longitudinal diam-

eters; b, d and f are the anteroposterior diameters.

Gastric emptying can be monitored by determining anteroposterior and longitudinal diameters of a single section of the stomach at an intermediate level that corresponds to the scanning plane passing through the superior mesenteric vein. This method is simpler than measuring the body-antral tract at various levels. This method has been validated by showing that gastric diameter (measured by ultrasound at the antral-body junction level) decreased linearly after introduction of a meal, and returned to the fasting level when the meal was emptied from the stomach.[4] Care is taken to perform basal and postprandial scans during the intervals between peristaltic waves.

PARAMETERS
The Empty Stomach

The stomach is empty when the section's area or the antral volume return to baseline values and persist unchanged for at least 30 minutes, and when a complete absence of food particles within the antrum is observed for 30 minutes. Final emptying time is calculated in relation to the start of the meal.

Maximum increase in gastric measurements from fasting to the end of the meal (DDMax) is measured as follows: DDmax = Dmax - Df. Dmax is the mean value of gastric measurements taken at the end of meal ingestion; DF is the mean value of the same measurements computed at the baseline before the meal.

The difference between the value measured at each observation (Dn) and that measured at baseline is calculated and called DDn, where DDn = Dn - Df. When DDn is 0 (ie, Dn = Df), gastric emptying is considered finished.

Fig. 20.3 Ultrasonographic view of the gastric antrum above the superior mesenteric vein. Anteroposterior and longitudinal diameters are clearly indicated.

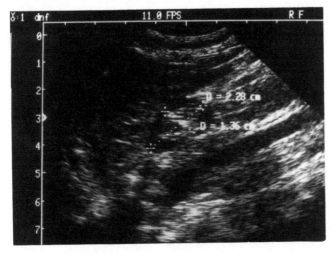

Antral Contractions

During ultrasonography it is possible to observe propulsive waves, grinding, and retropulsion. The frequency of antral contractions is defined as the number of contractions during a 2-minute interval. Scanning begins approximately 15 minutes after the end of the meal. The amplitude of antral contractions is defined as the maximal contraction-induced reduction of the antral areas (ie, the difference between relaxed and contracted areas) as a fraction of the relaxed area (Δ A/A).

To evaluate antral contractions, the probe is positioned vertically so that the antrum, superior mesenteric vein, and aorta can be visualized simultaneously. These vessels serve as landmarks to standardize the position of the scan.

Motility

The motility index is defined as amplitude × frequency. Antroduodenal coordination is expressed as the percentage of peristaltic cycles in which antral contractions are followed synchronously by a contraction of the duodenal bulb. Duodenogastric reflux is defined as the number of visible reflux episodes during 2-minute intervals.

Movement of intraluminal contents can be assessed by simultaneously visualizing the motor activity of the distal stomach, pyloric channel, and proximal duodenum using a transverse scan of the abdomen at the transpyloric plane. The latter is defined as a transverse plane situated halfway between the xiphisternum and the umbilicus. The pylorus lies deep to the midpoint of this plane. The transpyloric motion of echogenic bran particles in orange juice is scanned. These particles range in size from particulate to 1.5 mm. They should not aggregate into larger clumps and should remain suspended in the liquid phase.[6]

Gastric Emptying

Gastric contents are emptied as the terminal antrum, pylorus, and duodenum relax. This emptying pattern contradicts the standard view that gastric emptying of liquids either occurs as gushes that are related to the pumping action of the antral peristaltic contractions, or as a steady flow which is probably due to a gastroduodenal pressure gradient. The episodes of forward flow often end abruptly and are sometimes immediately followed by a period of retrograde flow. Short episodes of retrograde flow across the pylorus occur in normal subjects, usually while the antral wave is approaching the pylorus and remains nonocclusive. The remaining episodes occur after relaxation of the terminal antrum and pylorus, when their lumen is still patent. Many of the retrograde flow episodes through the pylorus occur immediately following episodes of flow from the stomach to the duodenum. It is possible, therefore, that these episodes of retrograde flow do not represent true duodenogastric reflux, since the refluxed fluid is not mixed with bile or pancreatic secretions.

Simultaneous ultrasonographic and scintigraphic studies of gastric emptying of liquid meals have resulted in similar values.[4,7] The parameters of gastric emptying as detected by scintigraphy significantly correlated with those obtained by ultrasound. The value for half emptying time ($T_{1/2}$) derived from ultrasonography correlated with the $T_{1/2}$ that was calculated by anterior scintigraphy (geometric mean). Comparison with x-ray contrast studies of the stomach has also shown that ultrasound reliably establishes the presence or absence of food particles in the gastric lumen.

INDICATIONS

Ultrasound measurement of gastric emptying can be performed as a first-line approach in patients presenting with symptoms that suggest upper gastrointestinal dysfunction (eg, nausea, vomiting, abdominal pain, early satiety, bloating, or anorexia). This syndrome is commonly referred to as nonulcer or functional dyspepsia. The diagnosis and treatment of nonulcer dyspepsia represent a formidable challenge for the research worker and the clinician. Clinical features suggesting gastroparesis or disturbed motility of the upper intestinal tract (excluding the esophagus) are particularly evident in the functional dyspepsia subgroup called

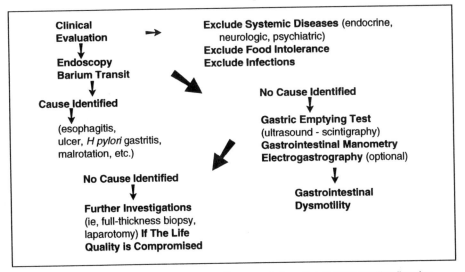

Fig. 20.4 Diagnostic investigation of children with suspected gastrointestinal motility disorder.

stasis, or dysmotility-associated dyspepsia.[8]

Figure 20.4 depicts a proposed algorithm for investigating children with symptoms of functional dyspepsia that suggest a gastrointestinal motor disorder. Since gastric emptying tests are more readily available and less invasive than gastrointestinal manometry, they are used far more frequently. In nonulcer dyspepsia, manometry and tests of gastric emptying might give complementary information.

Nonulcer dyspepsia has been reported to be associated with a significant delay in gastric emptying[3] or with inappropriate antral distention that appears to be related to the severity of dyspeptic complaints.[9] Gastric emptying studies by real-time ultrasound in 86 patients (age range: 3-16 years) referred for functional dyspepsia symptoms during the period of 1989-1991, revealed a higher prevalence of gastroparesis in the group with gastrointestinal dysmotility and/ or dysrhythmia (85%) than in other subsets of patients (40% in patients with *H pylori* gastritis, 78% in patients with pathogenic gastroesophageal reflux) and in 28% of patients with so-called idiopathic dyspepsia in whom no abnormalities had been identified.[10]

In patients with severe intestinal neuromuscular disease and symptoms of chronic intestinal pseudo-obstruction, gastric empty-ing assessment can be used to document gastric involvement. It should be emphasized, however, that although gastric emptying tests provide information on the functional aspects of motor disorders, their diagnostic range is limited because they provide only scanty data on the nature of the underlying pathophysiology.

Ultrasound may be used to evaluate the effect of drug treatment in patients with gastroparesis. A recent study by ultrasound scanning of gastroduodenal motility has shown that prostaglandin E_2 analog administered before ingestion of meals induced antroduodenal hypomotility with reduced, poorly coordinated peristaltic contractions and an open pylorus.[11]

Ultrasound can evaluate the transpyloric movement of gastric luminal contents (antroduodenal coordination) and the strength of antral contractions. It can also measure gastric emptying in patients with gastroparesis reflux disease. Radioscintigraphy used to be the most popular technique for evaluating gastric emptying in reflux disease. Recently, however, ultrasonographic measurement of gastric emptying time has been used in infants with gastroesophageal reflux disease.[12] Prolonged gastric emptying time was detected only in a minority of patients, but most (even those with a normal final emptying time) showed an excessive dilation of the antral area. Correlation with other variables detected by currently accepted investigative tools for gastroesophageal reflux disease (ie, pH metry, manometry) was not studied.

Preoperative evaluation of patients with gastroesophageal reflux can also be performed with ultrasonography. The presence of gastroparesis would suggest performing pyloromyotomy in addition to an antireflux procedure.[13]

CONCLUSION

Real-time ultrasonography of the stomach can reliably measure gastric emptying time and provide useful information on gastric diameters, antral contractions, and flow of chyme. Because studying gastric motility by manometric techniques is difficult, gastric ultrasonography will probably be further developed. The technique is still too new for a conclusive critique, but is of interest mainly because of its noninvasive character and the new information it provides by correlating gastric contractions with flow through the pylorus.

REFERENCES

1. Bateman DN, Whittingham TA. Measurement of gastric emptying by real time ultrasound. *Gut* 1982;23:524-7.

2. Mamtora H, Thompson DG. Gastric ultrasound. In: Read NW, ed, *Gastrointestinal Motility: Which Test?* Sheffield, England: Wrightson Biomedical Publishing, 1989;99-104.

3. Bolondi L, Bortolotti M, Santi V, Calletti T, Gaiani S, Labo G. Measurement of gastric emptying time by real-time ultrasonography. *Gastroenterology* 1985;89:752-9.

4. Marzio L, Giacobbe A, Conoscitore P, Facciorusso D, Frusciante V, Modoni S. Evaluation of the use of ultrasonography in the study of liquid gastric emptying. *Am J Gastroenterol* 1989;84:496-500.

5. Ricci R, Bontemp I, Corazziari E, La Bella A, Torsoli A. Real time ultrasonography of the gastric antrum. *Gut* 1993;34:173-6.

6. King PM, Adam RD, Pryde A, McDicken WN, Heading RC. Relationship of human antroduodenal motility and transpyloric fluid movement: noninvasive observations with real-time ultrasound. *Gut* 1984;25:1384-91.

7. Holt S, Cervantes J, Wilkinson AA, Kirk Wallace JH. Measurement of gastric emptying rate in humans by real-time ultrasound. *Gastroenterology* 1986;90:918-23.

8. Collin-Jones DG, Bloom B, Bodemar G, et al. Management of dyspepsia: report of a working party. *Lancet* 1988;1:576-9.

9. Bortolotti M, Bolondi L, Santi V, Brunellia F, Sarti P, Barbara L. Inappropriate antral distention rather than gastric stasis seems to be marker of dysmotility-like dyspepsia. *J Gastrointest Motil* 1993;5:182.

10. Cucchiara S. Advances in gastrointestinal motility disorders. In: Buts JP, Sokal EM, eds. *Management of Digestive and Liver Disorders in Infants and Children.* New York, NY: Elsevier Science Publishers, 1993;63-85.

11. Hausken T, Odegaard S, Berstad A. Antroduodenal motility studied by real-time ultrasonography. *Gastroenterology* 1991;100:59-63.

12. LiVoti G, Tulone V, Bruno R, Cataliotti F, Iacono G, Cavatalo F, Balsamo V. Ultrasonography and gastric emptying: evaluation in infants with gastroesophageal reflux. *J Pediatr Gastroenterol Nutr* 1992;14:397-9.

13. Fonkalsrud EW. The role of surgery in the treatment of gastroesophageal reflux and gastric dysmotility disorders in childhood. In: Ashcraft KW, Holder TM, eds. *Pediatric Esophageal Surgery.* Orlando, FL: Grune and Stratton, 1986:217-30.

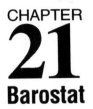

21
Barostat

PAUL E. HYMAN

The barostat is an electromechanical, computer-driven air pump used for measuring compliance and sensation within a hollow organ. When a balloon attached to the barostat is placed into the lumen of a hollow organ, the barostat maintains a constant pressure within the balloon by injecting or withdrawing an appropriate volume of air that is determined by an electronic feedback mechanism. Changes in the volume of air provide an indirect measure of contraction and relaxation in the wall of the viscus.

Although by definition this instrument responds to physiologic changes to keep the pressure constant, it is also possible to switch to different modes. The device measures contraction and relaxation as 1) changes in volume as a function of pressure, or 2) changes in pressure as a function of volume. Pressure and volume-regulated modes are programmed to evaluate continuous or discontinuous changes in pressure or volume, depending on the investigator's automated protocol.

INDICATIONS

In adults, the barostat has been used to evaluate gastric,[1-3] small-bowel,[4] colonic,[5] and rectal[6] sensation and motility. In pediatrics, experience is limited. The barostat may be most useful clinically for assessing chronic visceral pain because it can differentiate between pain arising from a hollow viscus and pain originating from the central nervous system. Individual differences in perceptions of visceral sensation may be the basis for some enteric neuromuscular disorders. In children with chronic incapacitating

abdominal pain, nausea, and early satiety not explained by abnormalities in gastrointestinal motility, the gastric barostat test may serve two purposes: 1) to determine the intragastric volume needed for first sensation, fullness, discomfort, and unbearable pain; and 2) to determine the ability of the stomach to stretch and fill. The rectal barostat study may be most helpful when symptoms of abdominal pain can be elicited by rectal distention.

EQUIPMENT

The barostat consists of a digitally controlled air-displacement servo, pressure transducer, analog-to-digital converter, and computer (Fig. 21.1). The air-displacement servo utilizes a bellows or syringe, and this unit is connected to a tube with a balloon at the end, which is placed into a hollow viscus. Pressure within the viscus is measured by a transducer within the apparatus, and is converted to a digital signal for computer analysis. The computer may be programmed to report volume changes at a fixed pressure (barostat), pressure changes with increasing or decreasing volumes, or a timed sequence of increases and decreases in pressure or volume.

Safety features include overpressure sensors, and volume sensors that prevent overfilling. Programs may incorporate push-button signals on a hand-held response paddle or physiologic signals, such as pulse or blood pressure, to modify the responses of the computer driven air-displacement servo. Software for data analysis may be included in the computer. A

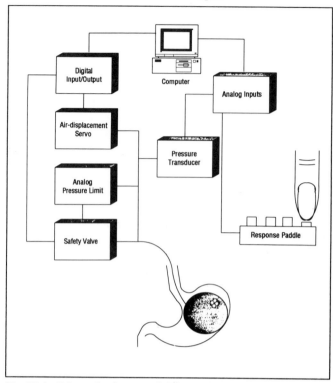

Fig. 21.1 Schematic diagram of the barostat. (Courtesy of UCLA Biomedical Instruments Facility; drawing by Tom Frew)

the intubation is accomplished with minimal discomfort through the gastrostomy. In neonates, the tube is swallowed with no more than a single gag.[7] Neonates rest comfortably or sleep during the barostat test. It may not be possible, however, to execute a satisfactory study in anxious or uncooperative children who do not have a gastrostomy.

The rectal barostat test is similar to anorectal manometry, and patient preparation is also similar. The study cannot be interpreted with confidence if the patient cannot or will not cooperate.

graphics program and printer facilitate clinically useful data presentations.

For adults, balloons are fashioned from condoms tied to the end of nasogastric tubes, or custom-manufactured "gastric distending balloons" may be used (Mak-La Co., Thousand Oaks, CA). For infants, the last 3 to 5 cm of a cut condom can be tied with silk suture over the end of an 8 Fr, 42-inch infant feeding tube.

APPROACH TO THE PEDIATRIC PATIENT

The gastric barostat test requires gastric intubation and a relaxed, cooperative patient. If a psychologist has previously established a therapeutic alliance with the child, it is helpful to have the psychologist at the child's side as the test is explained and performed. In patients with gastrostomy tubes, establishing an atmosphere of trust and cooperation is not a problem, because

STUDY EXECUTION

Gastric test sessions begin after an overnight fast, and last about an hour. After the balloon is attached to the tube, it is inflated outside the body at atmospheric pressure to obtain pressure readings that are due to the distention of the balloon alone. These data will be subtracted from pressures obtained when the balloon is in the stomach. Next, the tube and balloon are passed either through a gastrostomy or the mouth, and into the stomach. In cases of orogastric tube placement, the balloon is inflated 20 to 30 ml by a hand-held syringe. The tube is gently withdrawn until resistance is encountered, indicating that the proximal portion of the balloon is in the gastric cardia. Thereafter, individual protocols are begun.

One useful program involves increasing the balloon volume at a fixed rate (eg, 60 ml/min), as the pressures within the system are recorded continuously. The patient is given a hand-held paddle with four buttons, and is instructed to press the first button after feeling the first abdominal sensation, the second after feeling full, the third if there is discomfort, and the fourth if the discomfort becomes unbearable. Pressing the fourth button automatically and completely deflates the balloon. This program is repeated at least six times. To ascertain if responses are learned, or if false reporting occurs, the patient is unaware that the tube is disconnected from the pump during one of every three test runs during each part of the test session, so that no air enters the balloon. Sensations reported during these sham runs are related to central nervous system abnormalities, such as factitious disorder, or to anxiety about potentially noxious stimuli, which may cause the patient to disregard instructions. At the end of the test session, the tube is removed quickly and easily. There should be no after effects from the test, and the child may resume full activity immediately. The rectal barostat test involves similar procedures, except that the balloon is placed into the rectum.

The risks and discomforts of the barostat sensory evaluation include gagging and discomfort if the tube is passed through the mouth. The inflation of the balloon may cause vomiting or pain.

Subjective responses to balloon distention are influenced by personality, past experience, and cues from the environment (see Chapter 10). The ambiance and verbal as well as nonverbal communications should be standardized. Consistency in test conditions throughout individual sessions and for all studies will improve the reliability of the test.

DATA ANALYSIS

Data are digitized so that each point of time has a corresponding pressure and volume. Pressure-volume relationships can be plotted or expressed as compliance, which is the amount of volume per unit of pressure. In the stomach, compliance conveys information that depends on both gastric volume and its capacity for receptive relaxation. In the rectum, compliance may be most related to its potential volume. Instances when the buttons were pressed to note changes in

visceral sensation are plotted to correspond with the appropriate pressure and volume. The quality of the discomfort, whether it is similar or identical to the subjects' symptoms, and whether discomfort persists during sham runs can be assessed in the verbal, cooperative child.

Normal Values

No normal values for healthy children are available. Preliminary data on gastric compliance show that the stomachs of healthy, term, day-old infants were less compliant than those of adults (Fig. 21.2).

Abnormal Results

Since no normal values have been established for children, each test requires individual interpretation.

Example 1. A 13-year-old girl with a 3-year history of chronic nausea, early satiety, and weight loss following a viral-type acute illness had normal contrast studies, endoscopy, and antroduodenal manometry. Her personality was inconsistent with anorexia nervosa. During the barostat study, pressure rose continuously with each increase in gastric volume (ie, a "stiff stomach"). The compliance curve generated by increasing the balloon volume at a fixed rate was a straight line. She consistently retched in pain or pressed the fourth (escape) button when the balloon volume reached 260 to 280 ml, but she did not press buttons during sham runs. The study suggested that the patient had reduced or absent receptive relaxation of the gastric fundus, and hyperalgesia to distention.

Example 2. A 7-year-old boy repeatedly demonstrated conscious sensitivity at 30 ml, fullness at 60 ml (validating his mother's claim that 60 ml was the most he would volunteer to drink), pain after 90 ml, and pain sufficient to stop the test by 150 ml. Two features of the test were inconsistent with the child's report. First, although he claimed severe pain, there were no changes in heart rate, facial expression, or body position to corroborate his report. Second, on several sham tests the child pressed buttons to indicate feeling full even though the tub-

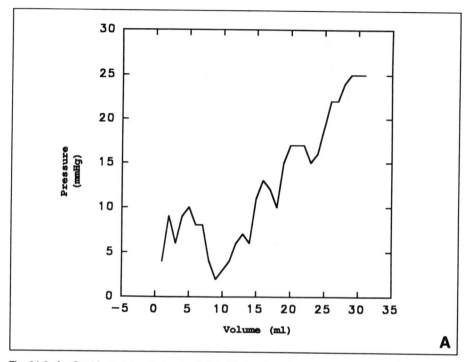

Fig. 21.2 **A,** Gastric pressure-volume relationship in a healthy, term, newborn infant. **B,** Gastric pressure-volume relationship in a healthy adult. Note the difference in volume and pressure scales as compared with **A**. The perpendicular lines at the top of the graph indicate when the subject first noted sensation and fullness. (Courtesy of Emeran Mayer, MD)

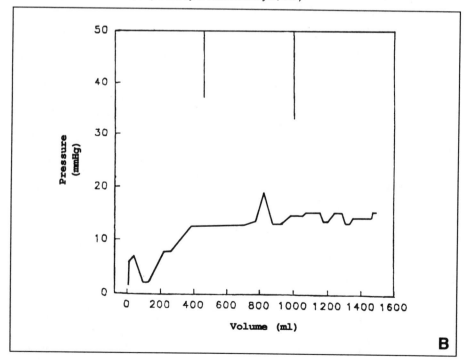

ing was disconnected and the balloon was flaccid. This study was interpreted to mean that the child experienced both gastric hypersensitivity to distention and an expectation for pain that caused him to exaggerate his sensory perceptions.

CLINICAL USEFULNESS

Causes for abdominal pain are rarely demonstrated with intestinal manometry, but the barostat's instrumentation can reproduce painful abdominal sensations, so that pain may be related to distention. When pain arises after amounts of distention that are less than expected, visceral hyperalgesia may be a contributing mechanism. When the pain report is inconsistent with physiologic parameters such as increases in pulse, blood pressure, sweating, facial expression, and body position, exaggeration due to psychologic conditioning or malingering is suggested.

REFERENCES

1. Azpiroz F, Malagelada J-R. Gastric tone measured by an electronic barostat in health and postsurgical gastroparesis. *Gastroenterology* 1987;92:934-43.

2. Mearin F, Cucala M, Azpiroz F, Malagelada J-R. The origin of symptoms on the brain-gut axis in functional dyspepsia. *Gastroenterology* 1991;101:999-1006.

3. Khan MI, Read NW, Grundy D. Effect of varying the rate and pattern of gastric distension on its sensory perception and motor activity. *Am J Physiol* 1993;264:G824-7.

4. Azpiroz F, Malagelada J-R. Isobaric intestinal distension in humans: sensorial relay and reflex gastric relaxation. *Am J Physiol* 1990;258:G202-7.

5. Steadman CJ, Phillips SF, Camilleri M, Haddad AC, Hanson RB. Variation of muscle tone in the human colon. *Gastroenterology* 1991;101:373-81

6. Bell AM, Pemberton JH, Hanson RB, Zinsmeister AR. Variations in muscle tone of the human rectum: recordings with an electromechanical barostat. *Am J Physiol* 1991;260:G17-25.

7. Di Lorenzo C, Mertz H, Alvarez S, Mori C, Mayer EA, Hyman PE. Gastric receptive relaxation is absent in newborn infants. *Gastroenterology* 1993;33:A595.

22

Pathology of Enteric Neuromuscular Disorders

MICHAEL D. SCHUFFLER

The majority of pediatric motility disorders are associated with structural abnormalities of either the muscularis propria or myenteric plexus. Many of these disorders, such as the aganglionosis of Hirschsprung's disease, clinically manifest in infancy. Others, such as familial visceral myopathies or some visceral neuropathies, present later in childhood. Structural abnormalities can often be discerned by conventional light microscopy if the tissue biopsies are properly processed and studied by an experienced histopathologist. Light microscopy may be the key to diagnosing a particular child's motility disorder.

NEUROMUSCULAR ANATOMY OF THE GUT

Knowledge of the normal structure of the gut's neuromuscular apparatus is necessary to understand the pathology of the enteric nervous system and muscularis propria. In conventional perpendicular sections of the bowel wall, the muscularis mucosa lies immediately beneath the lamina propria and separates it from the submucosa. Immunohistochemistry should reveal a rich innervation of the muscularis mucosa and submucosa that can be visualized by utilizing antibodies to various neural and glial cell markers, such as neuron-specific enolase (NSE), vasoactive intestinal peptide (VIP), substance P, and S-100. This innervation cannot be visualized by conventional hemotoxylin and eosin (H&E) microscopy.

The submucosa has a very rich innervation, which is organized into the submucosal plexus of Meissner. There are two major components of this plexus, one located just beneath the muscularis mucosae and the other just above the muscularis propria. Most ganglia are located in these two areas and contain numerous neurons and axons, which can be visualized on H&E stains. Because the superficial part of the submucosal plexus is close to the mucosa, suction biopsies of the rectum usually permit visualization of submucosal ganglia and neurons. Ganglia contain anywhere from one to seven neurons. Axons are arranged around the neurons, but are not well defined by H&E. A variable number of nerve trunks course through the submucosa outside this mesh. These are best visualized by immunohistochemistry.

The muscularis propria lies beneath the submucosa. It is organized into inner circular and outer longitudinal muscle layers in the esophagus, small intestine, and colon. The organization of the smooth muscles of the stomach is more complex due to an additional, oblique layer of muscle in the fundus and body. The longitudinal muscle of the colon contains the three taenia, which are thickened subdivisions of the muscle that extend the length of the colon to the rectum.

The smooth-muscle cells in each layer are arranged parallel to one another and form sheathlike coats in conventional sections. The smooth-muscle fibers of the circular muscle have distinct borders that vary from round to irregular, depending on the state of contractility at the time of fixation. Relaxed borders are round; contracted borders are irregular. The muscle fibers of the longitudinal muscle are of variable length and are smooth to irregular in contour. There may be thin strands of collagen within the muscle layers, dividing them loosely into bundles. The amount of collagen visualized by specialized stains is minimal. Diffuse collagen deposition is always abnormal.

Morphologic study of the smooth-muscle layers requires optimal fixation. Bouin's and Hollande's fixatives provide optimal morphology if the sections are cut at a thickness of 4 μm. The disadvantage of Hollande's fixative is that it does not lend itself to immunohistochemistry, which is important for study of the enteric nervous system. An H&E stain intense in eosin accentuates the muscle cells and allows easier interpretation. In addition, some sections should always be stained with Masson's trichrome, which differentiates blue-staining collagen from scarlet-stained smooth-muscle cells.

Between the circular and longitudinal muscles lies the myenteric plexus, originally described by Auerbach in 1864 (Figs. 22.1, 22.2). The plexus is a meshlike network consisting of ganglia and nerve tracts linking the ganglia (Fig. 22.3). The ganglia contain neurons, axons, and glial cells but lack inflammatory cells, blood vessels, and connective tissue. Serial sections stained with H&E are used for semiquantification of neurons[1] in addition to the detection of inflammatory cells, neuronal intranuclear inclusions, neuronal degeneration, and abnormal proliferation of neurons and axons. Thus, the presence or absence of neurons, inflammatory cells, intranuclear inclusions, and gross degenerative changes are discerned by this method. Conventional microscopy, however, has a number of disadvantages. It cannot visualize dendrites or axons, and the morphology of neurons is suboptimal, making it difficult to assess neuronal degeneration. Also, because the sections are cut perpendicular to the plexus, the meshlike architecture of the plexus cannot be visualized.

Because of these problems, Barbara Smith, a neuropathologist, devised a technique in which a flattened, formalin-fixed piece of intestine is placed serosal side up on a base-sledge freezing microtome.[2,3] Frozen sections of 50 μm are cut parallel to the serosa so that longitudinal sections can be taken. These sections contain parts of the circular and longitudinal muscles, with the myenteric plexus sandwiched between. They are stained by a silver technique that clarifies the meshlike layout of the plexus, and allows the nerve tracts to be traced from one ganglion to another. This method is excellent for studying the morphology of neurons, dendrites, and axons (Fig. 22.4). Abnormalities are readily visualized, and glial-cell proliferation as a response to injury can be detected. This technique is not well suited for studying the submucosal plexus, which is not as compact and densely populated as the myenteric plexus.

With Smith's silver technique, neurons, dendrites, axons, and extrinsic nerve fibers appear dark tan to black. The background muscle stains brown. Neurons are classified as being either argyrophilic or argyrophobic. Because of their stain intensity, the argyrophilic neurons are readily visualized and can be semiquantified (Fig. 22.5). The argyrophobic neurons are less well visualized, and their neural processes remain unstained, making them difficult to quantify.

Argyrophilic neurons are heterogeneous in size, shape, number of processes, and the organization of the processes around the border of the neuron bodies. Their axons, along with a small contribution from extrinsic nerve fibers, form the nerve tracts which connect the ganglia. Ganglia usually contain from ten to fifteen argyrophilic neurons. The nerve tracts have anywhere from 25 to 100 axons.

Argyrophilia is derived from the presence of neurofilaments within the neurons and axons. Thus, a deficiency of neurofilaments secondary to either degeneration and neuron dropout or a qualitative defect of neurons leads to a deficiency of argyrophilic neurons. This is a key finding in some of the neuronal maturation disorders responsible for intestinal pseudo-obstruction in infants and children. Using immunohistochemistry, some of these cases are deficient in neurofilament immunoreactivity,[4] which correlates with deficiency of argyrophilia.

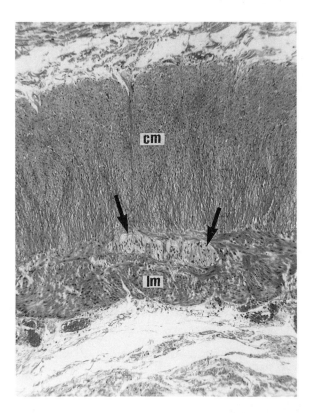

Fig. 22.1 Section of normal colon under H&E microscopy. Myenteric plexus (arrows) seen between the circular muscle (cm) and longitudinal muscle (lm). (Reprinted with permission from Krishnamurthy S, Schuffler M, 1987[5])

Fig. 22.2 Neurons (arrows), glial cell nuclei, and cross-sections of axons seen in a section of colonic myenteric plexus stained with H&E. (Reprinted with permission from Krishnamurthy S, Schuffler M, 1987[5])

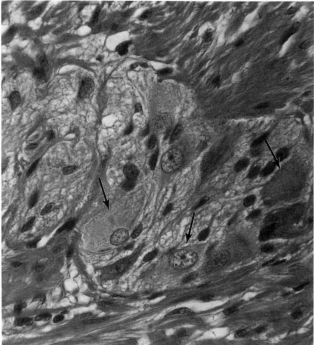

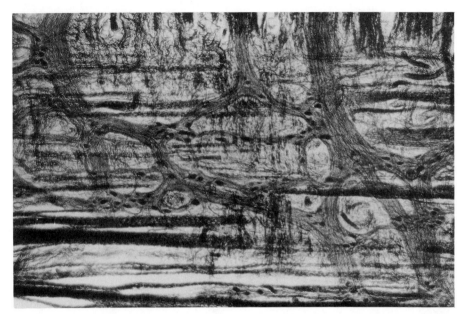

Fig. 22.3 Myenteric plexus of normal duodenum. The meshlike appearance of the plexus can be seen with neurons congregated in ganglia at intersections of the mesh. Strands of circular and longitudinal muscle can be seen around and between the nerve tracts interconnecting the ganglia (silver stain). (Reprinted with permission from Krishnamurthy S, Schuffler M, 1987[5])

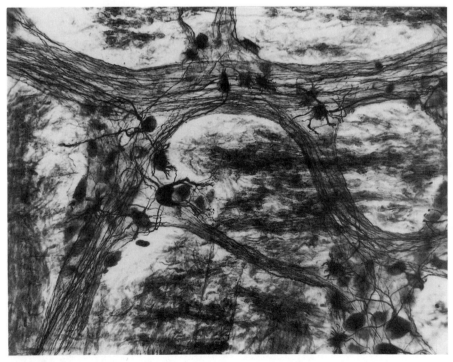

Fig. 22.4 Higher magnification of silver-stained ganglia and neurons from the small intestine.

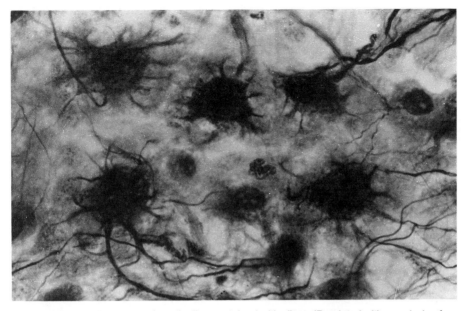

Fig. 22.5 Argyrophilic neurons from the ileum, stained with silver. (Reprinted with permission from Krishnamurthy S, Schuffler M, 1987[5])

Conventional light microscopy and silver stains can discern most abnormalities of the myenteric plexus. However, a major disadvantage is that an extra-large, full-thickness biopsy is necessary to sample the myenteric plexus. The sample must be between 1.5 and 2 cm in length and width to allow sectioning and staining. In some situations this is not a problem because the intestine is being resected for palliation, an ileostomy is being created, or the colon is being pulled down to treat Hirschsprung's disease. In other cases, however, laparotomy is done for the sole purpose of excluding mechanical obstruction and obtaining sufficient tissue for diagnosis. In this situation, two sites should be sampled to obtain enough tissue to process by Smith's technique.

The disadvantages of the H&E and silver techniques have led some investigators to rely on immunohistochemistry. Using antibodies to a variety of neural and glial-cell markers, immunohistochemistry readily visualizes the enteric nervous system and its innervation of the muscularis propria, submucosa, and mucosa. Markers include NSE, S-100, neurofilaments, PGP9.5, nitric oxide synthase, VIP, substance P, enkephalin, and

a variety of other neuropeptides. Immunohistochemistry can be performed on conventional full-thickness tissues, and most pathology laboratories worldwide can handle this technique. The only requirements are reactive antibodies to neural and glial-cell markers and some experience in interpreting the morphology with the use of each antibody. Unfortunately, few publications document and validate the use of these antibodies for diagnosis. Also, most pathologists have little experience in interpreting enteric neuropathology by this technique. While a variety of antibodies should be studied and validated, pathologists should acquire experience utilizing antibodies to NSE, S-100, and neurofilaments. It is possible that the use of antibodies to these three markers could allow diagnosis of most disorders of the enteric nervous system, as outlined below.

CLASSIFICATION AND DEFINITION

The pathology of neuromuscular disorders of the gastrointestinal tract is classified in Table 22.1. Disorders of the myenteric plexus are caused by either developmental

TABLE 22.1 Neuromuscular Disorders of the Gastrointestinal Tract in Infants and Children

Disorders of the Myenteric Plexus
Developmental abnormalities
  Hirschsprung's disease
  Total colonic aganglionosis—with or without small-intestinal aganglionosis
  Zonal aganglionosis
  Intestinal neuronal dysplasia
    with Hirschsprung's disease
    with neurofibromatosis
    with type IIb multiple endocrine neoplasia syndrome
    isolated to intestine, with none of the above
  Maturational arrest (hypoganglionosis, immaturity)
    Type I
    Type II
    Type III
  Infantile hypertrophic pyloric stenosis
Visceral neuropathies (primarily adults)
  Familial forms, both autosomal dominant and recessive
  Sporadic forms

Disorders of the Smooth Muscle
Primary
  Familial visceral myopathies
    Type I
    Type II
    Type III
  Sporadic visceral myopathies
    Type I childhood visceral myopathy
    Type II childhood visceral myopathy
Secondary
  Mitochondrial myopathy
  Progressive systemic sclerosis
  Progressive muscular dystrophy
  Ehlers-Danlos syndrome

problems or degeneration. Visceral neuropathies encompass degenerative disorders of the myenteric plexus[5] and are most often seen in adults. They are uncommon in the pediatric population. Visceral neuropathies are characterized by degeneration and loss of neurons and axons. Glial cells often proliferate in response to the injury. Visceral neuropathies are either familial or sporadic; most adult cases occur sporadically. Familial forms are transmitted as autosomal-dominant or -recessive traits. Although the vast majority are noninflammatory, some cases are characterized by inflammatory destruction of the myenteric plexus. Most of the latter in adults are associated with small-cell carcinoma of the lung (paraneoplastic visceral neuropathy), whereas others are idiopathic.

Developmental disorders of the myenteric plexus are the most frequent causes of severe dysmotility in infants and children. Hirschsprung's disease is the best recognized, while others include total colonic aganglionosis, small-bowel aganglionosis, intestinal neuronal dysplasia, and maturational arrest of the myenteric plexus.

Visceral Myopathies and Neuropathies

Visceral myopathy refers to degenerative disorders of the smooth muscle. It is characterized by degenerative changes of smooth-muscle cells, accompanied by proliferation of collagen within the muscularis propria.[6,7] Visceral myopathies may be primary to the intestinal and genitourinary tracts or secondary to systemic diseases that affect smooth muscle. The primary myopathies are characterized by muscle-cell degeneration, fragmentation, vacuolation, and fibrosis. These changes produce a characteristic honeycombed appearance of the muscle, which is easily recognized at low magnification on H&E and trichrome-stained sections. A continuum of change may result in the disappearance of all traces of degenerating muscle cells and vacuolation in the most severe areas, with only a few normal muscle cells and a large amount of collagen left behind. This appearance may be indistinguishable from systemic disorders that secondarily involve the smooth muscle, such as progressive systemic sclerosis and progressive muscular dystrophy. In some cases, it may be impossible to morphologically differentiate between primary visceral myopathy, progressive systemic sclerosis, and progressive muscular dystrophy.

The terms visceral neuropathy and visceral myopathy refer only to pathologic changes but not to a patient's clinical symptoms or the radiographic appearance of barium studies. Patients with visceral neuropathy and myopathy vary from being asymptomatic to having severe symptoms. There may be few changes on radiographic studies or the changes may be severe enough to produce a megaesophagus, megaduodenum, or megacolon.

Hirschsprung's megacolon is one type of colonic enlargement caused by absence of the intrinsic innervation of the rectosigmoid. Idiopathic megacolon may be secondary to either a visceral myopathy or visceral neuropathy throughout the colon. The presence of enlarged bowel may indicate an underlying structural abnormality of the smooth muscle or enteric nervous system. However, there are some cases of idiopathic megacolon in which structural abnormalities cannot be defined by either H&E or silver stains. Immunohistochemistry might define abnormalities of particular neural markers in such cases.

In addition to enlarging the bowel, visceral myopathies and neuropathies may result in diffuse small intestinal diverticulosis, ie, the presence of multiple diverticula in the jejunum or throughout the small intestine.[5] This occurs in visceral myopathies because focal areas of the intestinal wall are weakened by muscle atrophy and fibrosis and then protrude as diverticula. In contrast, the muscle in visceral neuropathies is usually very thick and, presumably because of hypercontractility, focal areas of the mucosa and submucosa are forced out through the bowel wall along the paths of penetrating blood vessels. Thus, in visceral myopathies the diverticula consist of the full thickness of the wall, whereas in visceral neuropathies they consist of mucosa and submucosa.

DEVELOPMENTAL DISORDERS OF THE ENTERIC NERVOUS SYSTEM
Hirschsprung's Disease

Hirschsprung's disease is characterized by the absence of the enteric nervous system within the distal colon.[8] This absence is usually limited to the rectum and rectosigmoid. In some cases, the absence of intrinsic innervation extends up to the splenic flexure and, rarely, to the entire colon. Theoretically, it is possible that when the entire colon is involved (total colonic aganglionosis) the pathogenesis of disease differs from classical Hirschsprung's disease. The absence of the intrinsic plexus in Hirschsprung's disease is caused by failure of neural crest cells to populate the distal colon. The cause of this failure in humans is unknown, but one theory is that the microenvironment of the smooth-muscle cells inhibits the ingrowth of neural crest cells.[9,10]

Although the intrinsic innervation is absent, the extrinsic innervation—consisting of the sympathetic and parasympathetic nerves that are derived from the spinal cord— is preserved and even increased. The theory is that developmental failure of the intrinsic plexus leads to a lack of feedback inhibition of ingrowth of extrinsic nerves. This results in enlarged bundles of extrinsic sympathetic and parasympathetic nerves coursing through the bowel wall. These nerve trunks can be visualized in the area between the circular and longitudinal muscles, but should not be mistaken for the myenteric plexus. They also course through the circular muscle and submucosa, where they provide branches to the muscularis mucosa and lamina propria.

These large nerve trunks can be identified on H&E sections. Whereas nerve tracts of the intrinsic nervous system are never surrounded by a supporting cell layer or perineurium, the extrinsic nerve trunks are encircled by a perineurium, which can be easily visualized (Fig. 22.6). Because these trunks contain acetylcholinesterase, histochemical methods were developed to more easily identify them, thereby aiding the diagnosis of Hirschsprung's disease.[11-13] Although immunohistochemistry and antibodies have been used to diagnose Hirschsprung's disease,[14-18] experience with these techniques is limited compared to the acetylcholinesterase method.

The acetylcholinesterase method requires excellent technique and careful interpretation.[13] Because false positive and negative results occur, careful attention to detail is important.[11-13] Classically, sections of aganglionic colon show intensely stained nerve trunks in the submucosa, muscularis mucosa, and lamina propria (Fig. 22.7). False-negative results may occur if the biopsy is taken from above the aganglionic zone, colonic aganglionosis is total, or the biopsy is taken at or proximal to the splenic flexure. This technique is more reliable after 3 weeks of age, when the acetylcholinesterase positive fibers have proliferated into the lamina propria. Before that, there may be large positive bundles in the muscularis mucosa and submucosa, but not in the lamina propria. Thus, a false negative could result from biopsies that are superficial and do not include the muscularis mucosa and submucosa. Lake reports that in rectal biopsies from 1556 patients, 324 of whom had Hirschsprung's disease, there was only one false negative—from a case of total colonic aganglionosis—and no false positives.[13] Lake emphasizes the need for a pseudocholines-

terase inhibitor to diminish background staining, and a delicate counterstain to define the presence of neurons without obscuring acetylcholinesterase-positive nerve trunks.

For optimal diagnosis, some sections should be stained with H&E and others with acetylcholinesterase. The literature reports that anywhere from one to four rectal suction biopsies should be obtained. Three biopsies are optimal; two for H&E, one for acetylcholinesterase. These should be taken 1.5 to 5 cm above the dentate line, with each biopsy extending into the submucosa so that the superficial component of the submucosal plexus can be sampled. All three biopsies should be carefully oriented on mesh, and two should be fixed in Bouin's or Hollande's solutions. The third specimen should be snap frozen, sectioned on a freezing microtome, then stained for acetylcholinesterase. The two fixed biopsies should be embedded in paraffin, serially cut to yield 60 sections each, and stained with H&E. A high-quality stain is necessary to detect the cytoplasm of submucosal neurons.

Classically, Hirschsprung's disease is diagnosed if the H&E serial sections—including adequate submucosa—fail to show a single neuron. Confirmation is obtained if the acetylcholinesterase stain is positive. Absence of neurons plus a negative acetylcholinesterase stain may indicate total colonic aganglionosis. The presence of submucosal neurons plus a positive acetylcholinesterase stain with positive nerve fibers in the lamina propria may indicate intestinal neuronal dysplasia. The latter diagnosis is strengthened if neurons are also present in the lamina propria and there is a hyperproliferation of submucosal ganglia and neurons.

If the diagnosis is inconclusive, a full-thickness rectal biopsy should be obtained to document the absence of the myenteric plexus. If immunohistochemistry is used, very little innervation of the circular muscle should be apparent. In most cases, three suction biopsies should confirm a diagnosis of Hirschsprung's disease.

Tissue should also be obtained during the operation to define the proximal margin of the aganglionic segment by frozen sections.

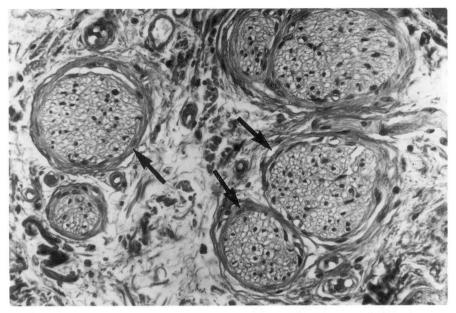

Fig. 22.6 Extrinsic nerve trunks with perineuriums (arrows) from a subserosal area of normal stomach, stained with H&E. (Reprinted with permission from Yoshida MM, et al, 1988[65])

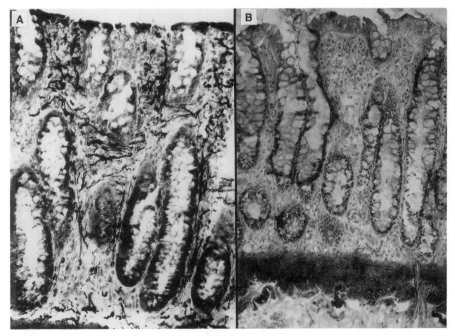

Fig. 22.7 **A,** Positive acetylcholinesterase stain shows a dark muscularis mucosa at the bottom and thick, irregular fibers throughout the entire width of the lamina propria. Note the presence of thick fibers on the luminal half of the biopsy specimen, many of which run parallel to the surface. **B,** Negative (non-Hirschsprung's disease) pattern of acetylcholinesterase stain with few thin fibers within the muscularis mucosa and rare thin fibers within the lamina propria. (Reprinted with permission from Schofield DE, et al, 1990[11])

Between the aganglionic and normal ganglionic colon there is a transition zone containing a deficient quantity of intrinsic innervation. The surgeon needs to be certain that normal ganglionic bowel is pulled through during the operation. Frozen sections should demonstrate normal ganglia before that bowel can be used for anastomosis.

The difficulties of the acetylcholinesterase method and the wide availability of immunohistochemistry in clinical pathology laboratories has enhanced interest in diagnosing Hirschsprung's disease with antibodies to neural- and glial-cell markers. For instance, in the normal colon an antineurofilament antibody produces only partial staining of some axon bundles in the plexuses. In Hirschsprung's disease, however, there are heavily stained hyperplastic nerve trunks.[4,19,20] Similarly, an S-100 antibody may show hypertrophied submucosal nerve trunks in the aganglionic colon, although the acetylcholinesterase stain may be more reliable in identifying nerve proliferation in the lamina propria.[14] A polyclonal antibody to PGP9.5 has also been used to demonstrate increased staining of nerve trunks in the lamina propria, muscularis mucosa, and submucosa of the aganglionic segment,[21] but it is not as sensitive as S-100 or acetylcholinesterase. An antibody against synaptic vesicles (antibody 171B5) is reported to differentiate between normal and aganglionic bowel.[15]

Recently, staining for nitric oxide synthase has been reported in Hirschsprung's disease.[22] Nitric oxide synthase is the enzyme that catalyzes the production of nitric oxide. In one study of six patients with Hirschsprung's disease, nitric oxide synthase was absent from both plexuses and the muscularis propria, whereas staining was moderate in abnormal large nerve bundles of the submucosa.[22]

Because enlarged nerve trunks in the submucosa, muscularis mucosa, and lamina propria are characteristic of Hirschsprung's disease, the question is which of the above methods can best visualize the trunks. Acetylcholinesterase has been more widely used than immunohistochemistry, but the question would be best answered by a prospective study comparing acetylcholinesterase with antibodies to a variety of neural and glial cell markers such as PGP9.5, S-100, neutropeptide Y, neurofilaments, 171B5, nitric oxide synthase, and other neural- and glial-cell markers. For now, a combination of H&E and acetylcholinesterase is most appropriate in the majority of pathology laboratories.

Total Colonic Aganglionosis

In approximately 5% to 10% of patients who present with clinical manifestations of Hirschsprung's disease, the enteric nervous system is absent throughout the entire colon. In some cases, varying lengths of the small intestine are also missing.[23-26] In the majority of the latter cases, the aganglionosis is limited to the ileum, but the entire small bowel may sometimes be involved. Intestinal aganglionosis may be associated with Waardenburg's syndrome,[27] the Smith-Lemli-Opitz syndrome,[28] and congenital failure of automatic control of ventilation (ie, Ondine's curse).[29] Rectal biopsies resemble those for Hirschsprung's disease, except for a lack of acetylcholinesterase staining. The extent of the aganglionosis can only be established at laparotomy. Multiple full-thickness biopsies must be performed to search for the myenteric plexus and the most proximal site of aganglionosis. Immunohistochemistry should not be necessary for diagnosis because the absence of neurons is readily apparent on conventional H&E sections.

A variant of this disorder is referred to as zonal aganglionosis.[30,31] A segment of aganglionic colon lies adjacent to the proximal and distal normal ganglionic areas. There may be one or two aganglionic areas in the colon and/or small bowel, and the rectum may be aganglionic or normally ganglionic. In the latter situation, rectal biopsies are normal.

In another variant, the myenteric plexus is markedly deficient, but the submucosal plexus is normal.[32] Rectal suction biopsy is misleading because normal neurons and nerve fibers are found in the submucosa. In contrast, full-thickness rectal biopsy is diagnostic. The proximal extent of the deficient myenteric plexus must be established at laparotomy.

Intestinal Neuronal Dysplasia

Intestinal neuronal dysplasia is characterized by hyperplasia of the enteric nerve plexuses and an abnormal distribution of neural elements.[33-38] It is also referred to as neuronal intestinal dysplasia, neuronal colonic dysplasia, pseudo-Hirschsprung's disease, and hyperganglionosis. A marked proliferation of the myenteric and submucosal plexuses is typical (Figs. 22.8, 22.9). Neurons may be found in the lamina propria, where normally they are extremely rare, and also within body of the smooth-muscle layers, where they are not normally found (Fig. 22.10). Acetylcholinesterase staining shows increased positive nerve fibers in the lamina propria and circular muscle.

Intestinal neuronal dysplasia can be difficult to diagnose. Submucosal neurons are not easily quantified. Unless the normal range is known, however, it may not be possible to determine whether neurons are abnormally increased in number. Ganglia within the normal submucosa may contain up to seven neurons. In addition, neurons are rarely found in the lamina propria of normal people. Even when neurons are present in the lamina propria in intestinal neuronal dysplasia, they are not usually numerous. Thus, diagnosis is less certain than in Hirschsprung's disease. It is best if multiple findings are present, such as neurons and acetylcholinesterase positive fibers in the lamina propria as well as enlargement and proliferation of ganglia and neurons within the submucosa. Histochemistry can be used to visualize submucosal neurons by staining them for lactic dehydrogenase and succinate dehydrogenase.[33] These stains may provide a more accurate diagnosis than H&E stain. Full-thickness rectal biopsy may be necessary for diagnosis, in which case proliferation of ganglia, neurons, and axons may be identified within the myenteric plexus, and neurons may be discerned within the body of the smooth muscles, especially the circular muscle.

Intestinal neuronal dysplasia may be associated with neurofibromatosis and type IIb multiple endocrine neoplasia syndrome. It may occur proximal to the aganglionic segment of Hirschsprung's disease, or exist as an isolated condition not associated with any of these disorders.

Intestinal neuronal dysplasia may be localized to the colon or disseminated throughout the small and large intestines. Distribution may be patchy, with normal bowel between areas of dysplasia. In some cases of small-bowel or proximal colonic involvement, where rectal biopsies might be inconclusive, laparotomy with full-thickness biopsies may be necessary for diagnosis. In those rare patients with aganglionosis of the colon and

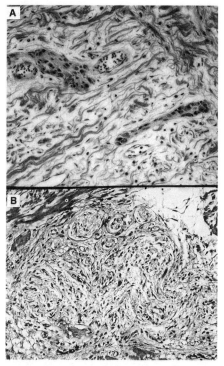

Fig. 22.8 **A,** Large, irregular submucosal ganglia in a patient with intestinal neuronal dysplasia. The muscularis mucosae is noted in the upper right-hand corner of the photograph. (Reprinted with permission from Schofield DE, Yunis EJ, 1992[37]) **B,** Marked enlargement of the myenteric plexus in a patient with intestinal neuronal dysplasia associated with neurofibromatosis. (Reproduced with permission from Feinstat T, et al, 1984[66])

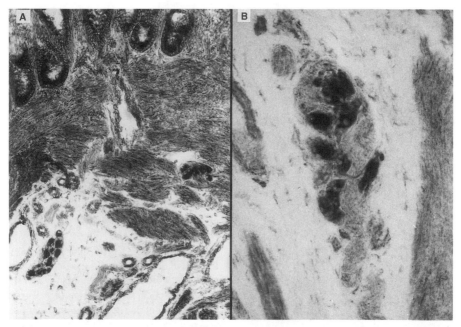

Fig 22.9 **A,** Colonic mucosa in intestinal neuronal dysplasia shows giant ganglia, some of which are located in the muscularis mucosa (lactic dehydrogenase). **B,** Single giant ganglion with nerve cells. Selective visualization by succinate dehydrogenase reaction. (**A, B:** Reprinted with permission from Meier-Ruge W, 1992[33])

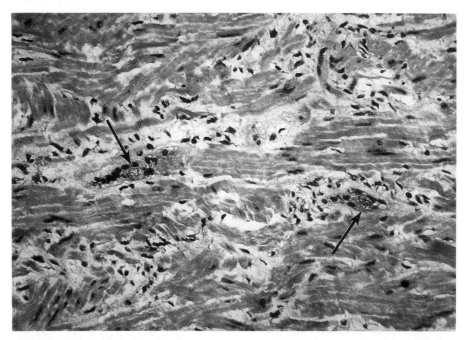

Fig. 22.10 Neurons (arrows) within the circular muscle of a case of intestinal neuronal dysplasia associated with neurofibromatosis (H&E stain). (Reprinted with permission from Feinstat T, et al, 1984[66])

terminal ileum, intestinal neuronal dysplasia may occur in the entire small bowel proximal to the ileum.[39]

Thus, intestinal neuronal dysplasia may be localized or disseminated throughout the gastrointestinal tract, associated with Hirschsprung's disease, and patchy in distribution. Histologic diagnosis may be difficult. Three rectal biopsies, processed as for Hirschsprung's disease, are the initial diagnostic steps, followed by full-thickness rectal biopsy if results are inconclusive. Laparotomy with full-thickness biopsies may be necessary if the rectal biopsies are inconclusive and there is evidence of more proximal disease. Because of scattered involvement and lack of diagnostic findings on some sections, multiple biopsies and serial sections are recommended.

Maturational Arrest of the Myenteric Plexus

Maturational arrest is sometimes referred to as "hypoganglionosis" or "immaturity" of the myenteric plexus. Patients with this disorder present with constipation, intestinal pseudo-obstruction, or recurrent constipation after surgical treatment for presumed Hirschsprung's disease.[40] A spectrum of abnormalities is identified in the myenteric plexus of different patients, varying from marked deficiency of all neural- and glial-cell elements to a deficiency of argyrophilic neurons.[40-45] These abnormalities usually exist throughout the small intestine and colon and require full-thickness tissue for diagnosis. Diagnosis is therefore usually made by obtaining full-thickness biopsies or resections at laparotomy. Three types of maturational arrest can be identified.[40]

Type I. Patients with type I maturational arrest exhibit a marked deficiency of all neural elements in both the myenteric and submucosal plexuses. This deficiency can be easily recognized on H&E sections. The normal meshwork of the myenteric plexus is absent on silver stains. There are only rare neurons between the circular and longitudinal muscles on H&E; although neurons are present in the submucosa, they are reduced in number and they appear immature.

Type II. In type II maturational arrest, submucosal neurons are present in normal numbers. However, semiquantification usually demonstrates a decrease in neurons between the circular and longitudinal muscles. Neurons are recognizable on H&E (Fig. 22.11A) but may sometimes appear immature, with large nuclei and scant cytoplasm. No argyrophilic neurons are present on silver stains (Fig. 11.11B), and because the axons are deficient, there are no nerve tracts and, therefore, no plexus. In some cases, the number of neurons in the H&E sections may appear normal at first glance. Smith's silver technique, which reveals absence of both argyrophilic neurons and a meshlike plexus, can provide the key to diagnosis.

Type III. In type III maturational arrest, numbers of neurons are normal on the H&E sections. Silver stains reveal a meshlike plexus. Although they often appear normal morphologically on H&E, neurons may have subtle abnormalities such as reduced cytoplasm and enlarged nuclei with prominent nucleoli and coarse chromatin (Fig. 22.12). In the vast majority of cases, biopsies stained only with H&E would be interpreted as normal. The silver technique, however, demonstrates that although a normal meshlike plexus is present, argyrophilic-staining neurons are deficient in number. Most normal ganglia contain 10 to 15 argyrophilic-staining neurons, but ganglia in this condition contain from 0 to 3 with only a few axons visible in the nerve tracts (Fig. 22.13). The ganglia and nerve tracts are filled with an abnormally large number of nuclei, probably representing glial cells and immature neurons that have not acquired argyrophilia. Thus, a normal number of neurons are seen on H&E, but they lack argyrophilia on silver stain.

The use of immunohistochemistry and antineurofilament antibodies may also demonstrate the abnormal myenteric plexus in this condition. Neurofilament-immunoreactivity is deficient in otherwise normal appearing axon bundles.[4,46] This deficiency

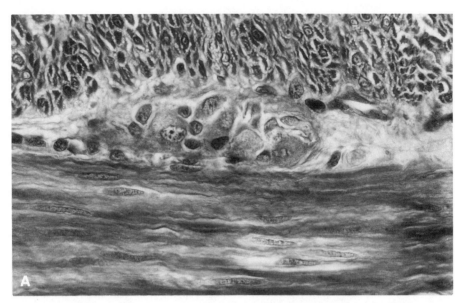

Fig. 22.11 Type II maturational arrest. **A,** A cluster of seemingly normal neurons can be seen between the circular and longitudinal muscles (H&E stain). **B,** No myenteric plexus is visible with silver staining. However, there are clusters of nuclei (arrows) and occasional axons (arrowhead) between the muscle layers. The nuclei are large and have prominent chromatin. (**A, B:** Reprinted with permission from Krishnamurthy S, et al, 1993[40])

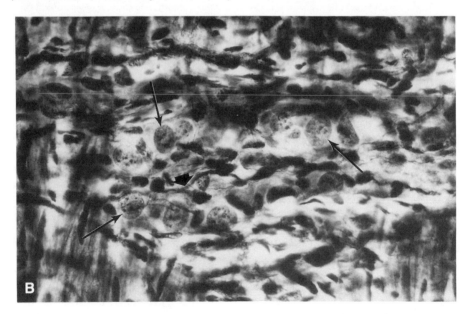

correlates with the lack of argyrophilia, since neurofilaments are necessary for argyrophilia. In type III maturational arrest, conventional H&E sections will miss the diagnosis. Either Smith's silver method or immunohis-tochemistry with an antineurofilament antibody is necessary for diagnosis. It is possible that antibodies to other neural- and glial-cell markers might also make the diagnosis. However, there has been almost no experience

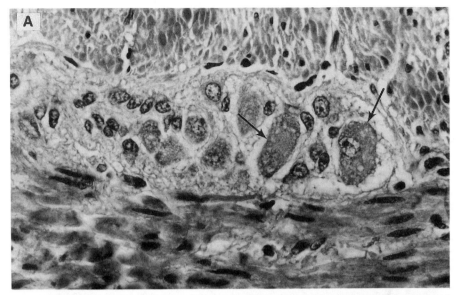

Fig. 22.12 **A,** A month-old control shows well-developed myenteric plexus between the circular and longitudinal muscles. Note mature neurons with prominent perikarya (arrows). The small nuclei represent glial cells (H&E stain). **B,** Type III maturational arrest. A 3-week-old girl with pseudo-obstruction. The myenteric plexus is present, but the two neuronal nuclei (arrows) have scant cytoplasm around them (H&E). (Reprinted with permission from Krishnamurthy S, et al, 1993[40])

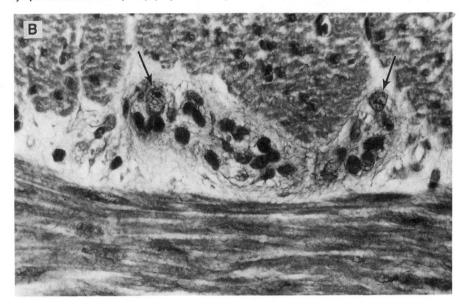

with other antibodies to diagnose this particular disorder.

Visceral Neuropathies

Visceral neuropathies are much more common in the adult population than in pediatric patients. A variety of familial and sporadic causes of visceral neuropathy exist.[5] Sporadic visceral neuropathy in children is characterized by degeneration and loss of neurons and axons in the absence of inflammatory cells.

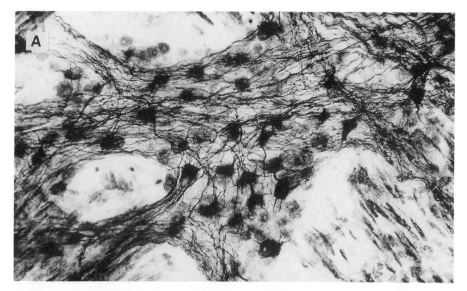

Fig. 22.13 **A,** Four-month-old control shows normal myenteric plexus with plentiful argyrophilic neurons and axons (silver stain). **B,** Type III maturational arrest. In this 4-month-old girl with pseudo-obstruction, a ganglionic area with a deficient number of argyrophilic neurons and many nuclei can be seen, some of which may represent nonrecognizable neuronal precursors. One unipolar argyrophilic nueron is present (arrow) on silver stain. (Reprinted with permission from Krishnamurthy S, et al, 1993[40])

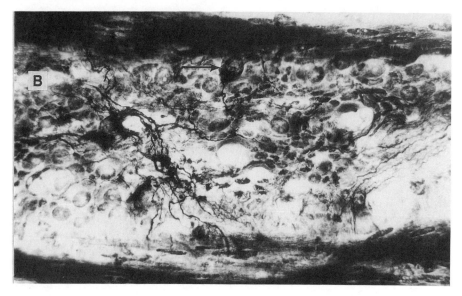

Infantile Hypertrophic Pyloric Stenosis

Hypertrophic pyloric stenosis is characterized by gastric outlet obstruction associated with marked thickening of the muscularis propria of the pylorus caused by hyper-trophy and hyperplasia of the smooth muscles.[47] The underlying pathology consists of an abnormality of the myenteric plexus of the pylorus.[48] The number of ganglia per unit area and the number of neurons in the ganglia are less than normal. Smith's silver technique demonstrates a marked deficiency of argyrophilic-staining neurons and axons,[2] which may represent a failure of development of the neurons of the pylorus, analogous to type III maturational arrest of the myenteric plexus. In hypertrophic pyloric stenosis, the abnormality is usually limited to the pylorus, although it may coexist in the small intestine of some infants who also have pseudo-obstruction associated with a short small bowel and malrotation.[45]

The deficiency of the myenteric plexus can also be demonstrated by using antibodies to neuropeptides.[49] Similarly, the use of methods for nitric oxide synthase demonstrate enlarged and distorted nerve fibers in the circular muscles of the pylorus, while the overall innervation of the myenteric plexus and smooth muscles is deficient.[50] Because nitric oxide mediates smooth-muscle relaxation, the lack of nitric oxide synthase may be responsible for the smooth-muscle spasm of the pylorus in hypertrophic pyloric stenosis.

VISCERAL MYOPATHIES

Visceral myopathies are much less frequent than enteric nervous system disorders in infancy and childhood. They are characterized by degeneration and fibrous replacement of the smooth muscles of the gastrointestinal tract, and in some cases, the urinary system as well (Fig. 22.14).[6,51,52] These structural abnormalities are similar in the various clinical syndromes of visceral myopathy (Fig. 22.15). Smooth-muscle cells have poorly staining cytoplasm and indistinct cell margins, producing a smudged appearance. Muscle-cell fragmentation and dropout create apparent spaces containing cell debris. This condition is associated with a variable amount of collagen, which is often deposited around individual or small groups of degenerating muscle cells, producing a honeycombed appearance that is easily recognized at low magnification. In general, the longitudinal muscle is more affected than the circular. In some areas it may be the only muscle affected. In others, the entire thickness of the muscularis propria may be completely replaced by collagen, and diverticula

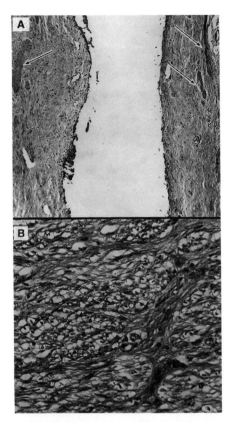

Fig. 22.14 **A,** Ureter from an infant with visceral myopathy. The wall of the ureter is replaced extensively by collagen, with only a small amount of smooth muscle left in this particular area (arrows). The mucosa is not well visualized secondary to traumatic artefacts (Masson's trichrome stain). **B,** In the bladder, there is prominent vacuolar degeneration and fibrosis of the smooth muscle (Masson's trichrome). (Reprinted with permission from Schuffler M, et al, 1988[6])

may form. Diffuse small intestinal diverticulosis may be an important part of the syndrome in some patients.[53] By electron microscopy, early changes are characterized by muscle-cell plasma membranes that are discontinuous, and disarrayed myofilaments that are no longer aligned with dense bodies.[52] The mitochondria are vacuolated and the cytoplasm is electron-lucent. Advanced changes consist of frank degeneration of the muscle cells, which then become widely separated by collagen. No abnormalities of the enteric nervous system are visible by

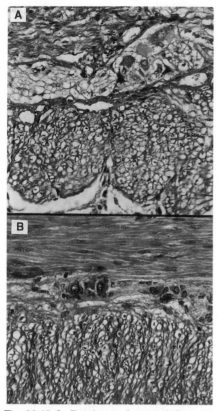

Fig. 22.15 **A,** Esophagus from an infant with visceral myopathy shows extensive vacuolar degeneration of the longitudinal muscle. Neurons are visible within the myenteric plexus just above this muscle (Masson's trichrome). **B,** Small intestine from an infant with visceral myopathy shows marked vacuolar degeneration of the longitudinal muscle and normal circular muscle. Neurons are visible within the myenteric plexus between the two muscle layers (Masson's trichrome stain). (Reprinted with permisson from Schuffler MD, et al, 1988[6])

either light or electron microscopy.

Visceral myopathies consist of several subtypes that are characterized by different patterns of involvement in the gastrointestinal and genitourinary systems, genetic transmission, and systemic involvement. Some are familial, whereas others occur sporadically.

Type I familial visceral myopathy is transmitted as an autosomal-dominant trait and is characterized by esophageal dilation, megaduodenum, a redundant ahaustral colon (or sometimes megacolon), and megacystis. In some patients, the entire small intestine may be involved. Type II familial visceral myopathy is transmitted as an autosomal-recessive trait.[53] It is characterized by gastric dilation and slight dilation of the entire small intestine, which contains numerous diverticula. In addition, patients have ptosis and external ophthalmoplegia, peripheral neuropathy, and deafness. Type III familial visceral myopathy is also transmitted as an autosomal-recessive trait.[54] It is characterized by marked dilation of the entire gastrointestinal tract from the esophagus to the rectum. There are no genitourinary or extraintestinal manifestations.

Visceral myopathy also occurs sporadically in infants and young children. Anuras has grouped these into types I and II childhood visceral myopathy.[55] Type I typically presents in infancy or very young childhood, and is characterized by involvement from the stomach to the rectum, with occasional esophageal peristalsis. Nearly all cases have megacystis and megaloureters.

Type II childhood visceral myopathy may manifest as the megacystis-microcolon-intestinal hypoperistalsis syndrome.[56] All patients have megacystis and some may have megaloureters. The patients present with intestinal pseudo-obstruction associated with a microcolon. The small intestine and colon may be shortened, and there may be malrotation of the microcolon. It is unlikely that all cases of megacystis-microcolon-intestinal hypoperistalsis syndrome are caused by visceral myopathy. Some are caused by maturational failure of the myenteric plexus.[57] Intestinal neuronal dysplasia and total colonic aganglionosis can also produce microcolon.

Chronic intestinal pseudo-obstruction has also been reported in association with mitochondrial myopathy,[58-60] a neurologic syndrome characterized by morphologic abnormalities of the mitochondria of striated muscle cells. Of the three patients reported with pseudo-obstruction, all had ophthalmoplegia. One had an intestinal biopsy which showed changes in the smooth muscle consistent with familial visceral myopathy.[60]

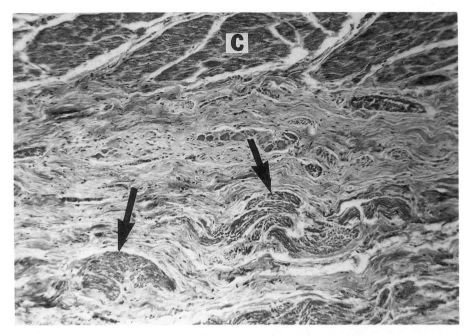

Fig. 22.16 H&E stain shows marked fibrosis of the oblique and longitudinal muscle of the stomach from a patient with muscular dystrophy (c, circular muscle). The arrows denote residual clusters of smooth-muscle cells. (Reprinted with permission from Leon S, et al, 1986[64])

SYSTEMIC DISORDERS INVOLVING SMOOTH MUSCLE

Progressive Systemic Sclerosis

Progressive systemic sclerosis frequently involves the gastrointestinal tract. The esophagus is involved in over 80% of cases, the small intestine in 50%, and the colon in 30%. Involvement of the muscularis propria may be patchy, with abrupt demarcations between normal and abnormal muscle.[61] The number of smooth-muscle cells is decreased, and the smooth-muscle layers are fibrotic and atrophied. In contrast to visceral myopathy, the muscle layers do not have a vacuolated, honeycombed appearance. The individual muscle cells are normal or small, without the degenerative features present in visceral myopathy.[61] The circular muscle is more involved than the longitudinal. The late stage of visceral myopathy may be indistinguishable from progressive systemic sclerosis, because both have atrophic fibrotic muscle. At times, it may be impossible to determine whether the patient has an end stage of visceral myopathy, progressive systemic sclerosis with absence of other systemic features of scleroderma, or a smooth-muscle disease that mimics progressive systemic sclerosis.[62,63]

Progressive Muscular Dystrophy

This condition may also involve the gastrointestinal tract.[64] The appearance of the muscularis propria may be identical to progressive systemic sclerosis (Fig. 22.16). Intestinal dilation and diverticula may form. The esophagus and stomach are more commonly involved than the small intestine and colon.

Ehlers-Danlos Syndrome

The Ehlers-Danlos syndrome may rarely involve the gastrointestinal tract and produce hypomotility, diverticula, and intestinal perforation. The morphologic abnormalities are patchy; focal areas of the muscularis propria are devoid of smooth muscle and have only small amounts of collagen.

The appearance may resemble progressive systemic sclerosis, but progressive systemic sclerosis is usually associated with much denser deposition of collagen. There is no muscle-cell degeneration characteristic of visceral myopathies.

DIAGNOSTIC APPROACH
Rectal Mucosal Biopsy

Suction biopsies of the rectum should be performed whenever Hirschsprung's disease or intestinal neuronal dysplasia is suspected. Three biopsies should be taken, two of which are processed for H&E, the third for acetylcholinesterase. The biopsies should reach into the superficial submucosa, including part of the submucosal plexus immediately beneath the muscularis mucosa. Each biopsy should be carefully oriented on monofilament nylon mesh, and 60 serial cross-sections should be taken from the central part of the biopsy and stained with H&E. Several frozen sections should be taken from the third biopsy and processed for acetylcholinesterase. The diagnosis of Hirschsprung's disease is justified when no neurons are found in any of the sections stained with H&E and acetylcholinesterase stain is positive, as manifested by reactive nerve trunks in the superficial submucosa, muscularis mucosae, and lamina propria. In very young children, however, the lamina propria may not yet have acetylcholinesterase-positive fibers.

Full-thickness Rectal Biopsy

Full-thickness rectal biopsy is indicated whenever mucosal biopsies are inconclusive. Perhaps no neurons were seen on the H&E sections, but the acetylcholinesterase stain was negative, or the biopsies were too superficial to ensure that the submucosal plexus was included. In this circumstance, full-thickness biopsy in Hirschsprung's disease should confirm the absence of myenteric plexus. It is best to orient the biopsy so that perpendicular sections are obtained all the way through the muscularis propria. Multiple sections should demonstrate absence of the myenteric plexus, although there may be large extrinsic nerve trunks between the circular and longitudinal muscles that could be mistaken for myenteric plexus. These can be easily recognized as extrinsic in origin by the presence of a perineurium. In addition, it may be easier to recognize intestinal neuronal dysplasia in full-thickness biopsies. The myenteric plexus may be enlarged, and neurons may be displaced into the body of the circular and/or longitudinal muscles. There may also be proliferation of ganglia and neurons in the submucosa, and neurons displaced into the lamina propria.

Full-thickness Small Intestinal and/or Colonic Biopsies

Full-thickness biopsies of the small intestine and/or colon are obtained whenever the diagnosis is in doubt and the patient has a diffuse intestinal motor disorder such as pseudo-obstruction, or when a pull-through operation for presumed Hirschsprung's disease did not result in remission of severe constipation. Clinical, manometric, and radiographic studies usually should result in a diagnosis of a diffuse motility disorder or pseudo-obstruction, but sometimes the diagnosis remains inconclusive. In such cases, exploratory laparotomy will exclude mechanical obstruction.

At the time of exploratory laparotomy, full-thickness biopsies should be obtained from the involved areas of the small intestine and colon. At least two biopsies are recommended because occasionally the abnormalities will be patchy. The biopsies should be fixed in Bouin's or Zamboni's solutions. The latter is preferable for immunohistochemistry. They should be well oriented, and serial sections should be cut for H&E staining to allow for semiquantification by counting neurons in every eighth serial section to derive a neuron score.[1,40] A deficiency of neurons characterizes many enteric nervous system disorders that produce pseudo-obstruction. Semiquantification will be meaningless, however, unless the pathologist can establish a normal range of neuron scores based on control studies of infants and children. Serial sections can visualize displaced neurons and hyperproliferation of the plexuses in intestinal neuronal dysplasia. Because neuronal dysplasia can be patchy, serial sections allow greater visualization of the intestinal wall.

Additional sections should be processed for immunohistochemistry with antibodies to NSE, S-100, and neurofilaments. Due to the variability of staining with different antineurofilament antibodies, several should be tested in control material. The one with the best immunoreactivity should be used in patients with motility disorders. An interested pathologist is necessary to interpret the results by building experience with these markers in control tissue. Unfortunately, very little experience has been reported with immunohistochemistry in the diagnosis of these disorders.

A variety of possible findings can be predicted by immunohistochemistry in disorders of the enteric nervous system. Where the system is grossly deficient in its development, there should be a deficiency of immunoreactivity for all three markers. Where there has been development of neurons but failure of expression of neurofilaments, NSE and S-100 staining will probably be normal and neurofilament immunoreactivity will be deficient. Where the glial-cell population is present but neurons are deficient, the S-100 staining should be normal, but both NSE and neurofilament immunoreactivity will be deficient. Because this is an evolving area that has had little investigation, a body of experience needs to be developed and reported with the use of these antibodies. In addition, other antibodies, such as those to PGP9.5, nitric oxide synthase, and tau, might be important to diagnosis and should also be investigated.

Immunohistochemistry provides better staining if the tissue is fixed in Zamboni's solution, with frozen sections rather than paraffin sections used for the staining. For that reason, some of the tissue should be processed into paraffin blocks and the rest saved in 30% sucrose for frozen sections.

CONCLUSION

Severe motility disorders of infancy and childhood are usually associated with structural abnormalities of either the enteric nervous system or muscularis propria. Micro-scopic diagnosis of these abnormalities may become less frequent in the future because of our greater knowledge of these syndromes and the ability of clinical findings, radiography, and manometry to diagnose them without tissue. However, whenever tissue becomes necessary for diagnosis, well-done light microscopy by an interested pathologist will remain important for diagnosis. H&E and trichrome stained sections are often sufficient for diagnosis without having to resort to more sophisticated methods, although additional techniques are necessary in selected cases. In the future, greater use should be made of immunohistochemistry, utilizing antibodies to a variety of neuronal and glial-cell markers.

REFERENCES

1. Schuffler M, Bird T, Sumi S, Cook A. A familial neuronal disease presenting as intestinal pseudo-obstruction. *Gastroenterology* 1978;75:889-98.

2. Smith B. *The Neuropathology of the Alimentary Tract.* London: Edward Arnold, 1972.

3. Schuffler M, Jonak Z. Chronic idiopathic intestinal pseudo-obstruction caused by a degenerative disorder of the myenteric plexus: the use of Smith's method to define the neuropathology. *Gastroenterology* 1982;82:476-86.

4. Kluck P, Tibboel D, Leendertse-Verloop K, van der Kamp A, ten Kate F, Molenaar J. Diagnosis of congenital neurogenic abnormalities of the bowel with monoclonal anti-neurofilament antibodies. *J Pediatr Surg* 1986;21:132-5.

5. Krishnamurthy S, Schuffler M. Pathology of neuromuscular disorders of the small intestine and colon. *Gastroenterology* 1987;93:610-39.

6. Schuffler M, Pagon R, Schwartz R, Bill A. Visceral myopathy of the gastrointestinal and genitourinary tracts in infants. *Gastroenterology* 1988;94:892-8.

7. Mitros F, Schuffler M, Teja K, Anuras S. Pathology of familial visceral myopathy. *Hum Pathol* 1982;13:825-33.

8. Doig C. Hirschsprung's disease: a review. *Int J Color Dis* 1991;6:52-62.

9. Parikh D, Tam P, Lloyd D, Van Velzen D, Edgar D. Quantitative and qualitative analysis of the extracellular matrix protein, laminin, in Hirschsprung's disease. *J Pediatr Surg* 1992;27:991-6.

10. Fujimoto T, Hata J, Yokoyama S, Mitomi T. A study of the extracellular matrix protein as the migration pathway of neural crest cells in the gut: analysis in human embryos with special references to the pathogenesis of Hirschsprung's disease. *J Pediatr Surg* 1989;24:550-6.

11. Schofield D, Devine W, Yunis E. Acetylcholinesterase-stained suction rectal biopsies in the diagnosis of Hirschsprung's disease. *J Pediatr Gastroenterol Nutr* 1990;11:221-8.

12. Athow A, Filipe M, Drake D. Problems and advantages of acetylcholinesterase histochemistry of rectal suction biopsies in the diagnosis of Hirschsprung's disease. *J Pediatr Surg* 1990;25:520-6.

13. Lake B, Malone M, Risdon R. Letter to the editor. *Pediatr Pathol* 1989;9:351-4.

14. Robey S, Kuhajda F, Yardley J. Immunoperoxidase stains of ganglion cells and abnormal mucosal nerve proliferations in Hirschsprung's disease. *Hum Pathol* 1988;19:432-7.

15. Yamataka A, Miyana T, Urao M, Mishiye H. Hirschsprung's disease: diagnosis using monoclonal antibody 171B5. *J Pediatr Surg* 1992;27:820-2.

16. Larsson L, Malmfors G, Ekblad E, Ekman R, Sundler F. NPY hyperinnervation in Hirschsprung's disease: both adrenergic and nonadrenergic fibers contribute. *J Pediatr Surg* 1991;26:1207-14.

17. Kato H, Yamamoto T, Yamamoto H, Ohi R, So N, Iwasaki Y. Immunocytochemical characterization of supporting cells in the enteric nervous system in Hirschsprung's disease. *J Pediatr Surg* 1990;25:514-9.

18. Larsson L, Sundler F. Neuronal markers in Hirschsprung's disease with special references to neuropeptides. *Acta Histochem* 1990;38:115-25.

19. Kluck P, van Muijen G, van der Kamp A, et al. Hirschsprung's disease studied with monoclonal antineurofilament antibodies on tissue sections. *Lancet* 1984;1:652-4.

20. Kluck P, ten Kate F, van der Kamp A, Tibboel D, Molenaar J. Pathologic explanation for postop-erative obstipation in Hirschsprung's disease revealed with monoclonal antibody staining. *Am J Clin Pathol* 1986;490-2.

21. Sams V, Bobrow L, Happerfield L, Keeling J. Evaluation of PGP9.5 in the diagnosis of Hirschsprung's disease. *J Pathol* 1992;168:55-8.

22. Vanderwinden J, DeLaet M, Schiffmann S, et al. Nitric oxide synthase distribution in the enteric nervous system of Hirschsprung's disease. *Gastroenterology* 1993;105:969-73.

23. Bickler S, Harrison M, Campbell T, Campell J. Long-segment Hirschsprung's disease. *Arch Surg* 1992;127:1047-51.

24. Careskey J, Weber T, Grosfeld J. Total colonic aganglionosis: analysis of 16 cases. *Am J Surg* 1982;143:160-8.

25. Boggs J, Kidd J. Congenital abnormalities of intestinal innervation: absence of innervation of jejunum, ileum, and colon in siblings. *Pediatrics* 1958;21:261-5.

26. Senyuz O, Buyukunal C, Danismend N, Erdogan E, Ozbay G, Soylet Y. Extensive intestinal aganglionosis. *J Pediatr Surg* 1989;24:453-6.

27. Farndon P, Bianchi A. Waardenburg's syndrome associated with total aganglionosis. *Arch Dis Child* 1983;58:932-3.

28. Zizka J, Maresova J, Kerekes Z, Juttnerova V, Balicek P. Intestinal aganglionosis in the Smith-Lemli-Opitz syndrome. *Acta Paediatr Scand* 1983;72:141-3.

29. Stern M, Hellwege H, Gravinghoff L, Lambrecht W. Total aganglionosis of the colon (Hirschsprung's disases) and congenital failure of automatic control of ventilation (Ondine's curse). *Acta Paediatr Scand* 1981;70:121-4.

30. Seldenrijk C, van der Harten H, Kluck P, Tibboel D, Moorman-Voestermans K, Meijer C. Zonal aganglionosis: an enzyme and immunohistochemical study of two cases. *Virchows Arch [A]* 1986;410:75-81.

31. Haney P, Hill J, Chen-Chih J. Zonal colonic aganglionosis. *Pediatr Radiol* 1982;12:258-61.

32. Mishalany H, Olson A, Khan F, Santos A. Deficient neurogenic innervation of the myenteric

plexus with normal submucous plexus involving the entire small and large bowel. *J Pediatr Surg* 1989;24:83-7.

33. Meier-Ruge W. Epidemiology of congenital innnervation defects of the distal colon. *Virchows Arch [A]* 1992;420:171-7.

34. Schofield D, Yunis E. Intestinal neuronal dysplasia. *J Pediatr Gastroenterol Nutr* 1991;12:182-9.

35. Stoss F, Meier-Ruge W. Diagnosis of neuronal colonic dysplasia in primary chronic constipation and sigmoid diverticulosis. Endoscopic biopsy and enzyme-histochemical examination. *Surg Endosc* 1991;5:146-9.

36. Athow A, Filipe M, Drake D. Hyperganglionosis mimicking Hirschsprung's disease. *Arch Dis Child* 1991;66:1300-3.

37. Schofield D, Yunis E. What is intestinal neuronal dysplasia? *Pathol Annu* 1992;27:249-62.

38. Munakata K, Morita K, Okabe K, Sueoka H. Clinical and histologic studies of neuronal intestinal dysplasia. *J Pediatr Surg* 1985;20:231-5.

39. Scharli A, Meier-Ruge W. Localized and disseminated forms of neuronal intestinal dysplasia mimicking Hirschsprung's disease. *J Pediatr Surg* 1981;16:164-70.

40. Krishnamurthy S, Heng Y, Schuffler M. Chronic intestinal pseudo-obstruction in infants and children caused by diverse abnormalities of the myenteric plexus. *Gastroenterology* 1993;104:1398-1408.

41. Puri P, Lake B, Nixon H. Adynamic bowel syndrome. *Gut* 1977;18:754-9.

42. Bughaighis A, Emery J. Functional obstruction of the intestine due to neurological immaturity. *Prog Pediatr Surg* 1971;3:37-52.

43. Mathe J, Khairallah S, Phat Vuoung N, Boccon-Gibod L, Rey A, Costil J. Dilation segmentaire du grele a revelation neonatale. *La Nouvelle Presse Medicale* 1982;11:265-6.

44. Navarro J, Sonsino E, Boige N, et al. Visceral neuropathies responsible for chronic intestinal pseudo-obstruction syndrome in pediatric practice: analysis of 26 cases. *J Pediatr Gastroenterol Nutr* 1990;11:179-95.

45. Tanner M, Smith B, Lloyd J. Functional intestinal obstruction due to deficiency of argyrophilic neurons in the myenteric plexus: familial syndrome presenting with short small bowel, malrotation, and pyloric hypertrophy. *Arch Dis Child* 1976;51:837-41.

46. Kluck P, Tibboel D, Leendertse-Verloop K, van der Kamp A, ten Kate F, Molenaar J. Disturbed defecation after colectomy for aganglionosis investigated with monoclonal antineurofilament antibody. *J Pediatr Surg* 1986;21:845-7.

47. Spicer R. Infantile hypertrophic pyloric stenosis: a review. *Br J Surg* 1982;69:128-35.

48. Spitz L, Kaufmann J. The neuropathological changes in congenital hypertrophic pyloric stenosis. *S Afr J Surg* 1975;13:239-42.

49. Wattchow D, Cass D, Furness J, et al. Abnormalities of the peptide-containing nerve fibers in infantile hypertrophic pyloric stenosis. *Gastroenterology* 1987;92:443-8.

50. Vanderwinden J, Mailleux P, Schiffmann S, Vanderhaeghen J, DeLaet M. Nitric oxide synthase activity in infantile hypertrophic pyloric stenosis. *N Engl J Med* 1992;327:511-5.

51. Nonaka M, Goulet O, Arahan P, Fekete C, Ricour C, Nezelof C. Primary intestinal myopathy, a cause of chronic idiopathic intestinal pseudo-obstruction syndrome (CIPS): clinicopathological studies of seven cases in children. *Pediatr Pathol* 1989;9:409-24.

52. Schuffler M, Lowe M, Bill A. Studies of idiopathic intestinal pseudo-obstruction: hereditary hollow visceral myopathy—clinical and pathological studies. *Gastroenterology* 1977;73:327-38.

53. Anuras S, Mitros F, Nowak P, et al. A familial visceral myopathy with external ophthalmoplegia and autosomal recessive transmission. *Gastroenterology* 1983;84:346-53.

54. Anuras S, Mitros F, Milano A, Kuminsky R, Decanio R, Green J. A familial visceral myopathy with dilatation of the entire gastrointestinal tract. *Gastroenterology* 1986;90:385-90.

55. Anuras S. Childhood visceral myopathies. In: Anuras S, ed. *Motility Disorders of the Gastrointestinal Tract.* New York, NY: Raven Press, 1992.

56. Puri P, Lake B, Gorman F, O'Donnell B, Nixon H. Megacystis-microcolon-intestinal hypoperistalsis syndrome: a visceral myopathy. *J Pediatr Surg* 1983;18:64-9.

57. Davis W, Allen R, Favara B, Slovis T. Neonatal small left colon syndrome. *Am J Roentgenol Radium Ther Nucl Med* 1974;120:322-9.

58. Cervera R, Bruix J, Bayes A, et al. Chronic intestinal pseudo-obstruction and ophthalmoplegia in a patient with mitochondrial myopathy. *Gut* 1988;29:544-7.

59. Li V, Hostein J, Romero N, et al. Chronic intestinal pseudo-obstruction with myopathy and ophthalmoplegia. *Dig Dis Sci* 1992;37:456-63.

60. Lowsky R, Davidson G, Wolman S, Jeejeebhoy K, Hegele R. Familial visceral myopathy associated with a mitochondrial myopathy. *Gut* 1993;34:279-83.

61. Schuffler M, Beegle R. Progressive systemic sclerosis of the gastrointestinal tract and hereditary hollow visceral myopathy: two distinguishable disorders of intestinal smooth muscle. *Gastroenterology* 1979;77:664-71.

62. Achandar J, Frank J, Jonas M. Isolated intestinal myopathy resembling progressive systemic sclerosis in a child. *Gastroenterology* 1988;95:1114-8.

63. Venizelos I, Shousha S, Bull T, Parkins R. Chronic intestinal pseudo-obstruction in two patients: overlap of features of systemic sclerosis and visceral myopathy. *Histopathology* 1988;12:533-40.

64. Leon S, Schuffler M. Intestinal pseudo-obstruction as a complication of Duchenne's muscular dystrophy. *Gastroenterology* 1986;90:455-9.

65. Yoshida MM, Schuffler MD, Sumi SM. There are no morphologic abnormalities of the gastric wall or abdominal vagus in patients with diabetic gastroparesis. *Gastroenterology* 1988;94:107-14.

66. Feinstat T, et al. Megacolon and neurofibromatosis: a neuronal intestinal dysplasia. *Gastroenterology* 1984;86:1573-98.

23

Personal Computers in Motility Testing

S. NARASIMHA REDDY

Computers have not had a dramatic impact on studies of gastrointestinal (GI) motility because visual analysis of motility signals is often satisfactory for clinical evaluations, and the evolution from chart recorder-based instruments to computerized motility systems has been slow. The one exception has been cutaneous electrogastrography (EGG), which requires computerized analysis to elicit useful information. This chapter deals with the application of personal computer (PC) technology for the acquisition, presentation, and analysis of clinical GI motility signals.

CLINICAL GI MOTILITY MEASUREMENTS

The smooth muscle of the GI system is characterized by an omnipresent, rhythmic electrical activity known as slow waves, basic electric rhythm, or electric control activity.[1] Slow waves resemble the electrocardiogram (EKG) in the stomach and small intestine. When recorded in vivo in the colon they are often random, as is the electroencephalogram (EEG).[2] When stimulated, this myogenic control system gives rise to spikes and/or other action potentials that result in a contraction. Transmucosal or serosal myoelectrical recordings, however, are not practical in most clinical settings. Cutaneous EGG appears to measure the underlying gastric slow waves. Because EGG is noninvasive, it is being explored as a diagnostic test (see Chapter 19).

Contractions can be recorded and easily interpreted. They may be phasic—occurring during the initial phase of the slow wave—or tonic—encompassing a longer duration. Phasic contractions may occur in recognizable groups like phase 3 of the migrating motor complex (MMC) or repetitive clusters, as in patients with mechanical obstruction. Other distinctive patterns include swallow-induced propagating contractions in the esophagus, mass contractions in the colon, and emetic contractions.

The most important features of the slow waves and contractions are:

1. *Amount of activity,* ie, the variation in power (amplitude squared) as a function of time for slow waves, amplitudes for single contractions, and motility index for a given length of contractile signal. Power is the standard measure of an AC signal such as myoelectric activity, and is a statistically stable quantification.[3]

2. *Duration of activity* of slow waves or of individual phasic contractions in the stomach and small intestine. Durations of specialized contractions and groups of contractions (eg, phase 3 of MMC) are important parameters that correlate with the underlying physiology (eg, normal peristaltic contractions versus those of nutcracker esophagus).

3. *Frequency*—the slow-wave frequency, which is normally 3 cpm in the stomach, 12 cpm in the small intestine, and varies in the colon. In the case of contractions, the frequency is $1/T$, where T is the interval between adjacent contractions. This quantification is known as the "instantaneous frequency." The maximum rate of contractions is the same as the maximum frequency of the underlying slow waves.

Variation in slow-wave rhythm is studied statistically, as the percentage of time during which specific frequencies occur among defined limits. For example, gastric slow-wave rhythms can be quantified into bradygastria (<2.5 cpm), normal (2.5-3.5 cpm), and tachygastria (>3.5 cpm). Variations in contractile rhythms are studied as histograms of contractile frequencies or intercontractile intervals.[4]

4. *Coupling or propagation,* ie, the amount and direction of slow-wave propagation. Usually slow waves appear to propagate aborad.[5] However, occasional disturbances in coupling cause them to propagate orad or to have no coupling relationships. Quantification of coupling is difficult and is limited in clinical applications.

Contractions may 1) propagate aborad to aid in the transit of the ingested material; 2) propagate orad to retard transit or to cause retrograde transit; 3) occur simultaneously to increase mixing, thus facilitating absorption of nutrients; or 4) occur independently and randomly, which results in a to-and-fro movement of the bolus and further absorption of nutrients. The amplitudes, directions, and velocities of propagating contractions form the parameters of the temporal nature of motility patterns.

Other clinical motility-related measurements include pH,[6] compliance in the gut wall as measured by barostat,[7] and transit as measured by scintigraphy.[8,9] These measurements can be obtained simultaneously with motility measurements or integrated on a PC later.

ROLE OF COMPUTERS

Increased computerization of motility studies is in line with recent attempts to improve the flow of information in clinical gastroenterology.[10] The PC is a powerful tool for the acquisition, analysis, and presentation of motility signals and related data, providing precise and reproducible quantifications. Computers save time by swiftly analyzing large amounts of data, and eliminate the observer bias which often accompanies unblinded visual analysis.[11,12]

Once quantified, the motility data can be assessed further, utilizing statistics or graphics software, and can be integrated into word processing. Both motility signals and results can be organized into a data base to establish normal and altered motility patterns.

A PC-based motility system, equipped with a solid-state catheter, is small enough to fit on a desktop. This is a real advantage in a hospital room, which is often crowded with equipment, health care professionals, and parents.

A complete desktop PC system, incorporating the latest technology, costs no more than $3000. Menu-driven software makes PCs easy to use. "Help" options reduce the need for computer literacy on the part of the operator.

IMPLEMENTATION

The hardware for a well configured PC system for clinical motility consists of a color monitor, memory, hard disk, tape storage, printer, and a fax-modem together with GI motility measurement equipment and software. The software must be menu-driven but allow complete user control so that critical decisions can be made during analysis. The optimal requirements of such software include: 1) ease of acquisition, 2) flexibility in displaying signals and presenting results, 3) preprocessing to minimize artefacts and noise, 4) appropriate analytic techniques, 5) data base and communication provisions, and 6) other nonmotility software such as word processing, statistics, and graphics.[13,14]

Acquisition

Until recently, the most common motility acquisition system was chart-based. Although this system set many recording and evaluation standards, it often did not consistently quantify the signals properly, as the recorded signals were often limited to less than 100 mm Hg in amplitude. Even though the chart-based systems are becoming obsolete, they can be computerized to obtain all the benefits of a PC-based system.

Computerized motility systems come with or without a chart-recorder. The minimal requirements are eight channels of multipurpose acquisition (pressure, pH, electromyograph, or compliance) and appropriate sampling rates with a provision for marking an event. Although technically not as sophisticated as PC-based motility systems, 24-hour ambulatory monitors can be used to record motility, with data later transferred to the PC for analysis and display. Often system-independent software allows importing or exporting of signals from an acquisition system to an analysis system.

Display

Since the integration of computers with biomedical equipment, the trend has been toward paperless recording. The simplicity of data storage on disks leads to enormous savings in effort, time, space, and cost. Paperless recording necessitates the proper display of signals during acquisition on the monitor and their presentation after recording in desired formats. In the absence of a chart recorder, the display can be printed as desired during recording.

Display during acquisition. In general, acquisition software offers a choice of "paper speeds" on the computer screen. Gastrointestinal motility signals fall into short- and long-duration displays.

Short-duration or rapid-speed display is the norm during recording of esophageal or anorectal motility, where responses to a stimulus (eg, swallow) and signals over shorter durations are explored. The length of time on the monitor screen can be set for 1 minute to follow the subtle features of the signals.

Long-duration or slow-speed display is often necessary during the recording of antroduodenal and colonic motility signals. These signals allow exploration of patterns such as those produced by the MMC during fasting or increases in motility after provocation with a meal or drug. In such cases, the duration on the screen is often set from 30 to 90 minutes.

Postacquisition display. Signals can be presented on-screen in several configurations: 1) the entire recording can be displayed in a compressed mode for a comprehensive view; 2) focus can be limited

to an interesting portion of the recording; 3) plotting can be performed in a scanned or random mode over precisely defined time limits; and 4) one plotted channel can be overlaid on another to explore duration and amplitude differences as well as propagation. Figure 23.1 shows an antroduodenal motility study covering 4 hours in a single display panel.

The amplitudes of recorded signals may be plotted as a function of space so that 1) all channels can be compared with respect to the most intense signal, known as global minimum and maximum limits; 2) all channels can be compared with a uniform scale, for example, 100 mm Hg maximum; or 3) each channel can be plotted with its own maximum and minimum, known as local minimum and maximum. Plotting the same signals as per global limits shows gradation of amplitudes of contractions, eg, from the antrum to the distal duodenum. Plotting on a uniform scale (eg, 80 or 100 mm Hg) provides a good visual display of signals limited to this range. Such evaluations contribute to the understanding of normal versus hyper- versus hypocontractility as a function of time and space.[15]

Analytic Techniques

Fast Fourier transform analysis. Fast Fourier transform (FFT) decomposes a complex signal into its basic frequency rhythms.[3] It provides power as a function of frequency, commonly known as smoothed power spectrum,[16] and is used for the frequency analysis of colonic slow waves and electrogastrography.[17] FFT analysis can be extended to study coupling among adjacent slow waves.

Period analysis. In this approach, the period (T) from cycle to cycle or from contraction to contraction is calculated. Peak detection is based on period, amplitude, duration, or slope-threshold criterion.[18] The period, its reciprocal ($1/T$), ie, instantaneous frequency, and time that an individual slow-wave cycle or contraction occurred can then be used to study waveform features, frequency, and propagation of contractions as well as the frequency of rhythmic slow waves.

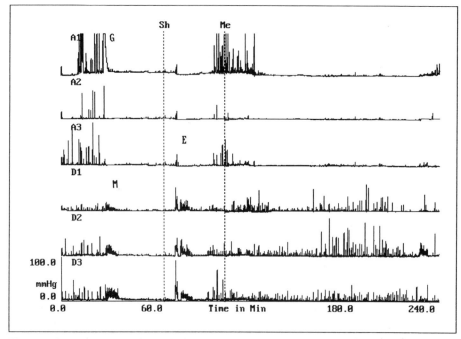

Fig. 23.1 Compressed plot of an entire antroduodenal motility study (4 h) shows the salient features of the study. A1-A3 and D1-D3 demonstrate recording sites in antrum and duodenum, respectively. (G, giant contraction; M, MMC phase 3; E, emetic contraction; Sh, sham feeding; Me, Meal)

Other analyses. Other approaches to analyzing motility signals employ digital signal processing algorithms[19] including filtering, mathematical operations such as the calculation of motility index, calculation of statistics, determination of area under the curve, and pattern-recognition techniques.[20,21]

The usual procedure for studying motility signals consists of preprocessing (if the signals are corrupted with noise and artefacts), analysis, and statistical evaluation. These techniques are implemented on the computer in an interactive dialog mode.

Preprocessing

Preprocessing refers to operator-controlled alterations in the recorded data prior to signal analysis. The requirement for preprocessing has often been perceived as a negative feature of computer analysis. However, preprocessing enhances the signal-to-noise ratio, improving the overall clarity of signals. The most important artefacts and their treatment are summarized below.

Movement. Artefacts can arise from the movement of either the patient or the catheter. Patient-related artefacts can be of any configuration, while those due to catheter movement tend to be sharp pulses. Some can be minimized by filtering; others must be removed before analysis. An artefact can be removed by defining its time limits (T_1 and T_2), then writing over the defined segment with interpolated signal values as per those at T_1 and T_2, or setting the signal values between these times to zero. Movement artefacts usually occur simultaneously at all sites; once defined on one channel, their elimination can be automatic on the other channels. Figure 23.2 demonstrates ileal contractile activity before and after removal of sharp artefacts which, if plotted differently, could be easily mistaken for contractions. The movement artefacts were eliminated by defining their time limits with a mouse and letting the software connect the points between these limits.

Baseline changes. Baseline changes in-

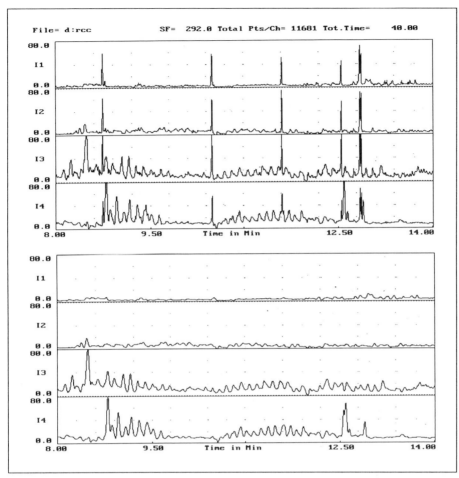

Fig. 23.2 Pressure activity in the ileum (11-14) before (top frame) and after (bottom frame) the removal of artefacts.

clude 1) abrupt, parallel shifts in baseline, known as offsets, such as those due to refilling of the perfusion system's water tank; 2) slowly decreasing or increasing baselines known as trends; and 3) drifts that may mimic tonic contractions but may be longer in duration. Offsets are compensated on the PC by defining the time limits and having the program automatically shift the baseline. Trendlike baseline changes are common in signal processing and are removed by linear detrend programs.[3] The long-duration toniclike baseline changes can be removed on the computer by defining the amount of tonic component.[22]

Respiration. Respiration creates undesir-

able artefacts with small intestinal and colonic manometry as well as EGG, as these signals tend to have frequency components common to respiration. Because respiration is recorded at all sites, the bias tends to be uniform across all channels. When evaluating the motility index (see page 355), the amplitude of the respiration signal (usually 5 mm Hg) can be determined on the computer, then subtracted from the motility index values at all channels. In the case of EGG, filtering frequencies to keep those below the respiratory rate reduces bias due to respiration, yet maintains the basic rhythms in the EGG.

Noise. Noise is mostly due to the sensors (electrodes and pressure transducers) and instrumentation. Signals captured from elsewhere in the body also constitute noise. Subtle transducer vibrations can give rise to noise. Most noise is composed of high-frequency signals not likely to be confused with motility signals. Proper low-pass filtering, which keeps low-frequency components, attenuates noise. Also, the sampling frequency for acquiring signals is too low (usually less than or equal to 10 Hz) to fully record such extraneous signals as the EKG, which has frequency components above those of pressure or slow waves. Figure 23.3 illustrates the EGG signal before and after filtering between 1 and 9 cpm. This effectively attenuated movement artefacts below the low-frequency limit as well as noise, EKG, and respiration above the high-frequency limit, resulting in a strikingly improved EGG signal. With both EGG and contractile signals, regions of activity unacceptably corrupted with noise and artefacts can be automatically eliminated from analysis by marking them with a mouse. The missing results can be interpolated from adjacent results or discarded from interpretation.

Analytic Examples

The following examples illustrate the scope of computer analysis of GI motility signals.

Visual analysis. One of the important requirements for motility analysis is to visually study and simultaneously quantify the signals. Such analysis can be implemented on the PC with a mouse in a "point-and-click" mode. The signal is plotted for the entire duration of recording and the portion of the signal to be analyzed is magnified. Once a particular time (T) is pointed out, it can provide the amplitude and time values of the signals across all channels. Defining a portion of the signal over times for T_1 and for T_2 can provide each channel with quantifications such as 1) minimum and maximum pressures, 2) area under the curve, 3) amplitude and duration, and 4) frequency and propagation across all channels. Such visual analysis is especially well suited for the study of esophageal and anorectal signals.

Propagation and coordination. Propagation in the esophageal body, colonic high-amplitude propagating contractions, and phase 3 of the MMC are easily recognized with direct vision. However, evaluation of antroduodenal coordination is more complex.

Antroduodenal coordination is an intriguing physiologic phenomenon. The antrum contracts at a maximal rate of 3 per minute while the duodenum contracts at a maximal rate of 12 per minute. These two dissimilar rhythmic activities, separated by the pylo-

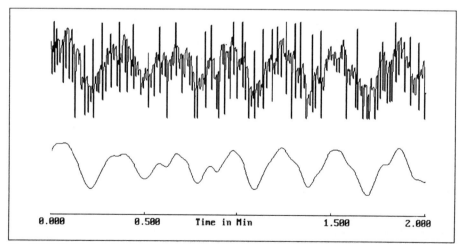

Fig. 23.3 EGG before (top tracing) and after (bottom tracing) filtering to remove noise, respiration, and EKG.

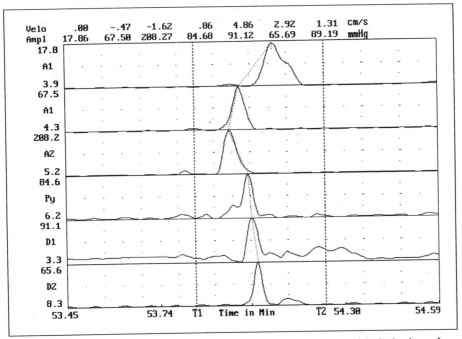

Fig. 23.4 Mouse-assisted visual analysis of antroduodenal coordination. Velocity is shown from previous channel to the next one; the last column shows average values. A1-A3 and D1-D3 refer to recording sites in the antrum and duodenum, respectively. D1 was near the pylorus.

rus, coordinate with each other. The antral contractions may propagate across the pylorus into the duodenum, enhance the duodenal contractions, or inhibit duodenal contractions partially or fully.[23] Variations in these coordinated activities can lead to increased or decreased gastric emptying. Duodenal contractions do not propagate into the antrum except during vomiting.

Automatic computer analysis of propagation and, hence, coordination is possible if the timing and propagation velocity limits are known.[24,25] Coordination can also be explored on the PC semiautomatically by visually inspecting the signals.[25] Once coordination is detected, computer analysis can be performed with a mouse, as previously discussed. One example of an interesting antroduodenal coordination is shown in Figure 23.4. The signal was preprocessed as described above. The portion of the signal showing coordination was marked at T_1 and T_2, enabling the software to provide amplitudes and velocities of the propagating contractions automatically. Both antral and du-

odenal contractions propagate from the pylorus with different antral and duodenal velocities of propagation.

Motility index. The motility index quantifies the amount of contractile activity during a selected length of recording time (T). Many definitions exist for the motility index, some of which are based only on the number and amplitude of contractions.[15] However, the area under the curve is the most appropriate definition[8] because area is a true measure of a varying DC signal, such as contractile activity;[3] other measurements are subsets of area measurements.

A contraction resembles a triangle; its area is represented by 0.5AB, where A is the height and B is the base (duration). In calculating the motility index, the constant 0.5 can be neglected. If B is also constant, the sum of amplitudes over T can represent the motility index. Such is the case in the antrum and small intestine because phasic contractions resemble triangles and tend to have constant durations. In this instance, a motil-

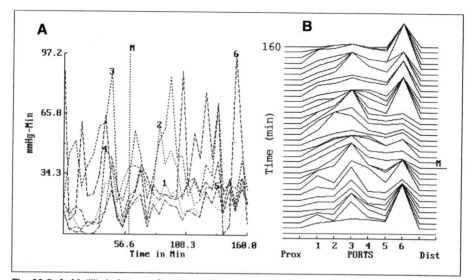

Fig. 23.5 **A**, Motility index as a function of time for each of six recording sites, extending from the transverse to the sigmoid colon. It is confusing to the eye, and difficult to interpret in a glance. (M, meal). **B**, Motility index plotted as a function of time and space (3-D motility index) provides ideas about both motility and pressure differences. The numbers 1 to 6 refer to recording sites extending from the transverse to the sigmoid colon. Visual analysis is simplified compared to **A**.

ity index based on amplitudes is adequate. However, contractions elsewhere in the gut, such as the fundus, ileum, and colon, are not always phasic and have different amplitudes and durations. The motility index as area is more appropriate in these and other cases.

The motility index may be presented as a function of time for each recording site (Fig. 23.5A). However, if it is presented as a function of space and time, resulting in a 3-dimensional motility index, more information can be gained. The computer technique involves plotting space (port locations) along the x-axis, time along the y-axis, and motility index values along the z-axis. Increases or decreases in motility as a function of time and space are thus illustrated, and varying pressure zones along the organ are also suggested.[26]

Figure 23.5B illustrates the 3-dimensional colonic motility index of a patient with constipation. After preprocessing, motility indexes were obtained as areas under the curve for every 5 minutes and plotted as a function of port locations (from transverse colon to the sigmoid) and time. There was no clearcut increase in motility after the meal. The

distribution of high- and low-pressure levels along the colon was clarified by the 3-dimensional figure, which shows that pressures were greatest in the sigmoid colon, and decreased elsewhere (except at port 3, corresponding to the splenic flexure). A favorable transit gradient is defined as higher pressure in the upper colon and lower pressure in the lower colon. The pressure gradient was higher in the sigmoid colon except for about 30 minutes after eating, when it was favorable for aboral transit. Such evaluation of motility and pressure gradients enables correlation of pressure gradients with the underlying pathophysiology.[26]

Frequency analysis of EGG. A precise quantification of EGG is possible only on the computer. The following clinical example shows the analysis of an EGG in a child with neuropathy. The signal was filtered to attenuate frequency components below 1 cpm and above 9 cpm to attenuate movement, artefacts, and noise. It was evaluated for power as a function of time and for frequencies by FFT analysis; the results were used to obtain statistics.

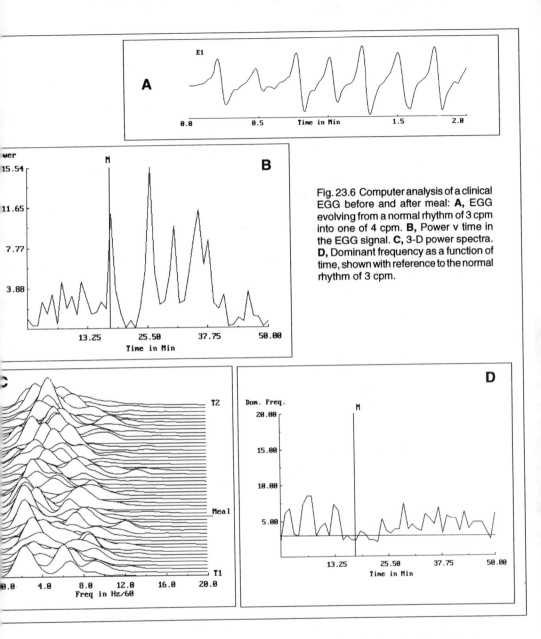

Fig. 23.6 Computer analysis of a clinical EGG before and after meal: **A,** EGG evolving from a normal rhythm of 3 cpm into one of 4 cpm. **B,** Power v time in the EGG signal. **C,** 3-D power spectra. **D,** Dominant frequency as a function of time, shown with reference to the normal rhythm of 3 cpm.

Figure 23.6A illustrates a normal 3-cpm EGG evolving into a 4-cpm activity (ie, tachygastria). This result was obtained by plotting the signal on the computer screen in a scan mode and printing the signal. Figure 23.6B demonstrates the power in the signal before and after the meal. Figure 23.6C shows the power spectra, plotted 3-dimensionally as a function of time and frequency. This result was obtained after normalizing power in each section of the signal so that the frequency peaks stand out irrespective of the EGG amplitude.[17] Peaks of around 3 cpm are distributed, not concentrated. Figure 23.6D shows the dominant frequency, obtained from the above result, as a function of time that corresponds to the highest peak in the power spectrum.

Statistics for the dominant frequency in Figure 23.6D were 4.4 ± 1.6 cpm. The incidence of normal rhythm was 16%, with bradygastria (1-2.5 cpm) accounting for 16%, while tachygastria (3.5-9 cpm) accounted for 68%. Usually these results form the basis of a clinical report on EGG (see below).

Data Base

Establishing a data base of normal and altered motility patterns based on past results helps classify diseases. Plots of important motility signals can also be a part of the data base. In each diagnostic class, patients and corresponding results are listed; an automatic update of average results in each class can be included. Other pertinent data include presence and severity of symptoms.

The procedure for diagnosis consists of examining the new patient's data, making an initial diagnosis, recalling similar cases from the data base to compare with the new data, and making the final diagnosis. Once classified, the particular class of disease in the data base should be updated with the new patient's data. Such approaches often take advantage of statistical pattern-recognition techniques.[20,21]

Clinical Motility Report

For clinical care, it is necessary to prepare a report with appropriate results and figures. While many normal ranges are known for esophageal and anorectal motility measurements, they are still being defined for colonic and antroduodenal motility patterns. The laboratory's "normal" results, therefore, may need to be enclosed with the report.

Procedure. A description of the catheter placement procedure, including selection and complications is necessary. Identifying the recording sites documents the extent of the organ tested. The protocol and times involved during recording, such as fasting, stimulus, and meal, as well as the equipment and software used, should be a part of this section.

Quality of signals. The nature of signals in general and whether they were recorded with minimal noise and artefacts is noted.

Motility in fasting state. The occurrence and characteristics of MMCs in the case of antroduodenal signals and quiescence in the case of colon signals, together with the nature of propagating contractions, if any, are described.

Motility after meal. A meal increases contractions in the stomach and duodenum.[15] It manifests as gastrocolonic response in the colon.[27] These factors, together with the occurrence of any propagating contractions, are mentioned.

Motility after a provocative test. The nature of motility to the stimulus, including any propagation, should be described.

Impressions. The above results usually provide a physiologic diagnosis which should be elucidated here.

Recommendations. In this section, treatment, any further testing, and suggestions for follow-up are included.

With appropriate figures, literature citation, and a relevant case, the report can be sent by fax-modem to the referring physician.

CONCLUSION

From acquisition to communication, every aspect of clinical motility can be implemented on the PC. All motility measurements—myoelectric activity, pressure, compliance, and pH—can be acquired simultaneously. Other measurements, such as 24-hour ambulatory signals and scintigraphic images, can be integrated with the motility signals on the PC after the study. Signals and results can be presented in any desired format. Computer-assisted analysis can be carried out quickly and precisely over large amounts of data. The results can be exported to a data base, spreadsheets, graphics, statistics, and desktop publication. Computerized communication can be set up with the referring physician. Advances in technology will lead to simultaneous acquisition, analysis, diagnosis, communication, and similar tasks on several motility measurements.

Computer-based motility acquisition and

analysis is no longer limited to research. Existing and emerging PC technology should lead to an enhanced understanding of clinical GI motility patterns in health and disease.

The author wishes to acknowledge Lynn Kirlin, Ed Daniel, and Bill Snape for making this chapter possible, Gabriele Bazzocchi for his helpful suggestions, and Jay Marks for constructive criticism of the manuscript. He also thanks his family for their support and understanding.

REFERENCES

1. Johnson LR, ed. *Physiology of the Gastrointestinal Tract.* New York, NY: Raven Press, 1981.

2. Daniel EE. Symposium on colonic function: electrophysiology of the colon. *Gut* 1975;16:298-306.

3. Bendat JS, Piersol AG. *Random Data: Analysis and Measurement Procedures.* New York, NY: J. Wiley & Sons, 1971.

4. Smoudt AJPM, ed. *Myoelectric Activity of the Stomach.* Amsterdam: Delft University Press, 1980.

5. Daniel EE, Sarna SK. The generation and conduction of activity in smooth muscle. *Ann Rev Pharm Toxicol* 1978;18:145-66.

6. Orr WC. Clinical applications of 24-hour esophageal pH monitoring. *Practical Gastroenterology* 1993; 17:10-21.

7. Steadman CCJ, Philips SF, Camilleri M, Haddad A, Hanson R. Variation of muscle tone in the human colon. *Gastroenterology* 1991;101:373-81.

8. Reddy SN, Chan S, Bazzocchi G, et al. Colonic motility and transit in health and ulcerative colitis. *Gastroenterology* 1991;101:1289-97.

9. Reddy SN, Di Lorenzo C, Yanni G, et al. A unified approach to the study of colonic scintigraphy and intraluminal pressure. *Gastroenterology* 1990;98:A383.

10. Williams JG, Ford DV, Yapp TR. Capturing clinical activity — coming to terms with information. *Gut* 1993;34:1651-2.

11. Castell J, Satell D. Computer analysis of human esophageal peristalsis and lower esophageal sphincter pressure. *Dig Dis Sci* 1986;31:1211-6.

12. Martin JB, Castillo FD, Wingate DL, Demetrakopolous J, Spyrou NM. The computer as referee in the analysis of human small bowel motility. *Am J Physiol* 1993;264:G645-54.

13. Reddy SN. Biomedical signal processing on the personal computer. *Proc. 9th Ann Conf IEEE Eng Med Biol Soc* 1987:1219-21.

14. Reddy SN. Multipurpose portable personal computer system for the acquisition and analysis of GI motility signals. *Gastroenterology* 1993;105:A569.

15. Malagelada J-R, Camilleri M, Stanghellini V. *Manometric Diagnosis of GI Motility Disorders.* Thieme, 1986.

16. Reddy SN, Kirlin RL. Spectral analysis of auditory evoked potentials with pseudorandom noise excitation. *IEEE Trans Biomed Eng* 1979;BME:26:479-87.

17. Reddy SN, Collins SM, Daniel EE. Frequency analysis of Gut EMG: an applied review. *CRC Critical Rev Biomed Eng* 1987;15:95-116.

18. Dumpala SR, Reddy SN, Sarna SK. An algorithm for the detection peaks in biological signals. *Comput Prog Biomed* 1982;14:249-56.

19. Mitra SK, Kaiser JF, eds. *Handbook of Digital Signal Processing.* New York, NY: J. Wiley & Sons, 1993.

20. Reddy SN, Dumpala SR, Sarna SK, Northcott P. Pattern recognition of canine duodenal contractile activity. *IEEE Trans Biomed Eng* 1981;BME:28:696-701.

21. Parker R, Whitehead WE, Schuster MM. Pattern recognition program for analysis of colonic myoelectric and pressure data. *Dig Dis Sci* 1987;32:953-61.

22. Zittel T, Reddy SN, Plopurde V, Raybould HE. Role of spinal afferents and CGRP in postoperative gastric ileus in anesthetized rats. *Ann Surg* 1994;219:79-87.

23. Reddy SN, Daniel EE. Neural control of duodenal motor inhibition by antral contractions in the dog. *Am J Physiol* 1990;G24-31.

24. Ehrlein H, Hiesinger E. Computer analysis of mechanical activity of gastroduodenal junction in unanesthetized dogs. *Q J Exp Physiol* 1982;67:17-29.

25. Mayer EA, Sytnik B, Reddy SN, van Deventer G, Tache Y. Corticotropin releasing factor (CRF) increases postprandial duodenal motor activity in humans. *J Gastrointest Motil* 1992;4:53-60.

26. Reddy SN, Lin HC, Lo S, et al. Colonic pressure gradient and transit in healthy subjects and patients with spastic colon. *J Gastrointest Motil* 1993:5:213.

27. Snape WJ, Mararazzo SA, Cohen S. Effect of eating and GI hormones on human colonic myo-electric and motor activity. *Gastroenterology* 1978;75:373-8.

Treatment of Enteric Neuromuscular Disorders

24

Nutritional Considerations in Pediatric Enteric Neuromuscular Disease

ERNEST SEIDMAN, MARJOLAIN PINEAULT

Chronic intestinal pseudo-obstruction (CIP) is a clinical syndrome resulting from ineffective bowel motility which is usually caused by a neuronal or muscular disorder. The clinical presentation is characterized by symptoms and signs of bowel obstruction in the absence of an occluding lesion. Typically, patients complain of variable degrees of abdominal distention, pain, and vomiting. Episodes of severe diarrhea and/or constipation are common, depending on the relative involvement of the small and large bowels, respectively. Symptoms are usually aggravated by eating. The combination of a dysfunctional bowel and these disabling symptoms often leads to malabsorption and anorexia. Consequently, malnutrition is frequently encountered in CIP patients of all ages. In the pediatric population, the additional metabolic costs of growth result in an even greater degree of malnutrition than in older patients. The associated nutritional deficits, when severe, lead to an increased morbidity and mortality. In this chapter, the pathogenesis, evaluation, and treatment of nutritional problems in pediatric patients with enteric neuromuscular disease will be reviewed.

PATHOPHYSIOLOGY OF MALABSORPTION

The physiologic processes underlying normal mucosal absorption of nutrients depend on the highly coordinated functions of the intestine, which include adequate gut motility (Fig. 24.1). The bowel is constantly faced with an enormous input of fluid and electrolytes, most of which is of endogenous origin (eg, salivary, gastric, pancreatic, or biliary). In infants, for example, approximately 250 to 300 cc/kg enter the small bowel daily, of which approximately 40% is derived from a dietary source. Yet normal infants excrete only 5 to 10 gm/kg of stool per day, representing an absorptive efficiency of approximately 97%.[1]

A number of mechanisms are potentially responsible for the maldigestion and malabsorption of nutrients, fluids, and electrolytes in intestinal motility disorders (Table 24.1). Altered transit can directly interfere with nutrient hydrolysis in the intestinal lumen. Asynchronous mixing of pancreatic and biliary secretions with chyme is an important cause of impaired lipolysis, and results in fat

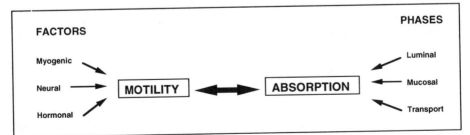

Fig. 24.1 The coordination of intestinal functions involves complex interactions between gut motility and absorption.

malabsorption. Rapid transit from motility disorders can cause malabsorption due to inadequate contact between hydrolytic enzymes and intraluminal carbohydrates. Undigested carbohydrates subsequently enter the colon and undergo bacterial fermentation, causing additional distention, diarrhea, borborygmi, and flatus. Bile-salt malabsorption and deconjugation by bacterial overgrowth may further impair fat solubilization. Bacterial dehydroxylation of unabsorbed bile acids can result in watery diarrhea by inducing colonic mucosal secretion. Cholestatic liver disease from prolonged use of total parenteral nutrition (TPN) may further impair biliary secretion, as discussed below.

Approximately half of total energy requirements are normally provided by carbohydrate ingestion. Major sources of digestible carbohydrate include starches derived from cereals and plants, as well as sugars derived from milk or infant formula, fruit and vegetables (sucrose, fructose, and glucose), processed foods (corn syrup, fructose, and polysaccharides), and table sugar (sucrose). The absorption of dietary carbohydrates is largely restricted to the uptake of hexose monomers across the brush-border membrane. This process requires the interaction between intraluminal digestive enzymes, such as salivary, gastric, and pancreatic amylase, and terminal digestion by brush-border hydrolases.[2] The resultant dietary monosaccharides (glucose, galactose, and fructose) are then absorbed by saturable carrier-mediated transport systems on enterocyte brush-border membranes.[3] The same transporter is responsible for the active conveyance of glucose and galactose, which act as a sodium cotransporter. The sodium pump (NaK ATPase) at the basolateral membrane generates a low intracellular sodium concentration. Sodium then crosses the apical membrane down its concentration gradient, along with a glucose or galactose molecule in a 1:1 molar ratio. Fructose absorption is accomplished by carrier-mediated absorption. The small intestinal enterocyte thus plays a critical role in the final stages of carbohydrate absorption. Intestinal pseudo-obstruction is one of many disorders of the

TABLE 24.1 **Mechanisms Underlying Malabsorption in Intestinal Motility Disorders**

Luminal Phase
Asynchronous mixing of pancreatico-biliary secretions and chyme
Inadequate contact between luminal hydrolases and carbohydrates
Bile-salt malabsorption or deconjugation*
Bacterial degradation of luminal nutrients*
Osmotic diarrhea

Mucosal Phase
Inadequate contact time between nutrients and enterocyte membrane
Villous atrophy (reduced absorptive surface)*
Impaired enterocyte function*
Brush-border enzyme deficiency*

Miscellaneous
Protein-losing enteropathy*
Malnutrition-induced villous atrophy
Disuse atrophy (inadequate enteral intake)

*Related to small intestinal bacterial overgrowth

small bowel which frequently result in damage to the brush-border membrane, probably due in part to bacterial overgrowth, as discussed below. A secondary loss of hydrolase activity is present, with lactase activity more susceptible to mucosal damage than other disaccharidases. The impaired enterocyte metabolic activity also includes inadequate intracellular lipid and peptide processing, leading to malabsorption of dietary fat and protein.

Intestinal pseudo-obstruction is not traditionally included in the differential diagnosis of intestinal villous atrophy. Nevertheless, the small intestinal bacterial overgrowth that frequently accompanies disorders of intestinal motility[4] is a well described cause of malabsorption.[5] This is attributed to a combination of the intraluminal effects of the proliferating bacteria and to enterocyte damage (see Table 24.1). Fat malabsorption results from bacterial alteration of bile salts.[6] Bacterial overgrowth is also associated with a patchy mucosal lesion of uncertain pathogenesis,[7] characterized by partial villous atrophy, enterocyte damage, and a nonspecific mixed inflammatory infiltrate in the lamina propria (Fig. 24.2). As a result, the surface area available for absorption is reduced. The malabsorption is compounded by diminished disaccharidase activity and decreased uptake of monosaccharides, amino acids, and fatty acids.[8] Hypoproteinemia may ensue from the combination of decreased mucosal transport of amino acids,[8] intraluminal degradation of protein by bacteria, as well as a protein-losing enteropathy[9]—all of which are related to bacterial overgrowth. Small-bowel bacterial overgrowth can also result in the specific malabsorption of vitamin B_{12}, due to bacterial uptake of cobalamin.[10] In contrast, small-bowel bacteria produce and release folate, leading to high folate levels in patients with bacterial overgrowth.

Other potential mechanisms of diarrhea attributable to bacterial overgrowth in patients with pseudo-obstruction include the production of organic acids. Together with carbohydrate malabsorption, this results in an increased osmolarity of the small-bowel contents and a decreased intraluminal pH. As mentioned above, byproducts of bacterial metabolism (bile acids, hydroxylated fatty acids, and organic acids) can induce a colonic secretory diarrhea. Furthermore, experimental bacterial overgrowth has been shown to disturb small-bowel motility.[11]

Patients with severe motility disorders are frequently malnourished. Malnutrition per se results in impaired intestinal absorption, due to morphologic and functional derangements of the gut.[12] Intestinal crypt cell renewal rates decrease, villi are blunted, and brush-border enzyme activities are reduced. In addition, experimental evidence suggests that malnutrition renders the small intestinal mucosa more susceptible to loss of brush-border hydrolase activity from bacterial overgrowth.[13] The coexistence of malnutrition and bacterial overgrowth may synergistically increase the magnitude of functional derangements in the gut of patients with motility disorders. Moreover, malnutrition itself may alter intestinal motility.

Inadequate enteral nutrition is an additional contributor to malabsorption in such patients (see Table 24.1). The importance of food as a trophic factor for normal gut mor-

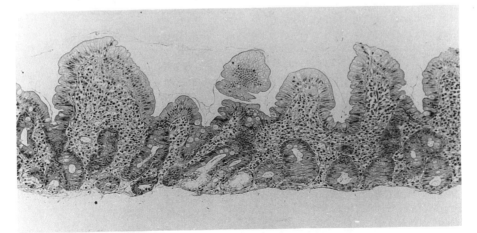

Fig. 24.2 Nonspecific enteritis in intestinal pseudo-obstruction. Duodenal biopsy in a 10-year-old boy with myenteric neuronal dysplasia presenting with abdominal distention, intermittent diarrhea, postprandial vomiting, anorexia, and growth failure. The biopsy reveals partial villous atrophy with an increased, mixed inflammatory cell infiltrate of the lamina propria. Bacterial overgrowth of small bowel fluid, as well as brush-border disaccharidase deficiency were documented. However, dietary restrictions, antibiotics, and nasojejunal feedings failed to improve the symptomatology, and the patient eventually required home TPN.

phology and function is well established.[14] Although the gut mucosa receives part of its nutrients from the systemic circulation, TPN does not restore normal gut function. Glutamine, the primary fuel for enterocyte metabolism, is lacking in standard TPN solutions. Patients with severely dysfunctional gastrointestinal systems who depend on TPN are thus likely to have disuse atrophy, which compounds the malabsorption.[15]

CLINICAL MANIFESTATIONS OF MALABSORPTION AND MALNUTRITION

Chronic intestinal pseudo-obstruction is a syndrome with multiple causes (see Chapter 7). Whether the primary cause is a disorder of smooth muscle or the nervous or endrocrine systems, the major symptoms relate to dysfunction of the digestive system. The clinical presentation relates more to the region of the gastrointestinal tract affected, rather than to the underlying cause. For example, patients with esophageal involvement usually present with dysphagia, pyrosis, regurgitation, reflux, and chest pain. Gastric involvement results in poor gastric emptying with nausea and vomiting, bloating and early satiety, as well as distention and pain. Small-bowel involvement is also associated with pain, distention, nausea, and vomiting, but is particularly characterized by diarrhea and malabsorption. Colonic involvement typically includes distention and constipation, which may alternate with periods of diarrhea. Pediatric patients tend to present more often with marked distention, whereas pain is more frequently reported in adults.[16,17]

The pain and distention in CIP may be almost continuous, whereas in other patients, periods of spontaneous improvement intervene. The gastrointestinal symptoms are often aggravated by food intake. The combination of gastrointestinal symptoms and malabsorption result in decreased food intake, weight loss, and malnutrition. In addition, iatrogenic or self-imposed dietary restrictions may worsen inadequate and unbalanced intake of nutrients. The multifactorial causes of malnutrition in patients with intestinal neuromuscular disorders are summarized in Table 24.2. Although malabsorption is a major factor, inadequate dietary intake is also of paramount importance. DiCecco[18] and co-workers performed a comparative study on oral nutritional intake in adult patients with gut failure requiring total parenteral nutrition (TPN). They noted that patients with CIP had the lowest intake (50% of energy requirements) of any group, compared to patients with radiation enteritis, Crohn's disease, or short-bowel syndrome.

Patients with small-bowel involvement are more likely to have bacterial overgrowth and nutrient malabsorption, as reviewed above. In a study of 26 pediatric cases with myenteric plexus disorders, 15 were found to have small-bowel bacterial overgrowth.[19] Severe malnutrition and growth failure, therefore, are more common in patients with small-bowel involvement. Such patients are also more likely to refuse hypercaloric supplements, less likely to tolerate enteral hyperalimentation, and thus more often require

---

TABLE 24.2 Causes of Malnutrition in Patients With Intestinal Motility Disorders

Inadequate Dietary Intake
Anorexia
Early satiety
Abdominal pain
Diarrhea
Iatrogenic (restrictive diets)

Malabsorption
Carbohydrates
Fat
Protein
Vitamins
Minerals

Excessive Bowel Losses
Bile-salt induced diarrhea
Osmotic diarrhea
Protein-losing enteropathy
Bacterial overgrowth

Subject Assessment	Laboratory Data
Detailed history	Complete blood count, red-cell morphology
Complete physical exam, pubertal staging	Serum albumin
Dietetic evaluation (3-day diary)	Serum Fe, total iron-binding capacity, ferritin
Anthropometry	Calcium, phosphorus, magnesium, alkaline phosphatase
Height, weight	Bone age, bone density
Growth velocity	Vitamins A, D, E, B_{12}, Folic acid
Height-for-age %, weight-for-height %	Prothrombin time, partial prothrombin time
Midarm circumference	Zinc
Tricipital skinfold thickness	Retinol binding protein
	24-h urinary Mg

parenteral nutritional support. The additional energy cost for growth is another important factor in the development of chronic malnutrition in children with enteric neuromuscular disorders.

NUTRITIONAL ASSESSMENT

A vicious cycle exists between impaired nutritional status and disease states. Any disorder associated with undernutrition may reduce the functional capacity of the gastrointestinal and immune systems. Gastrointestinal diseases such as motility disorders also commonly result in deterioration of the patient's nutritional status. Fundamental to the physician's capacity to offer proper pediatric care is the ability to correctly assess the nutritional status of their patients. Many patients with neuromuscular enteric disorders do not respond to medications, and nutritional therapy becomes essential to their management. In the pediatric age group, undernutrition is the principal cause of growth failure. It is also a significant risk factor for excess morbidity and mortality in children with various acute and chronic illnesses.[20]

A combination of relatively simple anthropometric, clinical, laboratory, and dietary methods form an integral part of the medical evaluation of the pediatric patient with a gut motility disorder (Table 24.3). The patient's rate of growth over time—or growth velocity—must be considered. A distinction should be made between undernutrition and a constitutionally delayed, but normal growth pattern. Using growth velocity charts, and correcting the incremental data for height change based on bone age rather than chronologic age, pathologic and normal but delayed patterns are easily distinguished.[21,22]

In patients with enteric neuromuscular disorders, it is helpful to classify malnutrition in terms of severity (Table 24.4). In acute malnutrition, a low weight-for-height is seen, whereas in chronic malnutrition there are frequently no clinical signs other than a low height-for-age.[23] Excessive morbidity and mortality related to malnutrition may be anticipated in patients with moderate or severe malnutrition.[20,24,25] Using this classification system, the treating physician can have objective measures for instituting aggressive nutritional interventions, whether enteral or parenteral. The simple calculation of percent of ideal weight-for-height and height-for-age can be repeated to monitor the response to nutritional support or other therapies.

TABLE 24.4 **Classification of Protein-calorie Malnutrition**				
Measure	**Malnutrition**	**Mild**	**Moderate**	**Severe**
Weight-for-height*	Acute, or wasting	80-89%	70-79%	<70%, or with edema
Height-for-age**	Chronic, or "stunting"	90-94%	85-89%	<85

*Weight-for-height deficit is calculated by dividing the patient's weight by the expected weight-for-height (50th percentile) x 100
** Height-for-age deficit is calculated by dividing the patient's height by expected height for age (50th percentile) x 100. (Reproduced with permission from Atlan P, Seidman E, 1990[22])

DIETARY MANAGEMENT

The goal in dietary management is to replace nutrient losses associated with malnutrition and to provide sufficient nutrients to promote positive energy and nitrogen balance for normal metabolic function. In the growing child, additional nutrients are necessary to restore weight and reestablish normal growth. Another important objective is to provide a nutritionally balanced diet that minimizes symptoms.

Methods for administering nutritional support include altering the diet, providing liquid hypercaloric supplements orally, tube feeding, or parenteral nutrition. Although CIP can be managed successfully with home parenteral nutrition,[26] the risk of complications is significant, as reviewed below. Practice guidelines have therefore been established for enteral and parenteral nutritional support in pediatric patients.[27] The advantages of using enteral feeding in terms of optimizing intestinal function are firmly established.[14] In a survey of pediatric patients with pseudo-obstruction by the North American Society of Pediatric Gastroenterologists, 15% required full parenteral nutrition, whereas 31% received both enteral and parenteral support.[16] The remainder were managed by diet. In another series of 26 cases, 21 required TPN at some point in their clinical course.[19] However, only 6 (23%) had severe malnutrition requiring home TPN.

The type of nutritional support depends on the severity and location of the motility disorder, more than the cause. Patients likely to benefit from specialized enteral or parenteral nutritional support are those with moderate to severe acute protein energy malnutrition or growth failure (see Table 24.4). Patients unable to maintain their weight and growth with dietary manipulations are candidates for enteral tube feedings.[27] Parenteral nutritional support should be reserved for patients who fail a trial of tube feeding.[27]

In intermittent or minimally symptomatic disease, patients may be able to resume a fairly normal oral diet after a period of bowel rest. During mild episodes, a temporary reduction of fat may improve gastric emptying. Generally, a lactose-free and low-sucrose diet is recommended for patients with malabsorption, particularly if small-bowel overgrowth is suspected. Dietary fiber or even solid foods may exacerbate obstructive symptoms and cause bezoars. A liquid enteral diet may be necessary.

The optimal choice of enteral formula used in patients with intestinal neuromuscular disorders is controversial. Preparations containing hydrolyzed proteins, fat, or amino acids may impair gastric emptying compared to casein- or other protein-based formulas. For infants below the age of 1 year, a semi-elemental formula such as Pregestimil (Mead Johnson, Evansville, IN) is often used. The casein hydrolysate is less antigenic than whole protein, which may sensitize the immune system if it crosses a compromised mucosal surface. The majority of the carbohydrate is glucose polymers, avoiding lactose or a high-sucrose content. Furthermore, 40% of the fat is in the form of medium-chain triglycerides, which do not require micelle formation, and so may be preferable in children with TPN- associated cholestatic liver disease. Neocate is an amino-acid based infant formula, with mostly long-chain triglycerides as a lipid source. Older patients may benefit from Vivonex Plus, a glutamine-enriched, amino-acid based formula with only 6% of calories as lipids. Peptamen is a partially hydrolyzed protein-based formula with 70% of its lipid content in the form of medium-chain triglycerides. Flavor packets that enhance palatability are also available.

Long-term compliance with these preparations can be difficult to maintain. Patients require motivation to take these nutritionally complete, but unappealing formulas. The nutritional support program must be tailored to meet the life-style requirements of each patient and family. Enteral nutritional support by tube feeding should be used in patients who are or will become malnourished, and in whom oral feedings and supplements are inadequate to maintain nutritional status and growth.[27] Recent advances in enteral hyperalimentation now afford a wide selection of liquid diets as well as delivery methods.[28] In general, the gastrointestinal tract should be accessed initially in the least invasive manner. Only patients who have been found to benefit from tube feedings over a significant period of observation should be considered for endoscopic gastrostomy tube placement. An additional benefit of such tubes is the ability to relieve abdominal distention by venting the gastrostomy.[29,30] Furthermore, feeding tubes can be advanced through gastrostomies into the small bowel, bypassing the paretic stomach.

USE OF TPN: INDICATIONS AND GUIDELINES

The decision to initiate TPN generally depends on malnutrition and severe dysfunction of the gastrointestinal tract.[31] As reviewed above, these criteria are often met in pediatric patients with enteric neuromuscular disease. The nutritional strategy must be individualized, taking into consideration clinical and nutritional status, the potential benefits of nutritional support, and the risks inherent in utilizing central venous alimen-

tation. A cumulative caloric deficit of 10,000 or more calories in adult surgical patients is associated with increased morbidity and mortality compared with those patients in positive caloric balance.[31] In critically ill patients, multiple organ failure is higher in those with marked cumulative caloric deficits. However, repletion of severe malnutrition may create metabolic and functional aberrations that can be detrimental or even fatal.[31-33] These risks, collectively referred to as the refeeding syndrome, are discussed below. A clear understanding of the indications, methods, and potential complications of nutritional support is essential.

Indications

The guidelines for the use of TPN in adult and pediatric patients with neuromuscular intestinal disorders have been reviewed by the American Society for Parenteral and Enteral Nutrition (ASPEN) Board of Directors.[27] Patients who are unable to gain weight or grow despite the use of maximal enteral nutritional support are candidates for parenteral nutrition. Patients generally not likely to require specialized nutritional support are those who have involvement limited to the large bowel, or those in whom the periods of distention and vomiting are intermittent and brief.[27] Such patients are much less likely to become malnourished or to manifest growth failure, so that the potential risks of TPN probably outweigh the benefits.

Refeeding and Overfeeding Syndromes

Once the decision to use TPN is made, the amount of nutrients prescribed may assume major importance with respect to patient outcome. The dangers of overfeeding the severely malnourished patient may be as harmful as not feeding at all. The first principle in nutritional support is to respect each patient's metabolic needs and tolerance, avoiding the refeeding and overfeeding syndromes. Standardized TPN solutions are inappropriate and potentially hazardous, particularly when initiating TPN. The major complications of TPN related to the refeeding syndrome are listed in Table 24.5. The functional complications of refeeding occur primarily in the gastrointestinal and cardiopulmonary systems, and may cause fatal arrhythmias, congestive heart failure, respiratory distress and hypercapnea.[31-33]

Overfeeding is associated with hepatic dysfunction and steatosis, sodium and fluid retention, prerenal azotemia, glucose intolerance, hypertriglyceridemia, hypercapnea, and respiratory dysfunction.[31] Chronic overfeeding can induce a hypermetabolic state, due to the thermogenic effect of feeding.[34]

It is difficult to set standard recommendations for energy and fluid requirements for pediatric patients on TPN. A number of factors influence each patient's needs, including the presence of enteric as well as third-space losses, activity level, and nutritional status. Initially, minimal requirements can be rapidly estimated as 1600 kcal or ml per m^2/d. Body surface is approximated as 4 times weight plus 7+ weight plus 90, where weight is expressed in kg. Calories and fluids must be increased judiciously, with careful monitoring (Table 24.6).

Optimizing Nutrients

Nitrogen requirements. The overall goal is to put the patient in positive nitrogen balance. To meet the patient's requirements, an optimal balance of nitrogen and caloric intake must be attained.[35] To achieve a nitrogen retention of 100 gm/kg/d in an adoles-

---

TABLE 24.5 **Potential Complications Related to the Refeeding Syndrome**

Hyperglycemia
Rebound hypoglycemia
Hypokalemia
Hyperkalemia
Hypophosphatemia
Hypomagnesemia
Hypocalcemia
Edema
Diarrhea
Nausea and vomiting
Arrhythmias
Cardiopulmonary failure

TABLE 24.6 **Monitoring of Malnourished Patients During Initiation of Nutritional Support**

Parameter	Frequency
Glycemia	A
BUN	A
Serum electrolytes (Na, K, Cl)	A
Magnesium	A
Phosphorus	A
Calcium (total + ionized)	A
Triglycerides; Blood gas	B
Liver function tests (ALT, AST, bilirubin, gamma GT, PT)	C
Vital signs; in & out	QID
Urinary density, reducing substances	TID
Weight	A
Nitrogen balance	C
Urinary electrolytes	B

A= Daily x 1 week, then 3 times weekly until stable intake
B= Three times weekly, then weekly
C= Weekly

QID= Four times daily
TID= Three times daily

cent, approximately 1.75 gm of amino acids per kg/d and an energy intake equivalent to 1.3 to 1.5 times energy expenditure should be provided. In an infant weighing about 10 kg, approximately 3 mg/kg of amino acids would be required, with an energy intake approaching 1.6 to 1.7 times expenditures. These intakes will result in calorie to nitrogen ratios of 130:150, which are associated with optimal utilization of nitrogen and avoidance of liver dysfunction, hyperlipidemia, and steatosis. It must be reemphasized that these represent optimal goals for the patient without metabolic complications. The initiation of TPN is best accomplished by the gradual progression of nutrients, according to the individual patient's tolerance. An initial feeding would generally be 1 gm/kg of amino acids daily. Biochemical parameters should be monitored carefully during the initial 2 weeks, as proposed in Table 24.6. Increases should be made progressively, to attain full nitrogen requirements as soon as possible.

Carbohydrates. Carbohydrates are a major energy source for enterally as well as parenterally nourished patients. Once again, individualization of the patient's needs must be attained, as malnutrition, infections, and various other disorders will affect glucose tolerance. In the malnourished patient, many of the metabolic complications (see Table 24.5) are compounded by carbohydrate administration that exceeds the patient's metabolic tolerance. Potassium and phosphorus are driven intracellularly, primarily as a result of their consumption for insulin-dependent activities. Without adequate supplementation, the resultant serum deficiencies may result in life-threatening myocardial dysfunction and arrhythmias.[31-33] Furthermore, excessive intravenous glucose administration increases the nonoxidative disposal of glucose via hepatic lipogenesis. Increasing the conversion of glucose to fat results in an increased respiratory quotient. The excess carbon dioxide produced accumulates and increases the respiratory workload, adversely affecting metabolic requirements and potentially causing respiratory distress and

growth problems. Finally, hyperglycemia also suppresses the chemotactic and phagocytic activities of immune cells.[31] Therefore, careful monitoring of blood-glucose levels, the presence of glucosuria, and serum electrolytes are essential while initiating TPN (see Table 24.6). Final glucose requirements in patients on long-term TPN vary according to age and energy expenditures. In infants, intakes approximating 12 to 16 gm/kg/d are generally well tolerated, whereas about 4 to 6 gm/kg/d are optimal for adolescents. Indirect calorimetry can be of enormous assistance for evaluating a patient's utilization of energy substrates.

Lipids. Lipid emulsions have the combined advantages of a high-energy coefficient, iso-osmolarity, and a metabolism that is independent of insulin activity. The use of intravenous fat emulsions as energy sources has reduced glucose requirements as nonprotein calories, and represents a significant advance in the provision of nutritional support. Intravenous lipids have been shown to decrease hepatic triglyceride synthesis, and consequently, hepatic steatosis. They also provide essential fatty acids.[36,37] As with other nutritional substrates, however, intravenous lipids must be used judiciously.[31] Adverse effects, such as nausea, vomiting, and fever generally occur when the fat is infused over too brief an interval. Furthermore, excessive long-chain triglyceride (LCT) infusion over short periods (<10 hours) may impair reticuloendothelial system function. Accumulation of LCTs in hepatic Kupffer's cells lining the sinusoids impair their ability to phagocytose bacteria.[31] Generally, 1.5 to 3 gm/kg/d (depending on age) of intravenous lipid is well tolerated over a 10- to 14-hour infusion in patients on home TPN. Clinical experience has shown that cycling of TPN over a 12-hour period is less likely to be associated with steatosis. Monitoring of lipid tolerance is best accomplished by following serum triglycerides, bearing in mind that the normal laboratory range is for patients in the fasting state. Lipid emulsions of 20% are generally better tolerated than 10% emulsions in view of increased clear-

TABLE 24.7 Daily Maintenance Requirements of Minerals and Trace Elements for Pediatric Patients on Long-term TPN*

Minerals		
Sodium (mEq)	2-4	
Potassium (mEq)	2-3	
Chloride (mEq)	2-3	
Calcium (mEq)	1-2 (max 30 mEq/d)	
Phosphorus (mg)	30-40 (max 700-1000 mg/d)	
Magnesium (mEq)	0.25	
Iron (µg)	50-100	

Trace Elements		Daily Maximum
Zinc (µg)	300	4000
Copper (µg)	40	500
Manganese (µg)	10	130
Selenium (µg)	2	25
Iodine (µg)	6	80
Chromium (µg)	0-0.05**	—

*Per kg/d
**TPN solutions generally deliver excessive amounts of chromium as a contaminant. Most patients will not require any supplementation.

TABLE 24.8 Daily Maintenance Vitamin Requirements for Pediatric Patients on Long-term TPN

Lipid-soluble Vitamins	<2 Years	≥2 Years
A (IU)	2300	2300-5000
D (IU)	400	400
E (IU)	7	7
K (µg)	200	200
Water-soluble Vitamins		
Folic acid (mg)	0.14	0.14-5
Pantothenic acid (mg)	5	5-15
Thiamin (B_1) (mg)	1.2	1.2-5
Riboflavin (B_2) (mg)	1.4	1.4-5
Niacin (B_3) (mg)	17	17
Pyridoxin (B_6) (mg)	1.0	1.0-5
Biotin (B_8) (µg)	20	20-60
Cobalamin (B_{12}) (µg)	1	2-12
Ascorbic acid (C) (mg)	80	80-500

ance from plasma (lower cholesterol and trig-lyceride concentrations for the same intake).

Micronutrients. Though not considered in energy requirements, micronutrients are essential elements of nutritional support due to their critical role as metabolic cofactors.[31] Micronutrient homeostasis is particularly challenging in patients with neuromuscular intestinal disorders, as the combination of malabsorption, malnutrition, and dependence on artificial nutritional support are risk factors for multiple deficiencies.[38] Requirements for minerals, trace elements, and vitamins for patients dependent on TPN are shown in Tables 24.7 and 24.8. The currently available multivitamin preparations were developed according to the recommendations of the Nutritional Advisory Group of the American Medical Association in the 1970s. One solution is available for pediatric patients below age 11, while the other is used for adolescents. Careful monitoring of patients for deficiencies upon initiation of nutritional support is critically important, in view of the risks of the refeeding syndrome (see Table 24.6). Patients who stabilize on home TPN subsequently require surveillance of growth and nutrient status on a less frequent basis (Table 24.9).

Any deficiencies or excesses due to diarrhea or coexisting conditions require tailoring of intake for individual patients. Patients who are not receiving any enteral nutrition, as well as those on antibiotics, require an additional 1 mg of vitamin K daily, administered over the period of infusion.[39] For iron-deficient patients, the parenteral iron can be increased to 250 µg/kg/d. Patients who are malnourished and hypoproteinemic, however, should not be given parenteral iron unless absolutely indicated, because increased free-iron levels raise the risk of sepsis. Increasing evidence suggests that TPN solutions are contaminated with chromium.[40] Most patients on long-term TPN have excessive serum chromium levels, without any overt consequences to date.

The mineral content of TPN must also be customized to maintain adequate acid-base balance by the proper use of chloride and acetate salts. The majority of malnourished

TABLE 24.9 **Monitoring Pediatric Patients on Long-term TPN**
Parameter Measured Monthly
Weight
Glucose
Serum electrolytes (Na, K, Cl)
Magnesium
Phosphorus
Calcium (total + ionized)
Triglycerides; cholesterol
Liver function
ALT
AST
bilirubin
gamma GT
PT
PTT
Albumin, total proteins
BUN, creatinine
Hemoglobin, RBC morphology, leukocytes, platelets
Uric acid
Parameter Measured Every Third Month*
Height; growth velocity
Midarm circumference; tricipital skinfold thickness
Vitamins A, D, E, Folate, B_{12}, Biotin
Zinc, Copper, Selenium, Chromium, Aluminum
Plasma lipoproteins; fatty acids
*In addition to monthly tests

patients are hypophosphatemic. However, increasing the concentration of phosphorus in TPN solutions will often cause precipitation of calcium phosphate. The use of monobasic phosphate increases the solubility of inorganic phosphorus by about 30% in TPN solutions, allowing the provision of up to 40 mg/kg/d. (M. Pineault, MD, unpublished data).

RISKS AND BENEFITS OF TPN

A significant proportion of patients with chronically active intestinal pseudo-obstruction do not tolerate enteral nutrition for prolonged periods and benefit from a regimen of little or no enteral intake, with TPN at home.[16,19,26] In a review of long-term home TPN use in 102 pediatric patients, CIP was the indication in 10% of cases.[41] At the Hôpital Ste-Justine in Montreal, inflammatory bowel disease is almost always managed with enteral hyperalimentation, and enteric neuromuscular disorders assume a much more prominent indication for home TPN. Malnutrition, micronutrient deficiencies, and growth failure can be overcome using long-term TPN.

Serious, potentially fatal complications may arise from the use of TPN via central venous catheters. The risks and benefits must be evaluated on an individual basis. Early complications relate mostly to the risks of catheter insertion and the refeeding syndrome. The latter metabolic and physiologic consequences of hyperalimentation in malnourished patients may also occur in patients receiving enteral nutritional support.[31-33] It is thus essential to recognize the patient at risk and to screen for electrolyte abnormalities before initiating nutritional support (see Table 24.6).

Long-term risks center primarily on septic complications and cholestatic liver disease. Catheter-related infections are the most common reason for catheter removal.[41] Patients with enteric neuromuscular disorders usually have a greater incidence of sepsis than other groups of patients. Sepsis and disseminated intravascular coagulation were reported to be the leading cause of death in pediatric patients with pseudo-obstruction.[16] In another series of 10 infants, all four deaths were TPN related.[42] Two each died of sepsis and hepatic failure.

Common organisms include *Staphylococcus epidermidis* (usually multiresistant strains requiring vancomycin) or *aureus, Candida, Klebsiella pneumonia, E coli, Pseudomonas, Streptococcus viridans,* or *Enterococci.* Catheter removal is routinely considered if sepsis arises. However, patients with severe neuromuscular enteric disorders often eventually develop difficulties with venous access for central catheter reinsertion. If the patient's clinical status permits, a conservative attitude should be considered. This strategy has been reported to save 86% of catheters in one series,[43] probably because many such infections are due to bacterial translocation across the bowel wall, rather than primary contamination of the catheter.[14,15,44] Recently, decreased rates of sepsis have been observed in two of three children with pseudo-obstruction on home TPN, utilizing oral glutamine supplementation.

Intrahepatic cholestasis with progressive liver failure remains the second most important cause of morbidity and mortality in patients on home TPN.[16,41,42] Cholelithiasis is another major problem on long-term TPN.[45] Biliary sludge is observed in 6% of patients after 3 weeks, and 100% after 6 weeks.[46] About half of those with sludge will proceed to cholelithiasis if TPN continues without enteral nutrition.[46,47] Risk factors for hepatobiliary disease include pediatric age group, the absence of enteral nutrients, increased duration of central TPN, the presence of dysfunctional or short bowel, infectious foci, micronutrient deficiencies, an unbalanced energy to nitrogen ratio, and the concomitant use of medications. Strategies to prevent TPN-related hepatobiliary disorders include maximizing enteral nutrition concomitant to TPN (>20% of calories, if possible), avoiding caloric overload, cycling TPN rather than delivering continuously, and providing a proper balance of nutrients. Recently, bile-acid displacement therapy with ursodeoxycholic acid has been utilized in pediatric patients with chronic cholestasis.[48] It remains to be determined whether ursodeoxycholic acid therapy can reverse or prevent biliary disease in pediatric patients on long-term TPN, or whether patients with enteric neuromuscular disorders will absorb this bile acid.

NUTRITIONAL SUPPORT: LONG-TERM OUTLOOK

Children afflicted with severe enteric neuromuscular disorders often have a distorted body image. Obviously, nutritional support via tube feedings or central lines may exacerbate these problems. The severe malnutrition, growth failure, and delayed puberty associated with these disorders can also be devastating to the patient's health and self-esteem. The aim of nutritional support is to help the patients achieve their full potential while normalizing their life-style as much as possible. Support from a multidisciplinary team is essential to educate the patient and family regarding safe technique. Diet, schooling, extracurricular activities, and behavior should be reevaluated regularly, along with growth and medical issues. The parameters used to follow and evaluate the safety and efficacy of nutritional support therapy are summarized in Table 24.9.

Enteric neuromuscular disorders represent a heterogeneous syndrome with a widely variable course. The need for TPN early on does not necessarily imply its long-term use.[42] Furthermore, TPN should be regarded as a supportive therapy that does not necessarily prevent symptomatic episodes.

Despite the obvious difficulties faced by families with a child on home TPN, most cope extremely well.[41] Nutritional support is an important adjunctive therapy, but does not alter the natural course of the disease process itself. The advent of small-bowel transplantation will probably have a major impact on the long-term prognosis in patients with severe enteric neuromuscular disorders.

REFERENCES

1. Rhoads JM, Powell DW. Diarrhea. In: Walker WA, Durie PR, Hamilton JR, Walker-Smith JR, Watkins JB, eds. *Pediatric Gastrointestinal Diseases.* Philadelphia, PA: BC Decker, 1991:62-3.

2. Tumberg LA, Riley SA. Digestion and absorption of nutrients and vitamins. In: Sleisenger MH, Fordtran JS, eds. *Gastrointestinal Disease,* 5th ed. Philadelphia, PA: WB Saunders, 1993:989-93.

3. Stevens BR, Kaunitz JD, Wright EM. Intestinal transport of amino acids and sugars: advances using membrane vesicles. *Ann Rev Physiol* 1984;46:417-33.

4. Parson AJ, Brzechwa-Adjukiewicz A, McCarthy CF. Intestinal pseudo-obstruction with bacterial overgrowth in the small intestine. *Am J Dig Dis* 1969;14:200-5.

5. Riley SA, Tumberg LA. Maldigestion and malabsorption. In: Sleisenger MH, Fordtran JS, eds. *Gastrointestinal Disease,* 5th ed. Philadelphia, PA: WB Saunders, 1993:1009-27.

6. Kim YS, Spritz N, Blum M, Terz J, Sherlock P. The role of altered bile acid metabolism in the steatorrhea of experimental blind loop. *J Clin Invest.* 1966;45:956-62.

7. Toskes PP, Giannella RA, Jervis HR, Rout WR, Takeuchi A. Small intestinal mucosal injury in the experimental blind loop syndrome. *Gastroenterology* 1975;68:193-203.

8. Giannella RA, Rout WR, Toskes PP. Jejunal brush border injury and impaired sugar and amino acid uptake in the blind loop syndrome. *Gastroenterology* 1974;67:965-74.

9. King CE, Toskes PP. Protein-losing enteropathy in the human and experimental rat blind-loop syndrome. *Gastroenterology* 1981;80:504-9.

10. Savage DC. Gastrointestinal microflora in mammalian nutrition. *Ann Rev Nutr* 1986;6:155-78.

11. Justus PG, Fernandez A, Martin JL, King CE, Toskes PP, Mathias JR. Altered myoelectric activity in the experimental blind loop syndrome. *J Clin Invest* 1983;72:1064-71.

12. Brunser O, Araya M, Espinoza J. The gut in malnutrition. In: Walker WA, Durie PR, Hamilton JR, Walker-Smith JR, Watkins JB, eds. *Pediatric Gastrointestinal Diseases.* Philadelphia, PA: BC Decker, 1991:722-7.

13. Sherman P, Wesley A, Forstner G. Sequential disaccharidase loss in rat intestinal blind loops: impact of malnutrition. *Am J Physiol* 1985;248:G626-32.

14. Seidman E. Gastrointestinal benefits of enteral nutrition. In: Baker S, Baker R, Davis A, eds. *Pediatric Enteral Nutrition.* Andover Medical Publishers, 1994 (In press).

15. Lacey JM, Wilmore DW. Is glutamine a conditionally essential amino acid? *Nutr Rev* 1990;48:297-309.

16. Vargas JH, Sachs P, Ament ME. Chronic intestinal pseudo-obstruction in pediatrics: results of a national survey by members of the North American Society for Pediatric Gastroenterology and Nutrition. *J Pediatr*

Gastroenterol Nutr 1988;7:323-32.

17. Stanghellini V, Camilleri M, Malagelada J-R. Chronic idiopathic intestinal pseudo-obstruction: clinical and intestinal manometric findings. *Gut* 1987;28:5-12.

18. DiCecco S, Nelson J, Burnes J, Fleming CR. Nutritional intake of gut failure patients on home parenteral nutrition. *J Parenter Enter Nutr* 1987;11:529-32.

19. Navarro J, Sonsino E, Boige N, et al. Visceral neuropathies responsible for chronic intestinal pseudo-obstruction syndrome in pediatric practice: analysis of 26 cases. *J Pediatr Gastroenterol Nutr* 1990;11:179-95.

20. Briend A, Dykewicz C, Graven K, Mazumder RN, Wojtyniak B, Bennish N. Usefulness of nutritional indices and classifications in predicting death of malnourished children. *Br Med J* 1986;293:373-5.

21. Seidman E, LeLeiko N, Ament M, Berman W, Caplan D. Nutritional issues in pediatric inflammatory bowel disease. *J Pediatr Gastroenterol Nutr* 1991;12:424.

22. Atlan P, Seidman E. Nutritional considerations in pediatric patients. *Can J Gastroenterol* 1990;4:41-4.

23. Waterlow JC. Classification and definition of protein-energy malnutrition. *WHO, Monograph Series* 1976;62:530-55.

24. Sommer A, Lowenstein MS. Nutritional status and mortality: a prospective validation of the QUAC stick. *Am J Clin Nutr* 1975;28:287-92.

25. McLaren DS, Shirajian E, Loshkajian H, Shadarevian S. Short-term prognosis in protein-calorie nutrition. *Am J Clin Nutr* 1969;22:863-70.

26. Warner E, Jeeheebhoy KN. Successful management of chronic intestinal pseudo-obstruction with home parenteral nutrition. *J Parenter Enter Nutr* 1985;9:173-8.

27. A.S.P.E.N. Board of Directors. Guidelines for the use of parenteral and enteral nutrition in adult and pediatric patients. *J Parenter Enter Nutr* 1993;17:1SA-52SA.

28. Mobarhan S, Trumbore LS. Enteral tube feeding: a clinical perspective on recent advances. *Nutr Rev* 1991;49:129-40.

29. Anuras S, Mitros FA, Soper RT, et al. Chronic intestinal pseudo-obstruction in young children. *Gastroenterology* 1986;91:62-70.

30. Pitt HA, Mann LL, Berquist WE, Ament ME, Fonkalsrud EW, DenBesten L. Chronic intestinal pseudo-obstruction: management with total parenteral nutrition and a venting enterostomy. *Arch Surg* 1985;120:614-8.

31. Driscoll DF, Blackburn GL. Total parenteral nutrition 1990: a review of its current status in hospitalized patients, and the need for patient-specific feeding. *Drugs* 1990;40:346-63.

32. Havala T, Shronts E. Managing the complications associated with refeeding. *Nutr Clin Prac* 1990;5:23-9.

33. Solomon SM, Kirby DF. The refeeding syndrome: a review. *J Parenter Enter Nutr* 1990;14:90-7.

34. Allard JP, Jeejheebhoy KN, Whitwell J, Pashutinski L, Peters WJ. Factors influencing energy expenditure in patients with burns. *J Trauma* 1988;28:199-202.

35. Elwyn DH, Kinney JM, Askanazi J. Energy expenditure in surgical patients. *Surg Clin North Am* 1981;61:545-56.

36. Bryan H, Shennan A, Griffin E, Angel A. Intralipid—its rational use in parenteral nutrition of the newborn. *Pediatrics* 1976;58:787-90.

37. Schreiner RL, Glick MR, Nordschow CD, Greshan EL. An evaluation of methods to monitor infants receiving intravenous lipids. *J Pediatr* 1979;94:197-200.

38. Kadowaki H, Ouchi M, Kaga M, et al. Problems of trace elements and vitamins during long-term total parenteral nutrition: a case report of idiopathic intestinal pseudo-obstruction. *J Parenter Enter Nutr* 1987;11:322-5.

39. Carlin A, Walker WA. Rapid development of vitamin K deficiency in an adolescent boy receiving total parenteral nutrition following bone marrow transplantation. *Nutr Rev* 1991;49:179-83.

40. Moukarzel AA, Song MK, Buchman Al, et al. Excessive chromium intake in children receiving

374

total parenteral nutrition. *Lancet* 1992;339:385-8.

41. Vargas JH, Ament ME, Berquist WE. Long-term home parenteral nutrition in pediatrics: ten years of experience in 102 patients. *J Pediatr Gastroenterol Nutr* 1987;6:24-32.

42. Bagwell CE, Filler RM, Cutz E, et al. Neonatal intestinal pseudo-obstruction. *J Pediatr Surg* 1984;19:732-9.

43. Nahata MC, King DR, Powell DA, Marx SM, Ginn-Pease ME. Management of catheter related infections in pediatric patients. *J Parenter Enter Nutr* 1988;12:58-9.

44. Freund HR, Rimon B. Sepsis during total parenteral nutrition. *J Parenter Enter Nutr* 1990;14:39-41.

45. Roslyn JJ, Pitt HA, Mann LL, Ament ME, DenBesten L. Gallbladder disease in patients on long-term parenteral nutrition. *Gastroenterology* 1983;84:148-54.

46. Messing B, Bories C, Kunstlinger F, Bernier JJ. Does total parenteral nutrition induce gallbladder sludge formation and lithiasis? *Gastroenterology* 1983;84:1012-9.

47. Gafa M, Sarli L, Miselli A, Pietra N, Peracchia A. Sludge and microlithiasis of the biliary tract after total gastrectomy and postoperative total parenteral nutrition. *Surg Gynecol Obstet* 1987;165:413-8.

48. Balistreri WF, A-Kader HH, Ryckman FC, Whitington PF, Heubi JE, Setchell KD. Biochemical and clinical response to ursodeoxycholic acid administration in pediatric patients with chronic cholestasis. In: Paumgartner G, Stiehl A, Gerok W, eds. *Bile Acids as Therapeutic Agents.* Boston, MA: Kluwer, 1991:323-33.

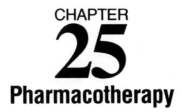

25

Pharmacotherapy

BRUCE B. GRILL, ALEJANDRO F. FLORES

Gastrointestinal motility disorders of childhood cause morbidity to the patient and often frustrate the physician. Motility disorders are treated with physical measures (eg, elevating the head of a prone infant with gastroesophageal reflux), dietary changes, and nutritional supplements. In the last 2 decades, the first useful drugs to improve motility and transit were developed in an explosion of basic and clinical research physiology and pharmacology. This chapter will describe drugs used specifically for their effects on gastrointestinal motility. The motility effects of selected drugs not primarily used to treat gastrointestinal disorders will also be described.

Since motility disorders of varying etiologies can cause identical symptoms, demonstrating the consistent effectiveness of motility drugs is often difficult.[1] A drug which is effective for one patient may have no effect in another with the same symptoms because different pathophysiologies underlie the common clinical presentation.[2] The results of in vitro studies of motility drugs cannot always be translated to clinical effectiveness. Factors such as diet, emotions, placebo effect, presence of systemic illness, interactions with other medications, and compliance cannot be readily controlled. Agents effective in vitro or in clinical studies that examine drug effects on specific, isolated motility phenomena (eg, sphincter pressure or contraction amplitude) may not relieve the symptoms of children.

Classifying pediatric motility disorders may help to better understand the role of individual agents. The most commonly encountered disorders are those associated with delayed esophageal or gastrointestinal transit, including gastroesophageal reflux, gastroparesis (idiopathic, postviral, or diabetic),[3] intestinal pseudo-obstruction, Hirschsprung's disease (upper-gut motility disturbances are present in 30-50% of cases after resection of the colonic aganglionosis[4]), the constipated form of irritable bowel syndrome (IBS), cyclic vomiting,[5] and slow-transit constipation. Disorders associated with accelerated intestinal transit include postsurgical gastric dumping syndrome, nonspecific diarrhea of infancy, and the diarrheal form of IBS (Table 25.1)

AGENTS THAT INCREASE MOTILITY

Bethanechol

Bethanechol is an ester derivative of choline (ie, quaternary ammonium) with direct cholinomimetic actions. It exerts its motility effect by binding to muscarinic cholinergic receptors and, like acetylcholine, increasing gastrointestinal smooth-muscle contractility.[6] It is absorbed slowly from the gastrointestinal tract and has its peak action 25 minutes after an oral dose, with effects lasting 60 to 120 minutes.[7] After a subcutaneous dose, the peak effects were seen at 10 minutes, with effects lasting 20 minutes.[8] It increased lower esophageal sphincter (LES) pressure, increased the amplitude and decreased the velocity of peristalsis in the esophageal body, and improved coordination of esophageal peristalsis.[9] The same study demonstrated that effects on the esophageal body were dose dependent; a 0.2 mg/kg dose was effective on

TABLE 25.1 **Pediatric Neuromuscular Disorders**
Associated With Delayed Gastrointestinal Transit
Achalasia
Gastroesophageal reflux
Intestinal pseudo-obstruction
Muscular dystrophies
Gastroduodenoparesis
Hirschsprung's disease
Neuronal intestinal dysplasia
Refractory constipation
Cyclic vomiting
Diabetic gastroparesis
Childhood visceral myopathy type II
megacystis
microcolon
intestinal hypoperistalsis syndrome
Fetal alcohol syndrome
Constipation type of irritable bowel syndrome (IBS)
Associated With Accelerated Gastrointestinal Transit
Dumping syndrome
Toddler's diarrhea
Diarrheal type of IBS
Hyperthyroidism
Hyperparathyroidism

all parameters, but a 0.1 mg/kg dose was effective only on LES pressure. Bethanechol shortened the esophageal acid clearance time and reduced the duration of reflux episodes.[10] Late postprandial reflux improved during chronic oral administration.[11]

Bethanechol has been used to treat infants with gastroesophageal reflux. In a double-blind crossover study, greater weight gain was seen in infants and children treated with bethanechol compared to placebo over 12 weeks.[12] Oral doses ranging from 0.125 mg to 0.25 mg/kg did not improve any parameter of reflux as determined by esophageal pH monitoring.[12] Bethanechol has minimal or no effect on gastric emptying or small intestinal or colonic transit.[13]

As expected from a cholinomimetic drug, bethanechol increases salivation and gastric secretion. While added salivation might buffer refluxed acid, the increased gastric acid could counteract this benefit or inhibit motility.

Side effects of bethanechol, which occur in 10% to 15% of patients, include abdominal cramping, blurred vision, fatigue, and increased urinary frequency. Bethanechol must be used with caution, if at all, in patients with bronchospasm or bladder outlet obstruction. The recommended oral dose in children is 2.9 mg/M^2 or 0.2 mg/kg given 20 to 30 minutes before a feeding four times a day.

Metoclopramide

Metoclopramide is a dopamine D$_2$ antagonist, and is a derivative of procainamide without cardiac or anesthetic actions.[14] Since dopamine is an inhibitory neurotransmitter in the gastrointestinal tract that causes smooth-muscle relaxation, metoclopramide enhances intestinal smooth-muscle tone.[15] Metoclopramide has a central antiemetic effect by dopamine D$_2$-receptor inhibition at the chemoreceptor trigger zone.[16] In addition, metoclopramide enhances acetylcholine release from postganglionic enteric motor neurons, therefore indirectly enhancing cholinergic tone.[17] It may also directly stimulate intestinal smooth muscle.[18] The combination of these actions results in accelerated gastric emptying.

The effects of metoclopramide diminish rapidly distal to the proximal small bowel, and are minimal on the colon.[19] The mechanisms for metoclopramide-mediated acceleration of gastric emptying may include increased antral motor activity and inhibition of fundic receptive relaxation. In two studies measuring its effects on esophageal pH in infants, there was no effect on any parameter of reflux either given orally or by injection. With doses of 0.3 mg/kg there was a decrease in postprandial reflux duration and frequency.[20,21]

In a randomized, prospective, 1-week, double-blind crossover study in infants less than 1 year of age, a 0.1 mg/kg dose of metoclopramide was superior to placebo in reducing the time that esophageal pH was less than 4.0, although this value remained above normal in most subjects.[22] Intravenous metoclopramide increased LES pressure, but most reflux parameters were not affected, as measured by pH monitoring over 24 hours after oral doses of 0.125 mg/kg.[22]

Metoclopramide accelerates gastric emptying. Patients with delayed emptying show greater improvement than normal subjects. In an open trial, ability to feed in premature infants with gastric stasis was promoted.[23] Metoclopramide, but not bethanechol, increased the fractional rate of gastric emptying following a 5% glucose meal in 10 infants with upper gastrointestinal motor disorders.[24] Peak serum concentrations were reached 1.5 hours after an oral dose of 0.15 mg/kg, suggesting that the common practice of administering the drug 30 minutes before feeding may not result in predictable effects.[25]

The oral dose is 0.1 mg/kg with a maximum of 0.5 mg/kg per day.[26] In clinical practice, however, many patients do not respond to this dosage and often require individual doses of 0.2 to 0.3 mg/kg or greater. The therapeutic index for metoclopramide is narrow, as doses required for efficacy often approach or exceed those that cause side effects.

Side effects occur in 20% to 30% of patients treated with effective doses. Side effects include somnolence, restlessness, and insomnia, but the most troubling are dystonic and extrapyramidal movements. Tremors, trismus, facial spasms, and oculogyric crises improve after withdrawal of the drug or administration of intravenous diphenhydramine 1 mg/kg. Tardive dyskinesias may not respond to drug withdrawal.[27] Metoclopramide is associated with increased serum concentration of prolactin, but gynecomastia and galactorrhea due to enhanced prolactin release are rare. [28] Although a low therapeutic index and effects limited to the upper gastrointestinal tract make it a less desirable first-line oral prokinetic than cisapride (see below), its parenteral dose form is helpful for both its antiemetic and prokinetic properties in hospitalized patients.

Domperidone

Domperidone is a benzimidazole derivative with dopamine-receptor antagonist properties. In contrast to metoclopramide, domperidone's higher molecular weight and lower lipid solubility limit its ability to cross the blood-brain barrier.[29] Its antiemetic effect is a result of an inhibition of the chemoreceptor trigger zone located on the blood side of the barrier. Domperidone increases LES pressure, inhibits relaxation of the gastric fundus, enhances contractility of the antrum, and improves antroduodenal coordination.[30]

In an open trial, 12 children with gastroesophageal reflux (mean age, 7.2 mo) were treated with 0.3 or 0.6 mg/kg of oral domperidone for 6 weeks. Domperidone decreased postprandial reflux time and improved symptoms. There was an increase in the percentage of normally conducted peristaltic sequences, frequency of gastric contractions, and a trend towards accelerated gastric emptying.[31] In a subsequent randomized placebo-controlled trial, 0.6 mg/kg oral domperidone was given four times a day for 4 weeks. Both domperidone and placebo improved the symptom score and acid clearance time, while placebo also improved the total reflux time.[32] Side effects were minimal in both studies. In a recent double-blind study, symptoms and objective parameters of reflux were studied before and after 4 weeks of domperidone (0.6 mg/kg) or placebo in infants. Although domperidone reduced postprandial reflux, symptoms did not improve. In a subset of patients continuing for an additional 4-week open-label trial, symptomatic improvement was noted, suggesting that a longer duration of therapy may be necessary—a phenomenon described for other prokinetic agents as well.[33] The lack of efficacy of domperidone over placebo in these studies may shed light on the confounding variables during clinical trials of prokinetics in children. Maturation of LES function, ad lib antacid therapy in the placebo groups, the placebo effect, and the inclusion of patients with varying severity of reflux may have all contributed to obfuscate the outcome.

In adults, domperidone improved idiopathic, postsurgical, and diabetic gastroparesis, possibly in a dose-related manner.[34] In fasting adults, peak plasma levels are reached 15 to 30 minutes after oral or intramuscular administration. High doses of H_2-histamine receptor antagonists may impair domperidone absorption. Side effects in children have been minimal, and have included transient diarrhea. Central nervous system (CNS) side effects have been reported in a few infants and in patients given more than 0.6 mg/kg.[35]

Domperidone may be an excellent choice for the treatment of nonulcer dyspepsia accompanied by nausea. It may be useful for some children with gastroparesis and in those with GER in whom side effects or lack of response make metoclopramide undesirable.

Cisapride

Cisapride is a substituted benzamide that acts as a serotonic $5HT_4$ agonist. Cisapride stimulates gastrointestinal motility by acting on myenteric cholinergic neurons to facilitate acetylcholine release.[36] In contrast to the dopamine antagonists metoclopramide and domperidone, radioligand binding studies indicate that cisapride has no direct interaction with dopaminergic receptors.

Oral cisapride is almost completely absorbed from the gastrointestinal tract. The absolute bioavailability of oral cisapride, however, is approximately 40% to 50%, indicating first-pass metabolism in the liver and/or gut wall. The bioavailability of a cisapride suppository is 30%. Peak plasma concentrations (C_{max}) are reached between 0.5 and 2 hours, with a plasma half-life ($T_{1/2}$) of 8 to 12 hours.[37] Steady-state plasma cisapride concentrations are achieved within 2 to 3 days. Bioavailability of cisapride is enhanced by food, although the rate of absorption is not altered. Cisapride is approximately 98% bound to plasma proteins, with albumin being the principal binding protein.[37] The elimination $T_{1/2}$ of cisapride is 7 to 10 hours.[37] In sheep, cisapride readily transfers across the placenta after intravenous administration. Sheep placenta is less permeable than human placenta; thus, cisapride may be transferred across the human placenta with even greater efficiency.[38] Cisapride is excreted in human breast milk in small amounts (approximately 0.1% of the original dose).[39] Cisapride enhances absorption of med-ications that are absorbed in the proximal intestine, including H_2-histamine receptor antagonists and diazepam. No interactions were observed with hepatic P450 enzymes.

Cisapride increased the LES pressure and the amplitude of esophageal contractions in infants with gastroesophageal reflux (GER).[40] It normalized the abnormal antroduodenal motility pattern in children with functional dyspepsia.[41] In a number of studies, cisapride accelerated gastric emptying in children with functional gastrointestinal symptoms or GER, and in preterm neonates with gastric stasis, but not in children with delayed gastric emptying secondary to progressive muscular dystrophy, or in those with chronic intestinal pseudo-obstruction (CIP).[42]

Cisapride is the first prokinetic drug to demonstrate efficacy for some cases of childhood CIP. A double-blind randomized trial of the effect of cisapride on antroduodenal motility and gastric emptying in 20 children with CIP showed that the drug increased the postprandial duodenal motility index, but did not alter gastric emptying.[43] In an open-label outpatient trial with 50 children, cisapride was most effective for CIP due to postprandial duodenal hypomotility. The drug was less effective in children lacking the migrating motor complex and those with dilated bowel. It facilitated a change from total parenteral nutrition or tube feeding to oral feeding in 7 of 50 children, and improved the symptom scores in an additional 17 of 50 children with CIP.[44]

In contrast to adults, constipated and encopretic children generally have a good clinical response to prolonged administration of cisapride, even when constipation is intractable and poorly responsive to high-dose laxatives. In most studies, stool consistency improved, the need for laxatives decreased, soiling episodes became significantly less frequent, and stool frequency increased. The thresholds for sensation of rectal distention and for elicitation of the rectoanal inhibitory reflex decreased during treatment with cisapride, whereas total transit time shortened.[45]

Its favorable side-effect profile in comparison to metoclopramide makes cisapride a first-line drug for treating pediatric motility disorders. Initial oral doses of 0.1 to 0.2 mg/kg three times daily are titrated up to 0.3 mg/kg four times daily to achieve maximal efficacy. Side effects may include transient diarrhea and behavioral changes, such as increased activity or irritability, in fewer than 5% of children.

Erythromycin

Dose-dependent antral contractions that resembled a naturally occurring migrating motor complex were induced by erythromycin in fasting dogs. These contractions were identical to those induced by intravenous infusion of motilin.[46] Similar results were found in humans,[47] but plasma motilin concentrations did not rise in humans as they did in dogs. Erythromycin acted as a motilin agonist on the gastric smooth-muscle cells, displacing radio-labeled motilin from its binding sites.[48] Erythromycin increased LES pressure but did not affect esophageal peristalsis.[49] Colonic and gallbladder motor activity may also be increased.[50] The molecular structure of the macrolide ring has been investigated, and it appears its specific physicochemical properties are responsible for its motilinlike activity.[48]

In adults, erythromycin was effective in diabetic gastroparesis, but tolerance developed.[51] Three children with diabetic gastroparesis had enhanced antral motor activity and two had improved gastric emptying after treatment.[52] In patients with gastric stasis syndrome, the response to intravenous drug predicts the clinical response to oral drug. If intravenous erythromycin induces repetitive antral contractions without nausea or emesis, those patients will respond with improved symptoms on chronic oral therapy using doses in the range of 1 to 6 mg/kg. Erythromycin may inhibit paroxysms of cyclic vomiting.[53]

Side effects due to enhanced motor activity (eg, nausea and vomiting) may occur, as may allergic reactions. At the doses used for motility effects, antibiotic effects are minimal. New macrolide derivatives are being developed for their prokinetic properties. Because erythromycin inhibits hepatic drug metabolism, it should be used with caution in patients taking methylxanthine derivatives.

A summary of mechanisms of action, major sites of action, and doses of the main prokinetic drugs for children is given in Table 25.2.

TABLE 25.2 **Prokinetic Drugs for Children**			
Drug	**Mechanism of Action**	**Major Sites of Action**	**Oral Dose**
Bethanechol	Muscarinic receptor agonist	Esophagus	0.1-0.3 mg/kg tid or qid
Metoclopramide	Dopamine antagonist	Esophagus and stomach	0.1-0.3 mg/kg tid or qid
Domperidone	Peripheral dopamine antagonist	Esophagus and stomach	0.3-0.6 mg/kg tid or qid
Cisapride	Serotonin (5-HT$_4$) receptor agonist	Entire gastrointestinal tract	0.1-0.3 mg/kg tid or qid
Erythromycin	Motilin receptor agonist	Gastric antrum	po 1-6 mg/kg bid or tid

Other Motility-enhancing Agents

Leuprolide. The gonadotropin-releasing factor antagonist leuprolide (Leupron, TAP Pharmaceuticals, North Chicago, IL) improves symptoms and manometric abnormalities in adolescent and adult women with enteric neuromuscular disease.[54,55] Its mechanisms of action in the gastrointestinal tract may involve altering membrane conductance in intrinsic and extrinsic myenteric nerves, and/or decreasing secretion of relaxin, a hormone that relaxes smooth muscle.[56] There is little experience with leuprolide in children with enteric neuromuscular disease.

Cathartic laxatives. The cathartic laxatives act by increasing colonic motor activity. Two classes within this group are the anthraquinones, exemplified by senna derivatives, and the polyphenolic drugs, which include bisacodyl and phenolphthalein. The anthraquinones, also known as anthracenes, are derived from plant products such as cascara, aloe, and senna. These laxatives are carried unabsorbed into the colon, where bacterial action converts them into an active form (ie, aglycon[57]) which enhances defecation by directly stimulating colonic peristalsis and inducing fluid secretion. The polyphenol bisacodyl induces high-amplitude peristaltic contractions that mimic the postprandial activity seen during colonic motility studies.[58] Polyphenols are effective in patients with slow-transit constipation. Prunes contain a derivative of a polyphenolic compound, suggesting a mechanism for their laxative effect.

Octreotide. This compound, a synthetic analog of the hormone somatostatin, has multiple gastrointestinal actions, primarily inhibitory, and will be discussed in more detail in the next section. The mean frequency of duodenal migrating motor complexes (MMC) in healthy volunteers significantly increased with low-dose octreotide (10 mg subcutaneously). In scleroderma patients who had no spontaneous migrating complexes, a dose of 100 mg induced MMC. Three weeks of administration of 50 mg at bedtime reversed abnormal breath hydrogen excretion and improved symptoms in patients with scleroderma and bacterial overgrowth.[59]

AGENTS THAT DIMINISH MOTILITY

Calcium Channel Blockers

These agents, typified by nifedipine, diltiazem, and verapamil, are well known for their hemodynamic and cardiac effects, as well as their use in achalasia. They stimulate ileal and colonic water and electrolyte absorption. They tend to relax gastrointestinal smooth muscle, perhaps by inhibiting the influx of extracellular calcium needed for smooth-muscle contraction.[60] In a rat model, nifedipine selectively inhibited spontaneous MMCs, but verapamil did not.[61] No clinical trials demonstrate the use of calcium channel blockers in conditions of rapid intestinal transit, but they have been used in spastic conditions of the esophagus (eg, diffuse esophageal spasm, noncardiac chest pain, and achalasia).[62]

Anticholinergics

Anticholinergic agents, such as atropine, have been used for many years as antisecretory agents. Before the advent of H_2-histamine receptor antagonists, they were the primary antisecretory therapy for peptic ulcer disease. They have been used as adjunctive therapy in IBS, especially where diarrhea or "smooth-muscle spasm" is a predominant component. They have also been used to treat esophageal motor disorders, bradycardia, and apparent chest pain associated with esophageal spasm in neonates.[63] Several cases of refractory bradycardia (without apnea) associated with either dysphagia or crying have been successfully treated with anticholinergic medication (atropine or glycopyrrolate). Preparations for pediatric use include dicyclomine, glycopyrrolate, and atropine singly or in combination with belladonna alkaloids. Significant potential side effects (eg, dry mouth, blurred vision, tachycardia, and sedation) limit their use in children.

Octreotide/Somatostatin. The mention of these agents properly belongs in a section on antimotility agents, since that is their predominant effect. Octreotide is an eight-peptide synthetic analog of native somatostatin, incorporating its active moiety.[62] These compounds have many gastrointestinal effects, mostly inhibitory (Table 25.3). Motility effects include inhibition of the late phase of gastric emptying, the gastric component of migratory motor complexes, and gallbladder contraction. Use in prepubertal and adolescent patients is limited by antigrowth hormone properties. In selected short-term usage, they have value in managing high-output secretory diarrhea such as that seen in enterocutaneous fistulae, AIDS, and some cases of short-bowel syndrome.[63] The adult dose usually ranges from 50 to 100 mg per day.

Ondansetron

The serotonin 5-HT$_3$ receptor antagonist ondansetron is effective for inhibiting chemotherapy-induced nausea and vomiting. Serotonin 5-HT$_3$ receptors control emesis by central and peripheral mechanisms.[64] Direct injury to or distention of the gastrointestinal tract, oncologic chemotherapy, and possibly even general anesthesia or abdominal surgery result in release of serotonin from intestinal enterochromaffin cells. This is turn stimulates vagal afferents. The exact mechanisms by which this stimulation induces emesis are unknown, but could involve 5-HT$_3$ receptors in the area of the brain near the projection of the afferent vagal fibers—the chemoreceptor trigger zone. In healthy volunteers, ondansetron slowed colonic transit, but there was no effect in diarrhea-predominant IBS patients.[65] In children, intravenous ondansetron has been a mainstay of treatment for chemotherapy-induced emesis. It has been used for paroxyms of cyclic vomiting (see Chapter 5). However, since the distribution and elimination of the compound do not differ for oral or intravenous administration, 0.1 to 0.2 mg/kg oral ondansetron may be used to treat abdominal pain in selected patients with functional gastrointestinal disorders with a component of pain or nausea who are not actively vomiting.

REFERENCES

1. Hyman PE, Tomomasa T, McDiarmid SV. Intestinal pseudo-obstruction in childhood. In: Milla PJ, Wilburn P, eds. *Disorders of Gastrointestinal Motility in Childhood.* Chichester, England: J Wiley & Sons, 1988;73-80.

2. Hyman PE, Napolitano JA, Diego A, et al.

TABLE 25.3 Biologic Actions of Somatostatin in the Gut

Inhibition of Exocrine Secretion
Stomach
  acid
  pepsinogen
Pancreas
  digestive enzymes
  bicarbonate
Liver
  bile acid independent bile flow
  ductular secretion
Salivary gland
  amylase

Inhibition of Endocrine Secretion
GI tract
  gastrin,
    cholecystokinin secretion
  VIP
  GIP
  motilin glucagon
Pancreas
  insulin
  glucagon
  pancreatic polypeptide

Motility
Inhibition
  late phase of gastric emptying
  gastric migrating motor
    complexes (MMCs)
  gallbladder contraction
Stimulation
  early-phase gastric emptying
  intestinal MMCs

Intestinal Transport
Inhibition
  secretion of fluid and bicarbonate
  absorption of calcium, glucose,
    galactose, xylose, fructose

Miscellaneous
Inhibition of splanchnic blood flow
Inhibition of tissue growth and proliferation

Antroduodenal manometry in the evaluation of chronic functional gastrointestinal symptoms. *Pediatrics* 1990;86:39-44.

3. Hillemeier ACC, Grill BB, McCallum RW, Grybowski J. Esophageal and gastric motor abnormalities in gastroesophageal reflux during infancy. *Gastroenterology* 1983;84:741-6.

4. Staiano A, Corazziari E, Andreotti MR, Clouse RE. Esophageal motility in children with Hirschsprung's disease. *Am J Dis Child* 1991;145:310-3.

5. Fleisher DR, Matar M. The cyclic vomiting syndrome: a report of 71 cases and literature review. *J Pediatr Gastroenterol Nutr* 113;17:361-9.

6. Koelle GB. Parasympathomimetic agents. In: Goodman LS, Gilman A, eds. *The Pharmacologic Basis of Therapeutics.* New York, NY: MacMillan, 1975:467-76.

7. Sondheimer JM, Mintz HL, Michaels M. Bethanecol treatment of gastroesophageal reflux in infants: effect on continuous esophageal pH records. *J Pediatr* 1984;104:128-31.

8. Sondheimer JM, Arnold GL. Early effects of bethanechol on the esophageal motor function of infants with gastroesophageal reflux. *J Pediatr Gastroenterol Nutr* 1986;5:47-51.

9. Strickland AD, Chang JH. Results of treatment of gastroesophageal reflux with bethanecol. *J Pediatr* 1983;103:311-5.

10. McCallum RW, Fink SM, Lerner E, Berkowitz DM. Effects of metoclopramide and bethanechol on delayed gastric emptying present in gastroesophageal reflux patients. *Gastroenterology* 1983;84:1573-7.

11. Euler AR. Use of bethanechol for the treatment of gastroesophageal reflux. *J Pediatr* 1980;96:321-4.

12. Orenstein SR, Lofton SW, Orenstein DM. Bethanechol for pediatric gastroesophageal reflux: a prospective, blind, controlled study. *J Pediatr Gastroenterol Nutr* 1986;5:549-55.

13. Reynolds JC, Putnam PE. Prokinetic agents. *Gastroenterol Clin North Am* 1992;21:567-96.

14. Schulze-Delrieu K. Drug therapy: metoclopramide. *N Engl J Med* 1981;305:28-33.

15. Eisner M. Gastrointestinal effects of metoclopramide in man: in vitro experiment with human smooth muscle preparation. *Br Med J* 1968;679-80.

16. Albibi R, McCallum RW. Metoclopramide: pharmacology and clinical application. *Ann Intern Med* 1983;98:86-95.

17. Jacoby HI, Brodie DA. Gastrointestinal actions of metoclopramide: an experimental study. *Gastroenterology* 1967;52:676-84.

18. Cohen S, Di Marino AJ. Mechanism of action of metoclopramide on opossum lower esophageal sphincter muscle. *Gastroenterology* 1976;71:996-8.

19. Pink SM, Lange RC, McCallum RW. Effect of metoclopramide on normal and delayed gastric emptying in gastroesophageal reflux patients. *Dig Dis Sci* 1983;28:1057-61.

20. Hyams JS, Leichtner AM, Zamett LO, Walters JK. Effect of metoclopramide on prolonged intraesophageal pH testing in infants with gastroesophageal reflux. *J Pediatr Gastroenterol Nutr* 1986;5:716-20.

21. Tolia V, Calhoun J, Kuhns L, Kauffman RE. Randomized, prospective double-blind trial of metoclopramide and placebo for gastroesophageal reflux in infants. *J Pediatr* 1989;115:141-5.

22. Machida HM, Forbes DA, Gall DG, Scott RB. Metoclopramide in gastroesophageal reflux in infancy. *J Pediatr* 1988;112:483-7.

23. Sankaran K, Yeboak EB, Bingham WT, Ninan A. Use of metoclopramide in preterm infants. *Dev Pharm Ther* 1982;5:114-9.

24. Hyman PE, Abrams C, Dubois A. Effect of metoclopramide and bethanechol on gastric emptying in infants. *Pediatr Res* 1985;19:1029-32.

25. Kearns GL, Butler HL, Lane JK, Carchman SH, Wright GH. Metoclopramide pharmacokinetics and pharmacodynamics in infants with gastroesophageal reflux. *J Pediatr Gastroenterol Nutr* 1988;19:965-8.

26. Harrington RA, Hamilton CW, Brogden RN, Linkewich JA, Romankiewicz JA, Heel RC. Metoclopramide: an updated review of its pharmacologic properties and clinical use. *Drugs* 1983;25:451-94.

27. Putnam PE, Orenstein SR, Wessel HB, Stowe

RM. Tardive dyskinesia associated with metoclopramide use in a child. *J Pediatr* 1992;121:983-5.

28. McCallum RW, Sowers JR, Hershman JM, Sturdevant RA. Metoclopramide stimulates prolactin secretion in man. *J Clin Endocrinol Metab* 1976;42:1148-52.

29. Brogden RN, Carmine AA, Heel RC, Speight TM, Avery GS. Domperidone: a review of its pharmacological activity, pharmacokinetics, and therapeutic efficacy in the symptomatic treatment of chronic dyspepsia and as an antiemetic. *Drugs* 1982;224:360-400.

30. Reyntjens AJ. Clinical pharmacology and therapeutics of domperidone. *Clin Res Rev* 1983;3:91-100.

31. Grill BB, Hillemeier AC, Semeraro LA, McCallum RW, Gryboski JD. Effects of domperidone therapy on symptoms and upper gastrointestinal motility in infants with gastroesophageal reflux. *J Pediatr* 1985; 106:311-6.

32. Grill BB, Logan LA, Schultz E. Prospective double-blind trial of domperidone versus placebo for gastroesophageal reflux in infants and children. *Pediatr Res* 1989;25:114A.

33. Bines JE, Quinlan JE, Treves S, Kleinman RE, Winter HS. Efficacy of domperidone in infants and children with gastroesophageal reflux. *J Pediatr Gastroenterol Nutr* 1992;14:400-5.

34. Champion MC, Harnett M, Yen M. Domperidone: a new dopamine antagonist. *Can Med Assoc J* 1986;135:457-61.

35. Steinherz R, Levy Y, Ban-Amati D, Shafrir Y, Nitzan M. Extrapyramidal reaction to domperidone [letter]. *Can Med Assoc* 1986;108:630-1.

36. McCallum RW, Prakash C, Campoli-Richards DM, Goa KL. Cisapride: a preliminary review of its pharmacodynamic and pharmacokinetic properties, and therapeutic use as a prokinetic agent in gastrointestinal motility disorders. *Drugs* 1988;36:652-81.

37. Van Peer A, Verlinden M, Woestenborghs R, Meuldermans W, Heykants J. Clinical pharmacokinetics of cisapride. In: Johnson AG, Lux G, eds. Progress in the Treatment of Gastrointestinal Motility Disorders: the Role of Cisapride. Amsterdam, The Netherlands: *Excerpta Medica.* 1988:23-9.

38. Veereman-Wauters G, Monbaliu J, Meuldermans W, Woestenborgs R, Verlinden M. Study of the placental transfer of cisapride in sheep: plasma levels in the pregnant ewe, the fetus, and the lamb. *Drug Metabolism and Disposition* 1991;19:168-72.

39. Hofmeyr GJ, Sonnendecker EW. Secretion of the gastrokinetic agent cisapride in human milk. *Eur J Clin Pharmacol* 1986;30:735-6.

40. Cucchiara S, Staiano A, Boccieri A, et al. Effects of cisapride on parameters of esophageal motility and on the prolonged intraesophageal pH tests in infants with gastro-esophageal reflux disease. *Gut* 1990;31:21-5.

41. Cucchiara S, Bortolotti M, Boccieri A, et al. Effects of cisapride on antroduodenal motility and on duodeno-gastric reflux in children with functional dyspepsia. *Ital J Gastroenterol* 1989;21:372.

42. Newell SJ. Cisapride: its use in children. *Br J Hosp Med* 1990;44:408-9.

43. Di Lorenzo C, Reddy SN, Villanueva-Meyer J, et al. Cisapride in children with chronic intestinal pseudo-obstruction: an acute double-blind, crossover, placebo-controlled trial. *Gastroenterology* 1991;101(6):1564-70.

44. Hyman PE, Di Lorenzo C, McAdams L, Flores AF, Tomomasa T, Garvey TQ. Predicting the clinical response to cisapride in children with chronic intestinal pseudo-obstruction. *Am J Gastroenterol* 1993;88:832-6.

45. Staiano A, Cucchiara S, Andreotti MR, Minella R, Manzi G. Effect of cisapride on chronic idiopathic constipation in children. *Dig Dis Sci* 1991;36:733-6.

46. Itoh Z, Nakaya M, Suzuki T, Arai H, Wakabayashi K. Erythromycin mimics exogenous motilin in gastrointestinal contractile activity in the dog. *Am J Physiol* 1984;247:G688-94.

47. Tomomasa T, Kuroume T, Arai H, Wakabayashi K, Itoh Z. Erythromycin induces migrating motor complex in human gastrointestinal tract. *Dig Dis Sci* 1986;31:157-61.

48. Peeters T, Matthis G, Depoortere I, Cachet T, Hoogmartens J, Vantrappen G. Erythromycin is a motilin receptor agonist. *Am J Physiol* 1989;257:G470-4.

49. Canatch SM, Fairclough PD. Erythromycin and the gut. *Gut* 1992;33:397-401.

50. Weber FH, Richards RD, McCallum RW. Erythromycin: a motilin agonist and gastrointestinal prokinetic agent. *Am J Gastroenterol* 1993;88:485-90.

51. Richards RD, Davenport K, McCallum RW. The treatment of idiopathic and diabetic gastroparesis with acute intravenous and chronic oral erythromycin. *Am J Gastroenterol* 1993;88(2):203-7.

52. Reid B, Di Lorenzo C, Travis L, Flores AF, Grill BB, Hyman PE. Diabetic gastroparesis due to postprandial antral hypomotility in childhood. *Pediatrics* 1992;90:43-6.

53. Vanderhoof J, Young R, Kaufman S, Ernst L. Treatment of cyclic vomiting in childhood with erythromycin. *J Pediatr Gastroenterol Nutr* 1993;17:387-91.

54. Mathias JR, Ferguson KL, Clench MH. Debilitating "functional" bowel disease controlled by leuprolide acetate, a gonadotropin-releasing hormone analogue. *Dig Dis Sci* 1989;34:761-6.

55. Mathias JR, Baskin GS, Reeves-Darby VG, et al. Chronic intestinal pseudo-obstruction in a patient with heart-lung transplant: therapeutic effect of leuprolide acetate. *Dig Dis Sci* 1992;37:1761-8.

56. Mathias JR, Clench MH, Reeves-Darby VG, Roberts PH, Smith LL. Effect of leuprolide acetate in patients with moderate-to-severe functional bowel disease: a double-blind placebo controlled study. *Gastroenterology* 1993;104:A548.

57. De Witte P, Lemli L. The metabolism of anthranoid laxatives. *Hepatogastroenterology* 1990;37:601-5.

58. Di Lorenzo C, Flores AF, Buie T, Hyman PE. Bisacodyl but not edrophonium stimulates high amplitude propagated colon contractions in children. *Gastroenterology* 1993;104:A498.

59. Soudah HC, Hasler WL, Owyang C. Effect of octreotide on intestinal motility and bacterial overgrowth in scleroderma. *N Engl J Med* 1991;325:1461-7.

60. Donowitz M, Levin S, Powers G, Elta G, Cohen P, Cheng H. Calcium channel blockers stimulate ileal and colon water absorption. *Gastroenterology* 1985;89:858-66.

61. Thollander M, Hellstrom PM, Svensson TH. Dihydropyridine calcium channel antagonists disrupt migrating myoelectric complexes and counteract intestinal disorders associated with morphine withdrawal diarrhea. *Scand J Gastroenterol* 1993;28:137-44.

62. Richter JE, Dalton CB, Bruice RG, Gastell DG. Nifedipine: a potent inhibitor of contractions in the body of the human esophagus. *Gastroenterology* 1985;89:549-54.

63. Fontan JP, Heldt GP, Heyman MB, Marin MS, Tooley WH. Esophageal spasm associated with apnea and bradycardia in an infant. *Pediatrics* 1984;73:52-5.

64. Battershill PE, Clissold SP. Octreotide: a review of its pharmacological and pharmacokinetic properties, and therapeutic potential in conditions associated with excessive peptide secretion. *Drugs* 1989;38:658-702.

65. Deivalle J. Application of somatostatin and its analogue octreotide in the therapy of gastrointestinal disorders. In: Wolfe MM, ed. *Gastrointestinal Pharmacotherapies*. Philadelphia, PA: WB Saunders, 1993;275-92.

26

Surgical Considerations: Upper Gastrointestinal Motility Disorders

J. BOIX-OCHOA, JOSEP M. CASASA, JOSEP M. GIL-VERNET, CLAUDIA MARHUENDA

This chapter covers the physiology, possibilities, limitations, and side effects of surgery on upper gastrointestinal motor disorders.

ESOPHAGEAL ATRESIA

Esophageal atresia is a congenital malformation that occurs in 1 of 3000 to 3500 newborns.[1] The most common type (87%) is atresia with a blind proximal pouch and a fistula from the distal segment to the trachea, or a bronchus. Pure esophageal atresia (ie, without fistula) is present in 8%, while tracheoesophageal fistula without atresia (the so-called H fistula) is present in 4%.[2]

The goal of surgery in esophageal atresia is to reestablish esophageal continuity. The most common surgical technique is ligation of the fistula and the end-to-end suture of both pouches by an extra- or transpleural approach, which is carried out during the neonatal period whenever possible. Gastrostomy is not the primary intervention, because it does not protect against anastomotic leaks and may delay gastric emptying and predispose to gastroesophageal reflux (GER).[3,4] Indications for gastrostomy include a distal obstruction (eg, duodenal atresia), postoperative incapacity for deglutition, and facilitation of repeated dilation of esophageal stricture.[5]

Cases with a great distance between segments (ie, "long-gap" atresia), are repaired using delayed end-to-end anastomoses: bougienage of the upper[6] or both pouches,[7] or circular myotomy of the upper segment according to Livaditis.[8] If these cannot be carried out, any technique of esophageal substitution by the colon, gastric tube, or small bowel may be performed, but these are the least satisfactory.[6]

Early complications include anastomotic leakage (20-30%), stricture of the suture line (20-40%), and recurrent fistula (5-10%).[3,5,9] Complications are found most frequently in long-gap atresia, in which excessive tension has been applied to create the anastomosis.[9]

Abnormal esophageal motility and consequent GER[10-12] may cause chronic symptoms such as regurgitation and vomiting, growth retardation, esophagitis, dysphagia, and a wide spectrum of respiratory manifestations.[13,14] Peristalsis is often absent because esophageal contractions tend to be simultaneous and feeble.[12] Inadequate contractions lead to a lack of peristalsis in the proximal esophagus or in a segment of the esophageal body,[11,15-17] or can result in a total incoordination of the motor waves in the proximal and distal esophagus.[10,18] With respect to the lower esophageal sphincter (LES), Romeo[10] found that the pressure and length of the sphincter was normal in 18 of 20 infants and relaxation was complete in all but one. Takano[18] found results within the normal range, although they were inferior in the group with GER. LeSouëf[17] found LES pressures within the normal range in 18 patients.

The etiology of motor disorders is controversial. In a postoperative manometric study there was total motor incoordination of the esophageal segments in all cases, suggesting that the alterations are part of the congenital malformation.[10] However, in contrast with Romeo's findings, in a pre- and postoperative study of a patient with esophageal atresia without a fistula, peristaltic contractions in the proximal esophagus during deglutition produced coordinated contractions of the distal segment and a reflex relaxation of the LES. In the postoperative study, simultaneous contractions and incomplete relaxation of the LES[19] suggested that dissection and mobilization during surgery may cause esophageal dysmotility in esophageal atresia.

The incidence of severe gastroesophageal reflux disease varies between 18%[3] and 35% and requires surgical intervention.[20] Shermeta[21] has suggested that severe GER might not be secondary to surgery, because vagotomy, sympathectomy, or esophageal transection and reanastomosis did not produce reflux in dogs. Moreover, two patients with a tracheoesophageal fistula without atresia presented with GER in the Parker series.[20] However, other authors have shown an incidence of GER eight times higher in patients with a long-gap esophageal atresia[9] and in those with early complications (eg, stenosis, recurrent fistula) requiring an esophageal resection.[22] This indicates that shortening the intra-abdominal esophagus and distorting the angle of His (produced by the dissection of the distal esophagus and the excessive tension on the suture line) can be important factors in the pathogenesis of GER.

Alterations in the motility of the esophageal body are practically universal in GER patients. Consequently, there is prolonged esophageal clearance predisposing to damage of the mucosa by gastric refluxate.

Indications for fundoplication in the treatment of GER for patients with esophageal atresia are similar to those for children with isolated GER: repeated pneumonia, apnea, growth retardation, or complications of esophagitis unresponsive to a vigorous medical treatment.[20,23-25] Respiratory manifestations (eg, bronchospasm, pneumonias) may be related to microaspiration. Alterations of esophageal motility, anastomotic stricture, recurrent fistula, tracheomalacia, congenital malformations of the heart, central nervous system, or the oropharynx are often associated with lung disease due to GER.[23] Persistent esophageal stenosis associated with GER is another indication for surgery. GER is most important in the first year of life, and is rarely diagnosed later in children with esophageal atresia.[22]

The most common surgery for reflux is Nissen's fundoplication. In most cases, the symptoms disappear and there are few complications.[3,20,24] Postoperative dysphagia is one possible complication. It may last several months and is probably produced by the incapacity of the anomalous esophagus to overcome the obstacle of the 360° fundoplication.[4,26] Failure of the fundoplication[27] with recurrence of reflux symptoms has an incidence of 33% in those patients with esophageal atresia, compared with the 10% who suffer isolated GER.

ACHALASIA

Achalasia of the esophagus is a motility disorder of unknown etiology, characterized by impaired or absent relaxation of the LES and failure of peristalsis in the body of the esophagus.[28] A few patients with achalasia present with aperistalsis alone and a completely relaxed LES,[29] but the basal pressure in the LES is usually increased. In some patients, high-amplitude, synchronous contractions are seen in the body of the esophagus. These patients have been described as having vigorous achalasia.[30]

The first case of muscular obstruction of the esophagus was described by the English anatomist Thomas Willis in 1674.[31] Hurst and Rake applied the term "achalasia" in 1930.[32]

Histopathologic and pharmacologic findings in patients suffering from achalasia indicate that its pathogenesis involves a denervation of the LES. This neurologic alteration can also be observed in the dorsal nuclei of the vagus and in the fibers of the vagus nerve. Some patients with achalasia lack ganglion cells and postganglionic fibers in the myenteric plexus of Auerbach.[33] Achalasia patients have a significantly reduced number of the nerve fibers that carry vasoactive intestinal polypeptide (VIP).[34] These fibers constitute nonadrenergic-noncholinergic inhibitory innervation. Decreased VIP has been related to the increased tone and incomplete relaxation of the LES, which characterizes achalasia. In a recent study[35] on muscle specimens from eight patients with achalasia and six controls, there was no detectable activity of nitric oxide synthase in the samples from patients with achalasia. Thus, the absence of nitric oxide synthase and VIP in the myenteric plexus may explain the functional abnormalities of the LES in achalasia.

The high frequency of achalasia in adults and older children suggests that it is an acquired disease. When it appears within the first 6 months of life, the existence of family cases and its association to genetic diseases suggests that it might be a congenital problem in some children.[36] One series showed a family occurrence of achalasia that affected several brothers, adults, and children.[37] An autosomal-recessive inheritance is suggested because the disorder affects equal numbers of males and females.[38]

Achalasia also may be associated with congenital alterations such as the triple-A syndrome (ie, achalasia, alacrima, and insensibility to adrenocorticotropic hormone),[39] Alport's syndrome,[40] or Rozycki syndrome (ie, deafness, vitiligo, small size, and muscular weakness).[41]

Symptoms

Achalasia is characterized by an insidious onset, in which symptoms present for months. Dysphagia or the sensation of something being "stuck" is the main symptom. It is sometimes more noticeable with liquids than with solids, and varies depending on the size and features of each swallow. The intensity of symptoms increases slowly but progressively. During the last stages of the disease, dysphagia is constant with both liquids and solids. Regurgitation of undigested food, the next most frequent symptom in achalasia,[42,43] is the initial symptom in children.[44] Regurgitations may cause pulmonary aspiration manifested by night cough or other pulmonary complications.

Pain defined as a feeling of a knot or spasm at a retrosternal level is usually an early symptom that tends to disappear as the esophagus dilates. Within the evolution of the disease, this symptom is more common in adults than in children.

Weight loss is directly related to the severity of dysphagia. The fear of eating, however, also causes weight loss because the patients' troubles are related to deglutition.

Symptoms in infants vary according to the patient's age. In small infants, respiratory problems and weight loss are predominant,[36] while symptoms in older children are similar to those of adults with dysphagia and regurgitation.

Diagnosis

The diagnosis is based on a detailed history. Confirmation is provided by radiology, esophageal manometry, isotopic studies, and esophageal endoscopy.

In radiologic studies, the barium swallow will show the absence of esophageal peristalsis, no relaxation of the LES, and dilation of the esophageal body. Esophageal images will vary according to the phase of the disease and the type of achalasia (ie, typical or vigorous). A discrete dilation in the esophagus might be observed in a patient suffering from typical achalasia in its initial phase, while more advanced stages of the disease may show greater esophageal dilation or, rarely, pseudosigmoidal pictures. In vigorous achalasia, tertiary contractions accompany a discrete esophageal dilation and a sharpening of the gastroesophageal union. This image has been compared to a pencil point and expresses insufficient or absent relaxation of the LES. Loss of the gastric air fluid level does not have a diagnostic value.

Esophageal manometry can demonstrate the complete loss of all peristaltic activity and the lack of relaxation of the LES (diagnostic data in achalsia). It can also determine whether achalasia is typical or vigorous. In typical achalasia, aperistalsis is found in the esophageal body. In vigorous achalasia, tertiary waves following swallows and the absence of LES relaxation are typical findings.

Isotopic studies of esophageal emptying may be useful for a quantitative assessment of efficacy after treatment.

Direct visualization of the esophageal muscosa by esophageal endoscopy is necessary to determine the presence or absence of ulcer, stricture, or tumor that caused symptoms and signs mimicking achalasia. Endoscopy should always be performed before any treatment for achalasia.

Differential Diagnosis

Scleroderma. Scleroderma is very rare in children. Sometimes the clinical and radiologic manifestations of esophageal scleroderma may be confused with achalasia. The skin and pulmonary manifestations of the scleroderma patient combined with the persistence of peristaltic waves in the proximal esophagus will be favorable data towards the diagnosis of progressive systematic sclerosis.

Chagas' disease. When a patient resides or has traveled in South America, particularly Brazil, or another country at risk, infection by Cruz's trypanosomiasis must be considered. In its chronic form, clinical manifestations may be similar to those of achalasia. Dilations of other structures, such as the megacholedochus, megaduodenum, or megacolon, are suggestive of this infection. Diagnosis is accomplished with a complement fixation test for Chagas' disease.

Treatment

Treatment should reduce LES pressure and thus minimize resistance to antegrade flow of food. This aim can be achieved with pharmacologic agents, forced dilation of the LES, or surgical cardiomyotomy.

Pharmacology. Pharmacologic treatment has been tried with different smooth-muscle relaxants, which are indicated when the clinical symptoms are caused by the presence of very powerful esophageal contractions or by incomplete relaxation of the LES.

Calcium antagonists reduce the pressure of the LES and the esophageal body, improving emptying and relieving the symptoms.[45] Its side effects are dizziness and skin rash. Sublingual nifedipine has been useful in the short-term management of achalasia in children.[46] Drug tolerance develops after weeks to months of use.

Dilation of the LES. The first description

of achalasia and its treatment through dilation is attributed to Thomas Willis.[31] In 1821, Ashley Cooper used bougies for the first time.

To obtain a clinical remission, it is necessary to make a sudden dilation of the esophageal union so that the resistance offered by the LES can be overcome and the transit of swallowed food through the esophagus is facilitated.[47,48] A passive dilation with mercury bougies produces a partial and transitory improvement of dysphagia.[49,50] A pneumatic dilation tries to tear the musculature of the LES.

A pneumatic dilation is performed with a guided catheter. Attached to its distal end is a polyurethane balloon 8 to 15 cm long, which expands to a maximum of up to 2 cm in diameter when inflated to the appropriate pressure. It may be placed under endoscopic control, although fluoroscopy is preferred because the balloon tends to displace itself. Fluoroscopy also allows insufflation of a contrast substance inside the ball, which permits direct observation of the dilation of the LES. Dilations last approximately 2 minutes, and progress until a diameter no larger than that of the esophageal body is reached, allowing 3 minutes' rest between dilations. The pneumatic dilation is a painful procedure and should be carried out under general anesthesia. A contrast study of the esophagus must always be performed 24 hours after dilation to assess complications such as perforations. Efficacy may be assessed by radiology, which demonstrates the decreased size of the esophagus, and by manometry, but the best measure of success is the disappearance of symptoms.[51-53]

Surgery. In 1913, Heller[54] devised a surgical intervention to treat a patient with achalasia who had not responded to dilation. He performed an extramucosal longitudinal myotomy carried out on the front and rear walls of the distal esophagus and the gastric cardia. Among the different modifications to this technique, the most popular is the esophagomyotomy proposed by Zaaijer in 1923.[55] The goal of myotomy is to relieve the barrier effect of the LES, which is responsible for the esophageal retention and, consequently, the dilation. Myotomy is accepted as the main principle in surgical treatment, but the best approach and myotomy's association with the antireflux procedure remain controversial. A left thoractomy is sometimes used[56-63] but most surgeons prefer the abdominal approach through a supraumbilical laparotomy up to the xyphoid.[63-70]

Successful isolated myotomy does not surpass 1 cm and respects the structures that attach the esophagus to the diaphragm.[56,58,64,65] The isolated esophagomyotomy decreases LES pressure, but the LES retains enough residual pressure to prevent GER, and even responds with pressure increases to the rise of intra-abdominal pressure. Underestimation will result in persistence of dysphagia. Overestimation causes GER. Twenty percent of patients with myotomy suffer from symptoms of GER.[71]

A wide and complete myotomy will diminish the tone of the LES so that it does not resist the passing of the bolus, necessitating an antireflux procedure,[72] as described below.

The first attempt to treat this disease should be pneumatic dilation. Surgical treatment should be used if the first two or three dilations fail. A long myotomy with the antireflux procedure is very successful, and eliminates reflux[72] after treatment. All treatments for achalasia—whether pharmacologic, dilatory, or surgical—are considered palliative, because they do not reestablish esophageal peristalsis and relaxation of the LES. However, recent studies by Cucchiara[73] show reestablishment of peristalsis and relaxation of the LES in children and adults after pneumatic dilation or surgical treatment. Posttreatment follow-up is necessary so that possible development of neoplasia can be detected. Functional recovery of the esophagus should be observed clinically, radiologically, and manometrically.

INDICATIONS AND CONTRAINDICATIONS FOR ANTIREFLUX SURGERY

The esophagogastric junction fulfills a double mission. On the one hand, it allows the free passage of ingested materials from the mouth to the stomach. On the other hand, it prevents the reflux of gastric contents back into the esophagus.

Fixation of the Esophagastric Union

It is vitally important to the proper functioning of the esophagastric union that its fixation to the neighboring structures be correct, so that the inferior segment of the esophagus is permanently in the abdomen.[74] Fixation depends on the integrity of a series of elements, the most important ones being the frenoesophageal membrane and the diaphragmatic hiatus. The tone of the diaphragmatic muscle is vital for the muscular hiatus to exactly adapt itself to the inferior esophagus, thus allowing the frenoesophageal membrane to remain tense and firm. A relaxed hiatus may leave too wide a hole, causing the frenoesophageal membrane to elongate, losing its resistance. Thus, the inferior esophagus and part of the tuberosity of the stomach may easily ascend to the thorax. When this happens, the valvular antireflux mechanism stops functioning; the LES may cause minimal opposition and, consequently, GER results. Hiatal tone is weak in patients with neurologic problems, Down syndrome, and those operated on because of diaphragmatic hernia. Loss of tone also may be acquired under other circumstances. For instance, the digestive troubles which provoke frequent vomiting in some unweaned babies may relax and open the hiatal zone due to the efforts of each vomit. Repetitive frequent coughing and exaggerated negative thoracic pressures (as in asthma and bronchopulmonary dysplasia) stress the anatomic relationships of the inferior esophagus. If the anatomy is disrupted, GER may result.

The esophagastric union must keep a perfect balance between the forces that can open it and those which keep it closed.[75] GER may cause emesis, pyrosis, retrosternal pain, or bronchospasm. It may also produce severe esophagitis with hemorrhage and stricture, especially if the refluxate is acidic.

Closing Mechanisms

Knowledge of the forces which close the esophagastric union and of those which favor its opening is indispensable to understanding the therapy for GER. Such knowledge can explain why medical treatment is so successful in many cases, and can help select the optimal surgical solution based on indications.

There are three different closing mechanisms: 1) the LES, 2) the intra-abdominal esophagus, and 3) the angle of His.

Lower esophageal sphincter. A high-pressure zone in the lower esophagus acts independently from other factors. Liebermann[76,77] demonstrated muscular thickening in this zone. A research study with cats revealed that this sphincter protected against GER even when the esophagus separated itself from its surrounding structures.[78] This high-pressure zone, however, does not function well during the first days of life. A rise of pressure in this zone is not influenced by birth weight or gestational age[79] and does not appear until children are 6 to 7 weeks of age. These findings can lead to a false conclusion that all reflux detected before 6 weeks of life is physiologic. It must be noted that the high-pressure zone of the lower esophagus is only one of the factors which act as barriers against reflux.

Intra-abdominal esophagus. The intra-abdominal segment is essential to the integrity of the gastroesophageal junction.[80,81] When intra-abdominal pressure increases, it is equally distributed throughout the abdominal esophagus and the stomach. The intra-abdominal segment then collapses, and flow stops due to the compression on the abdominal esophagus.

Because the pressure in a hollow viscus is inversely related to its radius, the narrower the tube, the less wall tension is required to close it. Assuming the ratio of the effective diameter of the esophagus to that of the stomach is 1:5, the pressure in the abdominal esophagus only needs to increase to 1/5 of the intragastric pressure for the esophagus to close. A long enough segment of abdominal esophagus is the best guarantee of a good barrier against reflux.

The negative pressure in the thoracic esophagus also produces a suctioning effect, emptying the abdominal segment and, in doing so, helps to keep the segment closed.[82] The intra-abdominal esophageal segment acts like a flutter valve. Although it is easy to blow through such a tube, it is impossible to suck back through it.

Angle of His. The acuteness of the gastroesophageal angle is important. When the patient attempts to vomit, more fluid strikes the fundus than escapes through the esophagus. The pressure of the fluid striking the fundus decreases the angle and squeezes the esophagus, closing it. If the angle is obtuse, however, the upper stomach is converted into a funnel and all the fluids are directed towards the esophagus.

Factors That Inhibit Closing

Abnormal esophageal motility. Without interfering with normal closing mechanisms per se, an alteration of esophageal transit may appear as a consequence of esophagitis or as a primary disorder, thus failing to effectively clear noxious refluxate from the esophagus.

Gastric retention. The fundus is essential for achieving a good peristaltic wave of gastric contraction, which propels the contents through the pylorus into the duodenum. The reconstruction of a good gastric fundus improves evacuation of the stomach, so that it is not necessary to perform pyloroplasty in addition to fundoplication.

Increased intra-abdominal pressure. When intra-abdominal pressure rises, intragastric pressure increases, putting more pressure on the gastroesophageal junction. This occurs in children who suffer from frequent attacks of coughing or in those who are constipated and expend great effort by contracting their abdominal muscles while defecating.

Lack of coordination between gastric peristalsis and opening of the pylorus is observed in infants who take antispasmodic medication. This type of medication should not be used in infants because it leads to serious iatrogenic abnormalities. Afflictions of the stomach such as gastritis, tumors, duplications, and ulcers can also cause uncoordinated movements.

Gastric wall tension. The first three factors discussed above produce retention and dilation. These in turn generate a force created by increasing tension of the gastric wall in the direction of the muscle fibers extending from the esophagus. The length of the sphincter is reduced until the sphincter opens. To illustrate, compare the stomach and the lower esophagus to a balloon. As the balloon is blown up, the neck (lower esophagus) shortens gradually. Similarly, competence is lost in the stomach and LES, thus allowing reflux. In a balloon, the pressure then decreases and the length of neck is restored. This demonstrates that the longer the intra-abdominal segment, the less important the gastric wall tension.[83]

Surgical Treatment

There are some basic principles to bear in mind:

1. GER often responds well to medical-postural treatment;

2. In infancy, GER tends to improve with age;

3. Surgery must only be used in special cases.

Circumstances that might modify the disposition towards surgery for GER include:

1. GER before the first year of life;

2. GER in infants over 1 year of age;

3. GER in patients with chronic respiratory disease;

4. GER in patients with Sandifer syndrome;

5. GER in patients with retardation and Down syndrome;

6. GER in patients with uncooperative families.

Surgery to prevent GER before the first year of life. During the first 6 weeks of life, GER can be due to the lack of maturity of the high-pressure zones of the inferior esophagus. Usually postural and medical treatment is effective and babies stop vomiting within a few weeks. These reasons are strong enough to avoid surgical intervention for most neonates.

After postural and medical treatment, when a baby affected with GER reaches the age of 12 to 14 months and is asymptomatic, studies should be initiated to see if GER persists silently or if it has disppeared. A radiologic test will show if it still persists. If so, 24-hour esophageal pH-metry and endoscopy must be performed. Surgical intervention is suggested if both tests are pathologic, although clinically the child might seem to recover.

GER therapy in children over 1 year of age. This pathology has a tendency to spontaneously evolve towards recovery. An undiagnosed child over 1 year of age who has digestive symptoms with repeated vomiting, dysphagia, or blood in the vomit has not evolved towards a spontaneous recovery. Endoscopy, esophageal biopsy, pH-metry tests confirm the aggressiveness of the GER and help determine whether surgery is appropriate.

GASTROESOPHAGEAL REFLUX AND OTHER PATHOLOGIES
Respiratory Problems

Gastroesophageal reflux has been considered an important cause of recurrent bronchitis, asthma, and sudden infant death syndrome (SIDS).[84,85] In the United States, particularly, infants admitted to hospital for apnea or "missed SIDS" routinely undergo evaluations for GER.

Some physicians believe that a 24-hour intraesophageal pH record demonstrating abnormal quantities of reflux in an infant with "missed SIDS" is sufficient criteria for fundoplication (see Chapter 4). In our opinion, GER rarely, if ever, causes "missed SIDS" or acid-induced reflex apnea; in the absence of a clear temporal relationship between GER and apnea, such infants should not receive operations.

Sandifer Syndrome

Surgical intervention is indicated in the presence of Sandifer syndrome.[86] The roentgenographic diagnosis of GER or a positive 24-hour pH-metry are sufficient documentation in the presence of the characteristic posturing.

Retardation or Down Syndrome

Gastroesophageal reflux in these children can be a constant cause of vomiting.[87] Surgical intervention is indicated.

Social Problems

It must be emphasized that postural and medical treatment is appropriate when the child's family understands and collaborates. If there is clear evidence of noncompliance, it is better to suggest surgical intervention to avoid any possible troubles caused by uncontrolled GER.

TREATMENT OF GER
Surgery

The best surgical technique is one which reinforces the closing mechanisms of the inferior esophagus. In 1951, Allison[88] reported that the abdominal esophagus could have an important role in GER.

In 1953, Duhamel[89] turned his attention towards the antireflux features of a good angle of His. He presented eight successful cases. In 1955, Boerema[90] proposed a simple procedure for babies, approached through the abdomen. A segment of the esophagus was placed into the abdomen, pulling it from the stomach downwards by fixing with stitches the minor curvature to the musculature of the anterior wall of the abdomen. He achieved excellent results, although among these children there was a high percentage who would have recovered without the intervention.

In 1959, Nissen[91] and Bettex[92] each reasoned that reinforcing the external esophagus through an external procedure would secure the closing mechanism of the esophagus. Nissen's proposal was fundoplication, which consisted of using the gastric fundus to surround the inferior esophagus, passing it by the back from left to right, joining it

with the gastric body at the front, and lacing it up with stitches. This technique became popular with most pediatric surgeons. The radiologic reflux disappeared and manometrics showed a good area of high pressure in the inferior esophagus.

Fundoplication is still a common technique, although its failures and complications are not insignificant. Thus, in 1981 Leonardi[93] reported 14 dysphagias, seven GER recurrences, two "gas bloat" syndromes, and two paraesophagic hernias out of 25 cases. In 1983, De Laet and Spitz[94] reported 8% reinterventions. In 1983, Negre[95] discovered that only 24% of 226 cases of adult fundoplications remained asymptomatic; many patients presented with dysphagia, deglutition problems, intestinal gas, or the inability to vomit. In 1986, Jolley[96] reported 6.1% of intestinal obstructions after a fundoplication, which he described as intestinal motility disorders that appear due to the intervention when the root of the mesentery is rotated. In 1987, Glick[97] presented two cases of gastric infarction; according to him they were produced by the inability of eructation and vomiting in the patients, which caused a sudden dilation of the stomach. In the same year, Idowu[98] published a report of visceral ischemia following gastric dilation which had appeared 2 years after fundoplication. Also in 1987, Dedinsky[99] recorded 69 complications among 429 postsurgical patients. Of these, 28 had to be reoperated. Wilkins and Spitz[100] also found 18 cases of intestinal obstruction in 16 of 156 operated patients. These authors had carried out 65 appendectomies and 13 sections of left anterior descending diagonal bands, taking advantage of a laparotomy. The obstructions occurred in patients who could not vomit. In 1988, Alrabeeah[101] presented 15 paraesophagic hernias as postoperative complications among 89 operated patients. In that same year, Low[102] presented a series of 116 cases of adults who had to be reoperated after the fundoplication. In 1990, Kiely[103] presented another case of intestinal occlusion aggravated by the fact that the child could not vomit.

Summarizing the above cases, the complications observed in patients receiving fundoplication are:

1. impossibility of burping or vomiting;
2. rise of the fundoplication to the thorax;
3. paraesophageal hernias;
4. gastric and intestinal infarction;
5. obstruction due to adhesions.

Despite good results, many[104-106] decided to modify the technique by loosening the fundoplication,[107,108] reducing it to half its size,[109,110] or fixing the esophagus to the hiatus.[111,112] The Thal modification[113,114] consists of mobilizing the esophagus, closing the hiatus at the back, and fixing the esophagus to the hiatus, leaving about 2 cm of posterior abdominal esophagus. The procedure is completed with an upward plicature towards the anterior wall of the fundus that covers the anterior wall of the esophagus.

Physiologic Treatment

In 1966, a surgical procedure was developed that would not modify the normal anatomy of the zone as fundoplication[115] does (Fig. 26.1). Basing the study on the physiopathology of the GER, the conclusion was reached that the key to the problem was to ensure an intra-abdominal esophagus, the cornerstone of the antireflux mechanism. With an intra-abdominal esophagus, the mucosal choke and the gastroesophageal angle (His) can act as antireflux factors.[116]

A good angle of His is important to hinder GER. This angle is formed by the esophagus and the fundus. The sharper it is, the more it opposes the reflux. As the stomach distends, its acuteness is accentuated, thus increasing its opposition to backward flow. The angle acts as a valve.

Another problem remained to be solved:

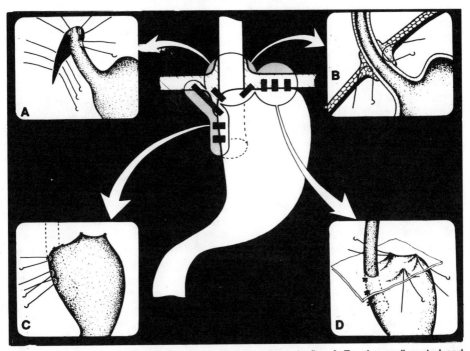

Fig. 26.1 Philosophy of surgical technique for gastroesophageal reflux. **A,** Esophagus dissected, and the length of the intra-abdominal esophagus restored. **B,** The esophagophrenic ligament and esophageal muscular wall are sutured to the edges of the crura and the crura behind the esophagus is tightened. **C,** The angle of His is restored by a suture taken from the fundus at the level of the highest short gastric level, which is sectioned, tied, and taken as reference point to the muscular rim of the hiatus superiorly and to the right. The reinforcing sutures maintaining the stomach in this position are placed between the fundus and the anterior esophageal wall. **D,** The fundus is unfolded by suspending sutures (three in a triangle) from the fundus to the diaphragm.

the gastric fundus had to be kept upwards and could not be left hanging loose in the abdomen. It had to be fixed to the inferior wall of the diaphragm so that it could maintain the security of the angle of His. The perfect anatomic location of the esophagus, the fundus, and angle of His was thus completed, as nature intended.

Later, as a security maneuver, the minor curvature of the stomach was fixed to the anterior abdominal wall, following Boerema's technique, to assure the length of the abdominal esophagus. This fixation is still advisable in those cases in which the GER affects children with psychomotor retardation or Down syndrome.

Summarizing the above, the physiologic technique achieves the following:

1. recovers the normal anatomy of the high-pressure zone;

2. improves esophageal motility because the esophagus is kept tractioned and free of undulations;

3. the rate of gastric emptying increases as the fundus is positioned upwards;

4. GER is avoided because the positive abdominal pressures are able to act on the inferior esophagus, due to the maximum severity of the angle of His;

5. there is no obstruction to interfere with the expulsion of gasses and the vomiting mechanism.

Gastrostomy

A patient who does not require gastrostomy for feedings or venting, but who has undergone a correct surgical intervention to treat GER, will not require a gastrostomy.

Some authors recommend it. Rohatgi et al,[117] for example, in 1971 practiced it in three out of 86 interventions so that the stomach was left well secured in the interior of the abdomen. In five other cases, gastrostomy was performed to carry out retrograde dilations and in another four to allow feeding. In 1983, Randolph[105] used it in all his operated patients under 3 months of age and in many older ones too. He left it for 3 months, considering it necessary for gastric decompression after fundoplication. In 1987, Wilkins and Spitz[100] practiced it 17 times in a series of 156 operated patients who were either dysmorphic or mentally retarded. Also in 1987, Dedinsky et al[99] practiced it in 385 out of 429 fundoplication interventions, for a total of 89%. This series is heterogeneous, comprising 297 neurologic patients whose ages ranged from 27-day-old babies to 18-year-olds.

Gastrostomy is useful for feeding children with esophageal strictures. These situations are rare thanks to the early diagnosis of GER and the possibility of postural and medical treatments during the first months of life.

Some neurologic patients who cannot be fed orally will require gastrostomy.[118] But in many of these patients, the condition that requires the gastrostomy is not GER, but impaired swallowing.

Pyloroplasty

The practice of performing pyloromyotomy in association with an antireflux procedure is common to achieve quicker gastric emptying. In 1963, Casten et al[119] ascertained that patients with hiatal hernias who presented with severe complications also suffered from duodenal ulcer. When they performed fundoplication, they sectioned the vagus to reduce gastric acid secretion. Pyloroplasty was associated with a double intention: they could directly inspect the antrum and the duodenum looking for peptic ulcers, and improve the rate of gastric emptying.

Some pediatric surgeons incorporated the pyloroplasty into their antireflux interventions,[117,120-122] but it is not necessary or even desirable. An antireflux technique will best respect the anatomic conditions of the zone. Pyloroplasty reduces coordination of gastric emptying between the stomach and duodenum. Thus, the digestive physiology is altered and "dumping" may result. When the fundus is fixed to the diaphragm through the upper gastropexy, its contraction capacity is increased—thus maximizing gastric emptying, especially with liquids.

No gastroduodenal peptic pathology concomitant in childhood GER has been found to justify a vagotomy and a pyloroplasty. Thus, it is preferable not to modify the antropyloroduodenal segment. Such a pathology does not naturally exist in children and should not be created.

Results

From 1966 to 1992, 2566 patients affected with GER were evaluated. In our series, there were 65 cases with large hiatal hernias. Surgery was performed on 244 (8.6%).

In a follow-up of 180 postsurgical cases, which ranged from 2-year-olds up to 18-year-olds, the clinical and radiologic results were excellent in 168, or 94.4% In 12, radiologic evidence of GER continued, but without any symptoms. In two cases treated during the first years, reoperation was necessary.

Complications included three intestinal obstructions by adhesions, five postoperative pneumonias, one mediastinitis due to perforation, and two persistent esophageal stenoses. There were two deaths in unweaned babies who had marasmus. This experience demonstrates that GER surgery is not an emergency procedure, but a last resort. The patient must have recovered from acute illness and failed trials of optimal medical treatment before definitive surgical intervention for GER is executed.

REFERENCES

1. Koch A, Rohr S, Plaschkes J. Incidence of gastroesophageal atresia. *Prog Pediatr Surg* 1986;19:103-13.

2. Cudmore RE. In: Lister J, Irving I, eds. *Neonatal Surgery,* 3rd ed. London, England: Butterworth, 1990.

3. Spitz L, Kiely E, Brereton RJ. Esophageal atresia: Five year experience with 148 cases. *J Pediatr Surg* 1987;22:103-8.

4. Wheatley MJ, Coran AG, Wesley JR. Efficacy of the Nissen fundoplication in the management of gastroesophageal reflux following esophageal atresia repair. *J Pediatr Surg* 1993;28:53-5.

5. Bishop PJ, Philippart KAI, Hixson DS, Hertzler JH. Transpleural repair of esophageal atresia without a primary gastrostomy: 240 patients treated between 1951 and 1983. *J Pediatr Surg* 1985;20:823-8.

6. Howard R, Myers WA. Esophageal atresia: A technique for elongation of the upper pouch. *Surgery* 1965;58:725-7.

7. Hays DM, Wooley MM, Snyder WH. Changing techniques in the management of esophageal atresia. *Arch Surg* 1966;92:611-16.

8. Livaditis A, Radberg L, Odensjö G. Esophageal end-to-end anastomosis. Reduction of anastomotic tension by circular myotomy. *Scand J Thorac Cardiovasc Surg* 1972;6:206-14.

9. Sillén U, Hagberg S, Rubenson A, Werkmäster K. Management of esophageal atresia: Review of 16 year's experience. *J Pediatr Surg* 1988;23:805-9.

10. Romeo G, Zuccarello B, Proietto F, Romeo C. Disorders of the esophageal motor activity in atresia of the esophagus. *J Pediatr Surg* 1987;22:120-4.

11. Schneeberger AL, Scott RB, Rubin SZ, Machida H. Esophageal function following Livaditis repair of long-gap esophageal atresia. *J Pediatr Surg* 1987;22:779-83.

12. Orringer MB, Kirsch MM, Sloan H. Long-term esophageal function following repair of esophageal atresia. *Ann Surg* 1977;186:436-43.

13. Shepard R, Fenn S, Sieber WK. Evaluation of esophageal function in postoperative esophageal atresia and tracheoesophageal fistula. *Surgery* 1966;59:608-17.

14. Burgess JN, Carlson HC, Ellis FH. Esophageal function after successful repair of esophageal atresia and tracheo-esophageal fistula. A manometric and cine-fluorographic study. *J Thorac Cardiovasc Surg* 1968;56:667-73.

15. Werlin SL, Dodds WJ, Hogan WJ, et al. Esophageal function in esophageal atresia. *Dig Dis Sci* 1981;26:796-800.

16. Winter HS, Madara JL, Stafford RJ, et al. Delayed acid clearance and esophagitis after repair of esophageal atresia *Gastroenterology* 1981;80:1317. Abstract.

17. LeSouëf PN, Myers NA, Landau LI. Etiologic

factors in long-term respiratory function abnormalities following esophageal atresia repair. *J Pediatr Surg* 1987;22:918-22.

18. Takano K, Iwafuchi M, Uchiyama M, et al. Evaluation of lower esophageal sphincter function in infants and children following esophageal surgery. *J Pediatr Surg* 1988;23:410-4.

19. Shono T, Suita S, Arima T, et al. Motility function of the esophagus before primary anastomosis in esophageal atresia. *J Pediatr Surg* 1993;28:673-6.

20. Parker AF, Christie DL, Cahill JL. Incidence and significance of GER following repair of esophageal atresia and tracheoesophageal fistula and the need for anti-reflux procedures. *J Pediatr Surg* 1979;14:5-8.

21. Shermeta DW, Whitington PF, Seto DA, Haller A. Lower esophageal sphincter dysfunction in esophageal atresia: Nocturnal regurgitation and aspiration pneumonia. *J Pediatr Surg* 1977;12:871-6.

22. Koch A, Rohr S, Plaschkes J, Bettex M. Incidence of gastroesophageal reflux following repair of esophageal atresia. *Prog Pediatr Surg* 1987;19:103-13.

23. Jolley SG, Johnson DG, Roberts CC, et al. Patterns of gastroesophageal reflux in children following repair of esophageal atresia and distal tracheosophageal fistula. *J Pediatr Surg* 1980;15:857-62.

24. Ashcraft KW, Goodwin C, Amoury RA, Holder TM. Early recognition and aggressive treatment of gastroesophageal reflux following repair of esophageal atresia. *J Pediatr Surg* 1977;12:317-21.

25. Montgomery M, Frenckner B. Esophageal pH monitoring for detecting gastroesophageal reflux in children with repaired esophageal atresia. *Pediatr Surg Int* 1991;6:304-5.

26. Curci MR, Dibbins AW. Problems associated with a Nissen fundoplication following tracheoesophageal fistula and esophageal atresia repair. *Arch Surg* 1988;123:618-20.

27. Lindahl H, Rintala R, Louhimo I. Failure of the Nissen fundoplication to control gastroesophageal reflux in esophageal atresia patients. *J Pediatr Surg* 1989;24:985-7.

28. Vantrappen G, Hellemans J. Achalasia. In: Vantrappen G, Hellemans J, eds. *Diseases of the Esophagus*. New York: Springer-Verlag;1975;287-354.

29. Katz PO, Richter JE, Cowan R, Castell DO. Apparent complete lower esophageal sphincter relaxation in achalasia. *Gastroenterology* 1986;90:978-83.

30. Goldenberg SP, Burrell M, Fette GG, Vos C, Traube M. Classic and vigorous achalasia: a comparison of manometric, radiographic, and clinical findings. *Gastroenterology*. 1991;101:743-8.

31. Willis T. Five diatribe de medicamentorum; operationibus in humano corpore. *Long Hauge-Comitis* 1674:18-9.

32. Hurst AF, Rake GW. Achalasia of the cardias. *Q J Med* 1930;23:491.

33. Csendes A, Smok G, Braghetto I, Ramirez C, Velasco N, Henriquez A. Gastroesophageal sphincter pressure and histological changes in distal esophagus in patients with achalasia of the esophagus. *Dig Dis Sci* 1985;30:941-5.

34. Aggestrup S, Uddman R, Sundler F, et al. Lack of vasoactive intestinal polypeptide nerves in esophageal achalasia. *Gastroenterology* 1983;84:924-7.

35. Mearin F, Mourelle M, Guarner F, et al. Patients with achalasia lack nitric oxide sinthase in the gastroesophageal junction. *Eur J Clin Invest* 1993;23:724-8.

36. Nihoul-Fékéte C, Bawab F, Lortat-Jacob S, Arhan P, Pellerin D. Achalasia of the esophagus in childhood: surgical treatment in 35 cases with special reference to familial cases and glucocorticoid deficiency association. *J Pediatr Surg*. 1989;24:1060-3.

37. Monning PJ. Familial achalasia in children. *Ann Thorac Surg* 1990;49:1019-22.

38. Tryhus MR, Davis M, Griffith JK, Ablin DS, Gogel HK. Familial achalasia in two siblings: significance of possible hereditary role. *J Pediatr Surg* 1989;24:292-5.

39. Tuck JS, Bisset RAL, Doig CM. Achalasia of the cardia in childhood and the syndrome of achalasia alacrima and ACTH insensitivity. *Clin Radiol* 1991;44:260-4.

40. Leichter HE, Vargas J, Cohen AH, Ament M, Salusky IB. Alport's syndrome and achalasia. *Pediatr Nephrol* 1988;2:312-4.

41. Rozycki DL, Ruben RJ, Rapin I, Spiro AJ. Autosomal recessive deafness associated with short stature, vitiligo, muscle wasting, and achalasia. *Arch Otolaryngol* 1971;93:194-7.

42. Ellis FH Jr, Olsen AM. *Achalasia of the Esophagus.* Philadelphia, PA: WB Saunders; 1969.

43. Mora F, Tomas-Ridocci M, Moreno-Osset E, et al. Valoración clinica en los trastornos motores esofágicos primarios (TMEP): analisis de 80 casos. *Gastroenterologia y Hepatologia* 1982;5:17-23.

44. Vantrappen G, Hellemens J. Motility disturbances of the esophagus: Achalasia. In: Vantrappen G, Hellemans J, eds. *Diseases of the Esophagus.* New York, NY: Springer-Verlag, 1974:287-354.

45. Hongo M, Traube M, McCallister R, McCallum RW. Effects of nifedipine on esophageal motor function in humans: correlation with plasma nifedipine concentration. *Gastroenterology* 1984;86:8-12.

46. Smith H, Buick R. The use of nifedipine for treatment of achalasia in children. *J Pediatr Gastroenterol Nutr* 1988;7:146.

47. Vantrappen G, Hellemans J. Treatment of achalasia and related motor disorders. *Gastroenterology* 1980;79:11-154.

48. Bennet JR. Treatment of achalasia: a review. *J R Soc Med* 1980;73:649-54.

49. Yon J, Christensen J. An uncontrolled comparison of treatment for achalasia. *Ann Surg* 1975;183:672-6.

50. Clouse RE. The esophagus-motor disorders. In: Sleisenger MH, Fordtran JS, eds. *Gastrointestinal Disease,* 4th ed. Philadelphia, PA: WB Saunders; 1989:559-93.

51. Vantrappen G, Hellemans J, Deloof W, Valembois P, Vandenbroucke J. Treatment of achalasia with pneumatic dilatations. *Gut* 1971;12:268-75.

52. Csendes A, Strauszer T. Long-term clinical, radiological, and manometric follow-up of patients with achalasia treated with pneumatic dilatation. *Digestion* 1974;11:127-8.

53. Heitmann P, Wienbeck M. The immediate effect of successful pneumatic dilatation on esophageal function in achalasia. *Scand J Gastroenterol* 1972;7:197-204.

54. Heller E. Extramuköse cardioplastik beim chronischen cardiospasmns mit dilatation des oesophagus. *Mitt Grenzgeb Med Chir* 1913;27:141.

55. Zaaijer JH. Cardiospasm in the aged. *Ann Surg* 1923;77:615-7.

56. Duranceau A, Lafontaine ER, Vallières B. Effects of total fundoplication on function of the esophagus after myotomy for achalasia. *Am J Surg* 1982;143:22-8.

57. Ellis FH Jr, Crozier RE, Watkins E Jr. Operation for esophageal achalasia: results of esophagomyotomy without an antireflux operation. *J Thorac Cardiovasc Surg* 1984;88:344-51.

58. Mansour KA, Symbas PN, Jones FL, Hatcher CR. A combined surgical approach in the management of achalasia of the esophagus. *Am Surg* 1979;42:192-5.

59. Murray GF. Operation for motor dysfunction of the esophagus. *Ann Thorac Surg* 1980;29:185-91.

60. Little AG, Soriano A, Ferguson MK, et al. Surgical treatment of achalasia: results with esophagomyotomy and Belsey repair. *Ann Thorac Surg* 1988;45:489-94.

61. Nelems JMB, Cooper JD, Pearson FG. Treatment of achalasia: esophagomyotomy with antireflux procedure. *Can J Surg* 1980;23:588-91.

62. Parrilla P, Ortiz A, Martinez de Haro LF, Aguayo JL, Morales G, Ramirez P. Assessment of gastroesophageal reflux following Heller's myotomy associated with a 270° posterior partial fundoplication. *Dig Surg* 1990;7:191-5.

63. Csendes A, Braghetto I, Mascaro J, Henriquez A. Late subjective and objective evaluation of the results of esophagomyotomy in 100 patients with achalasia of the esophagus. *Surgery* 1988;104:469-75.

64. Martinez de Haro LF, Soria T, Ortiz A, et al. Miotomía de Heller asociada a fundoplicatura par-

cialposterior como tratamiento de al acalasia de cardias. Valoración clínica y manométrica. *Cirugía Española* 1983;37:186-97.

65. Parrilla P, Martinez de Haro LF, Ortiz A, et al. Valoración clínica y manométrica de los resultados obtenidos con el tratamiento quirúrgico de al acalasia tipica y vigorosa de cardias. *Cirugía Española* 1987;412:197-205.

66. Menguy R. Management of achalasia by transabdominal cardiomyotomy and fundoplication. *Surg Gynecol Obstet* 1971;133:482-4.

67. Black J, Vorbach AN, Collis JL. Results of Heller's operation for achalasia of the esophagus: the importance of hiatal repair. *Br J Surg* 1976;63:949-53.

68. Jeckler J, Lhotha J. Modified Heller procedure to prevent postoperative reflux esophagitis in patients with achalasia. *Am J Surg* 1967;113:251-4.

69. Parrilla P, Martinez de Haro LF, Ortiz A, Aguayo J-L. Achalasia of the cardia: long-term results of oesophagomyotomy and posterior partial fundoplication. *Br J Surg* 1990;77:1371-4.

70. Ellis FH, Kiser JC, Schlegel JF, Earlam RJ, McVey JL, Olsen AM. Esophagomyotomy for achalasia of the esophagus: experimental, clinical, and manometric aspects. *Ann Surg* 1967;166:640-56.

71. Okike N, Payne WS, Neufeld DM, Bernatz PE, Pairolero PC, Sanderson DR. Esophagomyotomy versus forceful dilatation for achalasia of the esophagus: results in 899 patients. *Ann Thorac Surg* 1979;28:119-25.

72. Boix-Ochoa J, Casasa JM, Gil-Vernet JM. Une chirurgie physiologique pour les anomalies du secteur cardiohiatal. *Chir Pediatr* 1983;24:117-21.

73. Cucchiara S, Staiano A, Di Lorenzo C, et al. Return of peristalsis in a child with esophageal achalasia treated by Heller's myotomy. *J Pediatr Gastroenterol Nutr* 1986;5:150-2.

74. Boix-Ochoa J. Gastroesophageal reflux. In: Welch KJ, Randolph JG, Ravitch MH, et al. *Pediatric Surgery*. Chicago, IL: Year Book, 1986;712-20.

75. Boix-Ochoa J. Address of honored guest: the physiologic approach to the management of gastric esophageal reflux. *J Pediatr Surg* 1986;21:1032-9.

76. Liebermann D, Allgower M, Schmid P, et al. Muscular equivalent of the lower esophageal sphincter. *Gastroenterology* 1979;76: 31-8.

77. Liebermann D. Anatomie der gastroesophagealen verschluss organs. In: Blun AL, Siewert JR, eds. *Refluxterapie*. Berlin, Germany: Springer-Verlag, 1981.

78. Bardaji C, Boix-Ochoa J. Contribution of the His angle to the gastroesophageal antireflux mechanism. *Pediatr Surg Int* 1986; 1:172-5.

79. Boix-Ochoa J, Canals J. Maturation of the lower esophageal sphincter. *J Pediatr Surg* 1976;11:749-56

80. DeMeester TR, Wernly JA, Bryant CM, et al. Clinical and in vitro analysis of determinants of gastroesophageal competence: a study of principles of antireflux surgery. *Am J Surg* 1979;137: 39-46.

81. O'Sullivan GC, De Meester TR, Joelsson BE, et al. Interaction of LES pressure and length of sphincter in the abdomen as determinants of gastroesophageal competence. *Am J Surg* 1982;143:40-7.

82. Johnson HD. *The Antireflux Mechanism in the Cardia and Hiatus*. Springfield, IL: Charles C. Thomas, 1968:57.

83. Pettersson GB, Bombeck CT, Nyhus LM. The lower esophageal sphincter: mechanisms of opening and closure. *Surgery* 1980;88:307-14.

84. Leape L, Holder T, Franklin J, et al. Respiratory arrest in infancy secondary to gastroesophageal reflux. *Pediatrics* 1977; 60:924-8.

85. Christie DL. Respiratory disease associated with gastroesophageal reflux. *Pediatrics* 1979;63:344-5.

86. Murphy WJ, Gellis SS. Torticolis with hiatus hernia in infancy: Sandifer syndrome. *Am J Dis Child* 1977;131:564-5.

87. Schmitt M, Peiffert B, Pierre E, Barthelme H. L'intervention de Nissen chez l'enfant encephalopathe. *Chir Pediatr* 1986;27:138-42.

88. Allison PR. Reflux, esophagitis, sliding hiatal hernia and the anatomy of repair. *Surg Gynecol Obstet* 1951;92:419-31.

89. Duhamel D, Sauvegrain J, Masse NP. Les

hernies per l'hiatus esophagien et les malpositions cardiotubérositaires chez le nourisson et chez l'enfant. *Le Poumon.* 1953;1:33-45.

90. Boerema J. Hiatus hernia: Repair by right-side sub-hepatic anterior gastropexy. *Surgery* 1969;65:884-93.

91. Nissen R, Rossetti M. *Die behandlung von hiatus hernien und reflux esophagitis mit gastropexie und fundoplication.* Stuttgart, Germany: G Thieme Verlag, 1959.

92. Bettex M, Oesch I. The hiatus hernia saga. Ups and downs in gastroesophageal reflux: past, present, and future perspectives. *J Pediatr Surg* 1983;18:670-80.

93. Leonardi HK, Crozier RE, Ellis FH Jr. Reoperation for complications of the Nissen fundoplication. *J Thorac Cardiovasc Surg* 1981;81:50-6.

94. De Laet M, Spitz L. A comparison of Nissen fundoplication and Boerema gastropexia in the surgical treatment of gastroesophageal reflux in children. *Br J Surg* 1983;70:125-7.

95. Negre JB. Post-fundoplication symptoms. Do they restrict the success of Nissen fundoplication? *Ann Surg* 1983;198:698-700.

96. Jolley SG, Tunell WP, Hoelzer DJ, Smith EI. Postoperative small bowel obstruction in infants and children: a problem following Nissen fundoplication. *J Pediatr Surg* 1986;21:407-9.

97. Glick PL, Harrison MR, Adzick NS, et al. Gastric infarction secondary to small bowel obstruction: a preventable complication after Nissen fundoplication. *J Pediatr Surg* 1987;22:941-3.

98. Idowu J, Razzouk J, Georgeson K. Visceral ischemia secondary to gastric dilatation: a rare complication of Nissen fundoplication. *J Pediatr Surg* 1987;22:339-40.

99. Dedinsky GK, Vane DW, Black CTH, et al. Complication and reoperation after Nissen fundoplication in childhood. *Am J Surg* 1987;183:153-77.

100. Wilkins BM, Spitz L. Adhesion obstruction following Nissen fundoplication in children. *Br J Surg* 1987;77:774-9.

101. Alrabeeah A, Giacomantonio M, Gillis DA. Paraesophageal hernia after Nissen fundoplica-

tion: a real complication in pediatric patients. *J Pediatr Surg* 1988;23:766-8.

102. Low De, Mercer CD, James EC, Hill CD. Post-Nissen syndrome. *Surg Gynecol Obstet* 1988;167:1-5.

103. Kiely E, Spitz L. Is routine gastrostomy necessary in the management of esophageal atresia? *Pediatr Surg Int* 1987;2:6-9.

104. Bettex M Surgical treatment of hiatus hernia and cardioesophageal achalasia in infants and children. *Pediatrician* 1974;3:161-5.

105. Randolph J. Experience with the Nissen fundoplication for correction of gastroesophageal reflux in infants. *Ann Surg* 1983; 198:579-84.

106. Turnage RH, Oldham KT, Coran AG, Blane CE. Late results of fundoplication for gastroesophageal reflux in infants and children. *Surgery* 1989;105:457-64.

107. Bancewicz J, Mughal M, Marples M. The lower esophageal sphincter after floppy Nissen fundoplication. *Br J Surg* 1987;74: 162-4.

108. O'Hanrahan T, Marples M, Bancewicz J. Recurrent reflux and wrap disruption after Nissen fundoplication: detection, incidence and timing. *Br J Surg* 1990;77:545-7.

109. Ein SH, Shandling B, Stephens CA, Simpson JS. Partial gastric wrap-around as an alternative procedure in the treatment of hiatal hernia. *J Pediatr Surg* 1979;14:343-6.

110. Montupet PH, Gauthier F, Valayer J. Traitment chirurgical du reflux gastro-esophagien par hémivalve tubérositaire postérieur fixée. *Chir Pediatr* 1983;24:122-7.

111. Watson A, Jenkinson LR, Ball CS, et al. A more physiological alternative to total fundoplication for the surgical correction of resistant gastroesophageal reflux. *Br J Surg* 1991;78:1088-94.

112. Robie DK, Pearl RH. Modified Nissen fundoplication improved results in high risk children. *J Pediatr Surg* 1991;26:1268-71.

113. Thal AP. A unified approach to surgical problems of the esophagogastric function. *Ann Surg* 1968;168:542-50.

114. Ashcraft, KW. Gastroesophageal reflux. In: Ash-

craft KW, Holder TM, eds. *Pediatric Surgery*, 2nd ed. Philadelphia, PA: WB Saunders; 1993:270-88.

115. Boix-Ochoa J, Casasa JM, Gil-Vernet JM. Une chirurgie physiologique pour les anomalies due secteur cardiohiatal. *Chir Pediatr* 1983;24:117-21.

116. Boix-Ochoa J, Casasa JM. Surgical treatment of gastroesophageal reflux in children. *Surgery Annual* NYHUS ed. 1989;21:97-118.

117. Rohatgi M, Shandling B, Stephens CA. Hiatal hernia in infants and children: results in surgical treatment. *Surgery* 1971; 69:456-62.

118. Tovar JA, Morras I, Arana J, et al. El reflujo gastroesofaágico en enfermos neurologicos. *An Esp Pediatr* 1986;25:29-34.

119. Casten DF, Bernhang A, Nach RJ, Spinzia J. A physiological basis for the surgical treatment of sliding esophageal hiatal hernia. *Surg Gynecol Obstet* 1963;117:87-93.

120. Nihoul-Fekete C, Lortat Jacob S, Jehannin B, et al. Resultats de l'intervention de reposition Nissen-pyloroplastie et indications chirurgicales dans le traitement du reflux gastroesophagien et de la hernie hiatale du nourrisson et de l'enfant: a propos de 267 interventions. *Chirurgie* 1983;109:875-81.

121. Vaysse PH, Baunin CH, Guitard J, et al. Devenir a long terme des jonctions eso-gastriques operees pour correction d'un reflux gastro-esophagien. *Chir Pediatr* 1989;30:65-9.

122. Fonkalsrud EW, Ament Me, Vargas J. Gastric antroplasty for the treatment of delayed gastric emptying and gastroesophageal reflux in children. *Am J Surg* 1992;164:327-31.

27

Surgical Considerations: Lower Gastrointestinal Motility Disorders

ALBERTO PEÑA

The role of surgery in the treatment of children with lower gastrointestinal (GI) motility disorders varies from very well-defined, time-honored surgical interventions to empirical, ill-defined procedures. Examples of the first group include children suffering from the most common types of Hirschsprung's disease and congenital segmental dilation of the sigmoid. The results of surgical treatment for these conditions are rewarding and satisfactory. On the other extreme of the spectrum are patients suffering from lower GI disorders in which the indications for surgery are not well defined, the literature is controversial, and the operations are based on anecdotal, not scientific, evidence.

The surgical treatment of children with lower GI motility disorders is an evolving field. At present, surgery often relieves symptoms and occasionally provides a cure.

The surgeon may find a good correlation between the topography of the histologic abnormalities and the motility disorder, such as in most cases of Hirschsprung's disease. Unfortunately, in many other conditions the surgeon will encounter a lack of data to correlate symptoms, histology, and physiology. The surgeon, therefore, will have very poor guidelines for performing a bowel resection or diversion.

Surgeons who deal with these types of problems must constantly search for new descriptions of the intrinsic mechanisms of disease to be able to design appropriate techniques that will increase the rate of cure for these unfortunate children. Also, surgeons must investigate new descriptions of histo-logic abnormalities that can serve as accurate guidelines for resection or diversion. Bowel transplant is evolving from an experimental state into a clinical reality.

HIRSCHSPRUNG'S DISEASE
Primary Surgical Treatment

Operations designed for the treatment of Hirschsprung's disease vary, depending on the extent of the aganglionosis.

Ultrashort segment. Ultrashort segment is defined as the absence of ganglion cells in the most distal part of the rectum. This particular type of aganglionosis is not well described, and its existence is debated. The controversy is due to the fact that normal individuals have no ganglion cells in the most distal part of the rectum, in the so-called anal canal.[1-3] Efforts have been made to determine the length of the aganglionosis of the distal normal rectum for different age groups.[1]

Patients with ultrashort segment are clinically indistinguishable from those with severe idiopathic constipation. In patients with ultrashort segment Hirschsprung's disease, the funnel-shaped transition zone between healthy and aganglionic bowel is located in an area where normally there is a transition between the anal canal (which is normally closed) and the rectum (which is dilated in patients suffering from constipation). Biopsies in this area are frequently taken blindly with suction devices; the operators, therefore, cannot precisely determine the exact location of the biopsy site.

The surgical treatment for this ill-defined

condition is also empirical and has no satisfactory pathophysiologic basis. The operation is called posterior myotomy and is considered to be an internal sphincterotomy. Surgeons who advocate this technique[4-13] assume that they can resect a strip of smooth muscle from the posterior rectal wall, including the internal sphincter. The rectal mucosa must be preserved. The strip of smooth muscle is adequately oriented and submitted for histologic examination. Theoretically, it must show normal ganglion cells in its cephalad extreme and no ganglion cells in the distal or caudad portion. Significant controversy has been generated by the results obtained with this technique. In addition, some patients suffer from complications and even fecal incontinence after this type of operation. This procedure deserves further, careful investigation, but it is futile to design a rational surgical approach to a condition that still is ill defined.

Typical and long-segment types of Hirschsprung's disease. The majority of typical Hirschsprung's disease cases (80%) suffer from lack of ganglion cells in the rectum and most of the sigmoid.[14] Probably the next variety in frequency is the long-segment type, in which the aganglionic portion extends to the upper descending colon and may also affect the transverse colon. The basis for surgical treatment was established by Swenson[15] and consists of resecting the aganglionic segment and pulling through the normal ganglionic bowel to the preserved anal canal, thus creating an anastomosis between normal ganglionic bowel and the anal canal. Different techniques can achieve this goal, but all of them follow the basic principles established by Swenson.

Neonatal approach. Neonates with typical or long-segment Hirschsprung's disease suffer from obstipation, abdominal distention, and vomiting. They are frequently acutely ill and toxic. They often suffer from enterocolitis, which consists of severe toxemia and a proliferation of bacteria in the colonic lumen. Colonic irrigation with saline solution is a valuable, temporary, sometimes life-saving maneuver for the emergency treatment of enterocolitis. This treatment must be used only on a temporary basis, however, and should not replace a surgical decompression.

A colostomy is the most efficient method of decompression. Most surgeons open a colostomy immediately proximal to the transition zone. Simultaneously, biopsies are taken from the transition zone and from the nondilated distal bowel to confirm the absence of ganglion cells and the extent of the disease. Once the colostomy has been opened, the patient usually experiences a dramatic clinical improvement. The final operation must be performed at least 1 month after the colostomy.

Some surgeons prefer to open a transverse colostomy. At the time of the definitive procedure, the normal ganglionic bowel can be pulled down to the anal canal, leaving the transverse colostomy as a protection for the final repair. A third procedure will consist of closing the transverse colostomy. In cases in which the colostomy has been opened immediately above the transition zone, at the time of the definitive repair the surgeon has to pull the colostomy site down to the perineum, depriving the patient of the protection of a proximal diversion. The advantage of this approach, however, is that the patient will require only a two-stage procedure. Other surgeons[16] suggest a one-stage neonatal repair, which consists of an abdominoperineal pull-through without a protective colostomy. This last approach has been gaining acceptance recently. Each surgeon should perform the operation that is the safest in his or her own hands.

Final repair. After the original description of Swenson,[15] two important technical variations have been introduced in the surgical armamentarium. The first was described by Duhamel,[17] a French surgeon, and the other by Soave,[18] an Italian surgeon. Although a brief outline on these surgical techniques is given below, detailed descriptions are beyond the scope of this text and have been published elsewhere.[19]

In Swenson's technique, the aganglionic

segment located below the peritoneal reflection is dissected outside the bowel, but the surgeon stays as close as possible to the bowel wall to avoid pelvic nerve damage. Laterally, hemorrhoidal vessels are ligated. The entire dissected bowel is brought through the anus as an intussusception. The most dilated part of the normal ganglionic bowel is resected. The nondilated proximal bowel is mobilized in order to reach the perineum and is pulled through the space where the old aganglionic rectum had been located. The new colon is then anastomosed to the anal canal. The Swenson operation was still performed by 23% of American pediatric surgeons a decade ago.[20]

Duhamel's operation was designed to avoid extensive pelvic dissection. The main characteristic of this operation is that part of the aganglionic bowel is preserved. The colon is divided at the peritoneal reflection. The distal bowel is closed. The intraperitoneal aganglionic portion of the bowel and the most dilated normal ganglionic portion are resected. The nondilated, normal piece of colon is mobilized to reach the perineum. A dissection is then carried out between the posterior rectal wall and the anterior aspect of the sacrum. This seems to be a safe plane for dissection, since important nerves are located laterally. The posterior rectal wall is divided above the pectinate line. The piece of colon selected for the pull-through is then moved down through the presacral space and anastomosed to the opening of the posterior rectal wall. The anastomosis between the rectum and the pull-through colon is then created with a gastrointestinal anastomasis (GIA) stapler. The most common secondary negative effect of this procedure has been the accumulation of stool in the aganglionic rectal stump. However, those enthusiastic about this procedure insist that it is much simpler than the Swenson operation. Until recently, 30% of the American surgeons preferred the Duhamel operation.[20]

The Soave procedure is appealing, mainly because it guarantees no nerve damage in the pelvis. The entire dissection is carried out in an endorectal manner—between the mucosa and the smooth muscle of the bowel.

The colon is divided a few centimeters above the peritoneal reflection. The proximal aganglionic bowel and the most dilated normal ganglionic bowel are resected. A plane of dissection is created between the bowel mucosa and the seromuscular layer of the distal aganglionic bowel, usually beginning a few centimeters above the peritoneal reflection. The dissection is carried out distally to approximately 1 or 2 cm above the pectinate line. This dissection is usually completed from below, beginning above the anal canal with a circular incision that meets the dissection which began at the abdomen. The mucosal tube is resected and the mobilized normal-ganglionic colon is then pulled through the seromuscular cuff. According to the original Soave description, the pull-through bowel was left protruding outside the anus. Two or 3 weeks later, a separate operation excised the protruding bowel, and an anastomosis was carried out between the pull-through colon and the anal canal.[18] Boley[21] later proposed a modification consisting of a primary anastomosis of the pull-through rectum to the anal canal. Most surgeons presently perform a primary anastomosis. Until 1979, approximately 50% of pediatric surgeons in the United States preferred this operation, with or without Boley's modification.[20]

Protective colostomies are usually closed 1 month after the main operation. Probably more important than the choice of technique is the experience that each surgeon has with a specific operation.

Surgical treatment of total aganglionosis. In total aganglionosis, the entire colon is aganglionic and, therefore, nonfunctional. The normal ganglionic bowel is represented by the small bowel. Resecting the entire colon and performing an anastomosis between the terminal ileum and the anal canal is feasible, but produces important secondary effects such as severe chronic diarrhea, varying degrees of fecal incontinence, diaper rash, and sometimes dehydration. In an effort to avoid these complications, Lester Martin[22] described an ingenious technique for treating this condition. The basis of Martin's approach is to take advantage of the water-absorptive capacity of the aganglionic bowel, to decrease the number of bowel movements and give some consistency to the stool. This may help to make the diarrhea more manageable and, therefore, improve bowel control. Basically, the operation consists of mobilizing the ileostomy so as to reach the perineum. A presacral dissection is performed as described for the Duhamel operation. The normal ganglionic small bowel is pulled down and stapled to the posterior rectal wall, as described for the Duhamel procedure. A long, side-to-side anastomosis is performed between the distal ileum, the rectum, the sigmoid, and the aganglionic descending colon up to the level of the splenic flexure. The colon proximal to the splenic flexure is excised. More recently, Coran[23] proposed a straightforward end-to-end anastomosis between the terminal ileum and the rectum, claiming equally good results. Kimura[24] proposed a three-stage procedure to create a right colon patch, which is anastomosed to the aganglionic terminal ileum to take advantage of its demonstrated water-absorption capacity. Regardless of the technique used for the treatment of this type of aganglionosis, one must expect a rather stormy postoperative course in these patients since they lose a significant amount of water and electrolytes and have a difficult time trying to become toilet trained for stool.

A few very unfortunate patients are born with universal aganglionosis, in which ganglion cells are absent from the entire GI tract. There is no surgical treatment for this condition and all patients depend on parenteral nutrition for survival.

A posterior sagittal approach was used by the author in four patients with Hirschsprung's disease, including one case of total colonic aganglionosis. The posterior sagittal approach consists of exposing the rectum through a midsagittal incision between both buttocks, dividing all of the sphincteric mechanism. This allows a very precise resection of the rectum, with accurate preservation of the anal canal (including 2 cm of distal rectum) to guarantee preservation of the entire sphincteric mechanism and maintenance

of the exquisite sensation that resides in the anal canal. The rectum is dissected outside its wall, as described by Swenson, but in a retrograde manner. The abdominal approach is still necessary to mobilize the normal ganglionic part of the bowel and pull it down. The anastomosis between the normal ganglionic bowel and the anal canal is performed again with a posterior sagittal approach. This procedure seems to be easier than the previous operations and to have definite technical advantages. Further experience will determine its real value.

Secondary Surgical Treatment

Failed pull-throughs. Regardless of the type of technique used, a few patients may suffer catastrophic complications, including dehiscence of the pull-through bowel, severe rectal strictures, pelvic abscess, and chronic perineal fistulas. These complications can be successfully treated secondarily via the posterior sagittal approach. This approach allows the resection of strictured areas, mobilization of the proximal normal aganglionic bowel, and an accurate anastomosis with the anal canal.

Enterocolitis after pull-through for Hirschsprung's disease. Unfortunately, 2% to 15% of all patients operated on for Hirschsprung's disease still suffer from episodes of enterocolitis[20] in spite of a technically correct operation. The most prominent manifestations of this disorder include severe abdominal distention, periods of obstipation, and spontaneous or induced explosive, massive, deflating passage of liquid and gas bowel movements. The latter is followed by improvement of the patient's condition only to repeat the abdominal distention and obstipation. The colon shows mucosal ulcers, bacterial proliferation (particularly of the *Clostridium* type), and sometimes bowel perforation. This enterocolitis produces a very severe endotoxic condition that frequently kills the patient within a few hours. These patients improve dramatically when their colon is decompressed either by rectal irrigations or by the opening of a colostomy. This complication, unfortunately, occurs in spite of the presence of demonstrated normal ganglion cells in the pull-through bowel. A second pull-through is frequently necessary. The resection of bowel in these secondary procedures is performed, unfortunately, without specific histologic guidelines.

Neuronal Intestinal Dysplasia

The term neuronal colonic dysplasia was used to define a histologic entity that affects the colon, and was introduced by Meier-Ruge.[25] It refers to:

1. hyperplasia of the submucosa and myenteric plexus with formation of giant ganglia;

2. hypoplasia or aplasia of the sympathetic innervation of the myenteric plexus;

3. elevation of acetylcholinesterase activity in parasympathetic nerve fibers of the lamina propria and circular muscle;

4. isolated ganglion cells in the lamina propria and between the muscle layers of the muscularis mucosa and scattered smooth-muscle fibers in the lamina propria.

The current name, neuronal intestinal dysplasia (NID), was proposed by Scharli in 1981[26] and has been used by many others.[27-49] The described histologic findings are associated with a variety of symptoms, including constipation, diarrhea, abdominal distention, vomiting, and bloody stool. In addition, intestinal obstruction, enterocolitis, and a tendency for colon spasticity or megacolon formation are frequently mentioned. All of these symptoms create an enormous variety of clinical presentations. This condition is frequently found in association with Hirschsprung's disease.

Many types of empirical surgical interventions have been used to treat this condition, including partial or total resection of the affected bowel, resection of a coexistent aganglionic segment, sphincter myotomy, and the creation of short-term and long-term colostomies. Although the great variety of histologic findings, symptoms, types of treatments, and results in cases of NID[27-29] provoked significant waves of skepticism and debate in the pediatric surgical community, particularly in the United States, the concept

of NID as a new histologic abnormality is very attractive. It might explain many of the bowel motility disorders, including enterocolitis after operations for Hirschsprung's disease, for which we do not yet have a satisfactory explanation. As previously mentioned, a second pull-through in cases of severe enterocolitis after Hirschsprung's repair is performed by resecting a portion of normal ganglionic bowel, without histologic guidelines.

Theoretically, the presence of NID located proximal to the aganglionic bowel could explain the symptomatology seen in patients with enterocolitis, and could provide a rational basis for a new bowel resection, if the pathologist can establish the histologic diagnosis of NID as proposed by Meier-Ruge.[25] Also, the concept of a histologic entity such as NID suggests a spectrum of innervation disorders of the bowel. It represents hope for a more rational approach to different types of motility disorders. However, at present, surgeons face two great limitations when trying to perform operations based on these new histologic concepts:

1. conflicting evidence shows a striking inconsistency among histologic findings, clinical manifestations, medical and surgical treatments, clinical results, and long-term follow-up;[27-49]

2. the histologic techniques necessary to establish the diagnosis of NID have not been standardized and are not performed routinely in most hospitals.

NID deserves further investigation. A full understanding of its clinical implications, particularly for surgical treatment, must wait for more strict and systemized descriptions of this entity.

SEGMENTAL DILATION OF THE SIGMOID
Congenital

In 1953, Swenson[50] described a specific condition, seen in patients born with a very localized segmental dilation of the sigmoid, that provoked severe obstipation. Others soon reported on similar cases.[51-58] Interestingly, the resection of the dilated portion of the bowel, with an anastomosis between the normal-caliber proximal and distal colon, was followed by a complete remission of symptoms and permanent cure. The histologic analysis of the resected, massively distended bowel showed no abnormalities. It would be fascinating, of course, to examine those same specimens with the current histologic armamentarium. One of these cases is illustrated in Figure 27.1, which shows the radiologic appearance of the dilated sigmoid of a neonate. This condition is very unusual, but is 100% curable with an operation.[50-58]

Segmental Dilation of the Sigmoid Associated With Imperforate Anus

Most patients born with imperforate anus suffer from dilation of the most distal part of the bowel. This dilation seems to be more severe in patients who underwent the opening of a defective loop colostomy that allowed the passing of stool from the proximal limb into the distal one, provoking a chronic impaction in the distal blind rectal pouch. The dilation is also more severe in cases of transverse colostomy, as compared with cases of more distal types of colostomies. In transverse colostomies, it is more difficult to wash and irrigate the distal bowel than in cases of distal colostomies. Therefore, after the colostomy is opened and the patient is waiting for the final repair, the most distal part of the rectum remains very dilated and is frequently impacted with stool. There seems to be a direct correlation between the degree of dilation of the rectum, the length of time elapsed prior to the main repair, and the degree of constipation that these patients will eventually suffer.[59]

In addition to the congenital dilation of the rectosigmoid exhibited by these patients, this part of the bowel may enlarge even more if the patient does not receive proper care and is allowed to chronically carry a large amount of impacted stool inside the rectosigmoid. These patients cannot empty their rectum, which behaves like a floppy bag with very poor peristalsis. Interestingly, patients who were born with imperforate anus and were subjected to surgical repair that included resection of their original rectosigmoid—as was usually done during abdomino-

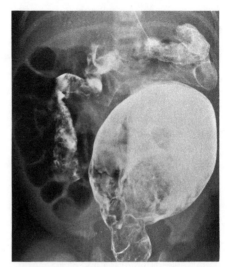

Fig. 27.1 The radiologic appearance of the dilated sigmoid of a neonate.

perineal procedures with endorectal dissections—suffer from constant passing of stool and a tendency to have diarrhea. This, of course, exacerbates their fecal incontinence and makes their management much more difficult.

Experimental evidence suggests that the chronic dilation of a hollow viscus may produce irreversible damage as well as permanent abnormalities in the peristalsis.[60-65] Clinically, this is frequently seen in cases of intestinal atresia. Pediatric surgeons have learned through experience to resect the most dilated part of the proximal blind-ended bowel prior to repairing these defects. Creating an anastomosis between the dilated proximal bowel and the distal microintestine generates multiple problems secondary to the malfunction of the anastomosis due to poor peristalsis of the dilated bowel.[60-65]

When the rectosigmoid becomes extremely dilated, the patients suffer from severe intractable constipation, in addition to possible encopresis or constant soiling. This creates a clinical dilemma since many patients who were born with imperforate anus suffer from fecal incontinence. The surgeon is then unable to determine whether to attribute the incontinence to a neuromuscular disorder associated with imperforate anus, or to overflow incontinence such as that seen in pa-

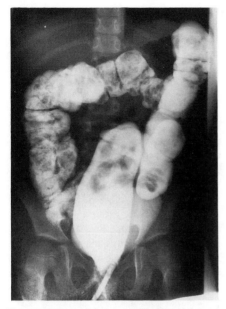

Fig. 27.2 A contrast enema without bowel preparation shows a characteristic segmental dilation of the rectosigmoid.

tients with functional fecal retention without imperforate anus (see Chapter 8). Anorectal malformations represent a spectrum of defects. Patients with good sacrum and good muscles have an excellent prognosis but those with poor sacrum, poor sphincteric mechanism, and very high defects have a poor prognosis.

The prognosis for bowel control can be predicted based on data obtained from the follow-up of a large series of patients.[59] Patients born with an anorectal defect of good prognosis who undergo technically correct surgical repair, but still suffer from fecal incontinence, may have severe constipation and chronic fecal impaction associated with encopresis. A contrast enema without bowel preparation shows a characteristic segmental dilation of the rectosigmoid (Fig. 27.2). The resection of the rectosigmoid above the peritoneal reflection, followed by the anastomosis of the normal-size descending colon to the dilated rectal ampulla, can cure constipation and make the patient fecally continent.[66]

An abdominoperineal complete resection of the rectosigmoid, as proposed by others,[67]

must be avoided. Such a procedure will certainly cure the constipation, but will render the patient fecally incontinent. One must remember that these patients seem to be fecally incontinent only because of the severe hypomotility disorder of their rectosigmoid. Since they were born with a good-prognosis type of anorectal defect, they have the necessary elements to have bowel control once the constipation problem is cured. This type of sigmoid resection also must not be performed in a patient who was born with a poor-prognosis type of anorectal defect (ie, very abnormal sacrum, poor sphincteric mechanism, and very high defect). The medical management of a patient with fecal incontinence and constipation by the use of enemas or colonic irrigations is much easier than when dealing with patients with fecal incontinence and loose stools. This last group of patients frequently requires a permanent colostomy to keep them clean and socially acceptable.

CONSTIPATION AND ENCOPRESIS

The experience obtained in children suffering from segmental dilation of the sigmoid associated with an anorectal malformation, as described above, becomes very useful when dealing with patients who suffer from severe constipation and encopresis without anorectal malformations. Ten children were subjected to a sigmoid resection as previously described. Eight patients experienced a dramatic improvement in their quality of life. Constipation disappeared or became easily manageable with a fiber-enriched diet. Two patients, however, remained constipated and still suffered from soiling after this operation. The retrospective analysis and comparison of those patients in whom the technique was very successful with those patients in whom it was not successful showed that the dilation of the rectosigmoid was more localized in the group of patients who were cured with the resection. The two patients who remained symptomatic after the procedure had a fairly uniform dilation of the entire colon. In fact, one of them was subjected to motility studies of the colon, and on the basis of these he was diagnosed as having colonic pseudo-obstruction. His symptoms were alleviated only by a diverting ileostomy.

The use of different types of colonic resections for the treatment of constipation does not represent a new concept. Many authors have performed these types of operations in adults, with variable clinical results.[68-74]

Constipation and encopresis seem to represent a spectrum of colonic motility disorders with different degrees of severity. Most cases can be successfully treated medically, but some are severe and do not respond to medical treatment. Many of these patients can be significantly helped by a sigmoid resection, particularly if the contrast study of the colon shows a segmental dilation of the sigmoid. The guidelines for the limits of the resection are empirical, however, since the most dilated part of the bowel is resected, assuming that the nondilated portion of the colon has a better functional capacity. A more objective and scientific surgical approach to this problem will occur after the development of new histologic techniques and motility studies that adequately differentiate between normal and abnormal peristalsis of the bowel.

Some surgeons[4-13] advocate the use of posterior sphincter myotomies for the treatment of severe intractable constipation and encopresis. As previously discussed, this is a controversial procedure because it has no scientific basis and the clinical results are inconsistent. In addition, the procedure is not free of complications, including infections and fecal incontinence.

The concept of an anterior anus has been proposed by others[75-79] as a cause of constipation. Presumably, the anterior location of an anus is accompanied by a posterior shelf in the rectal ampulla that interferes with the evacuation of feces. The surgical repositioning of the anus into a more posterior location supposedly corrects the presence of the posterior shelf and facilitates the passing of stool. The definition of an anterior anus has been rather arbitrary, except for one group of surgeons[79] who described a series of measurements that determine whether an anus is normally located or not. The concept that an anteriorly located anus and a posterior rectal shelf causes constipation does not stand the test of an objective critical analysis.

The presence of a rectal opening located anterior to the center of the external sphincter is well known and represents the simplest form of an anal malformation called perineal fistula. The orifice is abnormal, usually narrow, and is not surrounded by sphincter muscle, which is located in its normal position. These patients suffer from constipation. Treatment consists of performing an anoplasty to create a normally sized anal orifice located within the center of the external sphincter. Although the procedure alleviates constipation, most patients will still suffer some degree of constipation in the future. I have never seen a normal anus with a normal sphincter located anteriorly. Even assuming that one exists, moving it out of place would be risky because the sphincteric mechanism could be denervated and damaged.

Recently, an operation was developed to facilitate the irrigation of the colon in patients suffering from severe constipation or fecal incontinence.[80] A synthetic button can be implanted in the cecum, or the cecal appendix can be reimplanted with an antireflux mechanism in the cecum that is exteriorized through the skin in the lower right quadrant. A dry ministoma is created on the lower right quadrant. It does not allow the passing of stool, yet it is easily catheterizable for performing colonic irrigations in an antegrade manner. This operation has advantages for patients who refuse enemas and have problems in cleaning the entire colon every day.

INTESTINAL PSEUDO-OBSTRUCTION

The role of the surgeon in the management of a patient with pseudo-obstruction of the lower GI tract consists of helping the gastroenterologist obtain bowel specimens for the histologic diagnosis, and performing operations for the symptomatic treatment of this condition. Patients with a presumptive diagnosis of intestinal pseudo-obstruction of the lower GI tract often suffer from severe, intractable constipation. The surgeon is expected to divert the fecal stream, alleviate the symptoms, and take biopsies for a histologic diagnosis. The surgeon faces a serious problem when trying to determine the optimal location of the fecal diversion. In Hirschsprung's disease, bowel specimens sent to the pathology department will receive a considerably accurate diagnosis by frozen section that substantiates the presence or absence of ganglion cells. In dealing with intestinal pseudo-obstruction, however, the surgeon cannot expect this kind of diagnosis by frozen section. Even in permanent sections, the histologic diagnosis of intestinal pseudo-obstruction requires sophisticated special techniques, including silver stains, which are not routine in most hospitals. The surgeon must rely on the recommendations of the gastroenterologists, which are based on motility recordings and clinical manifestations. In addition, the surgeon will try to divert the fecal stream in a normal-looking bowel, generally proximal to the dilated, floppy, abnormal bowel. Therefore, it is not unusual in this type of patient to have a frustrating experience of opening a nonfunctional stoma. The surgeon must then open a new, more proximal fecal diversion under similarly vague guidelines.

Patients with intestinal pseudo-obstruction are well known for their tendency to suffer from prolonged ileus every time they are subjected to an abdominal operation. Therefore, the insertion of a Broviac or Hickman catheter is recommended in preparation for the use of parenteral nutrition for a patient who will remain incapable of receiving oral feedings for long periods of time.

REFERENCES

1. Adridge RT, Campbell PE. Ganglion cell distribution in the normal rectum and anal canal: a basis for the diagnosis of Hirschsprung's disease by anorectal biopsy. *J Pediatr Surg* 1968;3:475-90.

2. Weinberg AG. Hirschsprung's disease: a pathologist's view. *Perspect Pediatr Pathol* 1975;2:207-39.

3. Leutenegger F. Investigation of *m. sphincter ani* for ganglion cells. *Schweiz Med Wochenschr* 1969;99:1431-2.

4. Lynn HB. Personal experience with rectal myectomy in the treatment of selected cases of aganglionic megacolon. *Z Kinderchir* 1968;5:98-103.

5. Scobie WG, Mackinlay GA. Anorectal myectomy in treatment of ultrashort segment Hirschsprung's disease. *Arch Dis Child* 1977;52:713-5.

6. Thomas CG Jr, Bream CA, DeConnick P. Posterior sphincterotomy and rectal myotomy in the management of Hirschsprung's. *Ann Surg* 1970;171:796-809.

7. Bentley JFR. Posterior excisional ano-rectal myectomy in management of chronic fecal accumulation. *Arch Dis Child* 1966;41:144-7.

8. Shandling B, Desjardins JG. Anal myomyectomy for constipation. *J Pediatr Surg* 1969;4:115-8.

9. Nissan S, Bar-Maor JA, Levy E. Anorectal myectomy in the treatment of short segment Hirschsprung's disease. *Ann Surg* 1969;170:969-77.

10. Yoshioka K, Keighley MRB. Anorectal myectomy for outlet obstruction. *Br J Surg* 1987;74:373-6.

11. Lynn HB. Rectal myectomy in Hirschsprung's disease: a decade of experience. *Arch Surg* 1975;110:991.

12. Pinho M, Yoshioka K, Keighley MRB. Long-term results of anorectal myectomy for chronic constipation. *Br J Surg* 1989;76:1163-4.

13. Hata Y, Sasaki F, Uchino J. Sphincteromyectomy and sphincteroplasty in chronic constipation with megarectum. *J Pediatr Surg* 1988;23:141-2.

14. Ehrenpreis T. *Hirschsprung's Disease: Incidence.* Chicago, IL: Yearbook 57, 1970.

15. Swenson O, Bill AH. Resection of rectum and rectosigmoid with preservation of the sphincter for benign spastic lesions producing megacolon: an experimental study. *Surgery* 1948;24:212-20.

16. So HB, Schwartz DL, Becker J, et al. Endorectal "pull through" without primary colostomy in neonates with Hirschsprung's disease. *J Pediatr Surg* 1980;15:470-1.

17. Duhamel B. Retro rectal and transanal pull-through procedure for the treatment of Hirschsprung's disease. *Dis Colon Rectum* 1964;7:455-8.

18. Soave F. Hirschsprung's disease: a new surgical technique. *Arch Dis Child* 1964;39:116-24.

19. Peña A. Pediatric surgical problems: congenital megacolon or Hirschsprung's disease. In: Corman ML, ed. *Colon and Rectal Surgery*, 3rd ed. Philadelphia: JB Lippincott, 1993:337-47.

20. Kleinhaus S, Boley SJ, Sheran M, Sieber WK. Hirschsprung's disease: a survey of the members of the surgical section of the American Academy of Pediatrics. *J Pediatr Surg* 1979;14:588-97.

21. Boley SJ. New modification of the surgical treatment of Hirschsprung's disease. *Surgery* 1964;56:1015-7.

22. Martin LW. Surgical management of Hirschsprung's disease involving the small intestine. *Arch Surg* 1968;97:183-9.

23. Coran A. A personal experience with 100 consecutive total colectomies and straight ileoanal endorectal pull-through for benign disease of the colon and rectum in children and adults. *Ann Surg* 1990;212:242-8.

24. Kimura K, Nishijima E, et al. A new surgical approach to extensive aganglionosis. *J Pediatr Surg* 1981;16:840-3.

25. Meier-Ruge W. Cause of colon disorder with symptoms of Hirschsprung's disease. *Verh Dtsch Ges Pathol* 1971;55:506-9.

26. Scharli AF, Meier-Ruge W. Localized and disseminated neuronal intestinal dysplasia mimicking Hirschsprung's disease. *J Pediatr Surg* 1981;16:164-70.

27. Lassmann G, Wurning P. Lokale Ganglienzellhyperplasie in der submucosa am oralen ende des aganglionaren segmentes bei morbus Hirschsprung. *Z Kinderchir* 1973;12:236-43.

28. Gulotta F, Straaten G. Hirschsprungsche krankheit mit gleichzeitiger aganglionose und sogenannter neuronaler kolondysplasie (dysganglionosis colica). *Z Kinderchir* 1977;20:42-9.

29. Puri P, Lake BD, et al. Neuronal colonic dysplasia: an unusual association of Hirschsprung's disease. *J Pediatr Surg* 1977;12:681-5.

30. Klos I, Maier WA, Morger R, Schweitzer P. Die neuronale kolondysplasie (neuronal colonic dysplasia). *Kinderchir Grenzgebiete* 1973;23:53-4.

31. Fahr K, Nützenadel W. Die neuronale kolondysplasie. Therapiewoche 29. 1979:8717-20

32. MacMahon RA, Moore CCM, Cussen LJ. Hirschsprung-like syndromes in patients with normal ganglion cells on suction rectal biopsy. *J Pediatr Surg* 1981;16:835-9.

33. Sacher B, Briner J, Stauffer UG. Zur klinischen bedeutung der neuronalen in estinalen dysplasie. *Z Kinderchir* 1982;35:96-7.

34. Dickson JAS, Variend S. Colonic neuronal dysplasia. *Acta Paediatr Scand* 1983;72:635-7.

35. Fadda B, Maier W, Meier-Ruge W, Scharli A, et al. Neuronale intestinale displasie: eine kritische 10 jahres analyse klinischer und bioptischer diagnostik. *Z Kinderchir* 1983; 38:305-11.

36. Kessler S, Campbell J. Neuronal colonic dysplasia associated with short segment Hirschsprung's disease. *Arch Pathol Lab Med* 1985;109:532-3.

37. Munakata K, Morita K, Okabe I, et al. Clinical and histologic studies of neuronal intestinal dysplasia. *J Pediatr Surg* 1985;20:231-5.

38. Briner J, Oswald H, Hirsig J, et al. Neuronal intestinal dysplasia: clinical and histochemical findings and its association with Hirschsprung's disease. *Z Kinderchir* 1986;41:282-6.

39. Achem S, Owyang C, Schuffler M, et al. Neuronal dysplasia and chronic intestinal pseudo-obstruction: rectal biopsy as a possible aid to diagnosis. *Gastroenterology* 1987;92:805-9.

40. Fadda B, Pistor G, Meier-Ruge W, et al. Symptoms, diagnosis, and therapy of neuronal intestinal dysplasia masked by Hirschsprung's disease. *Pediatr Surg Int* 1987;2:76-80.

41. Pistor G, von Kap-herr H, Grussner R, et al. Neuronal intestinal dysplasia; modern diagnosis and therapy: report of 23 patients. *Pediatr Surg Int* 1987;87:352-8.

42. Rintaia R, Rapola J, Louhimo I. Neuronal

intestinal dysplasia. *Prog Pediatr Surg* 1989;24:186-92.

43. Bussman H, Roth H, Nützenadel W. Variabilität klinishcher symptome bei neuronaler intestinaler dysplasie. *Monatsschrift Kinderheilk* 1990;138:284-7.

44. Stoss F. Neuronal dysplasia. *Int J Color Dis* 1990;5:106-12.

45. Sacher P, Briner J, Stauffer UG. Unusual cases of neuronal intestinal dysplasia. *Pediatr Surg Int* 1991;6:225-6.

46. Schofield DE, Yunis EI. Intestinal neuronal dysplasia. *J Pediatr Gastroenterol Nutr* 1991;12:182-9.

47. Simpser E, Kahn E, Kenigsberg K, et al. Neuronal intestinal dysplasia: quantitative diagnostic criteria and clinical management. *J Pediatr Gastroenterol Nutr* 1991;12:61-4.

48. Scharli AF. Neuronal intestinal dysplasia. *Pediatr Surg Int* 1992;7:2-7.

49. Schofield DE, Yunis E. Intestinal neuronal dysplasia in a case of sigmoid stenosis. *Pediatr Pathol* 1992;12:275-80.

50. Swenson O, Rathauser F. Segmental dilation of the colon: a new entity. *Am J Surg* 1959;97:734-8.

51. De Lorimier AA, Benzian SR, Gooding CA. Segmental dilation of the colon. *Am J Roentgenol* 1971;112:100-4.

52. Brawner J, Shafer AD. Segmental dilation of the colon. *J Pediatr Surg* 1973;8:957-8.

53. Chiba T, Kokubo T. Congenital segmental dilation of the colon. *Arch Jpn Chir* 1976;45:45-7.

54. Etzioni A, Benderly A, Bar Maor JA. Segmental dilation of the colon: another cause of chronic constipation. *Dis Colon Rectum* 1980;23:580-2.

55. Helikson MA, Schapiro MB, Garfinkel DJ, et al. Congenital segmental dilation of the colon. *J Pediatr Surg* 1982;17:201-2.

56. Nguyen L, Shandling B. Segmental dilation of the colon: a rare cause of chronic constipation. *J Pediatr Surg* 1984;19:539-40.

57. Takehara H, Komi N, Hino M. Congenital segmental dilation of the colon: report of a case and review of the literature. *Pediatr Surg Int* 1988;5:66-8.

58. Martinez MA, Conde J, Bardaji C, et al. Dilatacion segmentaria congenita del colon. *Chir Pediatr* 1989;2:43-4.

59. Peña A. Posterior sagittal anorectoplasty: results in the management of 332 cases of anorectal malformations. *Pediatr Surg Int* 1988;3:94-104.

60. Benson CD, Lloyd JR, Smith JD. Resection and primary anastomosis in the management of stenosis and atresia of the jejunum and ileum. *Pediatrics* 1960;26:265-72.

61. Nixon HH. An experimental study of propulsion in isolated small intestine and applications to surgery in the newborn. *Ann R Coll Surg Engl* 1960;27:105-24.

62. Louw JH. Resection and end-to-end anastomosis in the management of atresia and stenosis of the small bowel. *Surgery* 1967;62:940-50.

63. Nixon HH, Tawes R. Etiology and treatment of small intestinal atresia: analysis of a series of 127 jejunoileal atresias and comparison with 62 duodenal atresias. *Surgery* 1971;69:41-51.

64. Tepas JJ, Wyllie RG, Shermeta DW, et al. Comparison of histochemical studies of intestinal atresia in the human newborn and fetal lamb. *J Pediatr Surg* 1979;14:376-80.

65. Pickard LR, Santoro S, Wyllie RG, et al. Histochemical studies of experimental fetal intestinal obstruction. *J Pediatr Surg* 1981;16:256-60.

66. Peña A, El Behery M. Megasigmoid: a source of pseudoincontinence in children with repaired anorectal malformations. *J Pediatr Surg* 1993;28:199-203.

67. Powell RW, Sherman JO, Raffensperger JE. Megarectum: a rare complication of imperforate anus repair and its surgical correction by endorectal pullthrough. *J Pediatr Surg* 1982;17:786-95.

68. Lane RH, Todd IP. Idiopathic megacolon: a review of 42 cases. *Br J Surg* 1977;64;305-10.

69. McCready RA, Beart RW. The surgical treat-

ment of incapacitating constiption associated with idiopathic megacolon. *Mayo Clin Proc* 1979;54:779-83.

70. Hughes ES, McDermott FT, Johnson WR, et al. Surgery for constipation. *Aust N Z J Surg* 1981;51:144-8.

71. Belliveau P, Goldberg SM, Rothenberger DA, et al. Idiopathic acquired megacolon: the value of subtotal colectomy. *Dis Colon Rectum* 1982;25:118-21.

72. Klatt GR. Role of subtotal colectomy in the treatment of incapacitating constipation. *Am J Surg* 1983;145:623-5.

73. Vasilevsky CA, Nemer FD, Balco EG, et al. Is subtotal colectomy a viable option in the management of chronic constipation? *Dis Colon Rectum* 1988;81:679-81.

74. Zenilman ME, Dunnegan DL, Soper NJ, et al. Successful surgical treatment of idiopathic colonic dysmotility: the role of preoperative evaluation of coloanal motor function. *Arch Surg* 1989;124:947-51.

75. Hendren WH. Constipation caused by anterior location of the anus and its surgical correction. *J Pediatr Surg* 1978;13:505-12.

76. Leape LL, Ramenofsky ML. Anterior ectopic anus: a common cause of constipation in children. *J Pediatr Surg* 1978;13:627-30.

77. Reisner SH, Sivan Y, Nitzan M, et al. Determination of anterior displacement of the anus in newborn infants and children. *Pediatrics* 1984;73:216-7.

78. Tuggle DW, Perkins TA, Tunnell WP, et al. Operative treatment of anterior ectopic anus: the efficacy and influence of age on results. *J Pediatr Surg* 1990;25:996-8.

79. Bar-Maor JA, Eitan A. Determination of the normal position of the anus (with reference to idiopathic constipation). *J Pediatr Gastroenterol Nutr* 1987;6:559-61.

80. Redel CA, Motil KJ, Bloss RS, et al. Intestinal button implantation for obstipation and fecal impaction in children. *J Pediatr Surg* 1992;27:654-6.

INDEX

Barr, R.G., 23
Barrett's esophagus
  associated with GERD, 62, 63
  diagnosis of, 73
Barrett's intestinal metaplasia, treatment, 77
Baseline changes, correcting for, 352-353
Basic electric rhythm. *See* Slow waves
Bayliss, M. 9
Beak deformity, 267
Behavior modification therapy. *See also*
  Biofeedback training
  for feeding disorders, 42-43
  for treating chronic constipation, 135, 139
Belching, LES relaxation during, 55, 57
Belt pneumograph, 308
Benzamides, for treating cyclic vomiting, 99
Benzodiazepines, use during catheter placement,
  222
Berde, C.B., 171
Bernstein, I.M., 258
Bernstein test, 257
  development of, 258-259
  for evaluating esophageal symptoms, 182
  for evaluating reflux-associated stridor and
    croup, 71, 74
  for evaluating wheezing, 69
Berseth, C.L., 8
Bethanechol
  dose, 377-378, **381**
  mechanism of action, 377, **381**
  side effects and contraindications, 378
  for treating GERD, 76
Bettex, M., 394
Bezoar, recurrent fecal, colonic motility pattern
  associated with, **224,** 225-226
Bicarbonate, labeled, for evaluating gastric transit
  times, 269
Bile-acid displacement therapy, 372
Bile acids
  determination of secretion rate of, 285
  reflux of, abnormal motility patterns associated
    with, 205
  role in GERD, 59
Bile-salt binding agents, for treating FAP, 112
Bile-salt malabsorption, 362
Bilirubin, determination of rate of secretion, 285
Biofeedback training
  outcome studies, 246
  prerequisites for, 248-249
  for treating chronic constipation, 137, 139
  for treating defecation disorders, 244-248, 252
  for treating visceral pain, 170-171
Bisacodyl, mechanism of action, 382
Bisacodyl stimulation test, 223, 224
Bloating. *See* Abdominal distention
Blood analysis, for evaluating transit disorders,
  266-267
Bloody stool, associated with intestinal neuronal
  dysplasia, 407
Body surface, formula for approximation of, 368
Boerema, J., 394
Boerema's technique for fixation of stomach, 396

Boldyreff, V.N., 196, 210
Boley modification, 405
Bolus-transport diagram, 293
Bontempo, I., 258
Booth, D.J., 258
Borderline respiratory function, associated with
  feeding disorders, 37
Bouin's fixative, 326, 332, 344
Bowel movement. *See* Defecation
Bradygastria, 308, 311, 357, 358
Brain stem glioma, differential diagnosis, 95
Bran
  particle size for ultrasonography, 316
  radio-labeled, 299
Breath analysis. *See* Hydrogen breath test
Brigham, K.L., 287
Brilliant blue, for evaluating transit disorders,
  266
Bronchopulmonary dysplasia, associated with
  CIP, 117
Bronchospasm, in response to GER, 60
Broviac catheter, 411
Brush-border membrane, role of, 362
Bulimia, delayed transit times associated with, **273**
Bulk clearance, abnormal, 58-59
Bupivacaine, for treating visceral pain, 172
Butyrophenones, for treating cyclic vomiting, 99

C
Cajal cells, 3
Calcium antagonists, for treating achalasia, 390
Calcium channel blockers, mechanism of action,
  382
Cannon, W.B., 195
Capsaicin cream, for treating referred pain, 171
Carbohydrates
  absorption and metabolism, 362
  effect on colonic motility, 217
  requirements, for patients on long-term TPN,
    369
Carmine red, for evaluating transit disorders, 266
Casten, D.F., 396
Catharsis, during office visit, 24
Cathartic laxatives, mechanism of action, 382
Catheter. *See also* Strain-gauge catheter
  for anorectal manometry, 231, 232
  for antroduodenal manometry, 198-200
  Broviac, 411
  for colonic manometry, 219, 221
  for esophageal manometry, 180-182
  Hickman, 411
  movement, data artefacts caused by, 352
  perfused, 199, 219
  radiopaque, polyvinyl, 222
  for TPN, infection risk with, 372
Catheter placement
  for antroduodenal manometry, 201-202
  in colonic manometry, 220-222
  for LES dilation, 390
  peroral, 222
Cavell, B., **283**
CCK. See Cholecystokinin

incidence, 89
management, 97-100
pathogenesis, 93-94
personality traits associated with, 93
recurrence rates, 90, **99**
somatizing with, 100
Cystic fibrosis, associated with neonatal
constipation, 150
Cytomegalovirus infection, associated with CIP,
117
Cywes, S., 244

D

Data analysis, by computer, 351-359
Data base, of normal and abnormal motility
patterns, 358
Davidson, M., 149, 150
Dawson, A.M., 146
Dedinsky, G.K., 394, 396
Defecation
biofeedback training for, 246
before birth, 218
normal and abnormal dynamics, 133, **238**
normal frequency of, 129, 130, 150
test for normal function, 236, 238, 239
Deglutition, response to, 2
De Laet, M., 394
Dent sleeve device, 232
Dermatomyositis, esophageal motor
abnormalities associated with, **189,** 190
Devos, P.G., 297
Devroede, G.J., 286
Dextrose, radio-labeled, 298
Diabetic motility disorders. *See also*
Gastroparesis, diabetic
abnormal motility pattern associated with, 206
Diagnosis, interview of patient and parents, 28
Diagnostic tests. *See also specific techniques*
avoidance of unnecessary, 165
for feeding disorders, 41-42
Diaphragm. *See* Crural diaphragm
Diarrhea, chronic. *See also* Toddler's diarrhea
abnormal motility pattern associated with,
207, 208
associated with CIP, 119
associated with cyclic vomiting, 91
associated with intestinal neuronal dysplasia,
407
associated with myelomeningocele, 242
associated with repaired imperforate anus, 408
causes, 362, 363
stress-related, 146
treatment, 112
Diarrhea, peas and carrots, 149
Diarrhea, postvagotomy, abnormal motility
pattern associated with, 208
Diarrhea, secretory, drug therapy, 383
Dairy products, elimination of, 109, 112
Diazepam
for treating cyclic vomiting, 98
use during catheter placement, 222
DiCecco, S., 364

Dicyclomine, 382
Dietary measures
for treating CIP, 122-123
for treating GERD, 75
for treating malnutrition, 366-367
for treating RAP, 108-109
Diethylene triamine pentacetic acid, 281, 299, 301
Dietl's crisis, 95
Diffuse esophageal spasm, 185-186
drug therapy, 382
Digestive motility patterns. *See also*
Interdigestive motility pattern
abnormal, 208-209
normal, **202, 203,** 205
Dilation
of lower esophageal sphincter, 390
visceral, associated with visceral myopathy,
341
Diltiazem, mechanism of action, 382
Direct influence procedures, 24
Disease, definition, 13, 17
Disimpaction, manual, for treating functional
fecal retention, 137
Distraction techniques, for treating visceral pain,
168-169
Diver Haber, A., 149
Diverticulosis, small intestinal
associated with visceral myopathy, 341, 342
causes of, 331
Doctor
accessibility of, 17
as patient's advocate, 27
role of, 13-17
school visits, 26
skills in managing malingering, 21
Doctor-patient relationship, 13-29
doctor's role in, 13-17
handling mental health referrals, 21-22
maintenance of, 100
models of, 14-16
Dodge, J.A., 148
Dog, colonic motility, 215
Domperidone
dose, 379-380, **381**
effect on gastric activity, 309
mechanism of action, 379, **381**
side effects, 380
use in manometric studies, 223
Dorsal horn, superficial layers, 157, 158
Double-balloon device, 231-232
Double sampling test meal method, 278, **281**
See also Gastric marker dilution test
Down syndrome, motility disorders associated
with, 63-64, 116-117, 291, 394, 396
Drossman, D.A., 146
Drug therapy, family beliefs about, 166
Dry needling, for treating visceral pain, 170
DTPA. *See* Diethylene triamine pentacetic acid
Duchenne muscular dystrophy, fecal incontinence
associated with, 244
Duhamel, B., 404
Duhamel, D., 394

Interdigestive motility pattern
   abonormal, 205-208
   normal, 215-218
Interview, diagnostic, 28
Intestinal atresia, complications, 408
Intestinal neuronal dysplasia
   associated with neurofibromatosis, 335, **336,**
      344-345
   cause of megarectum, 241
   diagnosis, 332, 335, **336,** 337, 344
   features of, 407
   histologic features, **335, 336**
   microcolon associated with, 342
   symptoms, 407
Intestinal pseudo-obstruction. *See* Chronic
   intestinal pseudo-obstruction
Intestinal transit time, with irritable bowel
   syndrome, 148-149
Intestinal transplantation, for treating CIP,
   125-126
Intraduodenal marker dilution test
   assumptions, 285-286
   indications for, 286
   principles, 284-285
Irritability
   associated with functional fecal retention, 132
   with regurgitation, 66
   as sign of GERD, 66, 67
Irritable bowel syndrome
   abnormal motility pattern associated with,
      206, 207, 208
   associated with cyclic vomiting, 93, 94
   associated with RAP, 108
   classification, 17, 105
   drug therapy, 382
   features of, 145
   intestinal transit time, 148-149
   pathogenesis, 145-146, 151
   postulated pathogenetic mechanism, 149
   symptoms, 146-151
Iwai, N., 243

J

Jejunum
   function, 195
   mean transit time, 285
Johansson, C., 285
Jolley, S.G., 394
Jonas, A., 149

K

Kantrowitz, P.A., 258
Kazem, I., 291
Ketamine, for treating pain, 173
Kiely, E., 394
Kimura, K., 406
Krypton, 268, 293

L

Lactase activity, effect of bacterial overgrowth
   on, 362
Lactic dehydrogenase staining, 335, **336**

Lactitol, 270, **271**
Lactose intolerance
   associated with toddler's diarrhea, 148
   as trigger for RAP, 109, 112
Lactose malabsorption, effect on hydrogen
   breath test, 271
Lactulose
   dose, in transit time studies, 270, **271**
   for treating chronic constipation, 136, 139
Lake, B., 332
Lamina propria, inflammatory infiltrate caused
   by bacterial overgrowth, **363**
Laparotomy, contraindications for, 117
Large bowel. *See* Colon
Laryngomalacia, 71
Laryngoscopy. *See* Endoscopy
Laryngospasm
   reflux-associated, 71
   in response to GER, 60
Larynx
   position of, 38-39
   reflux-associated inflammation of, 71, 72
Lask, B., 22, 23
Lawson, J.O., 150
Laxative, for treating functional fecal retention,
   prognosis, 240, 245, 246
Laxative treatment
   cathartic, mechanism of action, 382
   for constipation associated with
      neuromuscular diseases, prognosis, 244
LCT. *See* Triglyceride infusion
LeBaron, S., 169
Leonardi, H.K., 394
LES. *See* Lower esophageal sphincter
LeSouëf, P.N., 387
LESP. *See* Lower esophageal sphincter pressure
Leukocytosis, transient, associated with cyclic
   vomiting, 92, 96-97
Leuprolide, mechanism of action, 382
Levine, M.D., 23
Liebermann, D., 392
Light microscopy, for diagnosing motility
   disorders, 325-345
Livaditis, A., 387
Liver disease, TPN-related, 123, 369, 372
Loening-Baucke, V., 244
Loperamide, for treating toddler's diarrhea, 148
Lorazepam, for treating cyclic vomiting, 98
Low, D.E., 394
Lower esophageal sphincter, 40
   anatomy, 178
   assessment of relaxation, 183
   dilation of, 390
   effect of postural changes on, 57, 65
   evaluation of, 267-268
   function, 2, 178, 392
   innervation, 178
   involvement of, in achalasia, 188
   modulators of, 55, **56**
   myotomy of, 188-189
   physiology, 55-57, 178
   transient relaxations, 55, 57, 58, 74

Lower esophageal sphincter pressure
assessment, 181
basal, 2, 183
with CIP, 121
effect of drugs on, 377-378, 379, 380
during GER, 57-58
mechanisms, 2, 178
during phase 3, 55

M

MacGregor, I.L., 285
Magical thinking, associated with functional
fecal retention, 132
Magnesium salts, for treating functional fecal
retention, 136
Malabsorption
clinical manifestations, 364-365
pathophysiology, 361-364
underlying mechanisms, **362**
Malagelada, J-R., 284
Malingering, 21
Malnutrition
associated with CIP, 361, 362
causes of, **364**
classification, 365, **366**
clinical manifestations, 364-365
Malrotation
associated with CIP, 118
differential diagnosis, 109
Manometry. *See also* Anorectal
manometry; Antroduodenal manometry;
Esophageal manometry
respiration artefacts, **210**
Marker dilution tests, 277-287
principle, **279**
Marlett, J.A., 197
Martin, L.W., 405
Massage, for treating visceral pain, 166, 169-170
Mass movement, 216
Mastication, development of patterns of, 38
Mathieu, A., 278
Maturational arrest of myenteric plexus
classification, 337-339
histology, **338, 339, 340**
symptoms, 118, 337, 342
McLain, C.R., Jr., 1
MCT. *See* Colonic transit time, mean
Meal. *See* Test meal
Mechanical obstruction, abnormal motility
pattern associated with, 208, 209
Meckel's diverticulum, differential diagnosis, 109
Meconium, delayed passage of, 150, 218, **241**
Megacolon. *See also* Hirschsprung's megacolon
associated with myotonic dystrophy, 244
associated with visceral myopathy, 341
Megacystis, associated with visceral
myopathy, 341
Megacystis-microcolon-intestinal hypoperistalsis
syndrome, 118, 342
Megaduodenum, associated with visceral
myopathy, 341
Megaloureter, associated with visceral

myopathy, 342
Megarectum, after surgery for Hirschsprung's
disease, 241
Meier-Ruge, W., 407
Meissner's plexus, 3, 7
Melzack, R., 157, 162
Meningomyelocele. *See* Myelomeningocele
Mental disorder, definition, 23
Mental health referrals, 21-22, 24, 26, 169.
See also Psychiatric therapy
family beliefs about, 166
resistance to, 100
Metcalf, A.M., 271
Metoclopramide, **56**
dose, 378-379, **381**
mechanism of action, 378, **381**
side effects, 379
test for effectiveness, 203
for treating GERD, 76
use in manometric studies, 201, 203, 204, 223
Microaspiration, associated with GER, 388
Microcolloid, radio-labeled, 298
Microcolon
associated with CIP, 118
etiology, 342
Micronutrients, daily maintenance
requirements in TPN, **370,** 371
Midazolam, for treating pain, 173
Migraine
associated with cyclic vomiting, 93, 94
associated with RAP, 108, 110
Migrating motor complex, 3-6, 7. *See also*
Phase 1; Phase 2; Phase 3
developmental pattern, 118
discovery of, 196-197
drug therapy to increase, 382
in infants, 204-205
neural control of, 204
in normal adults, **203,** 204
Milk, types of, effects on gastric emptying, 298
Milla, P.J., 197
Mineral oil, for treating chronic constipation,
136, 137, 139
Minerals, daily maintenance requirements in
TPN, **370**
Ministoma, for treating constipation, 410
Mitochondrial myopathy, 342
Mixed dysrhythmias, 308
MMC. *See* Migrating motor complex
Mood, effect on appetite, 34
Moriarty, K.J., 146
Morphine, 158
for inducing phase 3, 204
Morris, F.H., 8
Mortensen, O., 112
Motilin, 3, 381
Motility
clinical measurements, 349-350
effects of laboratory stressors on, **146**
in normal gut, 195, 203-215
Motility disorders, classification, 377
Motility-enhancing agents, 377-382

428

Motility index
 agents for increasing, 223
 in CIP, 122
 of colon, 217
 definition, 355
 determined with ultrasonography, 316
 3-dimensional, **356**
 graphically represented as function of time,
  355, **356**
 and non-HAPC contractions, 218
 for predicting feeding intolerance in preterm
  infants, 197-198
Motility-suppressing agents, 382-383
Motion sickness
 associated with cyclic vomiting, 93, 94
 associated with gastric dysrhythmias, 311
Mouthing patterns, in utero, 37
Movement, data artefacts caused by, 352-354
Mucosal enzymes, levels of, in toddler's
  diarrhea, 148
Mucosal secretory disorder, 125
Mucus, of esophagus, function, 59-60
Munchausen's syndrome-by-proxy, features
  of, 119-120, 166-167
Muscular dystrophy
 associated with esophageal motor
  abnormalities, 190
 progressive, histology, **343**
Muscularis propria, visualization of neural
  components of, 325, **327, 328, 329**
Musculature
 of esophagus, 1, 2
 of stomach, 2-3
Musculocutaneous referred pain, management, 170
Mutual participation model, 14-15
Myelomeningocele
 anorectal functional abnormalities associated
  with, 242
 biofeedback training to improve defecation,
  247-248
 chronic constipation associated with,
  242, **272, 273**
 chronic diarrhea associated with, 242
Myenteric plexus
 abnormalities of, 206, 223, 407
 disorders associated with abnormal, 139,
  329, **330,** 364
 esophageal, 178
 involvement of, in achalasia, 186
 maturational arrest of, *see* Maturational arrest
 neural components of, 326, **327, 328, 329, 342**
Myenteric plexus neuropathy, in Down syndrome
  children, 116-117
Myoelectrography, limitations, 196
Myopathy. *See also* Visceral myopathy
 mitochondrial, 342
Myotherapy, for treating visceral pain, 170
Myotomy
 of LES, 188-189
 posterior, 404, 410
 for treating achalasia, 390-391
Myotonic dystrophy

abnormal motility pattern associated
 with, 206, 208
fecal incontinence associated with, 244

N

Nader, P.R., 26
Na K ATPase, 148
Nasal intubation, procedure, 181
Nausea
 assessed with barostat test, 319
 associated with cyclic vomiting, 91-93
 associated with gastric dysrhythmias, 311
 chronic, case history, 321
 drug therapy, 383
Negre, J.B., 394
Neocate, 367
Neonate
 anorectal manometry in, 236, 240, **241**
 antireflux operation, 393
 gastric emptying values, **283**
 normal motility pattern, **6,** 207-208
 pain memory, 160
 rectosphincteric reflex, 234, 236, 240
 stress response, 160
Neurofibromatosis, associated with intestinal
  neuronal dysplasia, 335, **336,** 344-345
Neurologic disease
 associated with GERD, 63-64, 78
 reflux-related diseases associated with, 190
Neuromuscular diseases. *See* Enteric
  neuromuscular disorders
Neuronal colonic dysplasia. *See* Intestinal
  neuronal dysplasia
Neuronal intestinal dysplasia. *See* Intestinal
  neuronal dysplasia
Neurons, gut, visualization of, 325-345
Neuron-specific enolase, histologic marker, 325
NID. *See* Intestinal neuronal dysplasia
Nifedipine
 mechanism of action, 382
 for treating achalasia, 390
Nipple, effect on feeding behavior, 37-38
Nissen, R., 394
Nissen fundoplication. *See* Fundoplication
Nitric acid, 9
Nitric oxide, **56,** 57
Nitric oxide synthase, 389
Nitric oxide synthase staining, 334
Nitrogen requirements, for total parenteral
  nutrition, 368-369
Noise, data artefacts caused by, 353-354
Nonabsorbable markers, for evaluating
  transit times, 266, 269, 278
Nonsteroidal anti-inflammatory agents,
  for treating visceral pain, 171
Nonulcer dyspepsia
 assessed by ultrasonography, 316-317
 classification, 105
 diagnostic algorithm for, 317
 drug therapy, 380
 EGG patterns, 309, **310**
 symptoms, 268, 316

functional fecal retention, 135
Plexus of Meissner, 325
Pneumonia, reflux-associated, 69
Polyethylene glycol, 281, 286
Polygraph, for anorectal manometry, 233, 252
Polyhydramnios, associated with in utero intestinal obstruction, 117
Polymyositis, esophageal motor abnormalities associated with, 190
Polyphenolic drugs, mechanism of action, 382
Position
changing, to relieve swallowing disorders, 43
effect on GER, 258
Positioning measures, for treating GERD, 75
Postenteritis syndrome, mucosal enzyme levels in, 148
Posterior myotomy. *See* Posterior sphincter myotomy
Posterior sagittal approach, for surgical treatment of Hirschsprung's disease
Posterior sphincter myotomy, for treating constipation, 404, 410
Postprandial duodenal hypomotility, features of, 119
Postprandial jiggle, 75
Posture. *See also* Positioning measures
role in GER, 63
Posturing
associated with reflux, 72
retentive, 132, **133**
Postvagotomy diarrhea, abnormal motility pattern associated with, 206, 208
Power
of AC signal, 349
of frequency band, defined, 308
as function of frequency, 351
Predischarge conference, 28-29
Pregnancy
cause of nausea and vomiting during, 311
GER associated with, 65
Preparatory phase, 33, **34**
Preprocessing of data, 352-354
Pressure inversion point, 182
Preterm infant
absence of MMC in, **202,** 204-205
gastric motility in, 3-5
prediction of feeding intolerance in, 197-198
pseudo-obstruction in, 117, 118
small intestinal motility in, 7, 8-9
Pritchard, J.A., 1
Proctocolectomy with ileal pouch anastomosis, abnormal motility pattern associated with, 207
Progesterone, effects on LES, 65
Prokinetic agents. *See also specific agents*
effect on colonic motility, 223
infant response to, 284
manometric studies of acute effects of, 198
mechanism of action and dose, 377-381, **381**
test for effectiveness, 203
for treating GERD, 76
use in manometric studies, 201-202, 203
withdrawal of, before manometry, 201

Propagation of slow wave, 350
recognition of signal of, 354-355
Propofol, for treating pain, 173
Propranolol, for treating cyclic vomiting, 99
Prostaglandins
role in chronic visceral pain, 171
role in toddler's diarrhea, 148
Prosthetic devices, to treat swallowing disorders, 43
Protein-losing enteropathy, associated with bacterial overgrowth, 363
Provocation tests
for antroduodenal manometry, 203
for colonic manometry, 223
for pH monitoring, 258-259
Prugh, D.G., 14
Pseudo-Hirschsprung's disease. *See* Intestinal neuronal dysplasia
Pseudo-obstruction. *See* Chronic intestinal pseudo-obstruction
Pseudo-three-dimensional plot, 307
Psychiatric illness, 18-19. *See also* Factitious disorders
Psychiatric skills, in pediatric practice, 21-22
Psychiatric therapy. *See also* Mental health referrals
for cyclic vomiting, 100
Psychogenic megacolon. *See* Functional fecal retention
Psychogenic symptom, 17
Psychologic therapy. *See also* Mental health referrals
family beliefs about, 166
hierarchical classification of, 24-26
Psychosomatic symptom, 17. *See also* Factitious disorders
Psychotherapy. *See* Mental health referral
Puborectalis muscle, 234, 236
Pudding, radio-labeled, 299
Pull-through operation, 151
complications, 406-407
failures, 344, 406
procedures, 404-406
Pull-through pressure, anal, 234
Pull-through technique, in esophageal manometry, 181-182, 183
Pyloric stenosis, infantile hypertrophic, diagnosis, 340-341
Pyloroplasty
efficacy of, 125
for treating GER, 396-397
Pylorospasm, gastric emptying pattern, 298
Pylorus, function of, 6

Q

Quinton-Rubin instrument, 74

R

Radiation dose
with scintigraphy, 268, 295, 301
in technetium contrast studies, 225
Radiography

reflux-related diseases associated with, 190
Retching, after fundoplication, 125
Retentive constipation. *See* Functional fecal retention
Retentive posturing, associated with functional fecal retention, 132, **133**
Reticular formation, 157
Retrograde flow, into stomach, 316
Richter, J.E., 146, 185
RMC. *See* Rectal motor complex
Rohatgi, M., 396
Romeo, G., 387
Rostral ventromedial medulla, 157, 158
Rotation, 66
Rotavirus infection
  associated with CIP, 117
  gastroenteritis, acute, gastric emptying values for, **283,** 284
Roux-en-Y anastomosis, 9
Roux-en-Y gastrojejunostomy, efficacy of, 125
Rozycki syndrome, 389
Rumination
  features of, 57
  treatment, 66, 67
Running spectral analysis of EGG signal, 307, **310**

S
Salazopyrine, for determining orocecal transit time, 267
Saline continence test, 232, 239
Saliva, role in esophageal clearance, 59
Salt preference, ontogeny, 34
Sandifer's syndrome
  features of, 72
  indication for surgical treatment, 393, 394
S-100 antibody staining, 325, 334
Savary's classification of esophageal epithelium, 74
Savilahti, E., 148
Scharli, A.F., 407
Schechter, N.L., 171
School phobia, 21, 111-112
Schuster's balloon instrument, 244
Scintigraphy. *See also* Radionuclides; Technetium
  compared with pH monitoring, 297
  for diagnosing aspiration during reflux, 69
  for evaluating esophageal function, 268, 291-295
  for evaluating gastric transit times, 269-270
  for evaluating reflux-associated symptoms, 73
  gastroesophageal, procedure, 295-297
  limitations, 313
  methods and data analysis, 291-295, 296-297, 298
  patient position, 291, 294, 296, 298, 299
  patient preparation, 291, 294, 295
  radiation dose, 268, 295, 301
  risks, 268
  sensitivity, 297
  sources of error, 299-300
Scleroderma

differential diagnosis, 390
  esophageal motor abnormalities associated with, 189, 190, 293, 294
Sclerosis. *See* Systemic sclerosis
Seizure disorder, cyclic vomiting as, 94
Senna derivatives
  mechanism of action, 382
  for treating fecal incontinence, 244
"Sensitive period," for learning specific oral skills, 38
Sensitization to pain. *See also* Hypersensitivity, visceral
  mechanism for development of, 161-163, 171
  treatment, 171
Separation anxiety disorder, 18
  case history, 19-21, 23-24
Sepsis, TPN catheter-related, 372
Serial test meal method, 278
Serotonin, role in pain modulation, 159
Sexual abuse
  anorectal trauma associated with, 243-244
  functional fecal retention associated with, 143
Shermeta, D.W., 388
Short-bowel syndrome
  abnormal motility pattern associated with, 206
  drug therapy, 383
Sickle cell disease, somatizing with, 18, 23
Sidebottom, R., **283**
SIDS. *See* Sudden infant death syndrome
Siegel, M., **283**
Sigmoid, segmental dilation of, surgical therapy, 407-409
Sigmoid resection, for treating constipation, 409-410
Silver stain, 326, **328, 329,** 337, 338, **340**
Single aspiration method, 277-278
Sinusitis, reflux-associated, 72
Skinner, D.B., 258
Sleeve sensor, for esophageal manometry, 180-181, 183, 184
Slow-transit constipation, 273
Slow waves, features of, 305, **306,** 309, 349-350
Small-bowel resection, for treating CIP, 125
Small-bowel tapering operation, for treating CIP, 125
Small-bowel transit time, 300-301
Small intestine
  effects of laboratory stressors on motility of, 146
  functional development, 7-9
  innervation, 7
  intrinsic rhythm of excitation, 9
  marker dilution tests, 286-287
  normal histology, **328**
  normal motility, 195, **202,** 203-215
  ontogeny of motility of, 7-9
  peristalsis in, 7-9
  structural development, 7
  transit times, **202,** 270-271, **271, 272,** 291, 300-301
Smith, B., 326
Smith-Lemli-Opitz syndrome, 334

Smooth muscle. *See also* Visceral myopathy
  disorders of, **329**
  systemic disorders involving, 343-344
Smooth-muscle relaxants, for treating
  achalasia, 390
Smooth power spectrum, 351
Sneezing, associated with GERD, 58
Soave, F., 404, 405
Soave procedure, 405
Soiling. *See* Fecal soiling
Somatizing
  case histories, 18, 23-24
  features of, 17-19, 23
  management difficulties, 21
  management goals, 26-27
Somatoform disorders, 18-19
Somatostatin, 3, 9
  biologic actions of, **383**
  effect on phase 2, 206
  for inducing phase 3, 203, 204
Sondheimer, J.M., 185
Spastic pelvic floor syndrome, 238
Sphincterotomy, internal, 404
Spikes, 305, 309
Spina bifida. *See also* Myelomeningocele
  constipation associated with, **272, 273**
Spinal afferent receptors, 161
Spinal cord, pain fibers in, 157
Spinal cord injury, treatment of associated
  constipation, 139
Spinomesencephalic tract, 157
Spinoreticular tract, 157
Spinothalamic tract, 157
Spitting of formula, treatment, 66
Spitz, L., 394, 396
Squeeze pressure, maximal
  associated with functional fecal retention, 239
  measurement of, 233-234
Starch intolerance, role in irritable bowel
  syndrome, 149
Starling, E.H., 9
Stasis, 317
Steatosis, associated with TPN, 369
Stomach. *See also* Gastric emptying; Gastric
  motility
  electrical dysrhythmias, 308-309
  fixation of, 395-396
  function, 195
  functional development, 3-7
  innervation, 3
  marker dilution tests, 277-284
  motor activity, 305-311
  musculature, 2-3
  retrograde flow into, 316
  structural development, 2-3
  transit times, **272**
Stool softeners, for treating chronic
  constipation, 136, 139
Strain-gauge catheter, 199
Strain-gauge transducer, for recording
  colonic motility, 219
Straining

associated with GERD, 58
  manometric results during, 238
  paradoxical contraction of pelvic floor during,
    238
Stress
  associated with cyclic vomiting, 93
  associated with RAP, 107-108
  effect on bowel motility, 145-146, 218
Stricture. *See* Esophageal stricture; Rectal stricture
Stridor, reflux-associated, 62, 70-72, 78
Subclavian artery, right, aberrant, manometric
  findings with, **186, 187**
Submucosa
  involvement of, in achalasia, 186
  visualization of neural components of, 325
Substance P, 9, 157, 171, 325
Substantia gelatinosa, **158,** 170
Succinate dehydrogenase staining, 335, **336**
Sucking movements
  disorders of, 38
  in utero, 37
Suction biopsy. *See* Esophageal suction biopsy;
  Rectal suction biopsy
Sudden infant death syndrome
  associated with GER, 393
  caused by sleeping position, 258
Sulfur colloid
  problems with, 281
  radio-labeled, 281, 291, 294, 295, 298, 299,
    301
Superior laryngeal nerve, 177, 178
Suppositories, for treating fecal incontinence, **244**
Surgical therapy. *See also specific procedures*
  for achalasia, 390-391
  for CIP, 120-121, 124-125
  for esophageal atresia, 387-388
  for gastroesophageal reflux, 391-397
  for lower gastrointestinal motility disorders,
    403-411
  for total aganglionosis, 405-406
  for upper gastrointestinal motility disorders,
    387-397
Sustaining procedures, 24
Swallowing. *See also* Esophageal transit time
  common disorders affecting, **35**
  by fetus, 1-2
  manometric studies of, 183-191
  mechanism, **179**
  neural pathways controlling, 39
  normal pattern, 177
  phases of, 36-40
  techniques for assessing, 41-42, 267-268
  therapeutic maneuvers for disorders of, 43
  in utero, 37
  velocity, 184
Sweets, preference for, 34
Swenson, O., 404, 407
Swenson procedure, 404-405
Synaptic vesicle antibody staining, 334
Systemic sclerosis
  abnormal motility patterns associated with,
    190, 205, 206, 208

GER associated with, 64
progressive, features of, 343
Szurszewski, J.H., 196

T

Tachybradyarrhythmia, 308
Tachycardia, associated with cyclic vomiting, 92
Tachygastria, 308, 309, **310**, 311, **357**, 358
Tachypnea, associated with feeding disorders,
37, 39
Takano, K., 387
Talley, N.J., 17
Tamarit Torres, J., 279
Team care
advantages and disadvantages, 22
for visceral pain, 155
Technetium, 73, 224-225, 268, 270, 281, 291, 294,
295, 298, 299, 301. *See also* Contrast studies
Technetium-indium ratio, 299
TENS. See Transcutaneous electrical nerve
stimulation
Test meal
for colonic manometry, 217-218, 223
double sampling method, 278, **281**
for electrogastrography, 308, 310
Ewald-Boas method, 277-278
for gastric motility studies, 267, 297-298, 299
radio-labeled eggs, 299
serial meal method, 278
technetium-labeled, 270
for ultrasonography, 318, **319**
Thal, A.P., 395
Thalamus, 157, 162
Thal modification, 395
Time-activity curve
of esophagus, 291, **292**, 294, **296,** 297
of gastric emptying, 298
of gastroesophageal reflux, **296,** 297
Toddler's diarrhea, 13
clinical presentation, 147
pathophysiology, 147-149
Tongue movements
for bolus movement, 38
for sucking, 37
TPN. *See* Parenteral nutrition, total
Trace elements, daily maintenance requirements
in TPN, **370**
Tracheoesophageal fistula, 291, 294
without atresia, 387
Transcutaneous electrical nerve stimulation, for
treating visceral pain, 170
Transit test, 265-273. *See also* Gastrointestinal
transit
techniques for, 265-267
Transit time. *See also* Esophageal transit time;
Gastric emptying time; Orocecal transit time
associated with eating disorders, **273**
gastrointestinal, normal, 129
radionuclide studies of, 291-301
total, determination of, 266
Transpyloric plane, 316
Trichrome staining, Masson's, **341, 342**

Tricyclic antidepressants, for pain management,
124
Trigeminus nerve, 177
Trigger-point injection, for treating visceral pain,
170
Triglyceride infusion, complications of, 369
Triple-A syndrome, 389
Tripp, J.H., 148
Trust of physician by patient, 14
Trypsin, role in GERD, 59
Tube feedings
advantages, 366
enteral, formula for, 366-367
gastrojejunal, 78
for treating CIP, 122, 124
visceral pain associated with, 172
Tuttle, S.G., 258
Tuttle test, 257, 258

U

UES. *See* Upper esophageal sphincter
Ulcer. *See also* Duodenal ulcer; Gastric ulcer;
Peptic ulcer
associated with RAP, 108
Ultrashort segment
features of, 403
surgical treatment, 403-404
Ultrasonography, 313-318
advantages and disadvantages, 266, 313
applications, 315-316
for diagnosing FAP, 109
for evaluating drug therapy, 317
for evaluating GERD, 317-318
indications for, 316-317
limitations, 195-196
principles, 313
procedures, 313-315
swallowing studies, 41
test meal, 318, **319**
Upper esophageal sphincter, 40
disorders of, 185
function, 39, 42, 60
physiology, 55-57, 177
relaxation, 177, 184
Upper esophageal sphincter pressure
assessment of, 182-183
basal, 184
normal, 55
Upper gastrointestinal series. *See* X-ray studies
Urine porphyrin determination, 110
Ursodeoxycholic acid therapy, 372

V

Vagal afferent receptors, 162
and visceral pain, 161
Vagal dysfunction, associated with GER, 65
Vagus nerve, 177, 178
involvement of, in achalasia, 186
modulator of phase 3, 204
Valori, R.M., 199
Vantrappen, G., 197, 271
Vasoactive inhibitory peptide, **56,** 57

Vasoactive intestinal peptide, 9, 325, 388
Vendel, S., 282, 284
Venereal warts, 134
Ventilation, 24
Verapamil, mechanism of action, 382
Vessel of disease model, 22-23
Videofluoroscopy
  for evaluating UES dysfunction, 185
  swallowing studies, 41
VIP. *See* Vasoactive intestinal peptide
Visceral feedback, 34
Visceral hyperalgesia. *See* Hyperalgesia
Visceral hypersensitivity. *See* Hypersensitivity,
  visceral
Visceral myopathy
  abnormal motility pattern associated with, 208
  classification, **330**, 342
  congenital, fecal incontinence associated with,
    244
  diagnosis, 196
  familial, 206
  features of, 330-331, 341
  GER associated with, 64
  histology, **341**
  incidence, 341
Visceral neuropathy
  classification, **330**
  computerized analysis of EGG, **357**
  features of, 330, 331, 339
  histology, **341**
Visceral pain, 155-173
  assessment of, 164, 319
  behavioral and psycholgic interventions,
    168-170
  case histories, 172
  development of pain systems, 159-163
  drug therapy, 171-172
  hypnotic control of, 168-169
  management, 165-173
  mechanical intervention, 169-170
Visual analysis, mouse-assisted, 354, **355**
Vitamin B absorption, 363
Vitamins, daily maintenance requirements in
  TPN, **370**
Vivonex Plus, 367
Vomiting. *See also* Cyclic vomiting
  associated with CIP, 115, 117, 119

associated with gastric dysrhythmias, 311
associated with GER, 63, 387
associated with Hirschsprung's disease, 404
associated with intestinal neuronal dysplasia,
  407
associated with RAP, 109-110
drug therapy, 383
evaluation of, with EGG, 309
and familial dysautonomia, 64
features of, 57
LES relaxation during, 55
in neonate, anorectal manometric results,
  240, **241**
as sign of brain tumor, 95
VSS. *See* Videofluoroscopy, swallowing studies

W

Waardenburg's syndrome, 334
Wall, P.D., 157
Wasserman, R., 149
Water drinking, compulsive, associated with
  cyclic vomiting, 92, 96-97
Weaver, L.T., 150
Weight-for-height deficit, calculation of, **366**
Weight loss
  associated with achalasia, 389
  associated with regurgitation, 66
Wheezing, reflux-associated, 60, 69-70
Whitehead, W.E., 247
Wiesenfeld-Hallin, Z., 163
Wilkins, B.M., 394, 396
Willis, T., 388, 390
Windup, 162

X

X-ray studies, for diagnosing FAP, 109-110

Y

Yaster, M., 171
Yu, V.Y.H., **283**

Z

Zaaijer, J.H., 390-391
Zamboni's fixative, 344, 345
Zeltzer, L.K., 169
Zighelboim, J., 17
Zonal aganglionosis, histologic features, 334-335